20
Li

D0401047

Pocket
Drug Guide
for Nurses

Amy M. Karch, RN, MS

Associate Professor of Clinical Nursing
University of Rochester School of Nursing
Rochester, New York

Wolters Kluwer

Philadelphia • Baltimore • New York • London
Buenos Aires • Hong Kong • Sydney • Tokyo

Publisher: Jay Abramovitz
Chief Nursing Officer: Judith A. Schilling McCann, RN, MSN
Product Director: David Moreau
Editor: Karen C. Comerford
Editorial Assistants: Jeri O'Shea and Linda K. Ruhf
Marketing Manager: Mark Wiragh
Art Director: Elaine Kasmer
Design: Joseph John Clark
Production Project Manager: Joan Sinclair
Manufacturing Manager: Kathleen Brown
Production Services: Aptara, Inc.

The clinical treatments described and recommended in this publication are based on research and consultation with nursing, medical, and legal authorities. To the best of our knowledge, these treatments reflect currently accepted practice. Nevertheless, they can't be considered absolute and universal recommendations. For individual applications, all recommendations must be considered in light of the patient's clinical condition and before administration of new or infrequently used drugs, in light of the latest package-insert information. The author and publisher disclaim any responsibility for any adverse effects resulting from the suggested treatments, from any undetected errors, or from the reader's misunderstanding of the text.

Printed in China.

LPDGN15011014

ISBN: 978-1-4698-5333-8

CIP data available on request from the publisher.

RRS1407

Contents

Preface

The number of clinically important drugs increases every year, as does the nurse's responsibility for drug therapy. No practitioner can memorize all the drug information necessary to provide safe and efficacious drug therapy. Compound the growing list of drugs with a continuing shortage of pharmacists and an anticipated shortage of nurses, and there is an ever-increasing risk of medication errors that lead to poor patient outcomes.

The *2015 Lippincott Pocket Drug Guide for Nurses* provides need-to-know information in an abbreviated format. Drugs are listed alphabetically. Monographs are concise. Each monograph provides the key information needed to ensure safe patient care:

- Drug class
- Pregnancy and Controlled Substance category
- Black box warning, if appropriate
- Indications and dosages
- Dosage adjustments that also alert you, when appropriate, to the need to consult a complete drug guide
- Most common and most critical adverse effects
- Key nursing and patient teaching points to ensure safe drug use.

The pocket size makes this book easy to carry into the clinical setting for a quick check before administering the drug.

Following the drug monographs, a new section on patient safety reviews the rights of medication administration, safety-oriented patient and family teaching, and other aspects of safe drug administration. Appendices cover biological agents, topical drugs, ophthalmic agents, laxatives, combination drugs, and contraceptives. There is also an appendix of common diseases, with the drugs used to treat each disease. To keep the book short and sweet, common abbreviations are used throughout; these are listed in the abbreviations list on pages ix–xi.

In the rush of the clinical setting, this guide will provide the critical information you need immediately. However, it is important to check complete facts and details as soon as time allows to ensure that the best outcomes are achieved for each patient.

Amy M. Karch, RN, MS

Guide to abbreviations

Abbreviations in headings

BBW	Black Box Warning
CLASS	Therapeutic/Pharmacologic Class
PREG/CONT	Pregnancy Risk Category/Controlled Substance Schedule
IND & DOSE	Indications & Dosages
ADJUST DOSE	Dosage Adjustment
ADV EFF	Adverse Effects
NC/PT	Nursing Considerations/Patient Teaching

Abbreviations in text

abd	abdominal	CAD	coronary artery disease
ABG	arterial blood gas	CABG	coronary artery bypass graft
ACE	angiotensin-converting enzyme	cAMP	cyclic adenosine monophosphate
ACT	activated clotting time	CBC	complete blood count
ACTH	adrenocorticotropic hormone	CDC	Centers for Disease Control and Prevention
ADH	antidiuretic hormone	CML	chronic myelogenous leukemia
ADHD	attention-deficit hyperactivity disorder	CNS	central nervous system
adjunct	adjunctive	conc	concentration
AHA	American Heart Association	COPD	chronic obstructive pulmonary disease
AIDS	acquired immunodeficiency syndrome	CK	creatine kinase
		CR	controlled-release
ALL	acute lymphocytic leukemia	CrCl	creatinine clearance
ALT	alanine transaminase	CSF	cerebrospinal fluid
a.m.	morning	CV	cardiovascular
AML	acute myelogenous leukemia	CVP	central venous pressure
		CYP450	cytochrome P-450
ANA	anti-nuclear antibodies	D_5W	dextrose 5% in water
ANC	absolute neutrophil count	DIC	disseminated intravascular coagulopathy
aPTT	activated partial thromboplastin time		
		dL	deciliter (100 mL)
ARB	angiotensin II receptor blocker	DR	delayed-release
		DVT	deep venous thrombosis
ASA	acetylsalicylic acid	dx	diagnosis
AST	aspartate transaminase	dysfx	dysfunction
AV	atrioventricular	ECG	electrocardiogram
bid	twice a day *(bis in die)*	ED	erectile dysfunction
BP	blood pressure	EEG	electroencephalogram
BPH	benign prostatic hypertrophy	ER	extended-release
		ET	endotracheal
BSA	body surface area	FDA	Food and Drug Administration
BUN	blood urea nitrogen		

ix

5-FU	fluorouracil	LHRH	luteinizing hormone-releasing hormone
5-HIAA	5-hydroxyindole acetic acid	m	meter
FSH	follicle-stimulating hormone	MAC	*Mycobacterium avium* complex
g	gram	maint	maintenance
GABA	gamma-aminobutyric acid	MAO	monoamine oxidase
GERD	gastroesophageal reflux disease	MAOI	monoamine oxidase inhibitor
GFR	glomerular filtration rate	max	maximum
GGTP	gamma-glutamyl transpeptidase	mcg	microgram
		mg	milligram
GI	gastrointestinal	mgt	management
G6PD	glucose-6-phosphate dehydrogenase	MI	myocardial infarction
GU	genitourinary	min	minute
HCG	human chorionic gonadotropin	mL	milliliter
		mo	month
Hct	hematocrit	MRSA	methicillin-resistant *Staphylococcus aureus*
HDL	high-density lipoprotein		
HF	heart failure	MS	multiple sclerosis
Hg	mercury	NA	not applicable
Hgb	hemoglobin	NG	nasogastric
Hib	*Haemophilus influenzae* type b	ng	nanogram
		NMJ	neuromuscular junction
HIV	human immunodeficiency virus	NMS	neuroleptic malignant syndrome
HMG-CoA	3-hydroxy-3-methylglutaryl coenzyme A	NRTI	nucleoside reverse transcriptase inhibitor
		NSAID	nonsteroidal anti-inflammatory drug
HPA	hypothalamic-pituitary axis	NSS	normal saline solution
hr	hour	n/v	nausea and vomiting
HR	heart rate	n/v/d	nausea, vomiting, and diarrhea
HSV	herpes simplex virus		
hx	history	OCD	obsessive-compulsive disorder
IBS	irritable bowel syndrome	oint	ointment
ICU	intensive care unit	OTC	over-the-counter
IHSS	idiopathic hypertrophic subaortic stenosis	P	pulse
		PABA	para-aminobenzoic acid
IM	intramuscular	PDA	patent ductus arteriosus
INR	International Normalized Ratio	PE	pulmonary embolus
		PEG	percutaneous endoscopic gastrostomy
IOP	intraocular pressure		
IV	intravenous	periop	perioperative
kg	kilogram	PFT	pulmonary function test
L	liter	PG	prostaglandin
lb	pound	pH	hydrogen ion concentration
LDL	low-density lipoprotein		
LFT	liver function test	PID	pelvic inflammatory disease
LH	luteinizing hormone		

p.m.	evening	T4	thyroxine (tetraiodothyronine)
PMDD	premenstrual dysphoric disorder	TB	tuberculosis
PMS	premenstrual syndrome	tbsp	tablespoon
PO	orally, by mouth (per os)	TCA	tricyclic antidepressant
postop	postoperative	temp	temperature
preop	preoperative	TIA	transient ischemic attack
PRN	when required (pro re nata)	tid	three times a day (ter in die)
PSA	prostate-specific antigen	TNF	tumor necrosis factor
pt	patient	TPA	tissue plasminogen activator
PT	prothrombin time	TPN	total parenteral nutrition
PTCA	percutaneous transluminal coronary angioplasty	TSH	thyroid-stimulating hormone
PTSD	post-traumatic stress disorder	tsp	teaspoon
PTT	partial thromboplastin time	tx	treatment
		unkn	unknown
PVCs	premature ventricular contractions	URI	upper respiratory (tract) infection
px	prophylaxis	USP	United States Pharmacopeia
q	every	UTI	urinary tract infection
qid	four times a day (quarter in die)	UV	ultraviolet
R	respiratory rate	VLDL	very–low-density lipoprotein
RBC	red blood cell	VREF	vancomycin-resistant Enterococcus faecium
RDA	recommended dietary allowance	w/	with
RDS	respiratory distress syndrome	WBC	white blood cell
		wk	week
RSV	respiratory syncytial virus	XR	extended-release
s&sx	signs and symptoms	yr	year
SA	sinoatrial		
SBE	subacute bacterial endocarditis		
sec	second		
SIADH	syndrome of inappropriate antidiuretic hormone secretion		
SLE	systemic lupus erythematosus		
sol	solution		
sp	species		
SR	sustained-release		
SSRI	selective serotonin reuptake inhibitor		
STD	sexually transmitted disease		
subcut	subcutaneous		
SWSD	shift-work sleep disorder		
s&sx	signs and symptoms		
sx	symptoms		
T3	triiodothyronine		

abacavir (Ziagen)
CLASS Antiviral, NRTI
PREG/CONT C/NA

BBW Risk of severe to fatal hypersensitivity reactions; increased w/ HLA-B*5701 allele. Monitor for lactic acidosis, severe hepatomegaly.
IND & DOSE *HIV infection (w/ other antiretrovirals).* **Adult:** 300 mg PO bid or 600 mg PO daily. **Child 3 mo–18 yr:** 8 mg/kg PO bid; max, 300 mg/dose.
ADJUST DOSE Mild hepatic impairment
ADV EFF Fatigue, headache, insomnia, malaise, **MI**, n/v/d, rash, **severe to fatal hepatomegaly, severe to fatal lactic acidosis, severe hypersensitivity reactions,** weakness
INTERACTIONS Alcohol
NC/PT Give w/ other antiretrovirals. Suggest use of barrier contraceptives. Monitor for s&sx of lactic acidosis, liver dysfx, hypersensitivity reactions.

abatacept (Orencia)
CLASS Antiarthritic, immune modulator
PREG/CONT C/NA

IND & DOSE *Tx of adult rheumatoid arthritis.* **Over 100 kg:** 1,000 mg/day IV. **60–100 kg:** 750 mg/day IV. **Under 60 kg:** 500 mg/day IV. After initial dose, give at 2 and 4 wk, then q 4 wk. *Tx of juvenile idiopathic arthritis in child 6 yr and older.* **75 kg or more:** Use adult dose; max, 1,000 mg/day. **Under 75 kg:** 10 mg/kg IV. After initial dose, give at 2 and 4 wk.
ADV EFF Headache, **hypersensitivity reactions and anaphylaxis, potentially serious infection**
INTERACTIONS Live vaccines; TNF antagonists (contraindicated)
NC/PT Monitor for s&sx of infection. Pretest for TB before beginning therapy. Do not give w/ TNF antagonists. Do not give live vaccines during or for 3 mo after tx.

abciximab (ReoPro)
CLASS Antiplatelet, glycoprotein IIb/IIIa inhibitor
PREG/CONT C/NA

IND & DOSE *Adjunct to percutaneous coronary intervention (PCI) to prevent cardiac ischemic complications in pt undergoing PCI.* **Adult:** 0.25 mcg/kg by IV bolus 10–60 min before procedure, then continuous IV infusion of 0.125 mcg/kg/min for 12 hr (max, 10 mcg/min). *Unstable angina not responding to conventional therapy when PCI is planned within 24 hr, w/ heparin and aspirin therapy.* **Adult:** 0.25 mcg/kg by IV bolus over at least 1 min, then 10 mcg/min by IV infusion for 19–24 hr, ending 1 hr after PCI.
ADV EFF Bleeding, edema, hypotension, n/v, pain, **thrombocytopenia**
INTERACTIONS Anticoagulants, antiplatelets, thrombolytics
NC/PT Provide safety measures to protect pt from bleeding and monitor for signs of bleeding. Monitor CBC. Give w/ heparin and aspirin therapy. Clearly mark chart that pt is on drug.

abiraterone (Zytiga)
CLASS Antineoplastic, CYP17 inhibitor
PREG/CONT X/NA

IND & DOSE *Tx of pts w/ metastatic castration-resistant prostate cancer who have received prior chemotherapy containing docetaxel, w/ prednisone.* **Adult:** 1,000 mg PO w/ 5 mg prednisone PO.
ADJUST DOSE Hepatic impairment
ADV EFF **Adrenocortical insufficiency,** arrhythmias, **cardiac toxicity,** cough, diarrhea, dyspepsia, dyspnea, edema, **hepatotoxicity,** hot flushes, hypertension, hypokalemia, nocturia, URI, UTI
INTERACTIONS CYP3A4 enzyme inducers, inhibitors; avoid use w/ CYP2D6 substrates

NC/PT Must be taken on empty stomach w/ no food 1 hr before or 2 hr after dosing. Not for use in pregnancy, breast-feeding. Monitor closely for cardiac toxicity, hepatotoxicity, adrenal insufficiency. Corticosteroids may be needed in stressful situations.

acamprosate calcium (Campral)
CLASS Antialcoholic, GABA analogue
PREG/CONT C/NA

IND & DOSE Maint of abstinence from alcohol as part of comprehensive psychosocial tx mgt program. *Adult:* 666 mg PO tid; begin as soon as abstinence achieved.
ADJUST DOSE Renal impairment
ADV EFF Diarrhea, suicidality
INTERACTIONS Alcohol
NC/PT Ensure pt is abstaining from alcohol and is in comprehensive tx program. Pt may take drug even if relapse occurs. Not for use in pregnancy, breast-feeding. Pt should report thoughts of suicide.

acarbose (Precose)
CLASS Alpha-glucosidase inhibitor, antidiabetic
PREG/CONT B/NA

IND & DOSE Monotherapy or adjunct to diet to lower blood glucose in pts w/ type 2 diabetes. *Adult:* 25 mg PO tid w/ first bite of meal. Max for pt 60 kg or less, 50 mg PO tid; over 60 kg, 100 mg PO tid. **Combination tx w/ sulfonylureas, metformin, or insulin to enhance glycemic control.** *Adult:* Adjust dose based on blood glucose levels in combination w/ dosage of other drugs used.
ADV EFF Abd pain, flatulence, hypoglycemia. n/v/d
INTERACTIONS Antidiabetics, celery, charcoal, coriander, dandelion root, digestive enzymes, digoxin, fenugreek, garlic, ginseng, juniper berries

NC/PT Give w/ food. Monitor blood glucose. Pt should follow diet and exercise program.

acebutolol hydrochloride (Sectral)
CLASS Antiarrhythmic, antihypertensive, beta-adrenergic blocker
PREG/CONT B/NA

IND & DOSE Tx of hypertension. *Adult:* 400 mg/day PO. Maint dose, 200–1,200 mg/day PO (larger dose in two divided doses). **Mgt of PVCs.** *Adult:* 200 mg PO bid. Range to control PVCs, 600–1,200 mg/day PO. Discontinue gradually over 3 wk.
ADJUST DOSE Renal, hepatic impairment; elderly pts
ADV EFF Arrhythmias (bradycardia, tachycardia, heart block), bronchospasm, constipation, decreased exercise tolerance, ED, flatulence, gastric pain, HF, n/v
INTERACTIONS Alpha blockers, aspirin, beta blockers, bismuth subsalicylate, calcium channel blockers, clonidine, insulin, magnesium salicylate, NSAIDs, prazosin
NC/PT Monitor apical P; do not use if P is less than 45. May give w/ food. Withdraw slowly over 3 wk after long-term therapy.

acetaminophen (Acephen, Ofirmev, Tylenol, etc)
CLASS Analgesic, antipyretic
PREG/CONT B/NA

IND & DOSE Temporary reduction of fever; temporary relief of minor aches and pains caused by common cold and influenza; headache, sore throat, toothache (pts 2 yr and older); backache, menstrual cramps, minor arthritis pain, muscle aches (pts over 12 yr). *Adult, child over 12 yr* (PO or rectal suppositories): 325–560 mg q 4–6 hr or 1,300 mg (ER) PO q 8 hr.

Adult, child 13 yr and older, 50 kg or more: 1,000 mg IV q 6 hr or 650 mg IV q 4 hr; max, 1,000 mg/dose IV or 4,000 mg/day IV. *Child 13 yr, under 50 kg:* 15 mg/kg IV q 6 hr or 12.5 mg/kg IV q 4 hr; max, 750 mg or 75 mg/kg/day. *Child 2–12 yr:* 15 mg/kg IV q 6 hr or 12 mg/kg IV q 4 hr; max, 75 mg/kg/day. May repeat PO or rectal doses four to five times/day; max, five doses in 24 hr or 10 mg/kg. PO doses: 11 yr, 480 mg/dose; 9–10 yr, 400 mg/dose; 6–8 yr, 320 mg/dose; 4–5 yr, 240 mg/dose; 2–3 yr, 160 mg/dose; 12–23 mo, 120 mg/dose; 4–11 mo, 80 mg/dose; 0–3 mo, 40 mg/dose. PR doses: 6–12 yr, 325 mg q 4–6 hr; 3–6 yr, 120 mg q 4–6 hr; 12–36 mo, 80 mg q 4 hr; 3–11 mo, 80 mg q 6 hr.
ADV EFF Hepatic failure, **hepato-toxicity, myocardial damage**
INTERACTIONS Alcohol, anticholin-ergics, barbiturates, charcoal, carbam-azepine, hydantoins, oral anticoagu-lants, rifampin, sulfinpyrazone, zidovudine
NC/PT Do not exceed recommended dosage. Avoid combining (many products contain acetaminophen). Administer IV over 15 min. Not rec-ommended for longer than 10 days. Overdose tx: acetylcysteine, possible life support.

---

acetazolamide (Diamox Sequels)
CLASS Antiepileptic, antiglaucoma, carbonic anhydrase inhibitor, diuretic
PREG/CONT C/NA

BBW Fatalities have occurred due to severe reactions; discontinue immediately if s&sx of serious reactions. Use caution if pt receiving high-dose aspirin; anorexia, tachypnea, lethargy, coma, death have occurred.
IND & DOSE Open-angle glaucoma. *Adult:* 250 mg–1 g/day PO, usually in divided doses, or 1 ER capsule bid

(a.m. and p.m.). Max, 1 g/day. **Acute congestive angle-closure glaucoma.** *Adult:* 500 mg (ER) PO bid or 250 mg PO q 4 hr. **Secondary glaucoma and preoperatively.** *Adult:* 250 mg PO q 4 hr, or 250 mg PO bid, or 500 mg PO bid (ER capsules), or 500 mg PO followed by 125–250 mg PO q 4 hr. May give IV for rapid relief of increased IOP: 500 mg IV, then 125–250 mg PO q 4 hr. **Diuresis in HF.** *Adult:* 250–375 mg PO (5 mg/kg) daily a.m. **Drug-induced edema.** *Adult:* 250–375 mg PO once q day or for 1 or 2 days alternating w/ day of rest. **Epilepsy.** *Adult:* 8–30 mg/kg/day PO in divided doses. Range, 375–1,000 mg/day. **Acute altitude sickness.** *Adult, child 12 yr and older:* 500 mg–1 g/day PO in divided doses.
ADV EFF Urinary frequency
INTERACTIONS Amphetamines, lithium, procainamide, quinidine, salicylates, TCAs
NC/PT Do not give IM. Make oral liquid by crushing tablets and sus-pending in sweet syrup (do not use alcohol or glycerin). Have IOP checked periodically. May cause dizziness, increased urination. Pt should report flank pain, bleeding, weight gain of more than 3 lb/day. Name confusion between *Diamox* and *Trimox* (ampicillin).

---

acetylcysteine (Acetadote)
CLASS Antidote, mucolytic
PREG/CONT B/NA

IND & DOSE Mucolytic adjuvant therapy for abnormal, viscid, or inspissated mucus secretions in acute and chronic bronchopulmona-ry disease. *Adult, child:* Nebulization w/ face mask, mouthpiece, tracheos-tomy: 3–5 mL of 20% sol or 6–10 mL of 10% sol tid or qid. Nebulization w/ tent, croupette: Up to 300 mL during a tx period. Direct or by tracheostomy: 1–2 mL of 10%–20% sol q 1–4 hr. Percutaneous intratracheal catheter:

1–2 mL of 20% sol or 2–4 mL of 10% sol q 1–4 hr. **To prevent or lessen hepatic injury that may occur after ingestion of potentially hepatotoxic dose of acetaminophen.** *Adult, child:* PO, 140 mg/kg loading dose, then 17 maint doses of 70 mg/kg q 4 hr, starting 4 hr after loading dose. IV, Loading dose, 150 mg/kg in 200 mL IV over 60 min; maint dose 50 mg/kg in 500 mL IV over 4 hr followed by second maint dose of 100 mg/kg in 1,000 mL IV over 16 hr. Total IV dose, 300 mg/kg over 21 hr.
ADV EFF Anaphylactoid reactions, bronchospasm, n/v, rhinorrhea
INTERACTIONS (in sol) Amphotericin B, erythromycin, hydrogen peroxide, lactobionate, tetracycline
NC/PT Use water to remove sol from pt's face. Monitor nebulizer for buildup of drug. Have suction equipment available. May mix 20% sol w/ soft drinks to concentration of 5%. Dilute oral sol w/ water if using gastric tube. Warn pt of possible disagreeable odor as nebulization begins. Pt should report difficulty breathing.

acitretin (Soriatane)
CLASS Antipsoriatic, retinoic acid
PREG/CONT X/NA

BBW Do not use in pregnancy; serious fetal harm possible. Males should not father a child during and for 3 mo after tx.
IND & DOSE Tx of severe psoriasis. *Adult:* 25–50 mg/day PO w/ main meal.
ADV EFF Hepatotoxicity
INTERACTIONS Methotrexate, phenytoin, retinoids, vitamin D
NC/PT Pt must have monthly negative pregnancy tests and agree to use two forms of contraception. Must have signed pt agreement in medical record. Pt may not donate blood for 3 yr after tx. Pt should swallow tablets whole and not cut, crush, or chew them; stop drug when lesions resolve; avoid sun exposure.

aclidinium bromide (Tudorza Pressair)
CLASS Anticholinergic, bronchodilator
PREG/CONT C/NA

IND & DOSE Long-term maint tx of bronchospasm associated w/ COPD. *Adult:* 400 mcg/actuation bid.
ADJUST DOSE Over 80 yr; under 60 kg; renal, hepatic impairment
ADV EFF Dry mouth, headache, nasopharyngitis, urine retention
INTERACTIONS Other anticholinergics; avoid this combination
NC/PT Ensure appropriate use of drug; use only w/ provided inhaler. Monitor for hypersensitivity. Stop drug w/ paradoxical bronchospasm. Monitor for glaucoma. Have pt void before each dose if urine retention occurs.

acyclovir (Zovirax)
CLASS Antiviral, purine nucleoside analogue
PREG/CONT B/NA

IND & DOSE Herpes genitalis. *Adult:* 5 mg/kg IV infused over 1 hr q 8 hr for 5 days. Herpes encephalitis. *Adult:* 10 mg/kg IV infused over 1 hr q 8 hr for 10 days. Herpes simplex (immunocompromised pts). *Adult:* 5 mg/kg IV infused over 1 hr q 8 hr for 7 days. Varicella zoster (immunocompromised pts). *Adult:* 10 mg/kg IV infused over 1 hr q 8 hr for 7 days. Initial genital herpes. *Adult:* 200 mg PO q 4 hr five times daily (1,000 mg/day) for 10 days. Long-term suppressive therapy. *Adult:* 400 mg PO bid for up to 12 mo. Recurrent therapy. *Adult:* 200 mg IV q 4 hr five times daily for 5 days. HSV infection. *Child under 12 yr:* 10 mg/kg IV infused over 1 hr q 8 hr for 7 days. Varicella zoster. *Child under 12 yr:* 20 mg/kg IV over 1 hr q 8 hr for 7 days. Shingles, HSV encephalitis. *Child 3 mo to 12 yr:* 20 mg/kg IV over 1 hr q 8 hr for

14–21 days. **Neonatal HSV.** 10 mg/kg IV infused over 1 hr q 8 hr for 10 days. *2 yr or older and 40 kg or less:* 20 mg/kg/dose PO q6h (80 mg/kg/day) for 5 days. *Over 12 yr, over 40 kg:* Give adult dose. **Ointment.** *All ages:* Apply sufficient quantity to cover all lesions six times/day (q 3 hr) for 7 days. 1.25-cm (0.5-in) ribbon of ointment covers 2.5 cm² (4 in²) surface area. **Cream.** *12 yr and older:* Apply enough to cover all lesions five times/day for 4 days.
ADJUST DOSE Elderly pts, renal impairment
ADV EFF Inflammation or phlebitis at injection sites, n/v/d, transient topical burning w/ topical use
INTERACTIONS Nephrotoxic drugs, probenecid, zidovudine
NC/PT Ensure pt well hydrated. Wear rubber glove or finger cot when applying topically. Drug not a cure and will not prevent recurrence. Pt should avoid sexual intercourse when lesions are present; use condoms to prevent spread.

---

adalimumab (Humira)
CLASS Antiarthritic, TNF blocker
PREG/CONT B/NA

BBW Risk of serious infection, activation of TB; risk of lymphoma and other potentially fatal malignancies in children, adolescents.
IND & DOSE Tx of rheumatoid arthritis, psoriatic arthritis, ankylosing spondylitis. *Adult:* 40 mg subcut every other wk. **Crohn's disease/ulcerative colitis.** *Adult:* Four 40-mg subcut injections in 1 day followed by 80 mg 2 wk later; 2 wk later begin 40 mg every other wk maint. **Plaque psoriasis.** *Adult:* 80 mg subcut, then 40 mg every other wk starting 1 wk later. **Juvenile idiopathic arthritis:** *Child 30 kg and over:* 40 mg subcut every other wk. *Child 15 to under 30 kg:* 20 mg subcut every other wk.

ADV EFF Anaphylaxis, headache, injection-site reactions, **malignancies, serious infections**
INTERACTIONS Anakinra, immunosuppressants, live vaccines
NC/PT High risk of infection; monitor pt, protect as appropriate. Monitor CNS for s&sx of demyelinating disorders. Advise pt to avoid pregnancy. Teach proper administration and disposal of syringes.

---

adefovir dipivoxil (Hepsera)
CLASS Antiviral, reverse transcriptase inhibitor
PREG/CONT C/NA

BBW Worsening hepatitis when discontinued. HIV resistance if used in undiagnosed HIV infection (test before use). Monitor for renal and hepatic toxicity. Withdraw drug and monitor if s&sx of lactic acidosis or steatosis.
IND & DOSE Tx of chronic hepatitis B. *Adult, child 12 yr and older:* 10 mg/day PO.
ADJUST DOSE Renal impairment
ADV EFF Asthenia, elevated LFTs, hepatitis exacerbation if discontinued, lactic acidosis, nephrotoxicity, severe hepatomegaly w/ steatosis
INTERACTIONS Nephrotoxic drugs
NC/PT Test for HIV infection before starting tx. Monitor for renal/hepatic dysfx, lactic acidosis, steatosis. Advise against use in pregnancy, breast-feeding. Drug does not cure disease; use precautions. Advise pt to not run out of drug; serious hepatitis can occur w/ sudden stopping.

---

adenosine (Adenocard, Adenoscan)
CLASS Antiarrhythmic, diagnostic agent
PREG/CONT C/NA

IND & DOSE Conversion to sinus rhythm from supraventricular

tachycardia (Adenocard). Pts over 50 kg: 6 mg IV bolus; may repeat within 1–2 min w/ 12-mg IV bolus up to two times. Pts under 50 kg: 0.05–0.1 mg/kg rapid IV bolus; may repeat in 1–2 min. Max single dose, 0.3 mg/kg. **Diagnosis of suspected CAD, w/ thallium** (Adenoscan): Adult: 140 mcg/kg/min IV over 6 min; inject thallium at 3 min.
ADV EFF Bronchoconstriction, *facial flushing,* **heart block**
INTERACTIONS Carbamazepine, digoxin, dipyridamole, theophylline, verapamil
NC/PT Do not refrigerate; discard unused portions. Have emergency equipment on standby and continuously monitor pt. Have methylxanthines on hand as antidote.

ado-trastuzumab
(Kadcyla)
CLASS Antineoplastic, microtubular inhibitor
PREG/CONT D/NA

> **BBW** Risk of hepatotoxicity, cardiac dysfunction, death. Can cause fetal harm.

IND & DOSE Tx of HER2-positive metastatic breast cancer in pts who have had prior tx or have developed recurrence during or within 6 mo of tx. Adult: 3.6 mg/kg as IV infusion every 3 wk until disease progression or toxicity.
ADV EFF Constipation, fatigue, headache, **hepatotoxicity, infusion reactions, left ventricular impairment,** musculoskeletal pain, neurotoxicity, **pulmonary toxicity,** thrombocytopenia
INTERACTIONS Strong CYP3A4 inhibitors; avoid this combination
NC/PT Ensure proper use; HER-2 testing required. Rule out pregnancy before starting tx (contraceptives advised); not for use in breast-feeding. Monitor LFTs (before and periodically during tx), cardiac output, respiratory function. Infusion reaction may

require slowing or interrupting infusion. Pt should: mark calendar for infusion dates; take safety precautions w/ neurotoxicity; report difficulty breathing, dark urine, yellowing of skin/eyes, abdominal pain, swelling, dizziness.

> **DANGEROUS DRUG**

afatinib (Gilotrif)
CLASS Antineoplastic, kinase inhibitor
PREG/CONT D/NA

IND & DOSE First-line tx of pts w/ metastatic non-small-cell lung cancer whose tumors have epidermal growth factor receptor exon 19 deletions or exon 21 substitution Adult: 40 mg/day PO at least 1 hr before or 2 hr after meal.
ADV EFF Abd pain, bullous/exfoliative skin disorders, dehydration, diarrhea, hepatotoxicity, keratitis, n/v/d, rash, stomatitis, weight loss
INTERACTIONS P-glycoprotein inducers/inhibitors
NC/PT Ensure proper dx. Monitor renal function/LFTs. Risk of dehydration. Pt should avoid pregnancy, breast-feeding; perform proper mouth care; eat small, frequent meals; report rash, difficulty breathing; severe n/v; urine, stool color changes.

aflibercept (Eylea)
CLASS Fusion protein, ophthalmic agent
PREG/CONT C/NA

IND & DOSE Tx of pts w/ neovascular (wet) age-related macular degeneration. Adult: 2 mg (0.05 mL) by intravitreal injection q 4 wk for first 3 mo, then 2 mg once q 8 wk.
ADV EFF Cataract, endophthalmitis, eye infections, eye pain, increased IOP, retinal detachment, **thrombotic events,** vision changes, vitreous floaters

NC/PT Monitor pt closely during and immediately after injection. Advise pt to immediately report eye redness, sensitivity to light, sudden vision changes.

agalsidase beta
(Fabrazyme)
CLASS Enzyme
PREG/CONT B/NA

IND & DOSE Tx of Fabry disease. *Adult:* 1 mg/kg IV q 2 wk at no more than 0.25 mg/min.
ADV EFF Anaphylaxis, potentially serious infusion reactions (chills, fever, dyspnea, n/v, flushing, headache, chest pain, tachycardia, facial edema, rash)
NC/PT Ensure appropriate supportive measures available during infusion. Premedicate w/ antipyretics; immediately discontinue if infusion reaction occurs.

albumin (human)
(Albuminar, Buminate, Plasbumin)
CLASS Blood product, plasma protein
PREG/CONT C/NA

IND & DOSE Plasma volume expansion related to shock, burns, nephrosis, etc. *Adult:* 5%—500 mL by IV infusion as rapidly as possible; additional 500 mg in 15–30 min; 20% or 25%—maintain plasma albumin conc at 2.5 ± 0.5 g/100 mL. *Child:* 0.6–1 g/kg, 25 g/day IV of 20% or 25%.
ADV EFF *BP changes*, chills, fever, flushing, HF, n/v, rash
NC/PT Monitor BP during infusion; discontinue if hypotension occurs. Stop infusion if headache, fever, BP changes occur; treat w/ antihistamine. Adjust infusion rate based on pt response.

albuterol sulfate
(AccuNeb, Proventil HFA, Ventolin, VoSpire ER)
CLASS Antiasthmatic, beta agonist, bronchodilator, sympathomimetic
PREG/CONT C/NA

IND & DOSE Relief, prevention of bronchospasm in COPD. *Adult:* 2–4 mg PO tid–qid or 4–8 mg ER tablets q 12 hr. *Child 6–12 yr:* 2 mg PO three to four times/day or 4 mg ER tablet PO q 12 hr. *Child 2–5 yr:* 0.1 mg/kg PO tid; max, 4 mg PO tid. Acute bronchospasm. *Adult:* 1–2 inhalations q 4–6 hr; max, 12 inhalations/day; 2.5 mg tid–qid by nebulization. *Child 2–12 yr, over 15 kg:* 2.5 mg bid–tid by nebulization; *under 15 kg:* 0.5% sol tid–qid by nebulization over 5–15 min. Exercise-induced bronchospasm. *Adult:* 2 inhalations 15–30 min before exercise.
ADJUST DOSE Elderly pts, pts sensitive to beta-adrenergic stimulation
ADV EFF Anxiety, apprehension, bronchospasm, cardiac arrhythmias, fear, flushing, n/v, pallor, sweating
INTERACTIONS Aminophylline, beta-adrenergics, digoxin, insulin, linezolid, QT-prolonging drugs, sympathomimetics
NC/PT Do not exceed recommended doses. Have beta blocker on standby. Pt should not cut, crush, or chew tablets. Dizziness may occur; use caution. Use inhalation for acute bronchospasm.

DANGEROUS DRUG
aldesleukin (Proleukin)
CLASS Antineoplastic, immune modulator
PREG/CONT C/NA

IND & DOSE Tx of metastatic renal carcinoma, metastatic melanoma. *Adult:* 600,000 international units/kg IV q 8 hr over 15 min for total of 14 doses; 9 days of rest, then repeat. Max, 28 doses/course.

ADV EFF Bone marrow suppression, cardiac arrhythmias, cardiac toxicity, hepatotoxicity, hypotension, n/v/d, nephrotoxicity, pulmonary toxicity
INTERACTIONS Bone marrow suppressants, cardiotoxic drugs, CNS depressants, dexamethasone, hepatotoxic drugs, nephrotoxic drugs
NC/PT Obtain baseline ECG. Protect pt from infection. Ensure proper mouth care. Pt should avoid pregnancy, breast-feeding; report s&sx of bleeding or infection.

alendronate sodium
(Binosto, Fosamax)
CLASS Bisphosphonate, calcium regulator
PREG/CONT C/NA

IND & DOSE Tx of postmenopausal osteoporosis; men w/ osteoporosis. *Adult:* 10 mg/day PO or 70 mg PO once a wk. **Prevention of osteoporosis.** *Adult:* 5 mg/day PO or 35 mg PO once wkly. **Tx of Paget disease.** *Adult:* 40 mg/day PO for 6 mo; may retreat after 6-mo tx-free period. **Tx of glucocorticoid-induced osteoporosis.** *Adult:* 5 mg/day PO (10 mg/day PO for postmenopausal women not on estrogen).
ADJUST DOSE Renal impairment
ADV EFF Bone pain, esophageal erosion, GI irritation, headache, n/v/d
INTERACTIONS Antacids, aspirin, calcium, iron, NSAIDs, ranitidine
NC/PT Give w/ full glass of water in a.m. at least 30 min before other food or medication; have pt stay upright for 30 min and until first food of day. Monitor serum calcium level; ensure pt has adequate calcium and vitamin D intake.

alfuzosin hydrochloride
(Uroxatral)
CLASS Alpha-adrenergic blocker, BPH drug
PREG/CONT B/NA

IND & DOSE Tx of s&sx of BPH. *Adult:* 10 mg/day PO after same meal each day.

ADV EFF Dizziness, orthostatic hypotension
INTERACTIONS Adrenergic blockers, antihypertensives, itraconazole, ketoconazole, phosphodiesterase inhibitors, protease inhibitors, ritonavir
NC/PT Ensure pt does not have prostate cancer. Monitor for orthostatic hypotension. Advise pt to change positions slowly, take safety precautions for dizziness. Pt should not cut, crush, or chew tablets; store tablets in dry place, protected from light.

alglucosidase alfa
(Lumizyme, Myozyme)
CLASS Enzyme, Pompe's disease drug
PREG/CONT B/NA

BBW Risk of life-threatening anaphylactic reactions; have medical support readily available. Potential for rapid disease progression. Pt must be part of limited access program *(Lumizyme)*. Risk of cardiorespiratory failure; monitor pts w/ cardiorespiratory disorders carefully *(Myozyme)*.
IND & DOSE To increase ventilator-free survival in pts w/ infantile-onset Pompe's disease *(Myozyme)*; tx of pts 8 yr and older w/ late-onset Pompe's disease without cardiac hypertrophy *(Lumizyme)*. *Adult, child:* 20 mg/kg IV infusion over 4 hr q 2 wk.
ADV EFF Anaphylaxis, **cardiopulmonary failure**, chest discomfort, dyspnea, flushing, neck pain, **rapid progression of disease**, rash, urticaria, v/d
NC/PT Have medical support readily available during administration. Begin infusion at 1 mg/kg/hr; increase by 2 mg/kg/hr to reach desired dose, carefully monitoring pt response. *Lumizyme* available only by limited access program. Monitor for disease progression.

aliskiren (Tekturna)
CLASS Antihypertensive, renin inhibitor
PREG/CONT D/NA

BBW Use during second, third trimesters of pregnancy can cause fetal injury or death.

IND & DOSE Tx of hypertension, alone or w/ other antihypertensives. *Adult:* 150–300 mg/day PO.
ADJUST DOSE Severe renal impairment
ADV EFF Angioedema w/ respiratory symptoms, cough, diarrhea, dizziness, dyspepsia, fatigue, GERD, headache, hypotension, URI
INTERACTIONS ACE inhibitors, ARBs, atorvastatin, furosemide, irbesartan, ketoconazole, thiazides
NC/PT Rule out pregnancy; not for use in breast-feeding. Monitor potassium levels. Store drug in dry place at room temp. Other drugs may also be needed to control BP.

allopurinol (Aloprim, Zyloprim)
CLASS Antigout, purine analogue
PREG/CONT C/NA

IND & DOSE Gout, hyperuricemia. *Adult:* 100–800 mg/day PO in divided doses. **Hyperuricosuria.** *Adult:* 200–300 mg/day PO. **Px of acute gouty attacks.** *Adult:* 100 mg/day PO; increase by 100 mg/day at wkly intervals until uric acid is 6 mg/dL or less. **Px of uric acid nephropathy in certain malignancies.** *Adult:* 600–800 mg/day PO for 2–3 days w/ high fluid intake. *Child 6–10 yr:* 300 mg/day PO. *Child under 6 yr:* 150 mg/day PO. **Recurrent calcium oxalate stones.** *Adult:* 200–300 mg/day PO. **Parenteral use.** *Adult:* 200–400 mg/day IV to max of 600 mg/day as continuous infusion or at 6-, 8-, 12-hr intervals. *Child:* 200 mg/m²/day IV as continuous infusion or at 6-, 8-, 12-hr intervals.

ADJUST DOSE Elderly pts, renal impairment
ADV EFF Drowsiness, headache, n/v/d, **serious to fatal skin reactions**
INTERACTIONS ACE inhibitors, amoxicillin, ampicillin, anticoagulants, cyclophosphamide, theophylline, thiazides, thiopurines
NC/PT Give after meals; encourage 2.5–3 L/day fluid intake. Check urine alkalinity. Pt should discontinue at first sign of rash; avoid OTC medications.

almotriptan malate (Axert)
CLASS Antimigraine, serotonin selective agonist, triptan
PREG/CONT C/NA

IND & DOSE Tx of acute migraines w/ or without aura. *Adult, child 12–17 yr:* 6.25–12.5 mg PO as single dose at first sign of migraine; may repeat in 2 hr. Max, 2 doses/24 hr.
ADJUST DOSE Hepatic, renal impairment
ADV EFF BP changes, dizziness, dry mouth, **MI**, nausea, pressure in chest
INTERACTIONS Antifungals, antivirals, ergots, ketoconazole, macrolides, MAOIs, nefazodone, SSRIs
NC/PT For acute migraine, not px. Ensure pt has not used ergots within 24 hr. Not for use in pregnancy. Pt should not take more than two doses/24 hr; discontinue if s&sx of angina; monitor environment.

alogliptin (Nesina)
CLASS Antidiabetic, DPP-4 inhibitor
PREG/CONT B/NA

IND & DOSE Adjunct to diet, exercise to improve glycemic control in type 2 diabetes. *Adult:* 25 mg/day PO.
ADJUST DOSE Renal impairment
ADV EFF Headache, **hepatotoxicity**, hypoglycemia, nasopharyngitis, **pancreatitis**, URI

NC/PT Ensure continued diet, exercise program. Monitor blood glucose, renal, liver, pancreatic function. May give w/ other antidiabetics. Pt should continue diet and exercise program, report uncontrolled blood glucose, all herbs/other drugs used.

alosetron (Lotronex)
CLASS 5-HT3 antagonist, IBS drug
PREG/CONT B/NA

BBW Only indicated for women with severe diarrhea-dominant IBS who have failed to respond to conventional tx. Ensure pt understands risks of use and warning signs to report. Discontinue immediately at signs of constipation, ischemic colitis.
IND & DOSE Tx of severe diarrhea-predominant IBS in women with chronic IBS, no anatomic or biochemical abnormalities of GI tract, and who have failed to respond to conventional therapy. *Adult:* 0.5–1 mg PO bid.
ADJUST DOSE Elderly pts, mild to moderate hepatic impairment
ADV EFF Constipation, **ischemic colitis**
INTERACTIONS Cimetidine, clarithromycin, fluoroquinolones, fluvoxamine, GI motility drugs, itraconazole, ketoconazole, telithromycin, voriconazole
NC/PT Ensure pt has signed physician-pt agreement. Give w/ or without food. Monitor for signs of constipation. Not for use in pregnancy. Regular follow-up required. Pt should report constipation.

alpha₁-proteinase inhibitor (Aralast NP, Prolastin, Zemaira)
CLASS Blood product
PREG/CONT C/NA

IND & DOSE Chronic replacement tx for pts w/ congenital alpha₁-antitrypsin deficiency; tx of pts with early evidence of panacinar emphysema. *Adult:* 60 mg/kg IV once wkly (Aralast NP, Prolastin). **Chronic augmentation and maint therapy of pts w/ alpha₁-proteinase inhibitor deficiency with emphysema.** *Adult:* 0.08 mL/kg/min IV over 15 min once a wk (Zemaira).
ADV EFF Dizziness, fever, flulike symptoms, light-headedness
NC/PT Warn pt that this is blood product and can carry risk of blood-borne diseases. Discontinue if s&sx of hypersensitivity. Pt should report fever, chills, joint pain.

alprazolam (Niravam, Xanax)
CLASS Anxiolytic, benzodiazepine
PREG/CONT D/C-IV

IND & DOSE Mgt of anxiety disorders; short-term relief of anxiety symptoms; anxiety associated w/ depression. *Adult:* 0.25–0.5 mg PO tid; adjust to max 4 mg/day in divided doses. **Panic disorder.** *Adult:* 0.5 mg PO tid; increase at 3- to 4-day intervals to 1–10 mg/day or 0.5–1 mg/day ER tablets. Range, 3–6 mg/day.
ADJUST DOSE Elderly pts, advanced hepatic disease, debilitation
ADV EFF Anger, apathy, confusion, constipation, crying, **CV collapse**, diarrhea, disorientation, drowsiness (initially), drug dependence (withdrawal syndrome when drug is discontinued), dry mouth, fatigue, hostility, lethargy, light-headedness, mild paradoxical excitatory reactions during first 2 wk of tx, restlessness, sedation
INTERACTIONS Alcohol, carbamazepine, cimetidine, digoxin, disulfiram, grapefruit juice, hormonal contraceptives, isoniazid, kava, ketoconazole, levodopa, omeprazole, valerian root, valproic acid
NC/PT Taper gradually when discontinuing. Pt should not cut, crush, or chew ER tablet; avoid alcohol, grapefruit juice; take safety measures w/

CNS effects. Name confusion w/ *Xanax* (alprazolam), *Celexa* (citalopram), and *Cerebyx* (fosphenytoin), and between alprazolam and lorazepam.

alprostadil (Caverject, Muse, Prostin VR Pediatric)
CLASS Prostaglandin
PREG/CONT Unkn/NA

BBW Apnea occurs in 10%–12% of neonates treated w/ alprostadil, particularly those weighing under 2 kg. Monitor respiratory status continuously; have ventilatory assistance readily available. Move neonate often during first hr of infusion.
IND & DOSE Tx of ED. *Adult:* Intracavernous injection, 0.2–60 mcg using 0.5-in, 27–30 gauge needle; may repeat up to three times/wk. Urogenital system, 125–250 mcg; max, 2 systems/24 hr. **Palliative tx to temporarily maintain patency of ductus arteriosus.** *Child:* 0.025–0.05 mcg/kg/min IV infusion; max, 0.4 mcg/kg/min if needed.
ADV EFF Apnea, bradycardia, **cardiac arrest,** flushing, hypotension, respiratory distress, tachycardia; w/ intracavernous injection: **penile fibrosis**
NC/PT Constantly monitor arterial pressure and blood gases w/ IV use. Use extreme caution. Teach pt injection technique, proper disposal of needles and syringes. Name confusion w/ *Prostin VR Pediatric* (alprostadil), *Prostin F₂* (dinoprost—available outside US), *Prostin E₂* (dinoprostone), and *Prostin 15M* (carboprost tromethamine).

DANGEROUS DRUG

alteplase recombinant (Activase, Cathflo Activase)
CLASS Thrombolytic enzyme, TPA
PREG/CONT C/NA

IND & DOSE Acute MI. *Adult over 67 kg:* 100 mg as 15-mg IV bolus fol-

lowed by 50 mg infused over 30 min; then 35 mg over next 60 min. *Adult 67 kg or less:* 15-mg IV bolus followed by 0.75 mg/kg infused over 30 min (max, 50 mg); then 0.5 mg/kg over next 60 min (max, 35 mg). For 3-hr infusion, 60 mg in first hr (6–10 mg as bolus); 20 mg over second hr; 20 mg over third hr. Pts under 65 kg should receive 1.25 mg/kg over 3 hr.
Pulmonary embolism. *Adult:* 100 mg IV infusion over 2 hr, followed immediately by heparin therapy when PTT or thrombin time returns to twice normal or less. **Acute ischemic stroke.** *Adult:* 0.9 mg/kg max, 90 mg total dose) infused over 60 min w/ 10% given as IV bolus over first min. **Restoration of function of central venous access devices.** *Adult:* 2 mg (*Cathflo Activase*) in 2 mL sterile water for injection; may repeat after 2 hr.
ADV EFF Bleeding, cardiac arrhythmias, intracranial hemorrhage, n/v, urticaria
INTERACTIONS Anticoagulants, aspirin, dipyridamole
NC/PT Discontinue heparin and alteplase if serious bleeding occurs. Monitor coagulation studies; apply pressure or pressure dressings as needed to control bleeding. Type and cross-match blood. Initiate tx within first 6 hr of MI, within 3 hr of stroke.

DANGEROUS DRUG

altretamine (Hexalen)
CLASS Antineoplastic
PREG/CONT D/NA

BBW Must be used under supervision of oncologist. Monitor blood counts regularly; monitor neurologic exams regularly for neurotoxicity.
IND & DOSE Palliative tx of pts w/ persistent or recurrent ovarian cancer following first-line therapy w/ cisplatin and/or alkylating agent–based combination. *Adult:* 260 mg/m²/day PO for 14 or 21 consecutive days of 28-day cycle w/ meals or at bedtime.

ADV EFF Bone marrow depression, neurotoxicity, n/v/d
INTERACTIONS Antidepressants, cimetidine, MAOIs, pyridoxine
NC/PT Not for use in pregnancy, breast-feeding. Monitor blood counts regularly. Perform neurologic exam before and regularly during tx. Give antiemetic if n/v severe.

aluminum hydroxide gel (generic)
CLASS Antacid
PREG/CONT Unkn/NA

IND & DOSE Hyperacidity, symptomatic relief of upset stomach associated w/ hyperacidity. *Adult:* Tablets/capsules, 500–1,500 mg three to six times/day PO between meals and at bedtime. Liquid, 5–10 mL between meals and at bedtime. *Child:* 5–15 mL PO q 3–6 hr or 1–3 hr after meals and at bedtime. Px of GI bleeding in critically ill infants. 2–5 mL/dose PO q 1–2 hr.
ADV EFF Constipation, intestinal obstruction
INTERACTIONS Benzodiazepines, corticosteroids, diflunisal, digoxin, fluoroquinolones, iron, isoniazid, oral drugs, penicillamine, phenothiazines, ranitidine, tetracyclines
NC/PT Do not give oral drugs within 1–2 hr of this drug. Monitor serum phosphorus levels w/ long-term therapy. Advise pt to chew tablets thoroughly and follow w/ water. Constipation may occur.

alvimopan (Entereg)
CLASS Peripheral mu-opioid receptor antagonist
PREG/CONT B/NA

BBW For short-term use in hospitalized pts only.
IND & DOSE To accelerate time to upper and lower GI recovery after partial large or small bowel resection surgery w/ primary anastomo-

sis. *Adult:* 12 mg 30 min–5 hr before surgery, then 12 mg PO bid for up to 7 days. Max, 15 doses.
ADJUST DOSE Renal, hepatic impairment
ADV EFF Anemia, back pain, constipation, dyspepsia, flatulence, hypokalemia, **MI**, urine retention
NC/PT Not for use w/ severe hepatic or renal dysfx. For short-term, in-hospital use only. Recent use of opioids may lead to increased adverse effects.

amantadine (Symmetrel)
CLASS Antiparkinsonian, antiviral
PREG/CONT C/NA

IND & DOSE Influenza A virus px or tx. *Adult:* 200 mg/day PO or 100 mg bid for 10 days. *Child 9–12 yr:* 100 mg PO bid. *Child 1–9 yr:* 4.4–8.8 mg/kg/day PO in one or two divided doses; max, 150 mg/day. Parkinsonism tx. *Adult:* 100 mg PO bid (up to 400 mg/day). Drug-induced extrapyramidal reactions. *Adult:* 100 mg PO bid, up to 300 mg/day in divided doses.
ADJUST DOSE Elderly pts, seizure disorders, renal disease
ADV EFF Dizziness, insomnia, n/d
INTERACTIONS Anticholinergics, hydrochlorothiazide, QT-prolonging drugs, triamterene
NC/PT Do not discontinue abruptly w/ Parkinson's disease. Dispense smallest amount possible. Safety precautions if dizziness occurs.

ambrisentan (Letairis)
CLASS Antihypertensive, endothelin receptor antagonist
PREG/CONT X/NA

BBW Rule out pregnancy before starting tx; may cause fetal harm. Pt should use two forms of contraception.
IND & DOSE Tx of pulmonary arterial hypertension to improve exercise ability and delay clinical worsening. *Adult:* 5–10 mg/day PO.

ADV EFF Abd pain, anemia, constipation, edema, flushing, **liver impairment**, nasal congestion, nasopharyngitis, sinusitis, reduced sperm count
INTERACTIONS Cyclosporine
NC/PT Available only through restricted access program. Not for use in pregnancy, breast-feeding; negative pregnancy test, use of two forms of contraception required. Pt should not cut, crush, or chew tablets.

amifostine (Ethyol)
CLASS Cytoprotective
PREG/CONT C/NA

IND & DOSE To reduce cumulative renal toxicity associated w/ cisplatin therapy in pts w/ advanced ovarian cancer; to reduce incidence of moderate to severe xerostomia in pts w/ postoperative radiation for head and neck cancer. *Adult:* 910 mg/m² IV daily over 15 min before chemotherapy, over 3 min before radiation therapy.
ADJUST DOSE Elderly pts, CV disease
ADV EFF Cutaneous reactions, dizziness, hypocalcemia, hypotension, n/v
INTERACTIONS Cyclosporine
NC/PT Premedicate w/ antiemetic, dexamethasone. Monitor BP carefully during tx. Discontinue at s&sx of cutaneous reaction.

amikacin sulfate (Amikin)
CLASS Aminoglycoside
PREG/CONT D/NA

BBW Monitor for nephrotoxicity, ototoxicity w/ baseline and periodic renal function and neurologic examinations. Risk of serious toxicity, including neuromuscular blockade and respiratory paralysis.
IND & DOSE Short-term tx of serious infections caused by susceptible strains of *Pseudomonas* sp, *Escherichia coli,* indole-positive and indole-negative *Proteus* sp, *Providencia* sp, *Klebsiella* sp, *Enterobacter* sp, *Serratia* sp, *Acinetobacter* sp, suspected gram-negative infections before susceptibility is known; initial tx of staphylococcal infection if penicillin contraindicated. *Adult, child:* 15 mg/kg/day IM or IV in two to three equal doses at equal intervals, not to exceed 1.5 g/day, for 7–10 days. UTIs. *Adult, child:* 250 mg IM or IV bid.
ADJUST DOSE Elderly pts, renal failure
ADV EFF Anorexia, **nephrotoxicity,** n/v/d, ototoxicity, pain at injection site, superinfections
INTERACTIONS Hetastarch in IV sol, NMJ blockers, ototoxic drugs, penicillin
NC/PT Culture before tx. Monitor renal function, length of tx. Ensure pt well hydrated. Give IM dose by deep injection. Pt should report loss of hearing. Name confusion between amikacin and anakinra.

amiloride hydrochloride (Midamor)
CLASS Potassium-sparing diuretic
PREG/CONT B/NA

BBW Monitor pt for hyperkalemia.
IND & DOSE Adjunctive tx for edema of HF or hypertension; to prevent hypokalemia in pts at risk. *Adult:* Add 5 mg/day PO to usual antihypertensive dose; may increase dose to 10–20 mg/day w/ careful electrolyte monitoring.
ADV EFF Anorexia, ED, n/v/d, weakness
INTERACTIONS ACE inhibitors, digoxin, potassium supplements, spironolactone, triamterene
NC/PT Give early in day w/ food. Monitor weight, edema, serum electrolytes. Advise pt to take early in day (so increased urination will not disturb sleep) and avoid foods high in potassium.

amino acids (Aminosyn, FreAmine, HepatAmine, ProcalAmine, Travasol, etc)
CLASS Calorie agent, protein substrate
PREG/CONT C/NA

IND & DOSE To provide nutrition to pts in negative nitrogen balance and unable to maintain in other ways.
Adult: 1–1.5 g/kg/day amino acid injection IV into peripheral vein; 250–500 mL/day amino acid injection IV mixed w/ appropriate dextrose, vitamins, and electrolytes as part of TPN sol. Must be individualized. **Hepatic encephalopathy.** *Adult:* 80–120 g amino acid/day; 500 mL HepatAmine w/ 500 mL 50% dextrose and electrolyte sol IV over 8–12 hr/day. **Child w/ renal failure.** 0.5–1 g/kg/day amino acid IV mixed w/ dextrose as appropriate. **Amino acids replacement.** *Adult, child 16 yr and older:* 1.5 g/kg/day IV. *Child 13–15 yr:* 1.7 g/kg/day IV. *Child 4–12 yr:* 2 g/kg/day IV. *Child 1–3 yr:* 2–2.5 g/kg/day IV.
ADV EFF Dizziness, headache, infection, n/v, pain at infusion site, **pulmonary edema**
INTERACTIONS Tetracyclines
NC/PT Use strict aseptic technique in preparation, administration. Individualize dose based on lab values. Replace all IV apparatus daily. Infuse slowly; monitor closely.

aminocaproic acid (Amicar)
CLASS Systemic hemostatic
PREG/CONT C/NA

IND & DOSE Tx of excessive bleeding due to systemic hyperfibrinolysis/urinary fibrinolysis. *Adult:* Initially, 5 g PO or IV followed by 1–1.25 g every hr to produce and sustain plasma levels of 0.13 mg/mL; do not give more than 30 g/day. **Acute bleeding.** *Adult:* 4–5 g IV in 250 mL diluent during first hr of infusion; then continu-ous infusion of 1 g/hr in 50 mL diluent. Continue for 8 hr or until bleeding stops. **Px of recurrence of subarachnoid hemorrhage.** *Adult:* 36 g/day PO or IV in six divided doses.
ADV EFF Abd cramps, dizziness, headache, malaise, n/v/d, **pulmonary embolism**, tinnitus
INTERACTIONS Estrogen, hormonal contraceptives
NC/PT Pt on oral therapy may need up to 10 tablets first hr and around-the-clock dosing. Orient, support pt if CNS effects occur. Monitor for s&sx of clotting.

aminolevulinic acid hydrochloride (Levulan Kerastick)
CLASS Photosensitizer
PREG/CONT C/NA

IND & DOSE Tx of nonkeratotic actinic keratosis of face and scalp w/ light therapy. *Adult:* 20% sol applied directly to lesions, followed by light therapy within next 14–18 hr; once q 8 wk if needed.
ADV EFF Local crusting, local erosion, itching, photosensitivity, scaling
NC/PT Clean and dry area; break ampule and apply directly to lesions. Light therapy must be done in 14–18 hr. May repeat in 8 wk.

aminophylline (generic)
CLASS Bronchodilator, xanthine
PREG/CONT C/NA

IND & DOSE Symptomatic relief or prevention of bronchial asthma, reversible bronchospasm associated w/ chronic bronchitis and emphysema; adjunct to inhaled beta$_2$-selective adrenergic agonists and systemic corticosteroids for tx of acute exacerbations of s&sx and reversible airflow obstruction associated w/ asthma. *Adult:* 300 mg PO in divided doses q 6–8 hr; after 3 days increase to 400 mg/day PO in divided doses q 6–8 hr; after 3 more days, if tolerated, 600 mg/day PO in divided doses q 6–8 hr; adjust dose based on peak theophylline levels. *Child:* Adjust dose based on response. *Child 1–15 yr:* Initially, 12–14 mg/kg/day PO in divided doses q 4–6 hr (max, 300 mg/day); after 3 days, 16 mg/kg/day PO in divided doses q 4–6 hr (max, 400 mg/day); after 3 more days, 20 mg/kg/day PO in divided doses q 4–6 hr (max, 600 mg/day). **IV infusion rate for rapid tx.** Loading dose, 5.7 mg/kg over 30 min. Then, *adult over 60 yr:* 0.3 mg/kg/hr (max, 400 mg theophylline/day); *healthy nonsmoking adult,* 0.4 mg/kg/hr (max, 900 mg theophylline/day); *adult w/ cardiac decompensation, cor pulmonale, hepatic impairment, sepsis w/ multiorgan failure, shock:* 0.2 mg/kg/hr (max, 400 mg theophylline/day, 17 mg/hr); *adolescent (nonsmoking) 12–16 yr:* 0.5 mg/kg/hr (max, 900 mg theophylline/day); *adolescent smokers/ child 9–12 yr:* 0.7 mg/kg/hr; *child 1–9 yr:* 0.8 mg/kg/hr; *infants 6–52 wk:* mg/kg/hr = 0.008 × age in wks + 0.21; *neonates over 24 days,* 1.5 mg/kg q 12 hr; *neonates 24 days or younger,* 1 mg/kg q 12 hr.

ADV EFF Related to serum theophylline levels: Anorexia, **brain damage, circulatory failure,** dizziness, irritability, n/v/d, **respiratory arrest, seizures,** tachycardia

INTERACTIONS Acyclovir, allopurinol, beta blockers, cimetidine, clindamycin, diltiazem, disulfiram, enoxacin, erythromycin, fluoroquinolones, fluvoxamine, hormonal contraceptives, nicotine, NMJ blockers, pentoxifylline, phenytoin, sympathomimetics, tetracyclines, thiabendazole, ticlopidine, verapamil, zileuton

NC/PT Maintain adequate hydration. Monitor serum theophylline levels carefully. Use in pregnancy only if clearly needed. Pt should avoid excessive intake of caffeinated beverages, report changes in smoking habits (smoking affects drug's effectiveness).

---

amiodarone hydrochloride
(Cordarone, Pacerone)
CLASS Adrenergic blocker, antiarrhythmic
PREG/CONT D/NA

BBW Reserve use for life-threatening arrhythmias; serious toxicity, including arrhythmias, pulmonary toxicity, possible.

IND & DOSE Tx of life-threatening recurrent ventricular arrhythmias. *Adult:* Loading dose, 800–1,600 mg/day PO in divided doses for 1–3 wk; reduce dose to 600–800 mg/day PO in divided doses for 1 mo; if rhythm stable, reduce dose to 400 mg/day PO in one to two divided doses for maint dose. Or, 1,000 mg IV over 24 hr: 150 mg IV loading dose over 10 min, followed by 360 mg IV over 6 hr at 1 mg/min, then 540 mg IV at 0.5 mg/min over next 18 hr. After first 24 hr, maint infusion of 0.5 mg/min (720 mg/24 hr) or less IV can be cautiously continued for 2–3 wk. Switch to PO form as soon as possible. Convert to PO dose based on duration of IV therapy: Less than 1 wk, initial PO dose is 800–1,600 mg; 1–3 wk, initial PO dose is 600–800 mg; more than 3 wk, initial PO dose is 400 mg.

ADV EFF Anorexia, ataxia, **cardiac arrest, cardiac arrhythmias,** constipation, corneal microdeposits, fatigue, **hepatotoxicity,** hyperthyroidism, hypothyroidism, n/v, photosensitivity, **pulmonary toxicity**

INTERACTIONS Azole antifungals, beta blockers, calcium channel blockers, digoxin, ethotoin, fluoroquinolones, grapefruit juice, macrolide antibiotics, phenytoin, quinidine, ranolazine, simvastatin, thioridazine, trazodone, vardenafil, warfarin, ziprasidone

NC/PT Monitor cardiac rhythm continually and pulmonary function w/

periodic chest X-ray. Regular blood tests and serum-level checks needed. Obtain baseline ophthalmic exam, then periodically. Not for use in pregnancy. Pt should avoid grapefruit juice, report vision or breathing changes.

amitriptyline hydrochloride (generic)

CLASS Antidepressant, TCA
PREG/CONT D/NA

BBW Increased risk of suicidality in children, adolescents, young adults; monitor carefully.
IND & DOSE Relief of sx of depression (endogenous). Adult, hospitalized pts: Initially, 100 mg/day PO in divided doses; gradually increase to 200–300 mg/day as needed. Outpt: Initially, 75 mg/day PO in divided doses; may increase to 150 mg/day. Maint dose, 40–100 mg/day (may give as single bedtime dose). Child 12 yr and older: 10 mg PO tid, then 20 mg at bedtime. Chronic pain. Adult: 75–150 mg/day PO.
ADJUST DOSE Elderly pts
ADV EFF Anticholinergic effects, confusion, constipation, disturbed concentration, dry mouth, **MI**, orthostatic hypotension, photosensitivity, sedation, **stroke**
INTERACTIONS Anticholinergics, barbiturates, cimetidine, clonidine, disulfiram, ephedrine, epinephrine, fluoxetine, furazolidone, hormonal contraceptives, levodopa, MAOIs, methylphenidate, nicotine, norepinephrine, phenothiazines, QT-prolonging drugs, thyroid medication
NC/PT Restrict drug access in depressed or suicidal pts; make major portion at bedtime. Pt should be aware of sedative effects and avoid driving, etc, not mix w/ other sleep-inducing drugs, avoid prolonged exposure to sun or sunlamps, report thoughts of suicide.

amlodipine besylate (Norvasc)

CLASS Antianginal, antihypertensive, calcium channel blocker
PREG/CONT C/NA

IND & DOSE Tx of chronic stable angina, Prinzmetal's angina; to reduce angina risk and need for revascularization procedures in pts w/ CAD without HF; tx of essential hypertension. Adult: Initially, 5 mg/day PO; may gradually increase dose over 7–14 days to max 10 mg/day PO. Tx of hypertension. Child 6–17 yr: 2.5–5 mg/day PO.
ADJUST DOSE Elderly pts, hepatic impairment
ADV EFF Dizziness, fatigue, flushing, headache, lethargy, light-headedness, nausea, peripheral edema
INTERACTIONS Anticholinergics, barbiturates, cimetidine, clonidine, disulfiram, ephedrine, epinephrine, fluoxetine, furazolidone, hormonal contraceptives, levodopa, MAOIs, methylphenidate, nicotine, norepinephrine, phenothiazines, QT-prolonging drugs, thyroid medication
NC/PT Monitor closely when adjusting dose; monitor BP w/ hx of nitrate use. Monitor cardiac rhythm during initiation and periodically during tx. Name confusion between Norvasc (amlodipine) and Navane (thiothixene).

ammonium chloride (generic)

CLASS Electrolyte, urine acidifier
PREG/CONT C/NA

IND & DOSE Tx of hypochloremic states and metabolic alkalosis; urine acidification. Adult: Dosage determined by pt's condition and tolerance. Monitor dosage rate and amount by repeated serum bicarbonate determinations. IV infusion should not exceed conc of 1%–2% of ammonium chloride

ADV EFF Ammonia toxicity, hepatic impairment, pain at injection site

INTERACTIONS Amphetamine, chlorpropamide, dextroamphetamine, ephedrine, flecainide, methadone, methamphetamine, mexiletine, pseudoephedrine

NC/PT Give IV slowly. Monitor for possible fluid overload, acidosis; have sodium bicarbonate or sodium lactate available in case of overdose.

---

amoxapine (generic)
CLASS Anxiolytic, TCA
PREG/CONT C/NA

BBW Increased risk of suicidality in children, adolescents, young adults; monitor carefully.

IND & DOSE Relief of sx of depression; tx of depression w/ anxiety or agitation. *Adult:* Initially, 50 mg PO bid–tid; gradually increase to 100 mg PO bid–tid by end of first wk if tolerated; increase above 300 mg/day only if dosage ineffective for at least 2 wk. Usual effective dose, 200–300 mg/day.

ADJUST DOSE Elderly pts

ADV EFF Anticholinergic effects, confusion, constipation, disturbed concentration, dry mouth, **MI**, orthostatic hypotension, photosensitivity, sedation, **stroke**

INTERACTIONS Anticholinergics, barbiturates, cimetidine, clonidine, disulfiram, ephedrine, epinephrine, fluoxetine, furazolidone, hormonal contraceptives, levodopa, MAOIs, methylphenidate, nicotine, norepinephrine, phenothiazines, QT-prolonging drugs, thyroid medication

NC/PT Restrict drug access in depressed or suicidal pts; give major portion at bedtime. Pt should be aware of sedative effects and avoid driving, etc, should not mix w/ other sleep-inducing drugs, should avoid prolonged exposure to sun or sun-lamps, report thoughts of suicide.

---

amoxicillin trihydrate
(Amoxil, Moxatag, Trimox)
CLASS Antibiotic, penicillin-type
PREG/CONT B/NA

IND & DOSE Tx of tonsillitis and pharyngitis caused by *Streptococcus pyogenes* (ER tablet); infections due to susceptible strains of *Haemophilus influenzae, Escherichia coli, Proteus mirabilis, Neisseria gonorrhoeae, Streptococcus pneumoniae, Enterococcus faecalis,* streptococci, non-penicillinase-producing staphylococci; *Helicobacter pylori* infection in combination w/ other agents; postexposure px against *Bacillus anthracis. Adult, child over 40 kg:* URIs, GU, skin and soft-tissue infections, 250 mg PO q 8 hr or 500 mg PO q 12 hr; severe infection, 500 mg PO q 8 hr or 875 mg PO q 12 hr; postexposure anthrax px, 500 mg PO tid to complete 60-day course after 14–21 days of a fluoroquinolone or doxycycline; lower respiratory infection, 500 mg PO q 8 hr or 875 mg PO bid; uncomplicated gonococcal infections, 3 g amoxicillin PO as single dose; *C. trachomatis* in pregnancy, 500 mg PO tid for 7 days or 875 mg PO bid; tonsillitis/pharyngitis, 775 mg/day PO for 10 days w/ food (ER tablet); *H. pylori* infection, 1 g PO bid w/ clarithromycin 500 mg PO bid and lansoprazole 30 mg PO bid for 14 days. *Child 3 mo and older, under 40 kg:* URIs, GU infections, skin and soft-tissue infections, 20 mg/kg/day PO in divided doses q 8 hr or 25 mg/kg/day PO in divided doses q 12 hr; severe infection, 40 mg/kg/day PO in divided doses q 8 hr or 45 mg/kg/day PO in divided doses q 12 hr; postexposure anthrax px, 80 mg/kg/day PO divided in three doses to complete 60-day course after 14–21 days of fluoroquinolone or doxycycline tx. *Child 3 mo and older:* Mild to moderate URIs, GU infections, skin infections, 20 mg/kg PO daily in divided doses q 8 hr or 25 mg/kg PO in divided doses q 12 hr; acute otitis media, 80–90 mg/kg/day PO for 10 days (severe cases) or 5–7 days (moderate cases); gonorrhea in prepubertal children, 50 mg/kg PO w/ 25 mg/kg probenecid PO as single dose; lower respiratory infections/severe URI, GU, and skin infections, 40 mg/kg PO daily in divided doses q 8 hr or 45 mg/kg PO daily in divided doses q 12 hr. *Child up to 12 wk:* 30 mg/kg PO daily in divided doses q 12 hr.

ADJUST DOSE Renal impairment

ADV EFF Abd pain, **anaphylaxis,** fever, gastritis, glossitis, n/v/d, sore mouth, superinfections, wheezing

INTERACTIONS Chloramphenicol, hormonal contraceptives, probenecid, tetracyclines

NC/PT Culture before tx. Monitor for superinfections; n/v/d may occur. Pt should not cut, crush, or chew ER tablets; should continue until at least 2 days after s&sx resolve; complete full course.

DANGEROUS DRUG

**amphotericin B;
amphotericin B
cholesteryl sulfate;
amphotericin B,
liposome** (Abelcet, AmBisome, Amphotec)
CLASS Antifungal
PREG/CONT B/NA

BBW Reserve systemic use for progressive or potentially fatal infections. Not for use in noninvasive disease; toxicity can be severe.

IND & DOSE Tx of potentially fatal, progressive fungal infections not responsive to other tx. *Adult, child:* 5 mg/kg/day IV as single infusion at 2.5 mg/kg/hr (Abelcet). **Aspergillosis.** *Adult, child:* Initially, 3–4 mg/kg/day IV; Infuse at 1 mg/kg/hr (Amphotec). Or, 3 mg/kg/day IV over more than 2 hr (AmBisome). **Presumed fungal infection in febrile neutropenic pts.** *Adult, child:* 3 mg/kg/day IV (AmBisome). **Cryptococcal meningi-**

tis in HIV pts. *Adult, child:* 6 mg/kg/day IV (AmBisome). **Leishmaniasis.** *Adult, child:* 3 mg/kg/day IV, days 1–5, 14, and 21 for immunocompetent pts; 4 mg/kg/day IV days 1–5, 10, 17, 24, 31, and 38 for immunocompromised pts (AmBisome).

ADV EFF Cramping, dyspepsia, electrolyte disturbances, n/v/d, pain at injection site, **renal toxicity**

INTERACTIONS Antineoplastics, corticosteroids, cyclosporine, digitalis, nephrotoxic drugs, thiazide diuretics, zidovudine

NC/PT Dose varies among brand names; check carefully. Culture before tx. Monitor injection sites, electrolytes, kidney function. Use antihistamines, aspirin, antiemetics, meperidine to improve comfort, drug tolerance.

---

ampicillin (Principen)
CLASS Antibiotic, penicillin
PREG/CONT B/NA

IND & DOSE Tx of bacterial infections caused by susceptible strains; tx of GU infections: *Adult:* 500 mg IM, IV, PO q 6 hr. **Tx of respiratory tract infections.** *Adult:* 250 mg IM, IV, PO q 6 hr. **Tx of digestive system infections.** *Adult:* 500 mg PO q 6 hr for 48–72 hr after pt asymptomatic or eradication evident. **Tx of STDs in pts allergic to tetracycline.** *Adult:* 3.5 g ampicillin PO w/ 1 g probenecid. **Prevention of bacterial endocarditis for dental, oral, or upper respiratory procedures in pts at high risk.** *Adult:* 2 g ampicillin IM or IV within 30 min of procedure. *Child:* 50 mg/kg ampicillin IM or IV within 30 min of procedure. Six hr later, 25 mg/kg ampicillin IM or IV or 25 mg/kg amoxicillin PO. **Tx of respiratory and soft-tissue infections.** *Adult, child 40 kg or more:* 250–500 mg IV or IM q 6 hr. *Under 40 kg:* 25–50 mg/kg IM or IV in equally divided doses at 6- to 8-hr intervals. *20 kg to 40 kg:* 250 mg PO q 6 hr. *Under 20 kg:* 50 mg/kg/day PO in equally divided doses q 6–8 hr. **Tx of GI and GU infections, including women w/ *N. gonorrhoeae*.** Adult, child over 40 kg: 500 mg IM or IV q 6 hr. 40 kg or less: 50 mg/kg/day IM or IV in equally divided doses q 6–8 hr. 20 kg to 40 kg: 500 mg PO q 6 hr. Under 20 kg: 100 mg/kg/day PO in equally divided doses q 6–8 hr. **Tx of bacterial meningitis.** Adult, child: 150–200 mg/kg/day by continuous IV drip, then IM injections in equally divided doses q 3–4 hr. **Tx of septicemia.** Adult, child: 150–200 mg/kg/day IV for at least 3 days, then IM q 3–4 hr.

ADJUST DOSE Renal impairment
ADV EFF Abd pain, **anaphylaxis,** fever, gastritis, glossitis, n/v/d, sore mouth, superinfections, wheezing
INTERACTIONS Atenolol, chloramphenicol, hormonal contraceptives, probenecid, tetracyclines
NC/PT Culture before tx. Give on empty stomach. Do not give IM injections in same site. Check IV site for thrombosis. Monitor for superinfections. Pt should use second form of contraception while on drug. May experience n/v/d.

anagrelide (Agrylin)
CLASS Antiplatelet
PREG/CONT C/NA

IND & DOSE Tx of essential thrombocythemia secondary to myeloproliferative disorders to reduce elevated platelet count and risk of thrombosis; to improve associated s&sx, including thrombohemorrhagic events. Adult: Initially, 0.5 mg PO qid or 1 mg PO bid; do not increase by more than 0.5 mg/day each wk. Max, 10 mg/day or 2.5 mg as single dose. Child: Initially, 0.5 mg/day–0.5 mg PO qid; do not increase by more than 0.5 mg/day each wk. Max, 10 mg/day or 2.5 mg in single dose.
ADJUST DOSE Moderate hepatic impairment

ADV EFF Abd pain, asthenia, **bleeding, complete heart block,** headache, **HF, MI,** n/v/d, palpitations, **pancreatitis,** thrombocytopenia
INTERACTIONS Grapefruit juice
NC/PT Obtain platelet count q 2 days for first wk, then wkly. Provide safety measures. Monitor for bleeding; mark chart for alert in invasive procedures. Not for use in pregnancy. Pt should not drink grapefruit juice; should take on empty stomach. Name confusion between *Agrylin* and *Aggrastat* (tirofiban).

anakinra (Kineret)
CLASS Antiarthritic, interleukin-1 receptor antagonist
PREG/CONT B/NA

IND & DOSE To reduce s&sx and slow progression of moderately to severely active rheumatoid arthritis in pts who have failed on one or more disease-modifying antirheumatic drugs. Adult 18 yr and older: 100 mg/day subcut at about same time each day.
ADJUST DOSE Renal impairment
ADV EFF Infections, injection-site reactions, sinusitis, URI
INTERACTIONS Etanercept, immunizations, TNF blockers
NC/PT Increased risk of serious infection w/ TNF blockers; monitor pt carefully. Store refrigerated, protected from light. Not for use in pregnancy. Rotate inject sites. Pt should dispose of syringes, needles appropriately. Other antiarthritics may also be needed. Name confusion between anakinra and amikacin.

DANGEROUS DRUG
anastrozole (Arimidex)
CLASS Antiestrogen, antineoplastic, aromatase inhibitor
PREG/CONT X/NA

IND & DOSE Tx of advanced breast cancer in postmenopausal women w/ disease progression following tamoxifen tx; first-line tx of post-menopausal women w/ hormone receptor–positive or hormone receptor–unknown locally advanced or metastatic breast cancer; adjuvant tx of postmenopausal women w/ hormone receptor–positive early breast cancer. *Adult:* 1 mg/day PO.

ADV EFF Asthenia, back pain, bone pain, decreased bone density, fractures, hot flashes, insomnia, n/v, pharyngitis

INTERACTIONS Estrogens, tamoxifen

NC/PT Monitor lipid levels periodically, bone density. Use analgesics for pain. Not for use in pregnancy.

anidulafungin (Eraxis)

CLASS Antifungal, echinocandin
PREG/CONT C/NA

IND & DOSE Tx of candidemia and other *Candida* infections. *Adult:* 200 mg by IV infusion on day 1, then 100 mg/day by IV infusion; generally for minimum of 14 days. **Tx of esophageal candidiasis.** *Adult:* 100 mg by IV infusion on day 1, then 50 mg/day by IV infusion for minimum of 14 days.

ADV EFF Liver toxicity, n/v/d
NC/PT Culture before tx. Monitor LFTs. Not for use in pregnancy, breast-feeding. Maintain fluid, food intake.

antihemophilic factor (Advate, Hemofil, Humate-P, ReFacto, Wilate, Xyntha)

CLASS Antihemophilic
PREG/CONT C/NA

IND & DOSE Tx of hemophilia A; short-term px (*ReFacto*) to reduce frequency of spontaneous bleeding; surgical or invasive procedures in pts w/ von Willebrand disease in whom desmopressin is ineffective

or contraindicated. *Adult, child:* Dose depends on weight, severity of deficiency, severity of bleeding; monitor factor VIII levels to establish dose needed. Follow tx carefully w/ factor VIII level assays. Formulas used as dosage guide:

$$\text{(\% of normal)} = \frac{\text{AHF/IU given} \times 2}{\text{weight in kg}}$$

$$\text{AHF/IU required} = \text{weight (kg)} \times \text{desired factor VIII increase (\% of normal)} \times 0.5$$

ADV EFF AIDS (from repeated use of blood products), bronchospasm, hemolysis, hepatitis, stinging at infusion site, tachycardia
NC/PT Monitor factor VIII levels regularly. Monitor pulse. Reduce rate of infusion w/ significant tachycardia. Pt should wear or carry medical alert information.

antithrombin, recombinant (ATryn)

CLASS Coagulation inhibitor
PREG/CONT C/NA

IND & DOSE Prevention of periop and peripartum thromboembolic events in pts w/ hereditary antithrombin deficiency. *Adult:* Individualize dose based on antithrombin level; loading dose over 15 min IV followed by maint dose to keep antithrombin activity levels 80%–120% of normal. Surgical pts, use formula 100 − baseline antithrombin activity ÷ 2.3 × body wt; maint, divide by 10.2. Pregnant women, 100 − baseline antithrombin activity ÷ 1.3 × body wt; maint, divide by 5.4.
ADV EFF Hemorrhage, infusion-site reactions
INTERACTIONS Heparin, low-molecular-weight heparin
NC/PT Not for use w/ allergy to goats or goat products. Follow clotting studies closely.

antithrombin III
(Thrombate III)
CLASS Coagulation inhibitor
PREG/CONT C/NA

IND & DOSE Tx of pts w/ hereditary antithrombin III deficiency in connection w/ surgical or obstetrical procedures or when suffering from thromboembolism; replacement tx in congenital antithrombin III deficiency.
Adult: Dosage units = desired antithrombin level (%) − baseline antithrombin level (%) × body wt (kg) ÷ 1.4 q 2–8 days IV.
ADV EFF Hemorrhage, infusion-site reactions
INTERACTIONS Heparin, low-molecular-weight heparin
NC/PT Frequent blood tests required. Dosage varies widely. Monitor for bleeding. Human blood product; slight risk of blood-transmitted diseases.

DANGEROUS DRUG
apixaban (Eliquis)
CLASS Anticoagulant, direct thrombin inhibitor
PREG/CONT B/NA

IND & DOSE Reduction of stroke, embolism in pts w/ nonvalvular atrial fibrillation. *Adult:* 5 mg PO bid.
ADJUST DOSE Elderly pts, severe renal impairment
ADV EFF Bleeding, rebound thrombotic events w/ discontinuation, severe hypersensitivity reactions
INTERACTIONS Carbamazepine, clarithromycin, itraconazole, ketoconazole, other drugs that increase bleeding, phenytoin, rifampin, ritonavir, St. John's wort
NC/PT Not for use w/ artificial heart valves. Monitor for bleeding; do not stop suddenly. Pt should avoid pregnancy, breast-feeding, OTC drugs that affect bleeding; ensure that drug is not stopped suddenly; take safety precautions to avoid injury; report increased bleeding, chest pain, headache, dizziness.

apomorphine (Apokyn)
CLASS Antiparkinsonian, dopamine agonist
PREG/CONT C/NA

IND & DOSE Intermittent tx of hypomobility "off" episodes caused by advanced Parkinson's disease.
Adult: 2 mg subcut; increase slowly to max of 6 mg. Give 300 mg trimethobenzamide PO tid for 3 days before starting to completion of 2 mo of tx.
ADV EFF Chest pain, dizziness, dyskinesia, edema, **fibrotic complications,** flushing, hallucinations, **hepatic impairment, melanoma,** n/v, **renal impairment,** rhinorrhea, sedation, somnolence, sweating, yawning
INTERACTIONS Antihypertensives, dopamine antagonists, 5-HT$_3$ antagonists (granisetron, ondansetron, etc), QT-prolonging drugs, vasodilators
NC/PT Give subcut injection in stomach, upper arm, or leg; rotate sites. Protect pt when CNS effects occur. Teach proper drug administration, disposal of needles and syringes; many CNS effects possible.

aprepitant (Emend),
fosaprepitant (Emend for Injection)
CLASS Antiemetic, substance P and neurokinin 1 receptor antagonist
PREG/CONT B/NA

IND & DOSE With other antiemetics for prevention of acute and delayed n/v associated w/ initial and repeat courses of moderately or highly emetogenic cancer chemotherapy.
Adult: Aprepitant, 125 mg PO 1 hr before chemotherapy (day 1) and 80 mg PO once daily in a.m. on days 2 and 3 w/ dexamethasone, ondansetron; or parenteral administration, fosaprepitant, 115 mg IV 30 min before chemotherapy on day 1 of antiemetic regimen; infuse over 15 min. *Child:* 115 mg IV 30 min before chemotherapy

infused over 15 min on day 1 of antiemetic regimen; 125 mg/day PO days 2 and 3. **Postop n/v.** *Adult:* 40 mg PO within 3 hr before anesthesia induction.
ADV EFF Anorexia, constipation, diarrhea, dizziness, fatigue
INTERACTIONS Docetaxel, etoposide, hormonal contraceptives, ifosfamide, imatinib, irinotecan, paclitaxel, pimozide, vinblastine, vincristine, vinorelbine, warfarin
NC/PT Give first dose w/ dexamethasone 1 hr before start of chemotherapy; give additional doses of dexamethasone and ondansetron as indicated as part of antiemetic regimen. Give within 3 hr before anesthesia induction if used to prevent postop n/v. Provide safety precautions, analgesics as needed. Not for use in pregnancy or breast-feeding. Pt should use caution if dizziness, drowsiness occur.

arformoterol tartrate
(Brovana)
CLASS Bronchodilator, long-acting beta agonist
PREG/CONT C/NA

BBW Increased risk of asthma-related death; alert pt accordingly. Contraindicated in asthma without use of long-term control medication.
IND & DOSE Long-term maint tx of bronchoconstriction in pts w/ COPD. *Adult:* 15 mcg bid (a.m. and p.m.) by nebulization. Max, 30 mcg total daily dose.
ADV EFF Asthma-related deaths, paradoxical bronchospasm
INTERACTIONS Beta-adrenergic blockers, diuretics, MAOIs, QT-prolonging drugs, TCAs
NC/PT Not for use in acute bronchospasm. Ensure pt continues other drugs to manage COPD, especially long-term control drugs. Not for use in pregnancy, breast-feeding. Teach proper use of nebulizer. Pt should have periodic evaluation of respiratory status.

argatroban (Argatroban)
CLASS Anticoagulant
PREG/CONT B/NA

IND & DOSE Px or tx of thrombosis in pts w/ heparin-induced thrombocytopenia, including pts at risk undergoing percutaneous coronary intervention (PCI). *Adult:* 2 mcg/kg/min IV; PCI, bolus of 350 mcg/kg IV over 3–5 min, then 25 mcg/kg/min IV.
ADV EFF Bleeding, cardiac arrest, chest pain, dyspnea, fever, headache, hypotension, n/v/d
INTERACTIONS Heparin, thrombolytics, warfarin
NC/PT Not for use in pregnancy, breast-feeding. Monitor for s&sx of bleeding.

aripiprazole (Abilify, Abilify Discmelt)
CLASS Atypical antipsychotic, dopamine/serotonin agonist and antagonist
PREG/CONT C/NA

BBW Elderly pts w/ dementia-related psychosis have increased risk of death if given atypical antipsychotics. Risk of suicidal ideation increases w/ antidepressant use, especially in children, adolescents, young adults; monitor accordingly.
IND & DOSE Oral sol may be substituted on mg-to-mg basis up to 25 mg of tablet. Pts taking 30-mg tablets should receive 25 mg if switched to sol. **Tx of schizophrenia.** *Adult:* 10–15 mg/day PO. Increase dose q 2 wk to max of 30 mg/day. *Child 13–17 yr:* Initially, 2 mg/day PO. Adjust to 5 mg/day after 2 days, then to target dose of 10 mg/day; max, 30 mg/day. **Tx of bipolar disorder.** *Adult:* 15 mg/day PO as one dose; maint, 15–30 mg/day PO. *Child 10–17 yr:* Initially, 2 mg/day PO; titrate to 5 mg/day after 2 days, then to 10 mg/day after another 2 days. Target dose, 10 mg/day; max, 30 mg/day. **Tx of major**

depressive disorder. *Adult:* Initially, 2–5 mg/day PO; maint, 2–15 mg/day as adjunct therapy. **Tx of agitation.** *Adult:* 5.25–15 mg IM; usual dose, 9.75 mg IM. May give cumulative doses of up to 30 mg/day PO. **Irritability associated w/ autistic disorder.** *Child 6–17 yr:* 2 mg/day PO; titrate to maint dose of 5–15 mg/day.

ADV EFF Hyperglycemia, **NMS, seizures** (potentially life-threatening), **suicidality**, weight gain

INTERACTIONS Alcohol, carbamazepine, CNS depressants, CYP2D6 inhibitors (fluoxetine, paroxetine, quinidine), CYP3A4 inhibitors (ketoconazole), lorazepam

NC/PT Dispense least amount possible to suicidal pts. Ensure pt well hydrated. Switch to oral sol w/ difficulty swallowing. Not for use in pregnancy, breast-feeding. Monitor weight; assess for hyperglycemia. May react w/ many medications; monitor drug regimen. Confusion between aripiprazole and proton pump inhibitors; use extreme caution.

armodafinil (Nuvigil)
CLASS CNS stimulant, narcoleptic
PREG/CONT C/C-IV

IND & DOSE To improve wakefulness in pts w/ excessive sleepiness associated w/ obstructive sleep apnea/hypopnea syndrome; narcolepsy. *Adult:* 150–250 mg/day PO as single dose in a.m. **Shift work sleep disorder.** *Adult:* 150 mg/day PO taken 1 hr before start of work shift.

ADJUST DOSE Elderly pts, severe hepatic impairment

ADV EFF Dizziness, headache, insomnia, nausea, **Stevens-Johnson syndrome**

INTERACTIONS Cyclosporine, ethinyl estradiol, hormonal contraceptives, midazolam, omeprazole, phenytoin, TCAs, triazolam, warfarin

NC/PT Rule out underlying medical conditions. Should be part of compre-hensive program for sleep. Provide safety measures if CNS effects occur. Not for use in pregnancy, breast-feeding. Pt should use barrier contraceptives, avoid alcohol.

arsenic trioxide (Trisenox)
CLASS Antineoplastic
PREG/CONT D/NA

BBW Extremely toxic and carcinogenic; monitor blood counts, electrolytes. Prolonged QT interval, arrhythmias; monitor ECG.

IND & DOSE Induction and remission of acute promyelocytic leukemia in pts refractory to retinoid or anthracycline chemotherapy w/ t(15:17) translocation or PML/RAR-alpha gene expression. *Adult:* Induction, 0.15 mg/kg/day IV until bone marrow remission; max, 60 doses. Consolidation, 0.15 mg/kg/day IV starting 3–6 wk after induction.

ADJUST DOSE Severe hepatic impairment

ADV EFF Abd pain, **APL differentiation syndrome, cancer, complete heart block,** cough, dizziness, dyspnea, edema, fatigue, headache, **hyperleukocytosis,** leukocytosis, n/v/d, **prolonged QT**

INTERACTIONS Cyclosporine, ethinyl estradiol, hormonal contraceptives, midazolam, omeprazole, phenytoin, TCAs, triazolam, warfarin

NC/PT Monitor CBC, ECG, electrolytes closely. Provide comfort measures for GI effects, safety measures for CNS effects. Not for use in pregnancy, breast-feeding.

asenapine (Saphris)
CLASS Atypical antipsychotic, dopamine/serotonin antagonist
PREG/CONT C/NA

BBW Elderly pts w/ dementia-related psychosis have increased

risk of death if given atypical antipsychotics. Risk of suicidal ideation increases w/ antidepressant use, especially in children, adolescents, young adults; monitor accordingly.
IND & DOSE Tx of schizophrenia. *Adult:* 5–10 mg sublingually bid.
Acute tx of manic or mixed episodes associated w/ bipolar I disorder; adjunctive therapy w/ lithium or valproate for acute tx of manic or mixed episodes associated w/ bipolar I disorder. *Adult:* 5–10 mg sublingually bid; may decrease to 5 mg/day if needed.
ADJUST DOSE Severe hepatic impairment
ADV EFF Akathisia, dizziness, extrapyramidal sx, **NMS, prolonged QT,** somnolence, **suicidality**
INTERACTIONS Alcohol, antihypertensives, CNS depressants, fluvoxamine, QT-prolonging drugs
NC/PT Monitor ECG periodically. Provide safety measures for CNS effects. Monitor weight gain and blood glucose. Not for use in pregnancy, breast-feeding. Pt should change positions slowly, take safety measures w/ CNS effects, report thoughts of suicide.

DANGEROUS DRUG

asparaginase Erwinia chrysanthemi (Erwinaze)
CLASS Antineoplastic
PREG/CONT C/NA

IND & DOSE Tx of pts w/ ALL who have developed sensitivity to asparaginase or pegaspargase. *Adult, child:* 25,000/m² international units IM for each scheduled dose of pegaspargase or asparaginase; limit volume to 2 mL/injection.
ADV EFF Anaphylaxis, arthralgia, **coagulation disorders, hyperglycemia,** n/v, **pancreatitis,** rash, seizures, urticaria
NC/PT Monitor for severe reaction, hyperglycemia, pancreatitis, coagula-

tion disorders. Not for use in pregnancy. Prepare calendar to keep track of appointments. Pt should have regular blood tests.

---

aspirin (Bayer, Bufferin, Heartline, Norwich, St. Joseph's, etc)
CLASS Analgesic, antiplatelet, antipyretic, salicylate
PREG/CONT D/NA

IND & DOSE Tx of mild to moderate pain, fever. *Adult:* 325–1,000 mg PO q 4–6 hr; max, 4,000 mg/day. SR tablets, 1,300 mg PO, then 650–1,300 mg q 8 hr; max, 3,900 mg/day. Suppositories, 1 rectally q 4 hr. *Child:* 10–15 mg/kg/dose PO q 4 hr, up to 60–80 mg/kg/day. Do not give to pts w/ chickenpox or flu symptoms. **Arthritis.** *Adult:* Up to 3 g/day PO in divided doses. *Child:* 90–130 mg/kg/24 hr PO in divided doses at 6- to 8-hr intervals. Maintain serum level of 150–300 mcg/mL. **Ischemic stroke, TIA.** *Adult:* 50–325 mg/day PO. **Angina, recurrent MI prevention.** *Adult:* 75–325 mg/day PO. **Suspected MI.** *Adult:* 160–325 mg PO as soon as possible; continue daily for 30 days. **CABG.** *Adult:* 325 mg PO 6 hr after procedure, then daily for 1 yr. **Acute rheumatic fever.** *Adult:* 5–8 g/day PO; modify to maintain serum salicylate level of 15–30 mg/dL. *Child:* Initially, 100 mg/kg/day PO, then decrease to 75 mg/kg/day for 4–6 wk. Therapeutic serum salicylate level, 150–300 mcg/mL. **Kawasaki disease.** *Child:* 80–100 mg/kg/day PO divided q 6 hr; after fever resolves, 1–5 mg/kg/day once daily.
ADV EFF Acute aspirin toxicity, bleeding, dizziness, difficulty hearing, dyspepsia, epigastric discomfort, nausea, occult blood loss, tinnitus
INTERACTIONS Alcohol, alkalinizers, antacids, anticoagulants, corticosteroids, furosemide, nitroglycerin, NSAIDs, urine acidifiers

NC/PT Do not use in children w/ chickenpox or flu symptoms. Monitor dose for use in children. Give w/ full glass of water. Pt should not cut, crush, or chew SR preparations; check OTC products for aspirin content to avoid overdose; report ringing in ears, bloody stools.

atazanavir sulfate (Reyataz)

CLASS Antiretroviral, protease inhibitor
PREG/CONT B/NA

IND & DOSE With other antiretrovirals for tx of HIV-1 infection.
Adult: Therapy-naïve, 300 mg/day PO w/ 100 mg ritonavir PO once daily; if unable to tolerate ritonavir, can give 400 mg PO once daily; therapy-experienced, 300 mg/day PO w/ 100 mg ritonavir PO taken w/ food. *Child 6–under 18 yr:* Therapy-naïve, base dose on weight, 150–300 mg/day atazanavir PO w/ 80–100 mg ritonavir daily PO; therapy-experienced, base dose on weight, 200–300 mg/day atazanavir PO w/ 100 mg ritonavir PO.
ADJUST DOSE Hepatic, renal impairment
ADV EFF Headache, liver enzyme elevation, nausea, rash, **severe hepatomegaly w/ steatosis** (sometimes fatal)
INTERACTIONS Antacids, bosentan, indinavir, irinotecan, lovastatin, proton pump inhibitors, rifampin, sildenafil, simvastatin, St. John's wort, warfarin. Contraindicated w/ ergot derivatives, midazolam, pimozide, triazolam
NC/PT Ensure HIV testing has been done. Monitor LFTs. Ensure pt takes drug w/ other antiretrovirals. Withdraw drug at s&sx of lactic acidosis. Not for use in pregnancy, breast-feeding. Does not cure disease. Pt should avoid St John's wort, report use to all health care providers.

atenolol (Tenormin)

CLASS Antianginal, antihypertensive, beta$_1$-adrenergic blocker
PREG/CONT D/NA

BBW Do not discontinue drug abruptly after long-term therapy; taper drug gradually over 2 wk w/ monitoring; risk of MI, arrhythmias.
IND & DOSE Hypertension. *Adult:* 50 mg PO once/day; after 1–2 wk, may increase to 100 mg/day. **Angina pectoris.** *Adult:* Initially, 50 mg/day PO; up to 200 mg/day may be needed. **Acute MI.** *Adult:* 100 mg/day PO or 50 mg PO bid for 6–9 days or until discharge.
ADJUST DOSE Elderly pts, renal impairment
ADV EFF Bradycardia, **bronchospasm**, cardiac arrhythmias, ED, exercise tolerance decrease, flatulence, gastric pain, **laryngospasm**, n/v/d
INTERACTIONS Ampicillin, anticholinergics, aspirin, bismuth subsalicylate, calcium salts, clonidine, hormonal contraceptives, insulin, lidocaine, prazosin, quinidine, verapamil
NC/PT Do not stop suddenly; taper over 2 wk. Pt should take safety precautions w/ CNS effects; report difficulty breathing.

atomoxetine hydrochloride (Strattera)

CLASS Selective norepinephrine reuptake inhibitor
PREG/CONT C/NA

BBW Increased risk of suicidality in children, adolescents. Monitor closely; alert caregivers of risk.
IND & DOSE Tx of ADHD as part of total tx program. *Adult, child over 70 kg:* 40 mg/day PO; increase after minimum of 3 days to target total daily dose of 80 mg PO. Max, 100 mg/day. *Child 6 yr and older, 70 kg or less:* 0.5 mg/kg/day PO; increase after

minimum of 3 days to target total daily dose of about 1.2 mg/kg/day PO. Max, 1.4 mg/kg or 100 mg/day, whichever is less.
ADJUST DOSE Hepatic impairment
ADV EFF Constipation, cough, dry mouth, insomnia, n/v, **sudden cardiac death, suicidality**
INTERACTIONS CYP3A4 substrates, fluoxetine, MAOIs (do not give within 14 days of atomoxetine), paroxetine, quinidine
NC/PT Ensure proper dx of ADHD; part of comprehensive tx program. Monitor growth. Provide drug vacation periodically. Give dose 6 p.m. to allow sleep. Not for use In pregnancy. Pt should avoid OTC drugs, herbs that may be stimulants.

atorvastatin calcium (Lipitor)
CLASS Antihyperlipidemic, HMG-CoA inhibitor
PREG/CONT X/NA

IND & DOSE Adjunct to diet to lower total cholesterol, serum triglycerides, LDL and increase HDL in pts w/ primary hypercholesterolemia, mixed dyslipidemia, familial hypercholesterolemia, elevated serum triglycerides; to prevent MI, CV disease in pts w/ many risk factors; to reduce risk of MI and CV events in pts w/ hx of CAD. *Adult:* 10–20 mg PO once daily without regard to meals; maint, 10–80 mg/day PO. *Child 10–17 yr:* 10 mg PO daily; max, 20 mg/day.
ADV EFF Abd pain, constipation, cramps, flatulence, headache, **liver failure, rhabdomyolysis w/ renal failure**
INTERACTIONS Antifungals, cimetidine, clarithromycin, cyclosporine, digoxin, diltiazem, erythromycin, fibric acid derivatives, grapefruit juice, hormonal contraceptives, nefazodone, niacin, protease inhibitors, tacrolimus
NC/PT Obtain baseline and periodic LFTs. Withhold drug in acute or seri-

ous conditions. Give in p.m. Ensure pt is using diet and exercise program. Not for use in pregnancy. Pt should report muscle pain. Name confusion between written orders for *Lipitor* (atorvastatin) and *Zyrtec* (cetirizine).

atovaquone (Mepron)
CLASS Antiprotozoal
PREG/CONT C/NA

IND & DOSE Prevention and acute oral tx of mild to moderate *Pneumocystis jiroveci* pneumonia in pts intolerant of trimethoprim-sulfamethoxazole. *Adult, child 13–16 yr:* Prevention of *P. jiroveci* pneumonia, 1,500 mg PO daily w/ meal. Tx of *P. jiroveci* pneumonia, 750 mg PO bid w/ food for 21 days.
ADJUST DOSE Elderly pts
ADV EFF Dizziness, fever, headache, insomnia, n/v/d
INTERACTIONS Rifampin
NC/PT Give w/ meals. Ensure drug is taken for 21 days for tx.

atropine sulfate (AtroPen, Isopto Atropine)
CLASS Anticholinergic, antidote, belladonna
PREG/CONT C/NA

IND & DOSE Antisialagogue, tx of parkinsonism, bradycardia, pylorospasm, urinary bladder relaxation, uterine relaxation. *Adult:* 0.4–0.6 mg PO, IM, IV, subcut. *Child:* Base dose on weight, 0.1–0.4 mg PO, IM, IV, subcut. **Bradyarrhythmia.** *Adult:* 0.4–1 mg (max, 2 mg) IV q 1–2 hr as needed. *Child:* 0.01–0.03 mg/kg IV. **Antidote for cholinergic drug overdose, organophosphorus insecticides; initial tx for nerve agent poisoning.** *Adult:* 2–3 mg parenterally; repeat until signs of atropine intoxication appear. Use of auto-injector recommended. **Ophthalmic sol for eye refraction.** *Adult:* 1–2 drops into eye 1 hr before refracting. **Ophthalmic sol**

for uveitis. *Adult:* 1–2 drops into eye tid.

ADJUST DOSE Elderly pts

ADV EFF Altered taste perception, bradycardia, decreased sweating, dry mouth, n/v, palpitations, **paralytic ileus,** predisposition to heat prostration, urinary hesitancy, urine retention

INTERACTIONS Anticholinergics, antihistamines, haloperidol, MAOIs, phenothiazines, TCAs

NC/PT Ensure adequate hydration. Provide temp control. Monitor heart rate. Pt should empty bladder before taking if urine retention occurs. Sugarless lozenges may help dry mouth.

---

auranofin (Ridaura)
CLASS Antirheumatic, gold salt
PREG/CONT C/NA

BBW Discontinue at first sign of toxicity. Severe bone marrow depression, renal toxicity, diarrhea possible.
IND & DOSE Mgt of pts w/ **active classic rheumatoid arthritis who have insufficient response to NSAIDs.** *Adult:* 3 mg PO bid or 6 mg/day PO; after 6 mo may increase to 3 mg PO tid. Max, 9 mg/day.
ADV EFF Angioedema, **bone marrow suppression, diarrhea,** eye changes, **GI bleeding,** gingivitis, **interstitial pneumonitis,** peripheral neuropathy, photosensitivity, rash, **renal failure,** stomatitis
NC/PT Monitor blood counts; renal, lung function. Corticosteroids may help w/ mild reactions. Pt should avoid ultraviolet light, use sunscreen or protective clothes.

---

avanafil (Stendra)
CLASS ED drug,
phosphodiesterase-5 inhibitor
PREG/CONT C/NA

IND & DOSE Tx of ED. *Adult:* 100 mg PO 30 min before sexual activity; range, 50–200 mg no more than once/day.
ADJUST DOSE Severe renal, hepatic impairment
ADV EFF Back pain, dyspepsia, flushing, headache, **MI,** nasal congestion, nasopharyngitis
INTERACTIONS Alcohol, alpha blockers, amprenavir, antihypertensives, aprepitant, diltiazem, fluconazole, fosamprenavir, grapefruit juice, itraconazole, ketoconazole, nitrates, ritonavir, verapamil
NC/PT Ensure proper dx. Does not prevent STDs; does not work in absence of sexual stimulation. Pt should not use w/ nitrates, antihypertensives, grapefruit juice, alcohol; report sudden loss of vision or hearing, erection lasting over 4 hr.

---

axitinib (Inlyta)
CLASS Antineoplastic, kinase inhibitor
PREG/CONT D/NA

IND & DOSE Tx of advanced renal cell cancer after failure of one prior systemic therapy. *Adult:* 5 mg PO bid 12 hr apart w/ full glass of water.
ADJUST DOSE Hepatic impairment
ADV EFF Anorexia, asthenia, constipation, diarrhea, dysphonia, fatigue, hand-foot syndrome, **GI perforation/fistula, hemorrhage, hepatic injury,** hypertension, **hypertensive crisis, hypothyroidism, proteinuria, RPLS, thrombotic events,** vomiting, weight loss
INTERACTIONS Strong CYP3A4/5 inhibitors or inducers (carbamazepine, dexamethasone, ketoconazole, phenobarbital, phenytoin, rifabutin, rifampin, rifapentine, St. John's wort); avoid these combinations
NC/PT Monitor closely for adverse reactions; have supportive measures readily available. Stop at least 24 hr before scheduled surgery. Not for use in pregnancy. Pt should take w/ full glass of water, report s&sx of

bleeding, severe headache, severe GI effects, urine/stool changes.

azacitidine (Vidaza)

CLASS Antineoplastic, nucleoside metabolic inhibitor
PREG/CONT D/NA

IND & DOSE Tx of myelodysplastic syndrome, including refractory anemias and chronic myelomonocytic leukemia. *Adult:* 75 mg/m²/day subcut for 7 days q 4 wk; may increase to 100 mg/m²/ day after two cycles if no response. Pt should have at least four cycles.
ADJUST DOSE Hepatic impairment
ADV EFF Bone marrow suppression, fever, **hepatic impairment**, injection-site reactions, n/v/d, pneumonia, **renal impairment**
NC/PT Not for use in pregnancy. Men on drug should not father a child. Monitor CBC, LFTs, renal function. Premedicate w/ antiemetic.

azathioprine (Azasan, Imuran)

CLASS Immunosuppressant
PREG/CONT D/NA

BBW Monitor blood counts regularly; severe hematologic effects may require stopping drug. Increases risk of neoplasia; adjust accordingly.
IND & DOSE Px of rejection w/ renal homotransplantation. *Adult:* 3–5 mg/kg/day PO or IV as single dose on day of transplant; maint, 1–3 mg/kg/day PO. Tx of classic rheumatoid arthritis not responsive to other therapy. *Adult:* 1 mg/kg PO as single dose or bid. May increase at 6–8 wk and thereafter by steps at 4-wk intervals; max, 2.5 mg/kg/day.
ADJUST DOSE Elderly pts, renal impairment
ADV EFF Carcinogenesis, hepatotoxicity, leukopenia, macrocytic anemia, n/v, **serious infection**, thrombocytopenia

INTERACTIONS Allopurinol, NMJ blockers
NC/PT Switch to oral form as soon as possible; monitor blood counts carefully. Give w/ food if GI upset a problem. Protect from infection.

azilsartan medoxomil (Edarbi)

CLASS Antihypertensive, ARB
PREG/CONT D/NA

BBW Rule out pregnancy before starting tx. Suggest use of barrier contraceptives during tx; fetal injury and death have been reported.
IND & DOSE Tx of hypertension, alone or w/ other antihypertensives. *Adult:* 80 mg/day PO. For pts on high-dose diuretics or who are volume-depleted, consider starting dose of 40 mg/day; titrate if tolerated.
ADV EFF Diarrhea
INTERACTIONS NSAIDs
NC/PT Rule out pregnancy; suggest use of barrier contraceptives. Monitor in situations that could lead to lower BP. Mark chart if pt is going to surgery; possible volume problems after surgery. Not for use in pregnancy, breast-feeding.

azithromycin (AzaSite, Zithromax, Zmax)

CLASS Macrolide antibiotic
PREG/CONT B/NA

IND & DOSE Tx of mild to moderate acute bacterial exacerbations of COPD, pneumonia, pharyngitis/tonsillitis (as second-line), uncomplicated skin and skin-structure infections. *Adult:* 500 mg PO as single dose on first day, then 250 mg PO daily on days 2–5 for total dose of 1.5 g or 500 mg/day PO for 3 days. Tx of nongonococcal urethritis, genital ulcer disease, cervicitis due to *Chlamydia trachomatis. Adult:* Single 1-g PO dose. Tx of gonococcal urethritis/cervicitis, mild to moderate acute bacterial sinusitis, community-acquired pneumonia. *Adult:* Single 2-g PO dose. *Child 6 mo and older:* 10 mg/kg/day PO for 3 days. **Disseminated MAC infections.** *Adult:* Prevention, 1,200 mg/m once wkly. Tx, 600 mg/day PO w/ ethambutol. **Tx of acute sinusitis.** *Adult:* 500 mg/day PO for 3 days or single 2-g dose of *Zmax*. **Tx of community-acquired pneumonia.** *Adult, child 16 yr and older:* 500 mg IV daily for at least 2 days, then 500 mg PO for 7–10 days. *Child 6 mo–15 yr:* 10 mg/kg PO as single dose on first day, then 5 mg/kg PO on days 2–5, or 60 mg/kg *Zmax* as single dose. **Tx of mild community-acquired pneumonia.** *Adult:* 500 mg PO day 1, then 250 mg PO for 4 days. **Tx of PID.** *Adult:* 500 mg IV daily for 1–2 days, then 250 mg/day PO for 7 days. **Tx of otitis media.** *Child 6 mo and older:* 10 mg/kg PO as single dose, then 5 mg/kg PO on days 2–5, or 30 mg/kg PO as single dose, or 10 mg/kg/day PO for 3 days. **Tx of pharyngitis/tonsillitis.** *Child 2 yr and older:* 12 mg/kg/day PO for days 1–5; max, 500 mg/day. **Tx of bacterial conjunctivitis.** *Adult, child:* 1 drop to affected eye bid for 2 days; then 1 drop/day for 5 days.

ADV EFF Abd pain, **angioedema,** diarrhea, superinfections

INTERACTIONS Aluminum- and magnesium-containing antacids, QT-prolonging drugs, theophylline, warfarin

NC/PT Culture before tx. Give on empty stomach 1 hr before or 2 hr after meals. Prepare sol by adding 60 mL water to bottle and shaking well; pt should drink all at once. May experience superinfections.

---

aztreonam (Azactam, Cayston)
CLASS Monobactam antibiotic
PREG/CONT B/NA

IND & DOSE Tx of UTIs. *Adult:* 500 mg–1 g IV or IM q 8–12 hr. **Tx of moderately severe systemic infec-** tion. *Adult:* 1–2 g IV or IM q 8–12 hr. *Child 9 mo and older:* 30 mg/kg IV or IM q 8 hr. **Tx of severe systemic infection.** *Adult:* 2 g IV or IM q 6–8 hr. *Child 9 mo and older:* 30 mg/kg IV or IM q 6–8 hr. **Tx of cystic fibrosis pts w/ *Pseudomonas aeruginosa* infections.** *Adult, child 7 yr and older:* 75 mg inhalation using Altera Nebulizer System tid for 28 days; space doses at least 4 hr apart. Then 28 days off.

ADJUST DOSE Renal impairment

ADV EFF Anaphylaxis, injection-site reactions, n/v/d, pruritus, rash

NC/PT Culture before tx. Discontinue, provide supportive tx if anaphylaxis occurs. Monitor for injection-site reactions. Use inhaled form only with provided nebulizer system.

---

bacitracin (Baci-IM)
CLASS Antibiotic
PREG/CONT C/NA

BBW Monitor renal function tests daily w/ IM tx; risk of serious renal toxicity.

IND & DOSE Pneumonia, empyema caused by susceptible strains of staphylococci in infants. *Over 2.5 kg:* 1,000 units/kg/day IM in two to three divided doses. *Under 2.5 kg:* 900 units/kg/day IM in two to three divided doses. **Px of minor skin abrasions; tx of superficial skin infections.** *Adult, child:* Apply topical ointment to affected area one to three times/day; cover w/ sterile bandage if needed. Do not use longer than 1 wk. **Superficial infections of conjunctiva or cornea.** *Adult, child:* Dose varies by product; see package insert.

ADV EFF Contact dermatitis (topical), **nephrotoxicity,** pain at injection site, superinfections

INTERACTIONS Aminoglycosides, NMJs

NC/PT Culture before tx. Reconstituted IM sol stable for 1 wk. Ensure adequate hydration. Monitor renal function closely (IM).

baclofen (Gablofen, Lioresal)

CLASS Centrally acting skeletal muscle relaxant
PREG/CONT C/NA

BBW Taper gradually to prevent rebound spasticity, hallucinations, possible psychosis, rhabdomyolysis, other serious effects; abrupt discontinuation can cause serious reactions.

IND & DOSE Alleviation of s&s x of spasticity from MS or spinal cord injuries (intrathecal). *Adult:* Testing usually done w/ 50 mcg/mL injected into intrathecal space over 1 min. Pt is observed for 4–8 hr, then 75 mcg/1.5 mL is given; pt is observed for 4–8 hr; final screening bolus of 100 mcg/2 mL is given 24 hr later if response still inadequate. Maint for spasticity of cerebral origin, 22–1,400 mcg/day; maint for spasticity of spinal cord origin, 12–2,003 mcg/day. **Spinal cord injuries, other spinal cord diseases** (oral). *Adult:* 5 mg PO tid for 3 days; 10 mg PO tid for 3 days; 15 mg PO tid for 3 days; 20 mg PO tid for 3 days. Thereafter, additional increases may be needed. Max, 80 mg/day.
ADJUST DOSE Elderly pts, renal impairment
ADV EFF Confusion, dizziness, drowsiness, fatigue, headache, hypotension, insomnia, urinary frequency, weakness
INTERACTIONS CNS depressants
NC/PT Use caution if spasticity needed to stay upright. Monitor implantable intrathecal delivery site, system. Taper slowly if discontinuing. Not for use in pregnancy. Pt should avoid OTC sleeping drugs and alcohol.

balsalazide disodium (Colazal, Giazo)

CLASS Anti-inflammatory
PREG/CONT B/NA

IND & DOSE Tx of mildly to moderately active ulcerative colitis. *Adult:* Three 750-mg capsules PO tid (total daily dose, 6.75 g) for up to 12 wk. Or, three 1.1-g tablets PO bid (total daily dose 6.6 g) for up to 8 wk. *Child 5–17 yr:* Three 750-mg capsules PO tid (6.75 g/day) for 8 wk, or one 750-mg capsule PO tid (2.25 g/day) for up to 8 wk.
ADV EFF Abd pain, cramps, depression, fatigue, flatulence, flulike symptoms, n/v/d
NC/PT Serious effects; use extreme caution. Maintain hydration. Observe for worsening of ulcerative colitis. Pt should take w/ meals, continue all restrictions and tx used for ulcerative colitis. Drug is high in sodium; monitor sodium intake. Name confusion between *Colazal* (balsalazide) and *Clozaril* (clozapine).

basiliximab (Simulect)

CLASS Immunosuppressant
PREG/CONT B/NA

BBW Only physicians experienced in immunosuppressive therapy and mgt of organ transplant pts should prescribe. Pts should be managed in facilities equipped and staffed w/ adequate laboratory and supportive medical resources.

IND & DOSE Px of acute rejection in renal transplant pts, w/ other immunosuppressants. *Adult:* Two doses of 20 mg IV—first dose 2 hr before transplant, second dose on day 4 posttransplant.
ADV EFF Abd pain, cramps, **hypersensitivity reactions,** hypertension, **infections,** n/v/d, pain
NC/PT Not for use in pregnancy, breast-feeding. Monitor for hypersensitivity reactions; protect pt from infections.

BCG intravesical (TheraCys, Tice BCG)

CLASS Antineoplastic
PREG/CONT C/NA

BBW Use precautions when handling. Contains live mycobacteria; infections can occur.

IND & DOSE Intravesical use in tx and px of carcinoma in situ of urinary bladder; px of primary or recurrent stage Ta and/or T1 papillary tumors after transurethral resection. *Adult:* 1 ampule in 50 mL diluent instilled via catheter into bladder by gravity.

ADV EFF Bone marrow suppression, chills, cystitis, dysuria, hematuria, infections, malaise, n/v, urinary urgency, UTI

INTERACTIONS Antibiotics, isoniazid

NC/PT Monitor for infection, local reactions. Pt should avoid fluids 4 hr before tx; empty bladder before instillation; lie down for first hr (turning side to side), then upright for 1 hr; try to retain fluid in bladder for 2 hr; empty bladder trying not to splash liquid; and increase fluid intake over next few hours.

---

beclomethasone dipropionate (OrbeShield, QNASL, QVAR), **beclomethasone dipropionate monohydrate** (Beconase AQ)
CLASS Corticosteroid
PREG/CONT C/NA

IND & DOSE Maintenance, control, prophylactic tx of asthma. *Adult, child 12 yr and older:* 40–160 mcg by inhalation bid; max, 320 mcg/bid. Titrate to response: "Low" dose: 80–240 mcg/day; "medium" dose: 240–480 mcg/day; "high" dose: Over 480 mcg/day. *Child 5–11 yr:* 40 mcg bid; max, 80 mcg bid. **Relief of s&s of seasonal or perennial and nonallergic rhinitis; prevention of recurrence of nasal polyps after surgical removal.** *Adult, child 12 yr and older:* 1–2 inhalations (42–84 mcg) in each nostril bid (total, 168–336 mcg/day). *Child 6–12 yr:* 1 inhalation in each nostril bid (total, 168 mcg). **Tx of GI acute radiation syndrome** (*OrbeShield*). *Adult:* 2 tablets PO as soon as possible after exposure.

ADV EFF Cushing's syndrome, epistaxis, headache, local irritation, nausea rebound congestion

NC/PT Taper oral steroids slowly in switching to inhaled forms. If using nasal spray, use nose decongestant to facilitate penetration of drug. If using other inhalants, use several min before using this drug. If using respiratory inhalant, allow at least 1 min between puffs; pt should rinse mouth after each inhalation.

---

bedaquiline (Sirturo)
CLASS Antimycobacterial, antituberculosis drug
PREG/CONT B/NA

BBW Increased risk of death; reserve for pts resistant to other effective therapy. Prolonged QT interval, risk of serious to fatal arrhythmias. Monitor ECG; avoid other QT-prolonging drugs.

IND & DOSE Tx of adults w/ multidrug-resistant pulmonary TB, w/ other antituberculosis drugs. *Adult:* 400 mg/day PO for 2 wk; then 200 mg/day PO three times/wk for 22 wk, w/ other antituberculosis drugs.

ADJUST DOSE Hepatic impairment, severe renal impairment

ADV EFF Arthralgia, headache, **hepatic impairment,** nausea, **prolonged QT interval**

INTERACTIONS Ketoconazole, lopinavir, QT-prolonging drugs, rifampin, ritonavir

NC/PT Obtain baseline ECG; monitor periodically. Monitor LFTs. Ensure proper use of drug and use w/ other antituberculosis drugs. Not for use in breast-feeding. Pt should mark calendar for tx days; swallow capsule whole and not cut, crush, or chew it; ensure also taking other drugs for TB; avoid alcohol; report urine/stool color changes; abnormal heartbeat.

belatacept (Nulojix)

CLASS T-cell costimulation blocker
PREG/CONT C/NA

BBW Increased risk of posttransplant lymphoproliferative disorder involving CNS, more likely without immunity to Epstein-Barr virus. Increased risk of cancers and serious infections.

IND & DOSE Px of organ rejection in pts w/ renal transplants, w/ other immunosuppressants. *Adult:* days 1 and 5, 10 mg/kg IV over 30 min; repeat end of wk 2, 4, 8, 12. Maint starting at wk 16 and q 4 wk thereafter, 5 mg/kg IV over 30 min.

ADV EFF Anemia, constipation, cough, edema, graft dysfx, headache, hyperkalemia, hypokalemia, **infections** (potentially fatal), **malignancies, posttransplant lymphoproliferative disorder, progressive multifocal leukoencephalopathy,** UTI

INTERACTIONS Live vaccines

NC/PT Not for use in liver transplants. Not for use in pregnancy, breast-feeding. Monitor blood counts, s&sx of infection, orientation, mood. Protect from infection. Encourage cancer screening exams.

belimumab (Benlysta)

CLASS B-cell activating factor inhibitor
PREG/CONT C/NA

IND & DOSE Tx of pts w/ active, antibody-positive SLE, w/ standard therapy. *Adult:* 10 mg/kg IV over 1 hr at 2-wk intervals for first three doses, then at 4-wk intervals.

ADV EFF Bronchitis, **death, depression/suicidality, hypersensitivity reactions, malignancies,** migraine, n/v/d, pain, pharyngitis, **serious to fatal infections**

INTERACTIONS Live vaccines

NC/PT Not for use in pregnancy, breast-feeding. Premedicate w/ antihistamines, corticosteroids. Do not use w/ acute infection; monitor for infections. Encourage cancer screening. Protect pt w/ suicidal thoughts.

benazepril hydrochloride (Lotensin)

CLASS ACE inhibitor, antihypertensive
PREG/CONT D/NA

BBW Rule out pregnancy; fetal abnormalities and death have occurred if used during second or third trimester. Encourage contraceptive measures.

IND & DOSE Tx of hypertension, alone or as part of combination therapy. *Adult:* 10 mg PO daily. Maint, 20–40 mg/day PO; max, 80 mg/day. *Child 6 yr and older:* 0.1–0.6 mg/kg/day; max, 40 mg/day.

ADJUST DOSE Renal impairment

ADV EFF Cough, **Stevens-Johnson syndrome**

INTERACTIONS Allopurinol, capsaicin, indomethacin, lithium, NSAIDs, potassium-sparing diuretics

NC/PT Use caution before surgery; mark chart. Protect pt w/ decreased fluid volume. Not for use in pregnancy. Cough may occur. Pt should change position slowly if dizzy, lightheaded.

DANGEROUS DRUG
bendamustine hydrochloride (Treanda)

CLASS Alkylating agent, antineoplastic
PREG/CONT D/NA

IND & DOSE Chronic lymphocytic leukemia. *Adult:* 100 mg/m² IV over 30 min on days 1 and 2 of 28-day cycle for up to six cycles. **Non-Hodgkin lymphoma.** *Adult:* 120 mg/m² IV over 60 min on days 1 and 2 of 21-day cycle for up to eight cycles.

ADJUST DOSE Hepatic, renal impairment

ADV EFF Fatigue, fever, infections, infusion reaction, **myelosuppression,** n/v/d, **rash to toxic skin reactions, tumor lysis syndrome**
INTERACTIONS Ciprofloxacin, fluvoxamine, nicotine, omeprazole
NC/PT Monitor blood counts closely. Protect pt from infection, bleeding. Monitor pt closely during infusion. Premedicate w/ antihistamines, antipyretics, corticosteroids. Assess skin regularly. Not for use in pregnancy, breast-feeding. Pt may feel very tired; should plan activities accordingly.

---

benzonatate (Tessalon, Zonatuss)
CLASS Antitussive
PREG/CONT C/NA

IND & DOSE Symptomatic relief of nonproductive cough. *Adult, child 10 yr and older:* 100–200 mg PO tid; max, 600 mg/day.
ADV EFF Constipation, dizziness, headache, nausea, rash, sedation
NC/PT Pt should not cut, crush, or chew capsules; must swallow capsule whole. Use caution if CNS effects occur.

---

benztropine mesylate (Cogentin)
CLASS Anticholinergic, antiparkinsonian
PREG/CONT C/NA

IND & DOSE Adjunct to tx of parkinsonism. *Adult:* Initially, 0.5–1 mg PO at bedtime; total daily dose, 0.5–6 mg at bedtime or in two to four divided doses; may give IM or IV at same dose. Control of drug-induced extrapyramidal disorders. *Adult:* 1–2 mg IM (preferred) or IV to control condition, then 1–4 mg PO daily or bid to prevent recurrences. Extrapyramidal disorders occurring early in neuroleptic tx. *Adult:* 2 mg PO bid to tid. Withdraw drug after 1 or 2 wk to determine continued need.

ADJUST DOSE Elderly pts
ADV EFF Blurred vision, constipation, decreased sweating, dry mouth, urinary hesitancy, urine retention
INTERACTIONS Alcohol, anticholinergics, haloperidol, phenothiazines, TCAs
NC/PT Pt should discontinue if dry mouth makes swallowing or speaking difficulty, use caution in hot weather when decreased sweating could lead to heat prostration, avoid alcohol and OTC drugs that could cause serious CNS effects, empty bladder before each dose if urine retention a problem; use caution if CNS effects occur.

---

beractant (natural lung surfactant) (Survanta)
CLASS Lung surfactant
PREG/CONT Unkn/NA

IND & DOSE Px for infants at risk for RDS. Give first dose of 100 mg phospholipids/kg birth weight (4 mL/kg) intratracheally soon after birth, preferably within 15 min. After determining needed dose, inject ¼ of dose into endotracheal (ET) tube over 2–3 sec; may repeat no sooner than 6 hr after dose. **Rescue tx of premature infants w/ RDS.** Give 100 mg phospholipids/kg birth weight (4 mL/kg) intratracheally. Give first dose as soon as possible within 8 hr of birth after RDS diagnosis is made and pt is on ventilator; may repeat after 6 hr from previous dose.
ADV EFF Bradycardia, hypotension, intraventricular hemorrhage, nonpulmonary infections, patent ductus arteriosus, sepsis
NC/PT Monitor ECG and O2 saturation continuously during and for at least 30 min after administration. Ensure ET tube is correctly placed. Suction immediately before dosing; do not suction for 1 hr after dosing.

betamethasone
(generic), **betamethasone dipropionate** (Diprolene AF, Maxivate), **betamethasone sodium phosphate and acetate** (Celestone Soluspan), **betamethasone valerate** (Beta-Val, Luxiq)
CLASS Corticosteroid
PREG/CONT C/NA

IND & DOSE Tx of primary or secondary adrenocortical insufficiency; hypercalcemia w/ cancer; short-term mgt of inflammatory and allergic disorders; thrombocytopenia purpura; ulcerative colitis; MS exacerbations; trichinosis w/ neurological or cardiac involvement. *Adult:* Oral (betamethasone), initially, 0.6–7.2 mg/day. IM (betamethasone sodium phosphate, betamethasone sodium phosphate and acetate), initially, 0.5–9 mg/day. Intrabursal, intra-articular, intradermal, intralesional (betamethasone sodium phosphate and acetate), 1.5–12 mg intra-articular (depending on joint size), 0.2 mL/cm³ intradermally (max, 1 mL/wk); 0.25–1 mL at 3- to 7-day intervals for foot disorders. Topical dermatologic cream, ointment (betamethasone dipropionate), apply sparingly to affected area daily or bid.
ADV EFF Aggravation of infection, headache, immunosuppression, increased appetite, local stinging and burning, masking of infection, vertigo, weight gain
INTERACTIONS Live vaccines
NC/PT Give oral dose at 9 a.m. Taper dosage when discontinuing. Pt should avoid overusing joints after injection; be cautious w/ occlusive dressings; do not stop drug suddenly; wear medical alert tag; apply sparingly if using topically; avoid exposure to infection; monitor blood glucose with long-term use.

betaxolol hydrochloride
(Betoptic S, Kerlone)
CLASS Antiglaucoma drug, antihypertensive, beta-selective blocker
PREG/CONT C/NA

IND & DOSE Hypertension, used alone or w/ other antihypertensives. *Adult:* 10 mg PO daily, alone or added to diuretic therapy. Tx of ocular hypertension and open-angle glaucoma alone or w/ other antiglaucoma drugs. *Adult:* 1 or 2 drops ophthalmic sol bid to affected eye(s).
ADJUST DOSE Elderly pts, severe renal impairment, dialysis pts
ADV EFF Allergic reactions, bradycardia, cardiac arrhythmias, decreased exercise tolerance, dizziness, HF, n/v/d, ocular itching/tearing (ophthalmic)
INTERACTIONS Anticholinergics, aspirin, hormonal contraceptives, insulin, prazosin, salicylates, verapamil
NC/PT Do not discontinue abruptly; taper over 2 wk. Protect eyes or joints from injury after dosing. Give eyedrops as instructed to avoid systemic absorption.

bethanechol chloride
(Urecholine)
CLASS Cholinergic, parasympathomimetic
PREG/CONT C/NA

IND & DOSE Acute postop and postpartum nonobstructive urine retention; neurogenic atony of urinary bladder w/ retention. *Adult:* 10–50 mg PO three/four times a day.
ADV EFF Abd discomfort, cardiac arrest, flushing, n/v/d, sweating
INTERACTIONS Cholinergics, ganglionic blockers
NC/PT Give on empty stomach 1 hr before or 2 hr after meals. Keep atropine on hand for severe response. Safety precautions if CNS effects occur.

DANGEROUS DRUG

bevacizumab (Avastin)
CLASS Antineoplastic, monoclonal antibody
PREG/CONT C/NA

BBW GI perforation, wound healing impairment, severe to fatal hemorrhage possible; monitor pt closely.
IND & DOSE Tx of metastatic cancer of colon/rectum, w/ 5-FU. *Adult:* 5–10 mg/kg IV q 14 days on progression; first infusion over 90 min, second over 60 min, then over 30 min. Tx of metastatic, unresectable or locally advanced nonsquamous, non-small-cell lung cancer. *Adult:* 15 mg/kg IV q 3 wk. Tx of glioblastoma. *Adult:* 10 mg/kg IV q 2 wk. Tx of metastatic renal cell carcinoma. *Adult:* 10 mg/kg IV q 2 wk w/ interferon alfa.
ADV EFF Arterial thrombotic events, back pain, epistaxis, exfoliative dermatitis, headache, hypertension, **infusion reactions**, non-GI fistula formation, proteinuria, ovarian failure, rectal hemorrhage, RPLS, rhinitis
NC/PT Do not initiate within 28 days of major surgery and until surgical wound is completely healed. Do not give as IV push or bolus. Monitor BP, wounds (for healing issues), during infusion (for infusion reactions). Not for use in pregnancy, breast-feeding. Pt should report rectal bleeding, high fever, changes in neurologic function.

DANGEROUS DRUG

bexarotene (Targretin)
CLASS Antineoplastic
PREG/CONT X/NA

BBW Not for use in pregnancy; fetal harm can occur.
IND & DOSE Cutaneous manifestations of cutaneous T-cell lymphoma in pts refractory to other tx. *Adult:* 300–400 mg/m²/day PO.

ADV EFF Abd pain, asthenia, dry skin, headache, **hepatic impairment**, hypothyroidism, lipid abnormalities, nausea, **pancreatitis**, photosensitivity, rash
INTERACTIONS Atorvastatin, carboplatin, gemfibrozil, paclitaxel, tamoxifen
NC/PT Rule out pregnancy before start of tx; ensure pt is using contraceptives. Monitor LFTs, amylase, lipids, thyroid function. Protect pt from exposure to sunlight. Pt should swallow capsules whole, not cut, crush, or chew them. Not for use in breast-feeding.

DANGEROUS DRUG

bicalutamide (Casodex)
CLASS Antiandrogen
PREG/CONT X/NA

IND & DOSE Tx of stage D2 metastatic carcinoma of prostate, w/ LHRH. *Adult:* 50 mg/day PO.
ADJUST DOSE Hepatic, renal impairment
ADV EFF Anemia, asthenia, constipation, diarrhea, dyspnea, edema, gynecomastia, hematuria, hot flashes, nausea, nocturia, pain, **severe hepatic injury to fatal hepatic failure**
INTERACTIONS Midazolam, warfarin
NC/PT Used w/ LHRH only. Monitor LFTs regularly, PSA levels, glucose levels. Not for use in pregnancy. Pt should report trouble breathing, blood in urine, yellowing of eyes or skin.

bismuth subsalicylate (Kaopectate, Pepto-Bismol, Pink Bismuth)
CLASS Antidiarrheal
PREG/CONT C (1st, 2nd trimesters); D (3rd trimester)/ NA

IND & DOSE To control diarrhea, gas, upset stomach, indigestion,

heartburn, nausea; to reduce number of bowel movements and help firm stool. *Adult, child 12 yr and older:* 2 tablets or 30 mL (524 mg) PO; repeat q 30 min–1 hr as needed (max, eight doses/24 hr). *Adult, child 12–17 yr:* 1 tablet or 15 mL PO. *Child 6–8 yr:* 2/3 tablet or 10 mL PO. *Child 3–5 yr:* 1/3 tablet or 5 mL PO. **Tx of traveler's diarrhea.** *Adult, child 12 yr and older:* 1 oz (524 mg) PO q 30 min for total of eight doses.
ADV EFF Darkening of stool
INTERACTIONS Antidiabetics, aspirin, methotrexate, sulfinpyrazone, tetracyclines, valproic acid
NC/PT Shake liquid well. Have pt chew tablets (not swallow whole). Pt should not take w/ drugs containing aspirin. Pt should report ringing in ears; stools may be dark.

bisoprolol fumarate (Zebeta)
CLASS Antihypertensive, beta-selective adrenergic blocker
PREG/CONT C/NA

IND & DOSE Mgt of hypertension, alone or w/ other antihypertensives. *Adult:* 5 mg PO daily, alone or added to diuretic therapy; 2.5 mg may be appropriate. Max, 20 mg PO daily.
ADJUST DOSE Renal, hepatic impairment
ADV EFF Bradycardia, bronchospasm, cardiac arrhythmias, constipation, decreased exercise tolerance, ED, fatigue, flatulence, headache, n/v/d
INTERACTIONS Anticholinergics, hormonal contraceptives, insulin, NSAIDs, prazosin, salicylates
NC/PT Do not discontinue abruptly; taper over 2 wk. Controversial need to stop before surgery. If diabetic pt, monitor glucose levels regularly. Pt should avoid OTC drugs. Name confusion with *Zebeta* (bisoprolol) and *DiaBeta* (glyburide).

bivalirudin (Angiomax)
CLASS Anticoagulant, thrombin inhibitor
PREG/CONT B/NA

IND & DOSE Pts w/ unstable angina undergoing PTCA. *Adult:* 0.75 mg/kg IV, then 1.75 mg/kg/hr during procedure. **Tx or px of heparin-induced thrombocytopenia in pts undergoing PTCA.** *Adult:* 0.75 mg/kg IV, then 1.75 mg/kg/hr during procedure; may continue for up to 4 hr, then 0.2 mg/kg/hr for up to 20 hr if needed.
ADJUST DOSE Renal impairment
ADV EFF Bleeding, fever, headache, thrombocytopenia
INTERACTIONS Heparin, thrombolytics, warfarin
NC/PT Used w/ aspirin therapy. Monitor for bleeding; could indicate need to discontinue.

bleomycin sulfate (BLM)
CLASS Antibiotic, antineoplastic
PREG/CONT D/NA

BBW Monitor pulmonary function regularly and chest X-ray wkly or bi-wkly for onset of pulmonary toxicity. Be alert for rare, severe idiosyncratic reaction, including fever, chills, hypertension, in lymphoma pts.
IND & DOSE Palliative tx of squamous cell carcinoma, lymphomas, testicular carcinoma, alone or w/ other drugs. *Adult:* 0.25–0.5 unit/kg IV, IM, or subcut once or twice wkly. **Tx of malignant pleural effusion.** *Adult:* 60 units dissolved in 50–100 mL NSS via thoracotomy tube.
ADJUST DOSE Renal impairment
ADV EFF Chills, dyspnea, fever, hair loss, hyperpigmentation, idiosyncratic reactions to **anaphylaxis**, pneumonitis, **pulmonary fibrosis**, stomatitis, striae, vesiculation, vomiting
INTERACTIONS Digoxin, oxygen, phenytoin

NC/PT Label reconstituted sol and use within 24 hr. Monitor LFTs, renal function tests, pulmonary function regularly; consult physician immediately if s&sx of toxicity. Not for use in pregnancy. Pt should mark calendar for injection dates, cover head w/ temp extremes (hair loss possible).

boceprevir (Victrelis)
CLASS Antiviral, protease inhibitor
PREG/CONT X/NA

IND & DOSE Tx of chronic hepatitis C in pts w/ genotype 1 infection, w/ peginterferon alfa and ribavirin. *Adult:* 800 mg PO tid w/ food for 28–48 wk; given w/ peginterferon alfa and ribavirin.

ADV EFF Anemia, dysgeusia, fatigue, headache, nausea, neutropenia
INTERACTIONS Alfuzosin, carbamazepine, dihydroergotamine, drospirenone, ergotamine, lovastatin, methylergonovine, midazolam, phenobarbital, pimozide, sildenafil, triazolam
NC/PT Must use w/ peginterferon alfa, ribavirin; start these drugs 4 wk before starting boceprevir. Interacts w/ many drugs; check full listing before administration. Protect from infection. Not for use in pregnancy. Pt can still transmit disease; should use precautions.

DANGEROUS DRUG

bortezomib (Velcade)
CLASS Antineoplastic, proteasome inhibitor
PREG/CONT D/NA

IND & DOSE Tx of multiple myeloma; tx of mantle cell lymphoma in pts who have received at least one other therapy. *Adult:* 1.3 mg/m² as 3–5 sec IV bolus or subcut for nine 6-day cycles (days 1, 4, 8, 11, then 10 days of rest, then days 22, 25, 29, 32).

ADV EFF Anemia, anorexia, asthenia, constipation, hypotension, leukopenia, neutropenia, n/v/d, **peripheral neuropathies, pulmonary infiltrates**
INTERACTIONS Ketoconazole, omeprazole, ritonavir, St John's wort
NC/PT Monitor for neurologic changes. Monitor CBC. Try to maintain hydration if GI effects are severe. Not for use in pregnancy, breast-feeding. Pt should use care when driving or operating machinery until drug's effects known.

bosentan (Tracleer)
CLASS Endothelin receptor antagonist, pulmonary antihypertensive
PREG/CONT X/NA

BBW Rule out pregnancy before starting tx; ensure pt is using two forms of contraception during tx and for 1 mo after tx ends. Verify pregnancy status monthly. Obtain baseline then monthly liver enzyme levels. Dose reduction or drug withdrawal indicated if liver enzymes elevated; liver failure possible.

IND & DOSE Tx of pulmonary arterial hypertension in pts w/ WHO class II–IV symptoms. *Adult, child over 12 yr:* 62.5 mg PO bid for 4 wk. Then, for pts 40 kg or more, maint dose is 125 mg PO bid. For pts under 40 kg but over 12 yr, maint dose is 62.5 mg PO bid.

ADJUST DOSE Hepatic impairment
ADV EFF Edema, flushing, headache, hypotension, **liver injury**, nasopharyngitis
INTERACTIONS Atazanavir, cyclosporine A, glyburide, hormonal contraceptives, ritonavir (serious toxicity), statins
NC/PT Available only through restricted access program. Obtain baseline Hgb, at 1 and 3 mo, then q 3 mo. Monitor LFTs. Do not use w/ cyclosporine or glyburide. Taper if discontinuing. Not for use in pregnancy (barrier contraceptives advised) or

breast-feeding. Pt should keep chart of activity tolerance to monitor drug's effects.

bosutinib (Bosulif)
CLASS Antineoplastic, kinase inhibitor
PREG/CONT D/NA

IND & DOSE Tx of accelerated blast phase Philadelphia chromosome–positive CML w/ resistance or intolerance to other tx. Adult: 500 mg/day PO, up to 600 mg/day.
ADJUST DOSE Hepatic impairment
ADV EFF Abd pain, anemia, fatigue, fever, **fluid retention, GI toxicity, hepatotoxicity, myelosuppression,** n/v/d, rash
INTERACTIONS CYP3A inhibitors/inducers (carbamazepine, dexamethasone, ketoconazole, phenobarbital, phenytoin, rifabutin, rifampin, rifapentine, St. John's wort), P-glycoprotein inhibitors; avoid these combinations. Proton pump inhibitors
NC/PT Monitor closely for bone marrow suppression, GI toxicity. Not for use in pregnancy. Pt should take once a day, report s&sx of bleeding, severe GI effects, **urine/stool** changes, swelling.

botulinum toxin type A
(Botox, Botox Cosmetic, Dysport, Xeomin)
CLASS Neurotoxin
PREG/CONT C/NA

BBW Drug not for tx of muscle spasticity; toxin may spread from injection area and cause s&sx of botulism (CNS alterations, trouble speaking and swallowing, loss of bladder control). Use only for approved indications.
IND & DOSE Improvement of glabellar lines. Adult: Total of 20 units (0.5 mL sol) injected as divided doses of 0.1 mL into each of five sites—two in each corrugator muscle, one in pro-

cerus muscle; repetition usually needed q 3–4 mo to maintain effect (Botox). Or, 50 units in five equal injections q 4 mo (Dysport). **Cervical dystonia.** Adult: 236 units (range, 198–300 units) divided among affected muscles and injected into each muscle in pts w/ known tolerance. In pts without prior use, 100 units or less, then adjust dose based on pt response (Botox), 120 units IM (Xeomin), or 250–1,000 units IM q 12 wk (Dysport). **Primary axillary hyperhidrosis.** Adult: 50 units/axilla injected intradermally 0.1–0.2 mL aliquots at multiple sites (10–15), about 1–2 cm apart. Repeat as needed. **Blepharospasm associated w/ dystonia.** Adult: 1.25–2.5 units injected into medial and lateral pretarsal orbicularis oculi of lower and upper lids. Repeat about q 3 mo. **Strabismus associated w/ dystonia.** Adult: 1.25–50 units injected in any one muscle. **Upper limb spasticity.** Adult: Base dose on muscles affected and severity of activity; electromyographic guidance recommended. Use no more than 50 units per site. **Chronic migraine.** Adult: 155 units IM as 0.1 mL (5 units) at each site; divide into seven head/neck muscle areas (Botox). **Blepharospasm in previously treated pts.** Adult: 35 units per eye (Xeomin). **Tx of urinary incontinence in pts w/ neurological conditions (Botox).** Adult: 200 units as 1-mL injection across 30 sites into detrusor muscle. **Tx of chronic migraines.** Adult: 155 units IM as 0.1 mL at each of seven sites in head/neck muscle area.
ADV EFF Anaphylactic reactions, dizziness, headache, local reactions, **MI, spread of toxin that can lead to death**
INTERACTIONS Aminoglycosides, anticholinesterases, lincosamides, magnesium sulfate, NMJ blockers, polymyxin, quinidine, succinylcholine
NC/PT Store in refrigerator. Have epinephrine available in case of anaphylactic reactions. Effects may not appear for 1–2 days; will persist for 3–4 mo. Not for use in pregnancy.

botulinum toxin type B
(Myobloc)

CLASS Neurotoxin
PREG/CONT C/NA

BBW Drug not for tx of muscle spasticity; toxin may spread from injection area and cause s&sx of botulism (CNS alterations, trouble speaking and swallowing, loss of bladder control). Use only for approved indications.

IND & DOSE Tx of cervical dystonia to reduce severity of abnormal head position and neck pain. *Adult:* 2,500–5,000 units IM injected locally into affected muscles.

ADV EFF Anaphylactic reactions, dry mouth, dyspepsia, dysphagia, spread of toxin that can lead to death

INTERACTIONS Aminoglycosides, anticholinesterases, lincosamides, magnesium sulfate, NMJ blockers, polymyxin, quinidine, succinylcholine

NC/PT Store in refrigerator. Have epinephrine on hand in case of anaphylactic reactions. Do not inject in area of skin infection; effects may not appear for 1–2 days; will persist for 3–4 mo. Not for use in pregnancy, breast-feeding. Pt should report difficulty swallowing, breathing.

brentuximab (Adcetris)

CLASS Monoclonal antibody
PREG/CONT D/NA

BBW Risk of potentially fatal progressive multifocal leukoencephalopathy (PML).

IND & DOSE Tx of Hodgkin lymphoma after failure of autologous stem-cell transplant; tx of systemic anaplastic large-cell lymphoma. *Adult:* 1.8 mg/kg IV over 30 min q 3 wk for max of 16 cycles.

ADV EFF Anaphylactic reactions, chills, cough, dyspnea, fever, infusion reactions, nausea, neutropenia, peripheral neuropathy, PML, Stevens-Johnson syndrome

INTERACTIONS Bleomycin, ketoconazole, rifampin

NC/PT Monitor pt during infusion. Monitor neutrophil count; dose adjustment may be needed. Protect pt w/ peripheral neuropathies. Not for use in pregnancy, breast-feeding. Pt should report mood or behavior changes, changes in vision or walking, weakness.

bromocriptine mesylate
(Cycloset, Parlodel)

CLASS Antidiabetic, antiparkinsonian, dopamine receptor agonist
PREG/CONT B/NA

IND & DOSE Tx of postencephalitic or idiopathic Parkinson's disease. *Adult, child 15 yr and older:* 11.25 mg PO bid. Assess q 2 wk, and adjust dose; max, 100 mg/day. **Tx of hyperprolactinemia.** *Adult, child 15 yr and older:* 1.25–2.5 mg PO daily; range, 2.5–15 mg/day. **Tx of acromegaly.** *Adult, child 15 yr and older:* 1.25–2.5 mg PO for 3 days at bedtime; add 1.25–2.5 mg as tolerated q 3–7 days until optimal response. Range, 20–30 mg/day. **Tx of type 2 diabetes.** *Adult:* 0.8 mg/day PO in a.m. within 2 hr of waking; increase by 1 tablet/wk to max 6 tablets (4.8 mg) daily (*Cycloset* only).

ADV EFF Abd cramps, constipation, dyspnea, fatigue, n/v/d, orthostatic hypotension

INTERACTIONS Erythromycin, phenothiazines, sympathomimetics

NC/PT Ensure proper diagnosis before starting tx. Taper dose if used in parkinsonism. Not for use in pregnancy, breast-feeding. Pt should take drug for diabetes once a day in a.m., use safety precautions if dizziness, orthostatic hypotension occur.

brompheniramine maleate (BroveX, J-Tan, Lo-Hist 12, Respa-AR, VaZol)

CLASS Antihistamine
PREG/CONT C/NA

IND & DOSE Relief of symptoms of seasonal rhinitis, common cold; tx of nonallergic pruritic symptoms. *Adult, child 12 yr and older:* Products vary. ER tablets, 6–12 mg PO q 12 hr. Chewable tablets, 12–24 mg PO q 12 hr (max, 48 mg/day). ER capsules, 12–24 mg/day PO. Oral suspension (*BroveX*), 5–10 mL (12–24 mg) PO q 12 hr (max, 48 mg/day). Oral liquid, 10 mL (4 mg) PO four times/day. Oral suspension 5 mL PO q 12 hr (max, two doses/day). *Child 6–12 yr:* ER tablets, 6 mg PO q 12 hr. Chewable tablets, 6–12 mg PO q 12 hr (max, 24 mg/day). ER capsules, 12 mg/day PO. Oral liquid, 5 mL (2 mg) PO four times/day. Oral suspension (*BroveX*), 5 mL (12 mg) PO q 12 hr (max, 24 mg/day). Oral suspension, 2.5 mL PO q 12 hr (max, 5 mL/day). *Child 2–6 yr:* Chewable tablets, 6 mg PO q 12 hr (max, 12 mg/day). Oral liquid, 2.5 mL (1 mg) PO 4 times/day. Oral suspension (*BroveX*), 2.5 mL (6 mg) PO q 12 hr up (max, 12 mg/day). Oral suspension 1.25 mL PO q 12 hr (max, 2.5 mL/day). *Child 12 mo–2 yr:* Oral suspension, 1.25 mL (3 mg) PO q 12 hr (max, 2.5 mL [6 mg]/day). Oral liquid, Titrate dose based on 0.5 mg/kg/day PO in equally divided doses four times/day.
ADJUST DOSE Elderly pts
ADV EFF Anaphylactic shock, disturbed coordination, dizziness, drowsiness, faintness, thickening bronchial secretions
INTERACTIONS Alcohol, anticholinergics, CNS depressants
NC/PT Double-check dosages; products vary widely. Pt should not cut, crush, or chew ER tablets; should avoid alcohol, take safety precautions if CNS effects occur.

budesonide (Entocort EC, Pulmicort, Rhinocort Aqua)

CLASS Corticosteroid
PREG/CONT B (inhalation); C (oral)/NA

IND & DOSE Nasal spray mgt of symptoms of allergic rhinitis. *Adult, child 6 yr and older:* 64 mcg/day as 1 spray (32 mcg) in each nostril once daily. Max for pts over 12 yr, 256 mcg/day as 4 sprays per nostril once daily. Max for pts 6 to under 12 yr, 128 mcg/day (given as 2 sprays per nostril once daily). **Maint tx of asthma as prophylactic therapy.** *Adult, child 12 yr and older:* 360 mcg by inhalation bid; max, 720 mcg bid. "Low" dose, 180–600 mcg/day; "medium" dose, 600–1,200 mcg/day; "high" dose, more than 1,200 mcg/day. *Child 5–11 yr:* 180 mcg by inhalation bid; max, 360 mcg/day. "Low" dose, 180–400 mcg/day; "medium" dose, 400–800 mcg/day; "high" dose, over 800 mcg/day. *Child 0–11 yr:* 0.5–1 mg by inhalation once daily or in two divided doses using jet nebulizer. Max, 1 mg/day. "Low" dose, 0.25–0.5 mg/day (0–4 yr), 0.5 mg/day (5–11 yr); "medium" dose, 0.5–1 mg/day (0–4 yr), 1 mg/day (5–11 yr); "high" dose, over 1 mg/day (0–4 yr), 2 mg/day (5–11 yr). **Tx, maint of clinical remission for up to 3 mo of mild to moderate active Crohn's disease involving ileum/ascending colon.** *Adult:* 9 mg/day PO in a.m. for up to 8 wk. May retreat recurrent episodes for 8-wk periods. Maint, 6 mg/day PO for up to 3 mo, then taper until cessation complete.
ADJUST DOSE Hepatic impairment
ADV EFF Back pain, cough, dizziness, fatigue, headache, lethargy, nasal irritation, pharyngitis
INTERACTIONS Erythromycin, grapefruit juice, indinavir, itraconazole, ketoconazole, ritonavir, saquinavir
NC/PT Taper systemic steroids when switching to inhaled form.

Ensure proper administration technique for nasal spray, inhalation. Monitor for potential hypercorticism. Pt should not cut, crush, or chew PO tablets.

bumetanide (generic)

CLASS Loop diuretic
PREG/CONT C/NA

BBW Monitor electrolytes, hydration, hepatic function w/ long-term tx; water and electrolyte depletion possible.

IND & DOSE Tx of edema associated w/ HF, renal and hepatic diseases. *Adult:* Oral, 0.5–2 mg/day PO; may repeat at 4- to 5-hr intervals. Max, 10 mg/day. Intermittent therapy, 3–4 days on, then 1–2 off. Parenteral, 0.5–1 mg IV/IM over 1–2 min; may repeat in 2–3 hr; max, 10 mg/day.
ADJUST DOSE Elderly pts, renal impairment
ADV EFF Anorexia, asterixis, drowsiness, headache, hypokalemia, nocturia, n/v/d, orthostatic hypotension, pain at injection site, polyuria
INTERACTIONS Aminoglycosides, cardiac glycosides, cisplatin, NSAIDs, probenecid
NC/PT Switch to PO as soon as possible. Monitor electrolytes. Give early in day to avoid disrupting sleep. Pt should eat potassium-rich diet, check weight daily (report loss/gain of over 3 lb/day).

DANGEROUS DRUG

buprenorphine hydrochloride (Buprenex, Butrans Transdermal)

CLASS Opioid agonist-antagonist analgesic
PREG/CONT C/C-III

IND & DOSE Relief of moderate to severe pain (parenteral). *Adult:* 0.3 mg IM or by slow (over 2 min) IV injection. May repeat once, 30–60 min after first dose; repeat q 6 hr. *Child*

2–12 yr: 2–6 mcg/kg body weight IM or slow IV injection q 4–6 hr. **Tx of opioid dependence** (oral). *Adult:* 8 mg on day 1, 16 mg on day 2 and subsequent induction days (can be 3–4 days). Maint, 12–16 mg/day sublingually (Suboxone). **Mgt of moderate to severe chronic pain in pts needing continuous, around-the-clock opioid analgesic for extended period** (transdermal). *Adult:* Initially, 5 mcg/hr, intended to be worn for 7 days; max, 20 mcg/hr.
ADJUST DOSE Elderly, debilitated pts
ADV EFF Dizziness, headache, hypotension, hypoventilation, miosis, n/v, sedation, sweating, vertigo
INTERACTIONS Barbiturates, benzodiazepines, general anesthetics, opioid analgesics, phenothiazines, sedatives
NC/PT Have opioid antagonists, facilities for assisted respiration on hand. Taper as part of comprehensive tx plan. Not for use in pregnancy, breast-feeding. Pt should place translingual tablet under tongue until dissolved, then swallow; apply transdermal patch to clean, dry area, leave for 7 days. Remove old patch before applying new one. Safety precautions if CNS effects occur.

DANGEROUS DRUG

buPROPion hydrobromide (Aplenzin), buPROPion hydrochloride (Wellbutrin, Zyban)

CLASS Antidepressant, smoking deterrent
PREG/CONT C/NA

BBW Monitor response and behavior; suicide risk in depressed pts, children, adolescents, young adults. Serious mental health events possible, including changes in behavior, depression, and hostility. *Aplenzin* not indicated for smoking cessation; risk of serious neuropsychiatric events, including suicide, when used for this purpose.

IND & DOSE *Tx of major depressive disorder.* Adult: 300 mg PO as 100 mg tid; max, 450 mg/day. SR, 150 mg PO bid. ER, 150 mg/day PO. Aplenzia, 174–348 mg/day PO; max, 522 mg/day. *Smoking cessation.* Adult: 150 mg (Zyban) PO daily for 3 days; increase to 300 mg/day in two divided doses at least 8 hr apart. Treat for 7–12 wk. *Tx of seasonal affective disorder.* Adult: 150 mg (Wellbutrin XL) PO daily in a.m.; max, 300 mg/day. Begin in autumn; taper off (150 mg/day for 2 wk before discontinuation) in early spring.

ADJUST DOSE Renal, hepatic impairment

ADV EFF Agitation, constipation, depression, dry mouth, headache, migraine, **suicidality**, tachycardia, tremor, weight loss

INTERACTIONS Alcohol, amantadine, cyclophosphamide, levodopa, MAOIs, paroxetine, sertraline

NC/PT Check labels carefully; dose varies. Avoid use w/ hx of seizure disorder. Monitor hepatic, renal function. Smoking cessation: Pt should quit smoking within 2 wk of tx. May be used w/ transdermal nicotine. Pt should avoid alcohol, take safety precautions if CNS effects occur, report thoughts of suicide.

---

busPIRone (generic)
CLASS Anxiolytic
PREG/CONT B/NA

IND & DOSE *Mgt of anxiety disorders; short-term relief of symptoms of anxiety.* Adult: 15 mg/day PO; may increase slowly to optimum therapeutic effect. Max, 60 mg/day.

ADV EFF Abd distress, dizziness, dry mouth, headache, insomnia, light-headedness, n/v/d

INTERACTIONS Alcohol, CNS depressants, erythromycin, fluoxetine, grapefruit juice, haloperidol, itraconazole, MAOIs

NC/PT Suggest sugarless lozenges for dry mouth, analgesic for headache. Pt should avoid OTC sleeping drugs, alcohol, grapefruit juice take safety measures if CNS effects occur.

---

busulfan (Busulfex, Myleran)
CLASS Alkylating agent, antineoplastic
PREG/CONT D/NA

BBW Arrange for blood tests to evaluate bone marrow function before tx, wkly during, and for at least 3 wk after tx ends. Severe bone marrow suppression possible.

IND & DOSE *Palliative tx of chronic myelogenous leukemia; tx of other myeloproliferative disorders, including severe thrombocytosis and polycythemia vera, myelofibrosis; bone marrow transplantation* (oral). Adult: Remission induction, 4–8 mg or 60 mcg/kg PO. Maint, resume tx w/ induction dosage when WBC count reaches 50,000/mm³; if remission shorter than 3 mo, maint of 1–3 mg PO daily advised to control hematologic status. Child: May give 60–120 mcg/kg/day PO, or 1.8–4.6 mg/m²/day PO for remission induction. *With cyclophosphamide as conditioning regimen before allogenic hematopoietic progenitor cell transplant for CML* (parenteral). Adult: 0.8 mg/kg IV of ideal body weight or actual body weight, whichever is lower, as 2-hr infusion.

ADJUST DOSE Hepatic impairment

ADV EFF Amenorrhea, anemia, hyperpigmentation, leukopenia, menopausal symptoms, n/v/d, ovarian suppression, **pancytopenia, pulmonary dysplasia, Stevens-Johnson syndrome**

NC/PT Arrange for respiratory function test before and periodically during tx; monitor CBC. Reduce dose w/ bone marrow suppression. Ensure pt is hydrated. Give IV through central venous catheter. Premedicate for IV tx w/ phenytoin, antiemetics. Not for use in pregnancy (barrier contraceptives advised) or breast-feeding. Pt should drink 10–12 glasses of fluid each day, report difficulty breathing, severe skin reactions.

DANGEROUS DRUG

butorphanol tartrate
(Stadol)

CLASS Opioid agonist-antagonist analgesic
PREG/CONT C (pregnancy); D (labor & delivery)/C-IV

IND & DOSE Relief of moderate to severe pain; preop or preanesthetic medication; to supplement balanced anesthesia. *Adult:* 2 mg IM q 3–4 hr or 1 mg IV q 3–4 hr; range, 0.5–2 mg IV q 3–4 hr. *During labor:* 1–2 mg IV/IM at full term during early labor; repeat q 4 hr. **Relief of moderate to severe pain** (nasal spray). 1 mg (1 spray/nostril); repeat in 60–90 min if adequate relief not achieved; may repeat two-dose sequence q 3–4 hr.
ADJUST DOSE Elderly pts; hepatic, renal impairment
INTERACTIONS Barbiturate anesthetics
ADV EFF Nausea, sedation, slow shallow respirations
NC/PT Ensure ready access to respiratory assist devices when giving IV/IM. Protect from falls; sedation, visual disturbances possible. Pt should not drive or perform other tasks requiring alertness.

C1-inhibitor (human)
(Cinryze)

CLASS Blood product, proteinase inhibitor
PREG/CONT C/NA

IND & DOSE Px against angioedema attacks in adults, adolescents w/ hereditary angioedema. *Adult, adolescent:* 1,000 units IV at 10 mL/min q 3–4 days.
ADV EFF Blood-related infections, headache, **hypersensitivity reactions,** n/v, rash, **thrombotic events**
NC/PT Have epinephrine available in case of severe hypersensitivity reactions. Slight risk of blood-related diseases. Not for use in pregnancy, breast-feeding. Pt should report difficulty breathing, hives, chest tightness.

---

cabazitaxel (Jevtana)
CLASS Antineoplastic, microtubular inhibitor
PREG/CONT D/NA

BBW Severe hypersensitivity reactions possible; prepare to support pt. Severe neutropenia, deaths have occurred; monitor blood counts closely. Not for use w/ hx of severe reactions to cabazitaxel or polysorbate 80.
IND & DOSE With oral prednisone for tx of pts w/ hormone-refractory metastatic prostate cancer previously treated w/ docetaxel. *Adult:* 25 mg/m² IV over 1 hr q 3 wk.
ADJUST DOSE Hepatic impairment
ADV EFF Abd pain, alopecia, anorexia, arthralgia, asthenia, **bone marrow suppression,** constipation, cough, dysgeusia, dyspnea, fever, **hepatic impairment, hypersensitivity reactions,** n/v/d, **neutropenia, renal failure**
INTERACTIONS Strong CYP3A inhibitors, inducers
NC/PT Premedicate w/ antihistamine, corticosteroid, and H₂ antagonist; antiemetic if needed. Always give w/ oral prednisone. Monitor blood count; dose adjustment needed based on neutrophil count. Monitor LFTs, renal function. Ensure hydration; tx w/ antidiarrheals may be needed. Not for use in pregnancy, breast-feeding. Pt should mark calendar w/ dates for tx, try to maintain food and liquid intake, report difficulty breathing, rash.

cabozantinib (Cometriq)

CLASS Antineoplastic, kinase inhibitor

PREG/CONT D/NA

BBW Risk of GI perforation, fistulas; monitor pt. Severe to fatal hemorrhage has occurred; monitor for s&sx of bleeding.

IND & DOSE Tx of progressive, metastatic medullary thyroid cancer. *Adult:* 140 mg/day PO.

ADJUST DOSE Hepatic impairment

ADV EFF Abd pain, anorexia, constipation, fatigue, hair color change, **hypertension**, n/v/d, **osteonecrosis of jaw, palmar-plantar erythrodysesthesia syndrome, proteinuria, RPLS, thromboembolic events**, weight loss, **wound complications**

INTERACTIONS Strong CYP3A4 inducers/inhibitors, grapefruit juice; avoid these combinations

NC/PT Monitor for s&sx of bleeding, GI perforation, drug interactions. Not for use in pregnancy, breast-feeding. Pt should take as directed on empty stomach, at least 2 hr before or after food; swallow capsule whole and not cut, crush, or chew it; avoid grapefruit juice; report s&sx of bleeding (bruising, coughing up blood, tarry stools, bleeding that won't stop); acute stomach pain; choking, difficulty swallowing; swelling or pain in mouth or jaw; chest pain, acute leg pain, difficulty breathing.

caffeine (Caffedrine, Enerjets, NoDoz, Vivarin), caffeine citrate (Cafcit)

CLASS Analeptic, CNS stimulant, xanthine

PREG/CONT C/NA

IND & DOSE Aid in staying awake; adjunct to analgesic preparations. *Adult:* 100–200 mg PO q 3–4 hr as needed. Tx of respiratory depression associated w/ overdose of CNS depressants. *Adult:* 500 mg–1 g

caffeine and sodium benzoate (250–500 mg caffeine) IM; max, 2.5 g/day. May give IV in severe emergency. **Short-term tx of apnea of prematurity in infants between 28 and 33 wk gestation.** *Premature infants:* 20 mg/kg IV over 30 min followed 24 hours later by 5 mg/kg/day IV over 10 min or PO as maint *(Cafcit).*

ADV EFF Diuresis, excitement, insomnia, restlessness, tachycardia, withdrawal syndrome (headache, anxiety, muscle tension)

INTERACTIONS Cimetidine, ciprofloxacin, clozapine, disulfiram, ephedra, guarana, hormonal contraceptives, iron, ma huang, mexiletine, theophylline

NC/PT Pt should avoid foods high in caffeine; not stop abruptly because withdrawal symptoms possible; avoid dangerous activities if CNS effects occur.

calcitonin, salmon (Calcimar, Miacalcin, Osteocalcin, Salmonine)

CLASS Calcium regulator, hormone

PREG/CONT C/NA

IND & DOSE Tx of Paget's disease. *Adult:* 100 units/day IM or subcut; maint, 50 units/day or every other day. Tx of postmenopausal osteoporosis. *Adult:* 100 units every other day IM or subcut or 200 units intranasally daily, alternating nostrils daily. **Emergency tx of hypercalcemia.** *Adult:* 4 units/kg q 12 hr IM or subcut. If response unsatisfactory after 1–2 days, increase to 8 units/kg q 12 hr; if response still unsatisfactory after 2 more days, increase to 8 units/kg q 6 hr.

ADV EFF Flushing of face or hands, local inflammatory reactions at injection site, n/v, rash, urinary frequency

NC/PT Before use, give skin test to pt w/ hx of allergies; give w/ calcium carbonate (1.5 g/day) and vitamin D (400 units/day) when treating osteoporosis. Monitor serum alkaline phosphatase and urinary hydroxyproline excretion before and during first 3 mo of therapy, then q 3–6 mo. Inject doses of more than 2 mL IM, not subcut. Store nasal spray in refrigerator until activated, then at room temperature. Alternate nostrils daily when using nasal spray. If self-administering, learn proper technique and proper disposal of needles, syringes.

calcium salts: calcium carbonate (Caltrate, Chooz, Tums), calcium chloride, calcium glubionate (Calcionate, Calciquid), calcium gluconate (Cal-G), calcium lactate (Cal-Lac)
CLASS Antacid, electrolyte
PREG/CONT C/NA

IND & DOSE **RDA** (carbonate or lactate). *Adult over 50 yr:* 1,200 mg/day PO. *Adult 19–50 yr:* 1,000 mg/day PO. *Child 14–18 yr:* 1,300 mg/day PO. *Child 9–13 yr:* 1,300 mg/day PO. *Child 4–8 yr:* 800 mg/day PO. *Child 1–3 yr:* 500 mg/day PO. *Child 7–12 mo:* 270 mg/day PO. *Child 0–6 mo:* 210 mg/day PO. *Pregnancy, breast-feeding, 19–50 yr:* 1,000 mg/day PO. *Pregnancy, breast-feeding, 14–18 yr:* 1,300 mg/ day PO. **Dietary supplement** (carbonate or lactate). *Adult:* 500 mg–2 g PO bid–qid. **Antacid.** *Adult:* 0.5–2 g PO calcium carbonate as needed. **Tx of hypocalcemic disorders.** *Adult:* 500 mg–1 g calcium chloride IV at intervals of 1–3 days. *Child:* 2.7–5 mg/kg or 0.027–0.05 mL/kg calcium chloride IV q 4–6 hr, or 200–500 mg/day IV (2–5 mL of 10% sol); for infants, no more than 200 mg IV (2 mL of 10% sol) in divided doses (calcium gluconate). **Tx of magnesium intoxication.** *Adult:* 500 mg calcium chloride IV promptly. **Cardiac resuscitation.** *Adult:* 500 mg–1 g IV or 200–800 mg calcium chloride into ventricular cavity.

ADV EFF Anorexia, bradycardia, constipation, irritation at injection site, hypercalcemia, hypotension, n/v, peripheral vasodilation, rebound hyperacidity, tingling
INTERACTIONS Fluoroquinolones, quinidine, salicylates, tetracyclines, thyroid hormone, verapamil
NC/PT Do not give oral drugs within 1–2 hr of antacid. Avoid extravasation of IV fluid; tissue necrosis possible. Monitor serum phosphate levels periodically. Monitor cardiac response closely w/ parenteral tx. Pt should take drug between meals and at bedtime; chew antacid tablets thoroughly before swallowing and follow w/ glass of water; not take w/ other oral drugs; space at least 1–2 hr after antacid.

calfactant (natural lung surfactant) (Infasurf)
CLASS Lung surfactant
PREG/CONT Unkn/NA

IND & DOSE **Prophylactic tx of infants at risk for developing RDS; rescue tx of premature infants up to 72 hr of age who have developed RDS.** Instill 3 mL/kg of birth weight in two doses of 1.5 mL/kg each intratracheally. Repeat doses of 3 mL/kg (to total of three doses) given 12 hr apart.
ADV EFF Bradycardia, hyperbilirubinemia, hypotension, intraventricular hemorrhage, nonpulmonary infections, patent ductus arteriosus, sepsis
NC/PT Monitor ECG and O2 saturation continuously during and for at least 30 min after administration. Ensure ET tube correctly placed; suction immediately before dosing. Do not suction for 1 hr after dosing. Maintain appropriate interventions for critically ill infant.

canagliflozin (Invokana)
CLASS Antidiabetic, sodium-glucose cotransporter 2 inhibitor
PREG/CONT C/NA

IND & DOSE W/ diet, exercise to improve glycemic control in type 2 diabetes. *Adult:* 100 mg/day w/ first meal of day; max, 300 mg/day.
ADJUST DOSE Severe renal impairment
ADV EFF Dehydration, genital yeast infections, hypoglycemia, hypotension, polyuria, UTI
INTERACTIONS Celery, coriander, dandelion root, digoxin, fenugreek, garlic, ginger, juniper berries, phenobarbital, phenytoin, rifampin
NC/PT Not for use with type 1 diabetes, pregnancy, breast-feeding. Monitor blood glucose, HbA1c, BP periodically; also monitor for UTI, genital infections. Pt should continue diet/exercise program, other antidiabetics as ordered; take safety measures w/ dehydration; report sx of UTI, genital infections.

canakinumab (Ilaris)
CLASS Interleukin blocker
PREG/CONT C/NA

IND & DOSE Tx of cryopyrin-associated periodic syndromes, including familial cold autoinflammatory syndrome and Muckle-Wells syndrome; tx of juvenile rheumatoid arthritis. *Adult, child 4 yr and older:* Over 40 kg, 150 mg subcut; 15 kg to under 40 kg, 2 mg/kg subcut; 15–40 kg w/ inadequate response, 3 mg/kg subcut. Injections given q 8 wk.
ADV EFF Diarrhea, flulike symptoms, headache, nasopharyngitis, nausea, **serious infections**
INTERACTIONS Immunosuppressants, live vaccines
NC/PT Use extreme caution in pts w/ infections; monitor for infections. Not for use in pregnancy, breast-feeding. Pt should report s&sx of infection.

candesartan cilexetil (Atacand)
CLASS Antihypertensive, ARB
PREG/CONT D/NA

BBW Rule out pregnancy before starting tx. Suggest barrier birth control; fetal injury and deaths have occurred. If pregnancy detected, discontinue as soon as possible.
IND & DOSE Tx of hypertension. *Adult:* 16 mg PO daily; range, 8–32 mg/day. *Child 6–under 17 yr:* Over 50 kg, 8–16 mg/day PO; range, 4–32 mg/day PO; under 50 kg, 4–8 mg/day PO; range, 4–16 mg/day PO. *Child 1–under 6 yr:* 0.20 mg/kg/day oral suspension; range, 0.05–0.4 mg/kg/day. Tx of HF. *Adult:* 4 mg PO; may be doubled at 2-wk intervals. Target dose, 32 mg/day PO as single dose.
ADJUST DOSE Volume depletion
ADV EFF Abd pain, diarrhea, dizziness, headache, URI symptoms
NC/PT If BP not controlled, can add other antihypertensives. Use caution if pt goes to surgery; volume depletion possible. Not for use in pregnancy (barrier contraception advised) or breast-feeding. Pt should use caution in situations that could lead to fluid volume loss; monitor fluid intake.

DANGEROUS DRUG
capecitabine (Xeloda)
CLASS Antimetabolite, antineoplastic
PREG/CONT D/NA

BBW Increased risk of excessive bleeding, even death, if combined w/ warfarin; avoid this combination. If combination must be used, monitor INR and PT levels closely; adjust anticoagulant dose as needed.
IND & DOSE Tx of breast and colorectal cancer. *Adult:* 2,500 mg/m²/day PO

in two divided doses 12 hr apart with-in 30 min after meal for 2 wk, followed by 1-wk rest period. Given in 3-wk cycles. **Adjuvant postsurgery Dukes C colon cancer.** *Adult:* 1,250 mg/m² PO bid, a.m. and p.m., within 30 min after meal for 2 wk, followed by 1 wk rest. Given as 3-wk cycles for eight cycles (24 wk).

ADJUST DOSE Elderly pts; hepatic, renal impairment

ADV EFF Anorexia, constipation, dermatitis, hand-and-foot syndrome, leukopenia, **MI,** n/v, **renal impairment,** stomatitis

INTERACTIONS Antacids, docetaxel, leucovorin (risk of severe toxicity, death), phenytoin, warfarin

NC/PT Obtain baseline and periodic renal function tests; monitor for s&sx of toxicity. Monitor nutritional status, fluid intake. Give frequent mouth care. Not for use in pregnancy (use of barrier contraceptives advised) or breast-feeding. Pt should mark calendar for tx days; avoid exposure to infection; report s&sx of infection.

---

capreomycin (Capastat Sulfate)

CLASS Antibiotic, antituberculotic
PREG/CONT C/NA

BBW Arrange for audiometric testing and assessment of vestibular function, renal function tests, and serum potassium before and regularly during tx; severe risk of renal failure, auditory damage. Drug's safety not established in children or pregnant women.

IND & DOSE Tx of pulmonary TB not responsive to first-line antituberculotics, as part of combination therapy. *Adult:* 1 g daily (max, 20 mg/kg/day) IM or IV for 60–120 days, followed by 1 g IM two to three times/wk for 12–24 mo.

ADJUST DOSE Elderly pts, renal impairment

ADV EFF Nephrotoxicity, ototoxicity
INTERACTIONS Nephrotoxic drugs, NMJ blockers

NC/PT Culture and sensitivity before tx. Use w/ other antituberculotics. Give by deep IM injection. Obtain audiometric testing regularly. Monitor renal function, potassium levels regularly.

---

captopril (generic)

CLASS ACE inhibitor, antihypertensive
PREG/CONT D/NA

BBW Rule out pregnancy; fetal abnormalities and death have occurred if used during second or third trimester. Encourage use of contraceptive measures.

IND & DOSE Tx of hypertension, alone or as part of combination therapy. *Adult:* 25 mg PO bid or tid. Range, 25–150 mg bid–tid; max, 450 mg/day. **Tx of heart failure.** *Adult:* 6.25–12.5 mg PO tid. Maint, 50–100 mg PO tid; max, 450 mg/day. **Left ventricular dysfx after MI.** *Adult:* 6.25 mg PO, then 12.5 mg PO tid; increase slowly to 50 mg PO tid starting as early as 3 days post-MI. **Tx of diabetic nephropathy.** *Adult:* Reduce dosage; suggested dose, 25 mg PO tid.

ADJUST DOSE Elderly pts, renal impairment

ADV EFF Agranulocytosis, aphthous ulcers, cough, dysgeusia, **HF, MI, pancytopenia,** proteinuria, rash, tachycardia

INTERACTIONS Allopurinol, indomethacin, lithium, probenecid

NC/PT Use caution before surgery; mark chart. Give 1 hr before meals. Protect pt in situations of decreased fluid volume. Not for use in pregnancy. Cough may occur. Pt should change position slowly if dizzy, lightheaded; avoid OTC preparations; consult prescriber before stopping drug.

carbamazepine
(Carbatrol, Equetro, Tegretol)

CLASS Antiepileptic
PREG/CONT D/NA

BBW Risk of aplastic anemia and agranulocytosis; obtain CBC, including platelet/reticulocyte counts, and serum iron determination before starting tx; repeat wkly for first 3 mo and monthly thereafter for at least 2–3 yr. Discontinue if evidence of marrow suppression. Increased risk of suicidality; monitor accordingly.

IND & DOSE Refractory seizure disorders. *Adult:* 200 mg PO bid on first day. Increase gradually by up to 200 mg/day in divided doses q 6–8 hr, or 100 mg PO qid suspension; range, 800–1,200 mg/day. *Child 6–12 yr:* 100 mg PO bid on first day. Increase gradually by adding 100 mg/day at 6- to 8-hr intervals until best response achieved; max, 1,000 mg/day. *Child under 6 yr:* Optimal daily dose, less than 35 mg/kg/day PO. **Tx of trigeminal neuralgia.** *Adult:* 100 mg PO bid on first day. May increase by up to 200 mg/day, using 100-mg increments q 12 hr as needed. Range, 200–1,200 mg/day; max, 1,200 mg/day. **Tx of bipolar 1 disorder.** *Adult:* 400 mg/day PO in divided doses; max, 1,600 mg/day (*Equetro* only).

ADJUST DOSE Elderly pts
ADV EFF Bone marrow suppression, CV complications, dizziness, drowsiness, hepatic cellular necrosis w/ total loss of liver tissue, hepatitis, HF, n/v, Stevens-Johnson syndrome, unsteadiness
INTERACTIONS Barbiturates, charcoal, cimetidine, danazol, doxycycline, erythromycin, isoniazid, lithium, MAOIs, NMJ blockers, phenytoin, primidone, valproic acid, verapamil, warfarin
NC/PT Use only for indicated uses. Taper dose if withdrawing; abrupt removal can precipitate seizures. Obtain

baseline and frequent LFTs, monitor CBC; dose adjustment made accordingly. Evaluate for therapeutic serum levels (usually 4–12 mcg/mL). Not for use in pregnancy (barrier contraceptives advisable). Pt should swallow ER tablets whole; wear medical alert tag; avoid CNS depressants (alcohol). May open *Equetro* capsule and sprinkle over food.

carbinoxamine maleate
(Karbinal ER)

CLASS Antihistamine
PREG/CONT C/NA

IND & DOSE Tx of seasonal/perennial allergic rhinitis; vasomotor rhinitis; allergic conjunctivitis; allergic skin reactions; dermatographism; anaphylactic reactions; allergic reactions to blood, blood products. *Adult, child 12 yr and older:* 6–16 mg PO q 12 hr. *Child 6–11 yr:* 6–12 mg PO q 12 hr. *Child 4–5 yr:* 3–8 mg PO q 12 hr. *Child 2–3 yr:* 3–4 mg PO q 12 hr.
ADV EFF Dizziness, drowsiness, dry mouth, epigastric distress, rash, thickened secretions, urine retention
INTERACTIONS CNS depressants, MAOIs; avoid this combination
NC/PT Ensure pt can tolerate anticholinergic effects; suggest increased fluids, humidifier. Not for use in pregnancy, breast-feeding. Pt should measure drug using mL measure provided; take safety measures w/ CNS effects; use humidifier, increase fluid intake; report difficulty breathing, fainting.

DANGEROUS DRUG
carboplatin (generic)

CLASS Alkylating agent, antineoplastic
PREG/CONT D/NA

BBW Evaluate bone marrow function before and periodically during tx; do not give next dose if marked bone marrow depression. Consult

physician for dosage. Ensure epinephrine, corticosteroids, antihistamines
readily available in case of anaphylactic reactions, which may occur within
min of administration.

IND & DOSE Initial, palliative tx of
pts w/ advanced ovarian cancer.
Adult: As single agent, 360 mg/m² IV
over at least 15 min on day
1 q 4 wk; adjust dose based on blood
counts.

ADJUST DOSE Elderly pts, renal
impairment

ADV EFF Abd pain, alopecia, asthenia, **anaphylactic reactions, bone
marrow suppression, bronchospasm, cancer,** constipation, electrolyte abnormalities, n/v/d, peripheral
neuropathies, renal impairment

INTERACTIONS Aluminum (IV form)

NC/PT Antiemetic may be needed.
Obtain CBC regularly; dose adjustment may be needed. Ensure emergency equipment available in case of
anaphylactic reaction. Not for use in
pregnancy. Hair loss, GI effects
possible.

carboprost tromethamine
(Hemabate)
CLASS Abortifacient,
prostaglandin
PREG/CONT C/NA

IND & DOSE Termination of pregnancy 13–20 wk from first day of last
menstrual period; evacuation of
uterus in missed abortion or intrauterine fetal death. *Adult:* 250 mcg
(1 mL) IM; give 250 mcg IM at 1.5- to
3.5-hr intervals. Max, 12 mg total
dose. **Tx of postpartum hemorrhage.**
Adult: 250 mcg IM as one dose; may
use multiple doses at 15- to 90-min
intervals. Max, 2 mg (eight doses).

ADV EFF Diarrhea, flushing, hypotension, nausea, **perforated uterus,
uterine rupture**

NC/PT Pretreat w/ antiemetics and
antidiarrheals. Give by deep IM injection. Ensure abortion complete; moni-

tor for infection. Ensure adequate hydration. Several IM injections may be
needed.

carfilzomib (Kyprolis)
CLASS Antineoplastic,
proteasome inhibitor
PREG/CONT D/NA

IND & DOSE Tx of multiple myeloma in pts w/ disease progression after at least two prior therapies.
Adult: Cycle 1: 20 mg/m²/day IV over
2–10 min on two consecutive days
each wk for three wk (days 1, 2, 8, 9,
15, 16) followed by 12-day rest period. Cycle 2 and beyond: Increase to
27 mg/m²/day IV over 2–10 min, following same dosing-days schedule.

ADV EFF Anemia, dyspnea, fatigue,
fever, **heart failure/ischemia,** hepatotoxicity, infusion reactions, **liver
failure,** n/v/d, **pulmonary complications, pulmonary hypertension,**
thrombocytopenia, **tumor lysis syndrome**

NC/PT Premedicate w/ dexamethasone; hydrate before and after tx.
Monitor for potentially severe adverse
reactions; arrange for supportive
measures, dosage adjustment. Not for
use in pregnancy. Pt should mark calendar for tx days; report difficulty
breathing, swelling, urine/stool color
changes, chest pain.

carglumic acid
(Carbaglu)
CLASS Carbamoyl phosphate
synthetase I activator
PREG/CONT C/NA

IND & DOSE Adjunctive/maint tx of
acute hyperammonemia due to hepatic *N*-acetylglutamate synthase deficiency. *Adult, child:* 100–250 mg/kg/day
PO in divided doses; may be made into
sol and given through NG tube.

ADV EFF Abd pain, anemia, fever,
headache, infections, nasopharyngitis, n/v/d

NC/PT Monitor ammonia levels during tx; dose adjustment may be needed. Restrict protein intake until ammonia level regulated. Not for use in pregnancy, breast-feeding. Store in refrigerator until opened, then room temp. Date bottle; discard after 1 mo.

carisoprodol (Soma)
CLASS Centrally acting skeletal muscle relaxant
PREG/CONT C/NA

IND & DOSE Relief of discomfort associated w/ acute, painful musculoskeletal conditions, as adjunct. *Adult, child over 16 yr:* 250–350 mg PO tid–qid. Pt should take last dose at bedtime for max of 2–3 wk.
ADJUST DOSE Hepatic, renal impairment
ADV EFF Allergic/idiosyncratic reaction, agitation, **anaphylactoid shock**, ataxia, dizziness, drowsiness, irritability, tremor, vertigo
NC/PT Monitor for idiosyncratic reaction, most likely w/ first doses. Provide safety measures w/ CNS effects. May become habit-forming; use caution. Pt should avoid other CNS depressants.

DANGEROUS DRUG
carmustine (BCNU)
(BiCNU, Gliadel)
CLASS Alkylating agent, antineoplastic
PREG/CONT D/NA

BBW Do not give more often than q 6 wk because of delayed bone marrow toxicity. Evaluate hematopoietic function before, wkly during, and for at least 6 wk after tx to monitor for bone marrow suppression. Monitor for pulmonary toxicity and delayed toxicity, which can occur yrs after therapy; death possible. Cumulative doses of 1,400 mg/m² increase risk.

IND & DOSE Palliative tx alone or w/ other agents (injection) for brain tumors, Hodgkin lymphoma, non-Hodgkin lymphoma, multiple myeloma. *Adult, child:* 150–200 mg/m² IV q 6 wk as single dose or in divided daily injections (75–100 mg/m² on 2 successive days); adjust dose based on CBC. **Adjunct to surgery for tx of recurrent glioblastoma as implantable wafer (w/ prednisone); tx of newly diagnosed high-grade malignant glioma** (wafer). *Adult, child:* Wafers implanted in resection cavity as part of surgical procedure; up to 8 wafers at a time.
ADV EFF Bone marrow suppression (may be delayed 4–6 wk), **cancer**, hepatotoxicity, local burning at injection site, **pulmonary fibrosis**, pulmonary infiltrates, **renal failure**, stomatitis
INTERACTIONS Cimetidine, digoxin, mitomycin, phenytoin
NC/PT Monitor CBC before and wkly during tx. Do not give full dose within 2–3 wk of radiation or other chemotherapy. Monitor pulmonary function; toxicity can be delayed. Monitor LFTs, renal function, injection site for local reaction. Premedicate w/ antiemetic. Not for use in pregnancy. Pt should try to maintain fluid intake, nutrition.

---

carvedilol (Coreg)
CLASS Alpha and beta blocker, antihypertensive
PREG/CONT C/NA

IND & DOSE Converting to once-daily CR capsules. 3.125 mg bid, give 10 mg CR; 6.25 mg bid, give 20 mg CR; 12.5 mg bid, give 40 mg CR; 25 mg bid, give 80 mg CR. **Mgt of hypertension, alone or w/ other drugs.** *Adult:* 6.25 mg PO bid; maintain for 7–14 days, then increase to 12.5 mg PO bid. Max, 50 mg/day. **Tx of mild to severe HF.** *Adult:* 3.125 mg PO bid for 2 wk, then may increase to 6.25 mg PO bid. Max, 25 mg/day if under 85 kg, 50 mg if over 85 kg. **Tx of left ventricular dysfx after MI.**

Adult: 6.25 mg PO bid; increase after 3–10 days to 25 mg PO bid.
ADJUST DOSE Hepatic impairment
ADV EFF Bradycardia, constipation, fatigue, flatulence, diarrhea, dizziness, gastric pain, **hepatic injury, HF**, hypotension, rhinitis, tinnitus, vertigo
INTERACTIONS Antidiabetics, clonidine, digoxin, diltiazem, rifampin, verapamil
NC/PT Do not discontinue abruptly; taper when discontinuing. Use caution if surgery planned. Use care in conversion to CR capsules. Monitor for orthostatic hypotension. Monitor LFTs. Provide safety measures. Pt should not cut, crush, or chew CR capsules; change position slowly if lowered BP occurs; if diabetic, should use caution and monitor glucose levels carefully.

caspofungin acetate (Cancidas)
CLASS Antifungal, echinocandin
PREG/CONT C/NA

IND & DOSE Tx of invasive aspergillosis; tx of esophageal candidiasis; tx of candidemia and other *Candida* infections; empirical tx when fungal infection suspected in neutropenic pts. *Adult:* Loading dose, 70 mg IV, then 50 mg/day IV infusion for at least 14 days. *Child 3 mo–17 yr:* Loading dose, 70 mg/m² IV, then 50 mg/m² IV daily for 14 days.
ADJUST DOSE Hepatic impairment, concurrent rifampin or inducers of drug clearance
ADV EFF Decreased serum potassium, diarrhea, fever, **hepatic damage**, hypersensitivity reactions, hypotension, increased liver enzymes
INTERACTIONS Cyclosporine, rifampin
NC/PT Monitor for IV complications. Monitor potassium levels; monitor LFTs before and during tx. Not for use in pregnancy, breast-feeding.

cefaclor (Ceclor)
CLASS Cephalosporin
PREG/CONT B/NA

IND & DOSE Tx of lower respiratory infections, URI, skin infections, UTIs, otitis media, pharyngitis caused by susceptible bacteria strains. *Adult:* 250 mg PO q 8 hr or 375–500 mg q 12 hr for 7–10 days; max, 4 g/day. *Child:* 20 mg/kg/day PO in divided doses q 8 hr; in severe cases, may give 40 mg/kg/day. Max, 1 g/day. For otitis media/pharyngitis, may divide dose and give q 12 hr.
ADV EFF Abd pain, **anaphylaxis**, anorexia, **colitis**, flatulence, n/v/d, rash, superinfections
INTERACTIONS Aminoglycosides, antacids, anticoagulants
NC/PT Culture before tx. Give w/ meals to decrease GI discomfort. Give oral vancomycin for serious colitis. Refrigerate suspension. Pt should not cut, crush, or chew ER tablets; complete full course of therapy; report diarrhea w/ blood or mucus.

cefadroxil (generic)
CLASS Cephalosporin
PREG/CONT B/NA

IND & DOSE Tx of pharyngitis/tonsillitis caused by susceptible bacteria strains. *Adult:* 1 g/day PO in single dose or two divided doses for 10 days. *Child:* 30 mg/kg/day PO in single or two divided doses; continue for 10 days. **Tx of UTIs caused by susceptible bacteria strains.** *Adult:* 1–2 g/day PO in single dose or two divided doses for uncomplicated lower UTIs. For all other UTIs, 2 g/day in two divided doses. *Child:* 30 mg/kg/day PO in divided doses q 12 hr. **Tx of skin, skin-structure infections caused by susceptible bacteria strains.** *Adult:* 1 g/day PO in single dose or two divided doses. *Child:* 30 mg/kg/day PO in divided doses.

ADJUST DOSE Elderly pts, renal impairment
ADV EFF Abd pain, **anaphylaxis,** anorexia, **bone marrow depression, colitis,** flatulence, n/v/d, rash, super-infections
INTERACTIONS Aminoglycosides, bacteriostatic agents, probenecid
NC/PT Culture before tx. Give w/ meals to decrease GI discomfort; give oral vancomycin for serious colitis. Refrigerate suspension. Pt should not cut, crush, or chew ER tablets; complete full course of therapy; report diarrhea w/ blood or mucus.

cefdinir (generic)
CLASS Cephalosporin
PREG/CONT B/NA

IND & DOSE Tx of community-acquired pneumonia, uncomplicated skin, skin-structure infections. *Adult, adolescent:* 300 mg PO q 12 hr for 10 days. **Tx of acute exacerbation of chronic bronchitis, acute maxillary sinusitis, pharyngitis, tonsillitis.** *Adult, adolescent:* 300 mg PO q 12 hr for 10 days or 600 mg PO q 24 hr for 10 days. **Tx of otitis media, acute maxillary sinusitis, pharyngitis, tonsillitis.** *Child 6 mo–12 yr:* 7 mg/kg PO q 12 hr or 14 mg/kg PO q 24 hr for 10 days; max, 600 mg/day. **Tx of skin, skin-structure infections.** *Child 6 mo–12 yr:* 7 mg/kg PO q 12 hr for 10 days.
ADJUST DOSE Renal impairment
ADV EFF Abd pain, **anaphylaxis,** anorexia, **colitis,** flatulence, n/v/d, rash, superinfections
INTERACTIONS Aminoglycosides, antacids, oral anticoagulants
NC/PT Culture before tx. Give w/ meals to decrease GI discomfort; give oral vancomycin for serious colitis. Arrange for tx of superinfections. Store suspension at room temp; discard after 10 days. Pt should complete full course of therapy; report diarrhea w/ blood or mucus.

cefditoren pivoxil (Spectracef)
CLASS Cephalosporin
PREG/CONT B/NA

IND & DOSE Tx of uncomplicated skin/skin-structure infections, pharyngitis, tonsillitis caused by susceptible bacteria. *Adult, child over 12 yr:* 200 mg PO bid for 10 days. **Tx of acute exacerbation of chronic bronchitis, community-acquired pneumonia caused by susceptible bacteria strains.** *Adult, child over 12 yr:* 400 mg PO bid for 10 days (chronic bronchitis) or 14 days (pneumonia).
ADJUST DOSE Renal impairment
ADV EFF Abd pain, **anaphylaxis,** anorexia, **colitis,** flatulence, **hepatotoxicity,** n/v/d, rash, superinfections
INTERACTIONS Antacids, oral anticoagulants
NC/PT Culture before tx. Do not give longer than 10 days; risk of carnitine deficiency. Give w/ meals to decrease GI discomfort; give oral vancomycin for serious colitis. Provide tx for superinfections. Not for pts w/ allergy to milk proteins. Pt should not take w/ antacids; should complete full course of therapy; report diarrhea w/ blood or mucus.

cefepime hydrochloride (generic)
CLASS Cephalosporin
PREG/CONT B/NA

IND & DOSE Tx of mild to moderate UTI. *Adult:* 0.5–1 g IM or IV q 12 hr for 7–10 days. **Tx of severe UTI.** *Adult:* 2 g IV q 12 hr for 10 days. **Tx of moderate to severe pneumonia.** *Adult:* 1–2 g IV q 12 hr for 10 days. **Tx of moderate to severe skin infections.** *Adult:* 2 g IV q 12 hr for 10 days. **Empiric therapy for febrile neutropenic pts.** *Adult:* 2 g IV q 8 hr for 7 days. **Tx of complicated intra-abdominal infections.** *Adult:*

2 g IV q 12 hr for 7–10 days. *Children over 2 mo, under 40 kg:* 50 mg/kg/day IV or IM q 12 hr for 7–10 days depending on infection severity. If treating febrile neutropenia, give q 8 hr (max, 2 g/day).

ADJUST DOSE Elderly pts, renal impairment

ADV EFF Abd pain, **anaphylaxis**, anorexia, **colitis**, disulfiram reaction w/ alcohol, flatulence, **hepatotoxicity**, n/v/d, phlebitis, rash, superinfections

INTERACTIONS Alcohol, aminoglycosides, oral anticoagulants

NC/PT Culture before tx. Have vitamin K available if hypoprothrombinemia occurs. Pt should avoid alcohol during and for 3 days after tx; report diarrhea w/ blood or and mucus.

cefotaxime sodium
(Claforan)
CLASS Cephalosporin
PREG/CONT B/NA

IND & DOSE Tx of lower respiratory tract, skin, intra-abdominal, CNS, bone and joint infections; UTIs; peritonitis caused by susceptible bacteria. *Adult:* 2–8 g/day IM or IV in equally divided doses q 6–8 hr; max, 12 g/day. *Child 1 mo–12 yr under 50 kg:* 50–180 mg/kg/day IV or IM in four to six divided doses. *Child 1–4 wk:* 50 mg/kg IV q 8 hr. *Child 0–1 wk:* 50 mg/kg IV q 12 hr. Tx of gonorrhea. *Adult:* 0.5–1 g IM in single injection. Disseminated infection. *Adult:* 1–2 g IV q 8 hr. Periop px. *Adult:* 1 g IV or IM 30–90 min before surgery. Cesarean section. *Adult:* 1 g IV after cord is clamped, then 1 g IV or IM at 6 and 12 hr.

ADJUST DOSE Elderly pts, renal impairment

ADV EFF Abd pain, **anaphylaxis**, anorexia, **bone marrow depression**, **colitis**, disulfiram reaction w/ alcohol, flatulence, **hepatotoxicity**, n/v/d, phlebitis, rash, superinfections

INTERACTIONS Alcohol, aminoglycosides, oral anticoagulants

NC/PT Culture before tx. Give IV slowly. Pt should avoid alcohol during and for 3 days after tx; report diarrhea w/ blood or mucus.

cefoxitin sodium
(generic)
CLASS Cephalosporin
PREG/CONT B/NA

IND & DOSE Tx of lower respiratory tract, skin, intra-abdominal, CNS, bone and joint infections; UTIs; peritonitis caused by susceptible bacteria. *Adult:* 2–8 g/day IM or IV in equally divided doses q 6–8 hr. *Child 3 mo and older:* 80–160 mg/kg/day IM or IV in divided doses q 4–6 hr. Max, 12 g/day. Tx of gonorrhea. *Adult:* 2 g IM w/ 1 g oral probenecid. Uncomplicated lower respiratory tract infections, UTIs, skin infections. *Adult:* 1 g q 6–8 hr IV. Moderate to severe infections. *Adult:* 1 g q 4 hr IV to 2 g q 6–8 hr IV. Severe infections. *Adult:* 2 g q 4 hr IV or 3 g q 6 hr IV. Periop px. *Adult:* 2 g IV or IM 30–60 min before initial incision, q 6 hr for 24 hr after surgery. Cesarean section. *Adult:* 2 g IV as soon as cord clamped, then 2 g IM or IV at 4 and 8 hr, then q 6 hr for up to 24 hr. Transurethral prostatectomy. *Adult:* 1 g before surgery, then 1 g q 8 hr for up to 5 days.

ADJUST DOSE Elderly pts, renal impairment

ADV EFF Abd pain, **anaphylaxis**, anorexia, **bone marrow depression**, **colitis**, disulfiram reaction w/ alcohol, flatulence, **hepatotoxicity**, n/v/d, phlebitis, rash, superinfections

INTERACTIONS Alcohol, aminoglycosides, oral anticoagulants

NC/PT Culture before tx. Give IV slowly. Have vitamin K available for hypoprothrombinemia. Pt should avoid alcohol during and for 3 days after tx; report diarrhea w/ blood or mucus.

cefpodoxime proxetil
(generic)

CLASS Cephalosporin
PREG/CONT B/NA

IND & DOSE Tx of upper and lower respiratory tract infections, skin and skin-structure infections, UTIs, otitis media caused by susceptible strains; STD caused by *Neisseria gonorrhoeae*. *Adult:* 100–400 mg PO q 12 hr depending on infection severity for 5–14 days. *Child:* 5 mg/kg/dose PO q 12 hr; max, 100–200 mg/dose for 10 days. **Tx of acute otitis media.** *Child:* 10 mg/kg/day PO divided q 12 hr; max, 400 mg/day for 5 days.
ADJUST DOSE Elderly pts, renal impairment
ADV EFF Abd pain, **anaphylaxis,** anorexia, **bone marrow depression, colitis,** flatulence, **hepatotoxicity,** n/v/d, phlebitis, rash, superinfections
INTERACTIONS Aminoglycosides, oral anticoagulants
NC/PT Culture before tx. Refrigerate suspension. Give oral vancomycin for serious colitis. Pt should take w/ food; complete full course of therapy; report diarrhea w/ blood or mucus.

cefprozil (generic)

CLASS Cephalosporin
PREG/CONT B/NA

IND & DOSE Tx of upper and lower respiratory tract infections, skin and skin-structure infections, otitis media, acute sinusitis caused by susceptible strains. *Adult:* 250–500 mg PO q 12–24 hr for 10 days. **Tx of acute otitis media, sinusitis.** *Child 6 mo–12 yr:* 7.5–15 mg/kg PO q 12 hr for 10 days. **Tx of pharyngitis, tonsillitis.** *Child 2–12 yr:* 7.5 mg/kg PO q 12 hr for 10 days. **Tx of skin and skin-structure infections.** *Child 2–12 yr:* 20 mg/kg PO once daily for 10 days.

ADJUST DOSE Elderly pts, renal impairment
ADV EFF Abd pain, **anaphylaxis,** anorexia, **bone marrow depression, colitis,** flatulence, **hepatotoxicity,** n/v/d, phlebitis, rash, superinfections
INTERACTIONS Aminoglycosides, oral anticoagulants
NC/PT Culture before tx. Refrigerate suspension. Give oral vancomycin for serious colitis. Pt should take w/ food; complete full course of therapy; report diarrhea w/ blood or mucus.

ceftaroline fosamil
(Teflaro)

CLASS Cephalosporin
PREG/CONT B/NA

IND & DOSE Tx of skin, skin-structure infections; community-acquired pneumonia caused by susceptible strains. *Adult:* 600 mg by IV infusion over 1 hr q 12 hr for 5–14 days (skin, skin-structure infections) or 5–7 days (community-acquired pneumonia).
ADJUST DOSE Renal impairment
ADV EFF *Clostridium difficile*–associated diarrhea, dizziness, **hemolytic anemia, hypersensitivity reactions,** injection-site reactions, rash, **renal failure**
NC/PT Culture before tx. Small, frequent meals may help GI effects. Monitor injection site, CBC. Not for use in pregnancy, breast-feeding. Pt should report severe diarrhea.

ceftazidime (Ceptaz, Fortaz, Tazicef)

CLASS Cephalosporin
PREG/CONT B/NA

IND & DOSE Tx of lower respiratory, skin and skin-structure, intra-abdominal, CNS, bone and joint infections; UTIs, septicemia caused by susceptible strains, gynecologic infections caused by *Escherichia coli*. *Adult:* Usual dose, 1 g (range,

250 mg–2 g) q 8–12 hr IM or IV; max, 6 g/day. *Child 1 mo–12 yr:* 30 mg/kg IV q 12 hr. *Child 0–4 wk:* 30 mg/kg IV q 12 hr. **Tx of UTIs caused by susceptible bacteria strains.** *Adult:* 250–500 mg IV or IM q 8–12 hr. **Tx of pneumonia, skin and skin-structure infections caused by susceptible bacteria strains.** *Adult:* 500 mg–1 g IV or IM q 8 hr. **Tx of bone and joint infections caused by susceptible bacteria strains.** *Adult:* 2 g IV q 12 hr. **Tx of gynecologic, intra-abdominal, life-threatening infections; meningitis.** *Adult:* 2 g IV q 8 hr.

ADJUST DOSE Elderly pts, renal impairment

ADV EFF Abd pain, **anaphylaxis,** anorexia, **bone marrow depression, colitis,** disulfiram-like reaction w/ alcohol, flatulence, injection-site reactions, n/v/d, pain, phlebitis, superinfections

INTERACTIONS Aminoglycosides, alcohol, oral anticoagulants

NC/PT Culture before tx. Do not mix in sol w/ aminoglycosides. Have vitamin K available if hypoprothrombinemia occurs. Pt should avoid alcohol during and for 3 days after tx; report diarrhea w/ blood or mucus.

---

ceftibuten (Cedax)

CLASS Cephalosporin
PREG/CONT B/NA

IND & DOSE Tx of acute bacterial exacerbations of chronic bronchitis, acute bacterial otitis media, pharyngitis, tonsillitis caused by susceptible strains. *Adult:* 400 mg PO daily for 10 days. *Child:* 9 mg/kg/day PO for 10 days; max, 400 mg/day.

ADJUST DOSE Renal impairment
ADV EFF Abd pain, **anaphylaxis,** anorexia, **bone marrow depression, colitis,** disulfiram-like reactions w/ alcohol, flatulence, **hepatotoxicity,** n/v/d, pain, superinfections

---

INTERACTIONS Aminoglycosides, alcohol, oral anticoagulants

NC/PT Culture before tx. Give w/ meals. Refrigerate suspension; discard after 14 days. Arrange tx for superinfections. Pt should avoid alcohol during and for 3 days after tx; complete full course of therapy; report diarrhea w/ blood or mucus.

---

ceftriaxone sodium
(Rocephin)

CLASS Cephalosporin
PREG/CONT B/NA

IND & DOSE Tx of lower respiratory tract, intra-abdominal, skin and skin-structure, bone and joint infections; acute bacterial otitis media, UTIs, septicemia caused by susceptible strains. *Adult:* 1–2 g/day IM or IV as one dose or in equal divided doses bid; max, 4 g/day. *Child:* 50–75 mg/kg/day IV or IM in divided doses q 12 hr; max, 2 g/day. **Tx of gonorrhea and PID caused by** *Neisseria gonorrhoeae. Adult:* Single 250-mg IM dose. **Tx of meningitis.** *Adult:* 1–2 g/day IM or IV as one dose or in equal divided doses bid for 4–14 days; max, 4 g/day. Loading dose of 100 mg/kg may be used. **Periop px.** *Adult:* 1 g IV 30–120 min before surgery.

ADV EFF Abd pain, **anaphylaxis,** anorexia, **bone marrow depression, colitis,** disulfiram-like reactions w/ alcohol, flatulence, **hepatotoxicity,** n/v/d, pain, superinfections

INTERACTIONS Aminoglycosides, alcohol, oral anticoagulants

NC/PT Culture before tx. Give w/ meals. Protect drug from light. Have vitamin K available if hypoprothrombinemia occurs. Do not mix w/ other antimicrobials. Arrange tx for superinfections. Pt should avoid alcohol during and for 3 days after tx; complete full course of therapy; report diarrhea w/ blood or mucus.

cefuroxime axetil (Ceftin), cefuroxime sodium (Zinacef)

CLASS Cephalosporin
PREG/CONT B/NA

IND & DOSE Tx of upper respiratory tract, skin and skin-structure infections; acute bacterial otitis media, uncomplicated gonorrhea, bacterial sinusitis, UTIs, early Lyme disease caused by susceptible strains. *Adult, child 12 yr and older:* 250 mg PO bid. For severe infections, may increase to 500 mg PO bid. Treat for up to 10 days. Or 750 mg–1.5 g IM or IV q 8 hr, depending on infection severity, for 5–10 days. *Child over 3 mo:* 50–100 mg/kg/day IM or IV in divided doses q 6–8 hr. **Tx of acute otitis media.** *Child 3 mo–12 yr:* 250 mg PO bid for 10 days. **Tx of pharyngitis/tonsillitis.** *Child 3 mo–12 yr:* 125 mg PO q 12 hr for 10 days **Tx of acute sinusitis.** *Child 3 mo–12 yr:* 250 mg PO bid for 10 days. **Tx of impetigo.** *Child 3 mo–12 yr:* 30 mg/kg/day (max, 1 g/day) in two divided doses for 10 days. **Uncomplicated gonorrhea.** *Adult:* 1.5 g IM (at two different sites) w/ 1 g oral probenecid. **Periop px.** *Adult:* 1.5 g IV 30–60 min before initial incision, then 750 mg IV or IM q 8 hr for 24 hr after surgery. **Tx of bacterial meningitis.** *Child:* 200–240 mg/kg/day IV in divided doses q 6–8 hr.
ADJUST DOSE Elderly pts, impaired renal function
ADV EFF Abd pain, **anaphylaxis**, anorexia, **bone marrow depression, colitis**, disulfiram-like reactions w/ alcohol, flatulence, **hepatotoxicity**, n/v/d, pain, superinfections
INTERACTIONS Aminoglycosides, alcohol, oral anticoagulants
NC/PT Culture before tx. Give w/ meals. Have vitamin K available for hypoprothrombinemia. Do not mix w/ other antimicrobials. Arrange for tx of superinfections. Have suspension made for children who cannot

swallow tablets. Pt should avoid alcohol during and for 3 days after tx; complete full course of therapy; report diarrhea w/ blood or mucus.

celecoxib (Celebrex)

CLASS Cox-2 specific inhibitor, NSAID
PREG/CONT C (1st, 2nd trimesters); D (3rd trimester)/NA

BBW Increased risk of CV events, GI bleeding; monitor accordingly.
IND & DOSE Tx of acute pain, dysmenorrhea; mgt of rheumatoid arthritis. *Adult:* 100 mg PO bid; may increase to 200 mg/day PO bid as needed. **Tx of osteoarthritis.** *Adult:* 200 mg/day PO. **Tx of ankylosing spondylitis.** *Adult:* 200 mg/day PO; after 6 wk, may try 400 mg/day PO for 6 wk. **Tx of juvenile rheumatoid arthritis.** *Child 2 yr and older:* Over 25 kg, 100 mg capsule PO bid. Ten kg to 25 kg or less, 50 mg capsule PO bid.
ADJUST DOSE Hepatic, renal impairment
ADV EFF Agranulocytosis, anaphylactoid reactions, dizziness, dyspepsia, headache, insomnia, **MI**, rash, somnolence, **stroke**
INTERACTIONS Alcohol, lithium, nicotine, warfarin
NC/PT Give w/ food if GI upset occurs. Use comfort measures to help relieve pain, safety measures if CNS effects occur. Name confusion w/ *Celebrex* (celecoxib), *Celexa* (citalopram), *Xanax* (alprazolam), and *Cerebyx* (fosphenytoin); use caution.

cellulose sodium phosphate (CSP) (Calcibind)

CLASS Antilithic, resin exchange drug
PREG/CONT C/NA

IND & DOSE Tx of absorptive hypercalciuria type 1 (calcium oxalate and calcium phosphate renal stones). *Adult:* 10–15 mg/day PO based on urine calcium level.

ADV EFF Abd discomfort, anorexia, dizziness, drowsiness, hypomagnesemia, muscle spasm, n/v/d

INTERACTIONS Ascorbic acid, calcium-containing drugs, milk products, oxalate-containing foods

NC/PT Suspend powder in water, soft drink, or fruit juice; give 1 hr before meal. Give w/ magnesium gluconate. Monitor serum calcium, magnesium, urine calcium, oxalate, PTH levels. Not for use in pregnancy, breast-feeding. Push fluids. Pt should limit calcium intake.

---

cephalexin (Keflex)
CLASS Cephalosporin
PREG/CONT B/NA

IND & DOSE Tx of respiratory tract infections, acute bacterial otitis media, bone infections, UTIs caused by susceptible strains. *Adult:* 1–4 g/day in divided doses; usual dose, 250 mg PO q 6 hr. *Child:* 25–50 mg/kg/day PO in divided doses. Tx of skin, skin-structure infections, uncomplicated cystitis, streptococcal pharyngitis. *Adult:* 500 mg PO q 12 hr. May need larger doses in severe cases; max, 4 g/day. *Child:* Divide usual daily dose; give q 12 hr. Tx of otitis media. *Child:* 75–100 mg/kg/day PO in four divided doses.

ADV EFF Abd pain, **anaphylaxis**, anorexia, **bone marrow depression, colitis,** disulfiram-like reactions w/ alcohol, flatulence, **hepatotoxicity,** n/v/d, pain, superinfections

INTERACTIONS Aminoglycosides, alcohol, oral anticoagulants

NC/PT Culture before tx. Give w/ meal. Pt should avoid alcohol during and for 3 days after tx; report diarrhea w/ blood or mucus.

---

certolizumab (Cimzia)
CLASS Immune modulator, TNF blocker
PREG/CONT C/NA

BBW Risk of serious infections, cancer, CNS demyelinating disorders. Prescreen for TB and hepatitis B; monitor pt carefully.

IND & DOSE To reduce s&sx of Crohn's disease; tx of moderately to severely active rheumatoid arthritis. *Adult:* 400 mg subcut repeated at 2 wk and 4 wk; maint, 400 mg q 4 wk (Crohn's), 200 mg q 4 wk (arthritis).

ADV EFF Anaphylaxis, lupus like syndrome, malignancies, serious to fatal infections, rash, URIs, UTIs

INTERACTIONS Abatacept, anakinra, live vaccines, natalizumab, rituximab

NC/PT Monitor carefully for s&sx of allergic reaction, infection. Not for use in pregnancy. Pt should report s&sx of infection.

---

cetirizine hydrochloride (Zyrtec)
CLASS Antihistamine
PREG/CONT B/NA

IND & DOSE Mgt of seasonal and perennial allergic rhinitis; tx of chronic, idiopathic urticaria. *Adult, child 6 yr and older:* 10 mg/day PO or 5 mg PO bid; max, 10 mg. *Child 6–11 yr:* 5 or 10 mg PO daily. *Child 2–6 yr:* 2.5 mg PO once daily; max,5 mg/day.

ADJUST DOSE Elderly pts; renal, hepatic impairment

ADV EFF Bronchospasm, sedation, somnolence

NC/PT Provide syrup or chewable tablets for children. Pt should maintain intake of fluids, use humidifier if secretions thicken; take safety precautions if sedation occurs. Name confusion between *Zyrtec* (cetirizine) and *Zyprexa* (olanzapine) and between *Zyrtec* (cetirizine) and *Zantac* (ranitidine); use caution.

cetrorelix acetate
(Cetrotide)

CLASS Fertility drug
PREG/CONT X/NA

IND & DOSE Inhibition of premature LH surges in women undergoing controlled ovarian stimulation. *Adult:* 3 mg subcut. If HCG not given within 4 days, continue 0.25 mg/kg/day subcut until HCG is given.
ADV EFF Headache, **hypersensitivity reactions**, injection-site reactions, nausea, ovarian overstimulation
NC/PT Part of comprehensive fertility program; many follow-up tests will be needed. Pt should learn proper administration of drug and disposal of syringes, needles.

DANGEROUS DRUG

cetuximab (Erbitux)

CLASS Antineoplastic, monoclonal antibody
PREG/CONT C/NA

BBW Serious to fatal infusion reactions, cardiac arrest, and sudden death have occurred. Closely monitor serum electrolytes during and after tx.
IND & DOSE Tx of advanced colorectal cancer, advanced squamous cell carcinoma of head and neck w/ radiation or as monotherapy after failure of platinum therapy. *Adult:* 400 mg/m² IV loading dose over 120 min, then 250 mg/m² IV over 60 min wkly.
ADV EFF Cardiac arrest, dermatological toxicity, diarrhea, headache, hypomagnesemia, infections, infusion reactions, pulmonary toxicity, rash, pruritus
NC/PT Premedicate w/ H₁ antagonist IV 30–60 min before first dose. Base future doses on clinical response. Do not infuse faster than 10 mg/min. Have emergency equipment on hand. Monitor electrolytes; assess lungs and skin for s&sx of

toxicity. Males and females should use contraception during and for 6 mo after tx; females should not breast-feed during or for 2 mo after tx. Pt should report s&sx of infection, difficulty breathing, rash.

cevimeline hydrochloride (Evoxac)

CLASS Parasympathomimetic
PREG/CONT C/NA

IND & DOSE Tx of dry mouth in pts w/ Sjögren's syndrome. *Adult:* 30 mg PO tid w/ food.
ADV EFF Cardiac arrhythmias, bronchial narrowing, dehydration, dyspepsia, excessive sweating, headache, n/v/d, URIs, visual blurring
INTERACTIONS Beta-adrenergic antagonists
NC/PT Give w/ meals. Monitor for dehydration. Pt should take safety precautions if visual changes occur.

charcoal, activated
(Actidose-Aqua, Liqui-Char)

CLASS Antidote
PREG/CONT C/NA

IND & DOSE Emergency tx in poisoning by most drugs and chemicals. *Adult:* 50–60 g or 1 g/kg PO, or approximately 8–10 times by volume amount of poison ingested, as oral suspension. Give as soon as possible after poisoning. With gastric dialysis, 20–40 g PO q 6 hr for 1–2 days for severe poisonings; for optimum effect, give within 30 min of poisoning. *Child 1–12 yr:* Over 32 kg, 50–60 g PO; 16–32 kg, 25–30 g PO; under 16 kg and under 1 yr, not recommended.
ADV EFF Black stools, constipation, diarrhea, vomiting
INTERACTIONS Laxatives, milk products, oral medications
NC/PT For use w/ conscious pts only. Take steps to prevent aspiration; have life-support equipment readily available. Pt should drink 6–8 glasses

of liquid/day to avoid constipation. Name confusion between *Actidose* (charcoal) and *Actos* (pioglitazone); use caution.

chenodiol (Chenodal)
CLASS Gallstone solubilizer
PREG/CONT X/NA

BBW Highly toxic to liver. Reserve use for select pts where benefit clearly outweighs risk.

IND & DOSE Tx of selected pts w/ radiolucent gallstones when surgery not an option. *Adult:* 250 mg PO bid for 2 wk, then 13–16 mg/kg/day in 2 divided doses a.m. and p.m. for up to 6–9 mo.

ADV EFF Colon cancer, diarrhea, hepatotoxicity, neutropenia
INTERACTIONS Clofibrate, warfarin
NC/PT Ensure correct selection of pt. Monitor LFTs carefully. Not for use in pregnancy (barrier contraceptives advised). Long-term therapy requires frequent tests. Diarrhea will occur.

DANGEROUS DRUG

chlorambucil (Leukeran)
CLASS Antineoplastic, nitrogen mustard
PREG/CONT D/NA

BBW Arrange for blood tests to evaluate hematopoietic function before and wkly during tx. Severe bone marrow suppression possible. Drug is carcinogenic; monitor pt regularly. Rule out pregnancy before starting tx. Encourage use of barrier contraceptives; drug is teratogenic. May cause infertility.

IND & DOSE Palliative tx of chronic lymphocytic leukemia (CLL); malignant lymphoma, including lymphosarcoma; giant follicular lymphoma; Hodgkin lymphoma. *Adult:* Initial dose and short-course therapy, 0.1–0.2 mg/kg/day PO for 3–6 wk; may give single daily dose. CLL alternative regimen, 0.4 mg/kg PO q 2 wk,

increasing by 0.1 mg/kg w/ each dose until therapeutic or toxic effect occurs. Maint, 0.03–0.1 mg/kg/day PO; max, 0.1 mg/kg/day.
ADV EFF Acute leukemia, alopecia, bone marrow depression
NC/PT Monitor CBC regularly. Rule out pregnancy. Do not give full dose within 4 wk of radiation or other chemotherapy. Divide dose w/ severe n/v; maintain hydration. Sterility can occur. Name confusion w/ *Leukeran* (chlorambucil), *Myleran* (busulfan), *Alkeran* (melphalan), and leucovorin; use caution.

chloramphenicol sodium succinate (generic)
CLASS Antibiotic
PREG/CONT C/NA

BBW Severe, sometimes fatal blood dyscrasias (in adults) and severe, sometimes fatal gray syndrome (in newborns, premature infants) possible. Restrict use to situations in which no other antibiotic effective. Monitor serum levels at least wkly to minimize toxicity risk (therapeutic conc: peak, 10–20 mcg/mL; trough, 5–10 mcg/mL).

IND & DOSE Severe infections caused by susceptible strains. *Adult:* 50 mg/kg/day IV in divided doses q 6 hr up to 100 mg/kg/day in severe cases. Severe infections and cystic fibrosis regimen. *Child:* 50–100 mg/kg/day IV in divided doses q 6 hr. Neonates, children w/ immature metabolic processes, 25 mg/kg/day IV; individualize doses at 6-hr intervals.

ADJUST DOSE Elderly pts; hepatic, renal impairment
ADV EFF Anaphylaxis, bone marrow depression, gray baby syndrome, n/v/d, superinfections
INTERACTIONS Bone marrow suppressants, glipizide, glyburide, phenytoins, tolazamide, tolbutamide, vitamin B$_{12}$, warfarin

NC/PT Culture before tx. Do not give IM. Monitor serum levels. Monitor CBC carefully. Change to another antibiotic as soon as possible.

chlordiazepoxide
(Librium)
CLASS Anxiolytic, benzodiazepine
PREG/CONT D/C-IV

IND & DOSE Mgt of anxiety disorders. *Adult:* 5 or 10 mg PO, up to 20 or 25 mg, tid–qid. *Child over 6 yr:* Initially, 5 mg PO bid–qid; may increase to 10 mg bid–tid. **Preop apprehension.** *Adult:* 5–10 mg PO tid–qid on days preceding surgery. **Alcohol withdrawal.** *Adult:* 50–100 mg PO, then repeated doses as needed (max, 300 mg/day).
ADJUST DOSE Elderly pts, debilitating disease
ADV EFF Apathy, confusion, constipation, **CV collapse**, depression, diarrhea, disorientation, drowsiness, drug dependence w/ withdrawal, fatigue, incontinence, lethargy, lightheadedness, restlessness, urine retention
INTERACTIONS Alcohol, aminophylline, cimetidine, disulfiram, dyphylline, hormonal contraceptives, smoking, theophylline
NC/PT Monitor LFTs, renal function, CBC periodically during long-term therapy. Taper gradually after long-term use. Not for use in pregnancy (barrier contraceptives advised). Pt should take safety precautions w/ CNS effects.

chloroquine phosphate
(Aralen Phosphate)
CLASS Amebicide, 4-aminoquinoline, antimalarial
PREG/CONT C/NA

IND & DOSE Tx of extraintestinal amebiasis. *Adult:* 1 g (600 mg base)/day PO for 2 days, then 500 mg

(300 mg base)/day for 2–3 wk. **Px and tx of acute malaria attacks caused by susceptible strains.** *Adult:* Suppression, 300 mg base PO once a wk on same day for 2 wk before exposure, continuing until 8 wk after exposure; acute attack, 600 mg base PO initially, then 300 mg 6–8 hr, 24 hr, and 48 hr after initial dose for total dose of 1.5 g in 3 days. *Child:* Suppression, 5 mg base/kg PO once a wk on same day for 2 wk before exposure, continuing until 8 wk after exposure; acute attack, 10 mg base/kg PO initially; then 5 mg base/kg 6 hr later; then third dose 18 hr later; then last dose 24 hr after third dose. Max, 10 mg base/kg/day or 300 mg base/day.
ADV EFF N/v/d, visual distortion, **permanent retinal changes**
INTERACTIONS Cimetidine
NC/PT Double-check child doses; child very susceptible to overdose. Give w/ food if GI effects occur. Arrange for ophthalmologic exam before and during long-term tx. Pt should take safety measures if vision changes.

chlorothiazide (Diuril), chlorothiazide sodium
(generic)
CLASS Thiazide diuretic
PREG/CONT C/NA

IND & DOSE Adjunctive tx for edema; tx of hypertension. *Adult:* 0.5–2 g daily PO or IV. *Child:* Generally, 10–20 mg/kg/day PO in single dose or two divided doses. *Child 2–12 yr:* 375 mg–1 g PO in two divided doses. *Child 6 mo–2 yr:* 125–375 mg PO in two divided doses. *Child under 6 mo:* Up to 30 mg/kg/day PO in two doses.
ADV EFF Agranulocytosis, anorexia, **aplastic anemia**, constipation, ED, n/v/d, nocturia, polyuria, vertigo
INTERACTIONS Alcohol, antidiabetics, cholestyramine, corticosteroids, diazoxide, digoxin, lithium, opioids
NC/PT Do not give IM or subcut. Monitor and record weight daily. Pt

should take w/ food if GI upset occurs, take early in day so sleep will not be disturbed. Increased urination will occur; pt should plan day accordingly.

chlorpheniramine maleate (Aller-Chlor, Allergy, Chlor-Trimeton Allergy, QDALL-AR)

CLASS Antihistamine
PREG/CONT C/NA

IND & DOSE Symptomatic relief of s&sx associated w/ perennial and seasonal allergic rhinitis; vasomotor rhinitis; common cold; allergic conjunctivitis. *Adult, child over 12 yr:* 4 mg PO q 4–6 hr; max, 24 mg in 24 hr (tablets, syrup). ER tablets, 16 mg w/ liquid PO q 24 hr. SR tablets, 8–12 mg PO at bedtime or q 8–12 hr during day. ER capsules, 12 mg/day PO; max, 24 mg/day. Caplets, 8–12 mg/day PO q 12 hr. *Child 6–12 yr:* 2 mg q 4–6 hr PO; max, 12 mg in 24 hr (tablets, syrup).
ADJUST DOSE Elderly pts
ADV EFF Anaphylactic shock, aplastic anemia, bronchial secretion thickening, disturbed coordination, dizziness, drowsiness, epigastric distress, sedation
INTERACTIONS Alcohol, CNS depressants
NC/PT Periodic CBC w/ long-term tx. Pt should take w/ food; not cut, crush, or chew SR/ER forms; avoid alcohol; take safety precautions w/ CNS effects.

chlorproMAZINE hydrochloride (generic)

CLASS Antiemetic, antipsychotic, anxiolytic, dopamine blocker, phenothiazine
PREG/CONT C/NA

BBW Risk of death in elderly pts with dementia-related psychoses; not approved for use.

IND & DOSE Tx of excessive anxiety, agitation. *Adult:* 25 mg IM; may repeat in 1 hr w/ 25–50 mg IM. Increase gradually in inpts, up to 400 mg q 4–6 hr. Switch to oral dose as soon as possible, 10 mg PO tid–qid; increase to 25 mg PO bid–tid. 25–50 mg PO tid for outpts; up to 2,000 mg/day PO for inpatients. *Child 6 mo–12 yr, outpts:* 0.5 mg/kg PO q 4–6 hr; 1 mg/kg rectally q 6–8 hr; 0.55 mg/kg IM q 6–8 hr; max, 40 mg/day (up to 5 yr) or 75 mg/day (5–12 yr). *Child, inpts:* 50–100 mg/day PO; max, 40 mg/day IM (up to 5 yr), 75 mg/day IM (5–12 yr). **Preop, postop anxiety.** *Adult:* Preop, 25–50 mg PO 2–3 hr before surgery or 12.5–25 mg IM 1–2 hr before surgery; intraop, 12.5 mg IM repeated in 30 min or 2 mg IV repeated q 2 min (up to 25 mg total) to control vomiting (if no hypotension occurs); postop, 10–25 mg PO q 4–6 hr or 12.5–25 mg IM repeated in 1 hr (if no hypotension occurs). *Child 6 mo–12 yr:* Preop, 0.55 mg/kg PO 2–3 hr before surgery or 0.55 mg/kg IM 1–2 hr before surgery; intraop, 0.25 mg/kg IM or 1 mg (diluted) IV, repeated at 2-min intervals up to total IM dose; postop, 0.55 mg/kg PO q 4–6 hr or 0.55 mg/kg IM, repeated in 1 hr (if no hypotension occurs). **Tx of acute intermittent porphyria.** *Adult:* 25–50 mg PO or 25 mg IM tid–qid until pt can take oral tx. **Adjunct tx of tetanus.** *Adult:* 25–50 mg IM tid–qid, usually w/ barbiturates, or 25–50 mg IV diluted and infused at 1 mg/min. *Child:* 0.55 mg/kg IM q 6–8 hr or 0.5 mg/min IV; max, 40 mg/day (up to 23 kg), 75 mg/day (23–45 kg). **Antiemetic.** *Adult:* 10–25 mg PO q 4–6 hr, or 50–100 mg rectally q 6–8 hr, or 25 mg IM. If no hypotension, give 25–50 mg q 3–4 hr. Switch to oral dose when vomiting ends. *Child:* 0.55 mg/kg PO q 4–6 hr, or 0.55 mg/kg IM q 6–8 hr. Max IM dose, 40 mg/day (up to 5 yr), 75 mg/day (5–12 yr). **Tx of intractable hiccups.** *Adult:* 25–50 mg PO tid–qid. If symptoms persist for 2–3 days, give

25–50 mg IM; if inadequate response, give 25–50 mg IV in 500–1,000 mL saline.

ADJUST DOSE Elderly pts

ADV EFF Anaphylactoid reactions, **aplastic anemia**, blurred vision, **bronchospasm**, **cardiac arrest**, **cardiomegaly**, drowsiness, dry mouth, extrapyramidal syndromes, **HF**, hypotension, **laryngospasm**, n/v/d, **NMS**, orthostatic hypotension, photophobia, **pulmonary edema**, urine retention, urticaria, vertigo

INTERACTIONS Alcohol, anticholinergics, barbiturate anesthetics, beta blockers, epinephrine, meperidine, norepinephrine

NC/PT Do not give by subcut injection; give slowly by deep IM injection into upper outer quadrant of buttock. If giving drug via continuous infusion for intractable hiccups, keep pt flat in bed; avoid skin contact w/ parenteral drug sol; monitor renal function, CBC; withdraw slowly after high-dose use. Aspiration risk w/ loss of cough reflex. Pt should avoid alcohol, take safety measures if CNS effects occur, protect from sun exposure. Name confusion between chlorpromazine, chlorpropamide, and clomipramine.

---

chlorproPAMIDE (generic)
CLASS Antidiabetic, sulfonylurea
PREG/CONT C/NA

IND & DOSE Tx of type 2 diabetes w/ diet and exercise. *Adult:* 100–250 mg/day PO; max, 750 mg/day.

ADJUST DOSE Elderly pts

ADV EFF Anorexia, **CV events**, disulfiram reaction w/ alcohol, dizziness, headache, hypoglycemia, n/v

INTERACTIONS Alcohol, beta blockers, MAOIs, miconazole, NSAIDs, salicylates, warfarin

NC/PT Monitor serum glucose; switch to insulin therapy in times of high stress. Not for use in pregnancy. Pt should take w/ food; continue diet and exercise program, avoid alcohol.

---

chlorthalidone (Thalitone)
CLASS Thiazide-like diuretic
PREG/CONT C/NA

IND & DOSE Adjunctive tx for edema. *Adult:* 50–100 mg/day PO or 100 mg every other day; max, 200 mg/day. Tx of hypertension. *Adult:* 25 mg/day PO; if response insufficient, increase to 50 mg/day. If needed, increase to 100 mg/day or add second antihypertensive.

ADV EFF Agranulocytosis, anorexia, **aplastic anemia**, constipation, dizziness, dry mouth, ED, nocturia, n/v/d, photophobia, polyuria, vertigo

INTERACTIONS Antidiabetics, cholestyramine, corticosteroids, diazoxide, digoxin, lithium

NC/PT Differentiate between Thalitone and other drugs; dosage varies. Monitor and record weight daily. Pt should take w/ food if GI upset occurs, take early in day so sleep will not be disturbed. Increased urination will occur; pt should plan day accordingly.

---

chlorzoxazone (Paraflex, Parafon Forte DSC, Remular-S)
CLASS Centrally acting skeletal muscle relaxant
PREG/CONT C/NA

IND & DOSE Relief of discomfort associated w/ acute, painful musculoskeletal conditions as adjunct to rest, physical therapy, other measures. *Adult:* 250 mg PO tid–qid; may need 500 mg PO tid–qid. Max, 750 mg tid–qid.

ADV EFF Anaphylaxis, dizziness, drowsiness, GI disturbances, **hepatic impairment**, light-headedness, orange to red urine

INTERACTIONS Alcohol, CNS depressants

NC/PT Use other measures to help pain. Pt should avoid alcohol and sleep-inducing drugs, take safety measures if CNS effects occur.

cholestyramine (Prevalite, Questran)

CLASS Bile acid sequestrant, antihyperlipidemic
PREG/CONT C/NA

IND & DOSE Adjunct to reduce elevated serum cholesterol in pts w/ primary hypercholesterolemia; pruritus associated w/ partial biliary obstruction. *Adult:* 4 g PO once to twice a day; w/ constipation, start w/ 4 g once a day; maint, 8–16 g/day divided into two doses. Max, 6 packets or scoopfuls (24 g/day). *Child:* 240 mg/kg/day PO in two to three divided doses; max, 8 g/day.

ADV EFF Constipation to fecal impaction, hemorrhoid exacerbation, increased bleeding tendencies

INTERACTIONS Corticosteroids, digitalis, diuretics, fat-soluble vitamins, thiazide preparations, thyroid medication, warfarin

NC/PT Mix packet contents w/ water, milk, fruit juice, noncarbonated beverages, soup, applesauce, pineapple; do not give in dry form. Monitor for constipation, which could be severe. Pt should take w/ meals, take other oral drugs 1 hr before or 4–6 hr after this drug.

choline magnesium trisalicylate (Tricosal)

CLASS NSAID, salicylate
PREG/CONT C/NA

IND & DOSE Tx of osteoarthritis, rheumatoid arthritis. *Adult:* 1.5–2.5 g/day PO; max, 4.5 g/day in divided doses. Tx of pain/fever. *Adult:* 2–3 g/day PO in divided doses.

Child: 217.5–652.5 mg PO q 4 hr as needed.

ADV EFF Anaphylactoid reactions, dizziness, drowsiness, GI bleeding, headache, heartburn, indigestion, n/v, sweating

INTERACTIONS ACE inhibitors, antidiabetics, carbonic anhydrase inhibitors, corticosteroids, insulin, meglitinide, methotrexate, valproic acid

NC/PT Pt should take w/ full glass of water and not lie down for 30 min after taking; take w/ food if GI effects are severe; use safety precautions if CNS effects occur.

chorionic gonadotropin (Novarel, Pregnyl)

CLASS Hormone
PREG/CONT X/NA

BBW Drug has no known effect on fat metabolism and is not for tx of obesity.

IND & DOSE Tx of prepubertal cryptorchidism not due to anatomic obstruction. *Adult, child over 4 yr:* 4,000 USP units IM three times/wk for 3 wk; then 5,000 USP units IM every second day for four injections; then 15 injections of 500–1,000 USP units over 6 wk; then 500 USP units three times/wk for 4–6 wk. If unsuccessful, start another course 1 mo later, giving 1,000 USP units/injection. Tx of hypogonadotropic hypogonadism in males. *Adult, child over 4 yr:* 500–1,000 USP units IM three times/wk for 3 wk; then same dose twice/wk for 3 wk; then 1,000–2,000 USP units IM three times/wk; then 4,000 USP units three times/wk for 6–9 mo. Reduce dose to 2,000 USP units three times/wk for additional 3 mo. Induction of ovulation and pregnancy. *Adult:* 5,000–10,000 units IM 1 day after last menotropins dose.

ADV EFF Gynecomastia, headache, irritability, ovarian cancer, ovarian hyperstimulation, pain at injection site

NC/PT Must give IM. Prepare calendar of tx schedule. Discontinue if s&sx of ovarian overstimulation. Provide comfort measures for headache, pain at injection site.

chorionic gonadotropin alfa (Ovidrel)
CLASS Fertility drug
PREG/CONT X/NA

IND & DOSE Ovulation induction in infertile women. *Adult:* 250 mcg subcut 1 day after last FSH dose.
ADV EFF Abd pain, injection-site pain, multiple births, n/v, ovarian enlargement, **ovarian hyperstimulation; pulmonary, vascular thromboembolic events**
NC/PT Part of comprehensive fertility program. Inject into abdomen. Risk of multiple births. Pt should report difficulty breathing, sudden abd or leg pain.

cidofovir (Vistide)
CLASS Antiviral
PREG/CONT C/NA

BBW Risk of severe renal impairment; monitor renal function closely. Risk of neutropenia; monitor CBC closely. Cancer, impaired fertility, teratogenic effects reported.
IND & DOSE Tx of CMV retinitis in AIDS pts. *Adult:* 5 mg/kg IV over 1 hr for 2 wk, then 5 mg/kg IV q 2 wk.
ADV EFF Decreased IOP, dyspnea, fever, infection, n/v, neutropenia, pneumonia, proteinuria, **renal failure**
NC/PT Use only for stated indication; not for other diseases. Give w/ PO probenecid (2 g before each dose, then 1 g at 2 and 8 hr after each dose). Monitor renal function, CBC. Protect pt from infection. Not for use in pregnancy, breast-feeding. Mark calendar for tx days.

cilostazol (Pletal)
CLASS Antiplatelet
PREG/CONT C/NA

BBW Do not give to pts w/ HF; decreased survival reported.
IND & DOSE To reduce s&sx of intermittent claudication, allowing increased walking distance. *Adult:* 100 mg PO bid at least 30 min before or 2 hr after breakfast and dinner; may not notice response for 2–12 wk.
ADV EFF Bleeding, diarrhea, dizziness, dyspepsia, flatulence, headache, **HF**, nausea, rhinitis
INTERACTIONS Azole antifungals, diltiazem, grapefruit juice, high-fat meal, macrolide antibiotics, omeprazole, smoking
NC/PT Not for use in pregnancy (barrier contraceptives advised). Pt should take on empty stomach 30 min before or 2 hr after breakfast and dinner, take safety precautions to prevent injury, avoid grapefruit juice, continue tx for up to 12 wk to see results.

cimetidine (Tagamet)
CLASS Histamine$_2$ antagonist
PREG/CONT B/NA

IND & DOSE Tx of heartburn, acid indigestion. *Adult:* 200 mg PO as s&sx occur; max, 400 mg/24 hr for max of 2 wk. Tx of active duodenal ulcer. *Adult:* 800 mg PO at bedtime or 300 mg PO qid w/ meals and at bedtime or 400 mg PO bid; continue for 4–6 wk. Intractable ulcers, 300 mg IM or IV q 6–8 hr. Maint, 400 mg PO at bedtime. Tx of active benign gastric ulcer. *Adult:* 300 mg PO qid w/ meals and at bedtime or 800 mg at bedtime for 8 wk. Tx of pathologic hypersecretory syndrome. *Adult:* 300 mg PO qid w/ meals and at bedtime or 300 mg IV or IM q 6 hr. Individualize doses as needed; max, 2,400 mg/day. Tx of

erosive GERD. *Adult:* 1,600 mg PO in divided doses bid–qid for 12 wk. **Prevention of upper GI bleeding.** *Adult:* 50 mg/hr continuous IV infusion for up to 7 days.

ADJUST DOSE Elderly pts, renal impairment

ADV EFF Cardiac arrhythmias, confusion, diarrhea, dizziness, hallucinations, ED

INTERACTIONS Alcohol, alkylating agents, benzodiazepines, beta-adrenergic blockers, carbamazepine, chloroquine, lidocaine, nifedipine, pentoxifylline, phenytoin, procainamide, quinidine, smoking, theophylline, TCAs

NC/PT Give w/ meals and at bedtime. Give IM undiluted into large muscle group. Pt should report smoking so dose can be regulated.

cinacalcet hydrochloride (Sensipar)
CLASS Calcimimetic, calcium-lowering drug
PREG/CONT C/NA

IND & DOSE Tx of hypercalcemia associated w/ parathyroid carcinoma or severe hypercalcemia in pts w/ primary hyperparathyroidism. *Adult:* Initially, 30 mg PO bid to maintain calcium levels within normal range; adjust dose q 2–4 wk in sequential doses of 60 mg bid, then 90 mg bid to max 90 mg tid–qid. **Tx of secondary hyperparathyroidism.** *Adult:* 30 mg/day PO. Monitor serum calcium and phosphorus levels within 1 wk; may increase dose 30 mg q 2–4 wk to max 180 mg/day. Target intact parathyroid hormone levels, 150–300 pg/mL.

ADV EFF Dizziness, hallucinations, hypocalcemia, myalgia, n/v, **seizures**
INTERACTIONS Amitriptyline, erythromycin, flecainide, ketoconazole, itraconazole, TCAs, thioridazine, vinblastine

NC/PT Monitor serum calcium levels before and regularly during tx. If

pt on dialysis, also give vitamin D and phosphate binders. Give w/ food. Not for use in breast-feeding. Pt should not cut, crush, or chew tablets, should take safety measures if CNS effects occur.

ciprofloxacin (Ciloxan, Cipro)
CLASS Antibacterial, fluoroquinolone
PREG/CONT C/NA

BBW Risk of tendinitis and tendon rupture; risk higher in pts over 60 yr, those on steroids, and those w/ renal, heart, or lung transplant. Avoid use in pts w/ hx of myasthenia gravis; drug may exacerbate weakness.

IND & DOSE Tx of uncomplicated UTIs. *Adult:* 250 mg PO q 12 hr for 3 days or 500 mg (ER tablets) PO daily for 3 days. **Tx of mild to moderate UTIs.** *Adult:* 250 mg PO q 12 hr for 7–14 days or 200 mg IV q 12 hr for 7–14 days. **Tx of complicated UTIs.** *Adult:* 500 mg PO q 12 hr for 7–14 days or 400 mg IV q 12 hr or 1,000 mg (ER tablets) PO daily q 7–14 days. **Tx of chronic bacterial prostatitis.** *Adult:* 500 mg PO q 12 hr for 28 days or 400 mg IV q 12 hr for 28 days. **Tx of infectious diarrhea.** *Adult:* 500 mg PO q 12 hr for 5–7 days. **Anthrax postexposure.** *Adult:* 500 mg PO q 12 hr for 60 days or 400 mg IV q 12 hr for 60 days. *Child:* 15 mg/kg/dose PO q 12 hr for 60 days or 10 mg/kg/dose IV q 12 hr for 60 days; max, 500 mg/dose PO or 400 mg/dose IV. **Tx of respiratory infections.** *Adult:* 500–750 mg PO q 12 hr or 400 mg IV q 8–12 hr for 7–14 days. **Tx of acute sinusitis.** *Adult:* 500 mg PO q 12 hr or 400 mg IV q 12 hr for 10 days. **Tx of acute uncomplicated pyelonephritis.** *Adult:* 1,000 mg (ER tablets) PO daily q 7–14 days. **Tx of bone, joint, skin infections.** *Adult:* 500–750 mg PO q 12 hr or 400 mg IV q 8–12 hr for 4–6 wk. **Tx of nosocomial pneumonia.** *Adult:* 400 mg IV q 8 hr for 10–14 days. **Tx of**

ophthalmic infections caused by susceptible organisms not responsive to other tx. *Adult:* 1 or 2 drops q 2 hr in affected eye(s) while awake for 2 days or q 4 hr for 5 days; or ½-inch ribbon ointment into conjunctival sac tid on first 2 days, then ½-inch ribbon bid for next 5 days. **Tx of acute otitis externa.** *Adult:* 4 drops in infected ear tid–qid, or 1 single-use container (0.25 mL) in infected ear bid for 7 days.

ADJUST DOSE Renal impairment

ADV EFF Headache, n/v/d, **tendinitis, tendon rupture**

INTERACTIONS Antacids, didanosine, foscarnet, St John's wort, sucralfate, theophylline, warfarin

NC/PT Avoid use in pts w/ hx of myasthenia gravis; may exacerbate weakness. Use cautiously w/ children; increased incidence of joint/tissue injury. Culture before tx. Give antacids at least 2 hr apart from dosing. Ensure hydration. Pt should not cut, crush, or chew ER form.

DANGEROUS DRUG

cisplatin (CDDP) (generic)
CLASS Alkylating agent, antineoplastic, platinum agent
PREG/CONT D/NA

BBW Arrange for audiometric testing before starting tx and before subsequent doses. Do not give if audiometric acuity outside normal limits. Monitor renal function; severe toxicity related to dose possible. Have epinephrine, corticosteroids available for anaphylaxis-like reactions.

IND & DOSE Tx of metastatic testicular tumors. *Adult:* Remission induction: Cisplatin, 20 mg/m²/day IV for 5 consecutive days (days 1–5) q 3 wk for three courses; bleomycin, 30 units IV wkly (day 2 of each wk) for 12 consecutive doses; vinblastine, 0.15–0.2 mg/kg IV twice wkly (days 1 and 2) q 3 wk for four courses. Maint: Vinblastine, 0.3 mg/kg IV q

4 wk for 2 yr. **Tx of metastatic ovarian tumors.** *Adult:* 75–100 mg/m² IV once q 4 wk. For combination therapy, give separately: Cisplatin, 75–100 mg/m² IV once q 3–4 wk; cyclophosphamide, 600 mg/m² IV once q 4 wk. Single dose: 100 mg/m² IV once q 4 wk. **Tx of advanced bladder cancer.** *Adult:* 50–70 mg/m² IV once q 3–4 wk; in heavily pretreated (radiotherapy or chemotherapy) pts, give initial dose of 50 mg/m² repeated q 4 wk. Do not give repeated courses until serum creatinine under 1.5 mg/dL, BUN under 25 mg/dL, or platelets over 100,000/mm³ or WBCs over 4,000/mm³. Do not give subsequent doses until audiometry indicates hearing within normal range.

ADJUST DOSE Renal impairment

ADV EFF Anaphylaxis-like reactions, anorexia, **bone marrow suppression, nephrotoxicity,** n/v/d, ototoxicity

INTERACTIONS Aminoglycosides, bumetanide, ethacrynic acid, furosemide, phenytoins

NC/PT Monitor renal function before and regularly during tx. Monitor hearing. Maintain hydration. Use antiemetics if needed. Monitor electrolytes regularly. Do not use needles containing aluminum. Use gloves when preparing IV. Not for use in pregnancy. Pt should report changes in hearing, difficulty breathing, unusual bleeding.

---

citalopram hydrobromide (Celexa)
CLASS Antidepressant, SSRI
PREG/CONT C/NA

BBW Increased risk of suicidality in children, adolescents, young adults; monitor accordingly.

IND & DOSE Tx of depression. *Adult:* 20 mg/day PO as single daily dose. May increase to 40 mg/day; max, 40 mg/day.

ADJUST DOSE Elderly pts; renal, hepatic impairment
ADV EFF Dizziness, dry mouth, ejaculatory disorders, insomnia, nausea, **prolonged QT interval,** somnolence, **suicidality,** tremor
INTERACTIONS Azole antifungals, beta blockers, citalopram, erythromycin, linezolid, macrolide antibiotics, MAOIs, pimozide, QT-prolonging drugs, St. John's wort, TCAs, warfarin
NC/PT Avoid doses over 40 mg; increased risk of prolonged QT interval. Limit drug to suicidal pts; monitor for suicidality. May take several wk to see effects. Not for use in pregnancy, breast-feeding. Pt should avoid St. John's wort, report thoughts of suicide. Name confusion w/ *Celexa* (citalopram), *Celebrex* (celecoxib), *Xanax* (alprazolam), and *Cerebyx* (fosphenytoin).

DANGEROUS DRUG

cladribine (generic)
CLASS Antimetabolite, antineoplastic, purine analogue
PREG/CONT D/NA

BBW Monitor complete hematologic profile, LFTs, renal function tests before and frequently during tx. Consult physician at first sign of toxicity; consider delaying dose or discontinuing if neurotoxicity or renal toxicity occurs.
IND & DOSE Tx of active hairy cell leukemia. *Adult:* Single course of 0.09–0.1 mg/kg/day by continuous IV infusion for 7 days.
ADV EFF Abnormal breath sounds, anorexia, arthralgia, **bone marrow suppression,** chills, cough, fatigue, fever, headache, **hepatotoxicity,** injection-site reactions, **nephrotoxicity, neurotoxicity,** n/v/d
NC/PT Use gloves when handling drug. Must be given by continuous infusion for 7 days. Monitor renal function, LFTs, CBC before and regularly

during tx. Not for use in pregnancy; pt should use contraception during and for several wk after tx ends. Pt should report numbness, tingling, pain at injection site.

---

clarithromycin (Biaxin)
CLASS Macrolide antibiotic
PREG/CONT C/NA

IND & DOSE Tx of pharyngitis, tonsillitis; pneumonia; skin, skin-structure infections; lower respiratory infections caused by susceptible strains. *Adult:* 250 mg PO q 12 hr for 7–14 days. *Child:* 15 mg/kg/day PO divided q 12 hr for 10 days. Tx of acute maxillary sinusitis, acute otitis media, lower respiratory infections caused by susceptible strains. *Adult:* 500 mg PO q 12 hr for 14 days or 1,000 mg (ER tablets) PO q 24 hr. Tx of mycobacterial infections. *Adult:* 500 mg PO bid. *Child:* 7.5 mg/kg PO bid; max, 500 mg PO bid. Tx of duodenal ulcers. *Adult:* 500 mg PO tid plus omeprazole 40 mg PO q a.m. for 14 days, then omeprazole 20 mg PO q a.m. for 14 days. Tx of community-acquired pneumonia. *Adult:* 250 mg PO q 12 hr for 7–14 days or 1,000 mg (ER tablets) PO q 24 hr for 7 days.
ADJUST DOSE Elderly pts, renal impairment
ADV EFF Abd pain, diarrhea, superinfections
INTERACTIONS Carbamazepine, grapefruit juice, lovastatin, phenytoin, theophylline
NC/PT Culture before tx. Arrange for tx of superinfections. Do not refrigerate suspension. Pt should take w/ food if GI upset occurs; avoid grapefruit juice; should not cut, crush, or chew ER tablets.

clemastine fumarate
(Dayhist-1, Tavist Allergy)
CLASS Antihistamine
PREG/CONT B/NA

IND & DOSE Symptomatic relief of s&sx of allergic rhinitis. *Adult:* 1.34 mg PO bid. Max, 8.04 mg/day (syrup), 2.68 mg/day (tablets). *Child 6–12 yr:* (syrup only) 0.67 mg PO bid; max, 4.02 mg/day. Tx of mild, uncomplicated urticaria and angioedema. *Adult:* 2.68 mg PO daily–tid; max, 8.04 mg/day. *Child 6–12 yr:* (syrup only) 1.34 mg PO bid; max, 4.02 mg/day.

ADJUST DOSE Elderly pts
ADV EFF Anaphylactic shock, bronchial secretion thickening, disturbed coordination, dizziness, drowsiness, epigastric distress, sedation
INTERACTIONS Alcohol, CNS depressants, MAOIs
NC/PT Use syrup if pt cannot swallow tablets. Give w/ food if GI upset occurs. Pt should drink plenty of fluids, use humidifier, avoid alcohol, report difficulty breathing/irregular heartbeat.

clevidipine butyrate
(Cleviprex)
CLASS Antihypertensive, calcium channel blocker
PREG/CONT C/NA

IND & DOSE To reduce BP when oral therapy not possible or desirable. *Adult:* 1–2 mg/hr IV infusion; titrate quickly by doubling dose q 90 sec to achieve desired BP; maint, 4–6 mg/hr; max, 21 mg/hr/24-hr.
ADV EFF Headache, **HF,** n/v
NC/PT Continuously monitor BP, ECG during administration. Taper beta blockers before use. Handle drug w/ strict aseptic technique. Use within 4 hr of puncturing stopper. Rebound hypertension possible within 8 hr of stopping drug; switch to oral antihypertensive as soon as possible.

clindamycin hydrochloride (Cleocin), clindamycin palmitate hydrochloride (Cleocin Pediatric), clindamycin phosphate (Cleocin T, Clindagel, ClindaMax)
CLASS Lincosamide antibiotic
PREG/CONT B/NA

BBW Serious to fatal colitis, including *Clostridium difficile*–associated diarrhea, possibly up to several wk after tx ends. Reserve use; monitor pt closely.

IND & DOSE Serious infections caused by susceptible bacteria strains. Reserve use for penicillin-allergic pts or when penicillin inappropriate. *Adult:* 150–300 mg PO q 6 hr (up to 300–450 mg PO q 6 hr in more severe infections) or 600–2,700 mg/day IV or IM in two to four equal doses (up to 4.8 g/day IV or IM for life-threatening situations). *Child:* Clindamycin hydrochloride, 8–16 mg/kg/day PO (serious infections) or 16–20 mg/kg/ day PO (more serious infections in three or four equal doses). *Child under 10 kg:* 37.5 mg PO tid as min dose. *Child older than 1 mo:* 20–40 mg/kg/day IV or IM in three or four equal doses or 350–450 mg/m²/day. *Neonates:* 15–20 mg/kg/day IV or IM in three or four equal doses.

Tx of bacterial vaginosis. *Adult:* 1 applicator (100 mg clindamycin phosphate) intravaginally, preferably at bedtime for 7 consecutive days in pregnant women and 3 or 7 days in nonpregnant women. Tx of acne vulgaris. *Adult:* Apply thin film to affected area bid.
ADJUST DOSE Renal impairment
ADV EFF Abd pain, **agranulocytosis,** anaphylactic reactions, anorexia, **cardiac arrest,** contact dermatitis, esophagitis, n/v/d, pain following

injection, **pseudomembranous colitis**, rash

INTERACTIONS Aluminum salts, kaolin, NMJ blockers

NC/PT Culture before tx. Give orally w/ full glass of water or food. Do not give IM injection of more than 600 mg; inject deeply into muscle. Monitor LFTs, renal function. Pt should avoid eye contact w/ topical sol, give intravaginally at bedtime, report severe or watery diarrhea.

clobazam (Onfi)
CLASS Benzodiazepine, antiepileptic
PREG/CONT C/C-IV

IND & DOSE Adjunct tx of seizures associated w/ Lennox-Gastaut syndrome. *Adult, child 2 yr and older:* Over 30 kg, initially 5 mg PO bid; increase to 10 mg PO bid starting on day 7; increase to 20 mg PO bid starting on day 14. 30 kg or less, initially 5 mg/day PO; increase to 5 mg PO bid starting on day 7; increase to 10 mg PO bid starting on day 14.

ADJUST DOSE Elderly pts, mild to moderate hepatic impairment, poor CYP2C19 metabolizers

ADV EFF Aggression, ataxia, constipation, drooling, dysarthria, fatigue, fever, insomnia, sedation, somnolence, **suicidality**

INTERACTIONS Alcohol, fluconazole, fluvoxamine, hormonal contraceptives, omeprazole, ticlopidine

NC/PT Taper drug after long-term use; dispense least amount feasible. Administer whole or crush and mix in applesauce. Not for use in pregnancy, breast-feeding. Dizziness, sleepiness possible. Pt should take bid, swallow whole or crush and take in applesauce, avoid alcohol, report thoughts of suicide, increase in seizure activity.

clofarabine (Clolar)
CLASS Antimetabolite, antineoplastic
PREG/CONT D/NA

IND & DOSE Tx of pts w/ ALL who relapsed after at least two other regimens. *Child 1–21 yr:* 52 mg/m² IV over 2 hr daily for 5 consecutive days of 28-day cycle; repeat q 2–6 wk.

ADV EFF Anxiety, **bone marrow suppression, capillary leak syndrome**, fatigue, flushing, headache, **hepatotoxicity**, hyperuricemia, infections, mucosal inflammation, n/v/d, pruritus, rash, **renal toxicity**

NC/PT Premedicate w/ antiemetic. Monitor LFTs, renal function, CBC regularly; dose adjustment may be needed. Protect pt from infection, injury. Not for use in pregnancy, breast-feeding.

clomiPHENE citrate (Clomid, Serophene)
CLASS Fertility drug, hormone
PREG/CONT X/NA

IND & DOSE Tx of ovulatory failure in pts w/ normal liver function, normal endogenous estrogen level. *Adult:* 50 mg/day PO for 5 days started anytime there has been no recent uterine bleeding. If no ovulation occurs, 100 mg/day PO for 5 days as early as 30 days after first. May repeat if no response.

ADV EFF Abd discomfort/distention, bloating, breast tenderness, flushing, multiple births, n/v, ovarian enlargement, ovarian overstimulation, visual disturbances

NC/PT Perform pelvic exam, obtain urine estrogen and estriol levels before tx. Discontinue if s&sx of ovarian overstimulation. Prepare calendar of tx days. Risk of multiple births. Failure after three courses indicates tx not effective and will be discontinued. Name confusion between *Serophene* (clomiphene) and *Sarafem* (fluoxetine).

clomiPRAMINE hydrochloride (Anafranil)

CLASS Anxiolytic, TCA
PREG/CONT C/NA

BBW Increased risk of suicidality in children, adolescents, young adults; monitor pt carefully.

IND & DOSE Tx of obsessions, compulsions in pts w/ OCD. *Adult:* Initially, 25 mg PO daily. Increase as tolerated to approximately 100 mg during first 2 wk; max, 250 mg/day. Maint, adjust dose to maintain lowest effective dose; effectiveness after 10 wk not documented. *Child:* Initially, 25 mg PO daily. Increase as tolerated during first 2 wk; max, 3 mg/kg or 100 mg, whichever smaller. Maint, adjust dose to maintain lowest effective dosage; effectiveness after 10 wk not documented.

ADV EFF Agranulocytosis, anticholinergic effects, confusion, constipation, disturbed concentration, dry mouth, **MI**, nasal congestion, orthostatic hypotension, photosensitivity, sedation, **stroke**

INTERACTIONS Anticholinergics, barbiturates, cimetidine, clonidine, disulfiram, ephedrine, epinephrine, fluoxetine, furazolidone, hormonal contraceptives, levodopa, MAOIs, methylphenidate, nicotine, norepinephrine, phenothiazines, QT-prolonging drugs, St. John's wort, thyroid medication

NC/PT Restrict drug access in depressed, suicidal pts. Give major portion at bedtime. Obtain periodic CBC w/ long-term therapy. Pt should not mix w/ other sleep-inducing drugs; avoid driving, etc, until drug's effects known; avoid St. John's wort, prolonged exposure to sun and sunlamps; report thoughts of suicide. Name confusion between clomipramine and chlorpromazine.

clonazepam (Klonopin)

CLASS Antiepileptic, benzodiazepine
PREG/CONT D/C-IV

IND & DOSE Tx of Lennox-Gastaut syndrome (petit mal variant); akinetic and myoclonic seizures. *Adult:* 1.5 mg/day PO divided into three doses; increase in increments of 0.5–1 mg PO q 3 days until seizures adequately controlled. Max, 20 mg/day. *Child at least 10 yr or 30 kg:* 0.01–0.03 mg/ day PO. Max, 0.05 mg/kg/day PO in two or three doses; maint, 0.1–0.2 mg/kg. Tx of panic disorder w/ or without agoraphobia. *Adult:* Initially, 0.25 mg PO bid; gradually increase to target dose of 1 mg/day.

ADV EFF Agranulocytosis, apathy, confusion, constipation, **CV collapse**, depression, diarrhea, disorientation, drowsiness, drug dependence w/ withdrawal, fatigue, incontinence, lethargy, light-headedness, restlessness, urine retention

INTERACTIONS Alcohol, aminophylline, cimetidine, digoxin, disulfiram, dyphylline, hormonal contraceptives, omeprazole, theophylline

NC/PT Monitor suicidal and addiction-prone pts closely. Monitor LFTs. Monitor for therapeutic level (20–80 ng/mL). Taper gradually after long-term tx. Pt should avoid alcohol, may wear or carry medical alert notice, take safety precautions if CNS effects occur. Name confusion between *Klonopin* (clonazepam) and clonidine.

clonidine hydrochloride (Catapres, Duraclon, Kapvay)

CLASS Antihypertensive, central analgesic, sympatholytic
PREG/CONT C/NA

BBW Epidural route not recommended for obstetric, postpartum, or periop pain because of risk of hemo-dynamic instability.

IND & DOSE **Tx of hypertension.** *Adult:* 0.1 mg bid PO. For maint, increase in increments of 0.1 or 0.2 mg to reach desired response; common range, 0.2–0.6 mg/day or 0.1-mg transdermal system (releases 0.1 mg/ 24 hr). If, after 1–2 wk desired BP reduction not achieved, add another 0.1-mg system or use larger system. More than two 0.3-mg systems does not improve efficacy. **Pain mgt.** *Adult:* 30 mcg/hr by epidural infusion. **Tx of ADHD.** *Child 6–17 yr:* 0.1 mg PO at bedtime; titrate at 0.1 mg/wk to total of 0.2 mg, w/ 0.1 mg in a.m. and 0.1 mg in p.m., then 0.1 mg in a.m. and 0.2 mg in p.m. Maint, 0.2 mg in a.m. and 0.2 mg in p.m. (*Kapvay* only).

ADV EFF Constipation, dizziness, drowsiness, dry mouth, local reactions to transdermal system

INTERACTIONS Alcohol, CNS depressants, propranolol, TCAs

NC/PT Taper when withdrawing to avoid rebound effects. *Kapvay* not interchangeable w/ other forms. Remove old patch before applying new to clean, dry skin; rotate skin sites. Remove transdermal patch before defibrillation and MRI. Pt should avoid alcohol, take safety precautions if CNS effects occur. Name confusion between clonidine and *Klonopin* (clonazepam).

clopidogrel bisulfate
(Plavix)
CLASS ADP receptor antagonist, antiplatelet
PREG/CONT B/NA

BBW Slow metabolizers may experience less effects, as drug is activated in liver by CYP2C19. Genotype testing for poor metabolizers suggested before tx.

IND & DOSE **Tx of pts at risk for ischemic events (recent MI, stroke, established peripheral arterial dis-**ease). *Adult:* 75 mg/day PO. **Tx of acute coronary syndrome.** *Adult:* 300 mg PO loading dose, then 75 mg/day PO w/ aspirin, at dose from 75–325 mg once daily.

ADV EFF Bleeding risk, dizziness, GI bleed, headache, rash
INTERACTIONS NSAIDs, warfarin
NC/PT Genotype testing before tx. Monitor for bleeding. May give w/ meals. Pt should report unusual bleeding.

clorazepate dipotassium bisulfate
(Tranxene-T-tab)
CLASS Antiepileptic, anxiolytic, benzodiazepine
PREG/CONT D/C-IV

IND & DOSE **Mgt of anxiety disorders.** *Adult:* 30 mg/day PO in divided doses tid. **Adjunct to antiepileptics.** *Adult:* Max initial dose, 7.5 mg PO tid. Increase dose by no more than 7.5 mg q wk; max, 90 mg/day. *Child 9–12 yr:* Max initial dose, 7.5 mg PO bid. Increase dose by no more than 7.5 mg q wk; max, 60 mg/day. **Acute alcohol withdrawal.** *Adult:* Day 1, 30 mg PO initially, then 30–60 mg in divided doses. Day 2, 45–90 mg in divided doses. Day 3, 22.5–45 mg PO in divided doses. Day 4, 15–30 mg PO in divided doses. Thereafter, gradually reduce dose to 7.5–15 mg/day PO; stop as soon as condition stable.

ADJUST DOSE Elderly pts, debilitating disease
ADV EFF Agranulocytosis, apathy, CV collapse, constipation, depression, diarrhea, disorientation, dizziness, drowsiness, dry mouth, lethargy, light-headedness, mild paradoxical excitatory reactions during first 2 wk
INTERACTIONS Alcohol, cimetidine, CNS depressants, digoxin, disulfiram, hormonal contraceptives, kava, omeprazole, theophylline

NC/PT Taper gradually after long-term use. Monitor for suicidality. Encourage use of medical alert tag. Not for use in pregnancy. Pt should avoid alcohol, take safety precautions for CNS effects. Name confusion between clorazepate and clofibrate; use caution.

clotrimazole (Cruex, Desenex, Gyne-Lotrimin, Lotrimin)
CLASS Antifungal
PREG/CONT B (topical/vaginal); C (oral)/NA

IND & DOSE Tx of oropharyngeal candidiasis; prevention of oropharyngeal candidiasis in immunocompromised pts receiving radiation, chemotherapy, steroid therapy (troche). *Adult, child 2 yr and older:* Dissolve lozenge in mouth five times daily for 14 days. For prevention, tid for duration of chemotherapy, radiation. **Local tx of vulvovaginal candidiasis (moniliasis).** *Adult, child 12 yr and older:* 100-mg suppository intravaginally at bedtime for 7 consecutive nights, or 200-mg suppository for 3 consecutive nights, or 1 applicator (5 g/day) vaginal cream, preferably at bedtime for 3–7 consecutive days. **Topical tx of susceptible fungal infections.** *Adult, child 2 yr and older:* Gently massage into affected area and surrounding skin bid in a.m. and p.m. for 14 days. Treat for 2–4 wk.
ADV EFF Abd cramps, abnormal LFTs, local reaction to topical forms, n/v, urinary frequency
NC/PT Culture before tx. Dissolve troche in mouth. Insert vaginal suppository or cream high into vagina using applicator; apply even during menstrual period. Apply topically to clean, dry area. Pt should take full course of tx. Name confusion between clotrimazole and co-trimoxazole; use caution.

clozapine (Clozaril, FazaClo)
CLASS Antipsychotic, dopaminergic blocker
PREG/CONT B/NA

BBW Use only when pt unresponsive to conventional antipsychotics. Risk of serious CV and respiratory effects, including myocarditis. Monitor WBC count wkly during and for 4 wk after tx; dosage must be adjusted based on WBC count. Potentially fatal agranulocytosis has occurred. Elderly pts w/ dementia-related psychosis are at increased risk for death; drug not approved for these pts. Monitor for seizures; risk increases in pts w/ hx of seizures and as dose increases.
IND & DOSE Mgt of severely ill schizophrenics unresponsive to standard antipsychotics; to reduce risk of recurrent suicidal behavior in pts w/ schizophrenia. *Adult:* 12.5 mg PO daily or bid. Continue to 25 mg PO daily or bid, then gradually increase w/ daily increments of 25–50 mg/day, if tolerated, to 300–450 mg/day by end of second wk; max, 900 mg/day. Maintain at lowest effective dose. Withdraw slowly over 2–4 wk when discontinuing.
ADV EFF Agranulocytosis, constipation, dizziness, drowsiness, dry mouth, fever, headache, hypotension, n/v, potentially fatal myocarditis, sedation, seizures, syncope
INTERACTIONS Caffeine; cimetidine; CYP450 inducers, inhibitors; ethotoin; phenytoin
NC/PT Obtain through limited access program. Monitor WBC closely. Monitor temp; report fever. Monitor for seizures. Ensure hydration in elderly pts. Not for use in pregnancy. Pt should empty bladder before taking, use sugarless lozenges for dry mouth, obtain wkly blood tests, report s&sx of infection. Name confusion between *Clozaril* (clozapine) and *Colazal* (balsalazide); dangerous effects possible.

coagulation factor VIIa (recombinant)
(NovoSeven RT)
CLASS Antihemophilic
PREG/CONT C/NA

BBW Serious thrombotic events associated w/ off-label use. Use only for approved indication.

IND & DOSE Tx of bleeding episodes in hemophilia A or B pts w/ inhibitors to factor VIII or IX. *Adult:* 90 mcg/kg as IV bolus q 2 hr until bleeding controlled. Continue dosing at 3- to 6-hr intervals after hemostasis in severe bleeds.

ADV EFF Arthralgia, edema, fever, headache, **hemorrhage, hypersensitivity reactions,** hypertension, hypotension, injection-site reactions, n/v, rash, **thromboembolic events**
INTERACTIONS Do not mix in sol w/ other drugs.
NC/PT Use only for approved indications. Monitor for hypersensitivity reactions, thrombotic events; alert pt to warning signs of each.

coagulation factor IX, recombinant (Rixubis)
CLASS Antihemophilic factor
PREG/CONT C/NA

IND & DOSE Control, prevention of bleeding w/ hemophilia B. *Adult:* International units (IU) needed = body weight (kg) × desired factor IX increase (% of normal) × reciprocal of observed recovery (IU/kg per IU/dL). **Routine px of hemophilia B.** *Adult:* 40–60 international units/kg IV twice weekly.

ADV EFF Hypersensitivity reactions, nephrotic syndrome, neutralizing antibody development, thrombotic events
NC/PT Ensure proper dx. Do not use with DIC, fibrinolysis, known hypersensitivity to hamster proteins, pregnancy, breast-feeding. Pt should take safety measures to prevent injury, blood loss; report difficulty breathing, rash, chest pain, increased bleeding.

codeine phosphate
(generic)
CLASS Antitussive, opioid agonist analgesic
PREG/CONT C (pregnancy); D (labor)/C-II

IND & DOSE Relief of mild to moderate pain. *Adult:* 15–60 mg PO, IM, IV, or subcut q 4–6 hr; max, 360 mg/ 24 hr. *Child 1 yr and older:* 0.5 mg/kg or 15 mg/m² IM or subcut q 4 hr. **Suppression of coughing induced by chemical or mechanical irritation.** *Adult:* 10–20 mg PO q 4–6 hr; max, 120 mg/24 hr. *Child 6–12 yr:* 5–10 mg PO q 4–6 hr; max, 60 mg/24 hr. *Child 2–6 yr:* 2.5–5 mg PO q 4–6 hr; max, 12–18 mg/day.

ADJUST DOSE Elderly pts, impaired pts
ADV EFF Cardiac arrest, clamminess, confusion, constipation, dizziness, floating feeling, lethargy, lightheadedness, n/v, sedation, **shock**
INTERACTIONS Barbiturate anesthetics, CNS depressants
NC/PT Do not give IV in children. Ensure opioid antagonist available during parenteral administration. Ensure perfusion of subcut area before injecting. Monitor bowel function. Use of laxatives advised. Breast-feeding women should receive drug 4–6 hr before next feeding and should monitor baby closely for signs of sedation or difficulty breathing. Pt should take safety precautions for CNS effects. Name confusion between codeine and *Cardene* (nicardipine); use caution.

colchicine (Colcrys)
CLASS Antigout drug
PREG/CONT C/NA

IND & DOSE Tx of acute gout flares. *Adult:* 1.2 mg PO at first sign of gout flare, then 0.6 mg 1 hr later; max, 1.8 mg over 1-hr period. **Px of**

gout flares. Adult, child 16 yr and older: 0.6 mg PO once or twice daily; max, 1.2 mg/day. **Tx of familial Mediterranean fever.** *Adult:* 1.2–2.4 mg/day PO in one or two divided doses; increase or decrease in 0.3-mg increments as needed. *Child older than 12 yr:* Use adult dosage. *Child 6–12 yr:* 0.9–1.8 mg/day PO. *Child 4–6 yr:* 0.3–1.8 mg/day PO.

ADJUST DOSE Hepatic, renal impairment

ADV EFF Abd pain, **bone marrow suppression,** n/v/d, rash, **rhabdomyolysis**

INTERACTIONS Amprenavir, aprepitant, atazanavir, atorvastatin, clarithromycin, cyclosporine, digoxin, diltiazem, erythromycin, fibrates, fluconazole, fluvastatin, fosamprenavir, gemfibrozil, grapefruit juice, indinavir, itraconazole, ketoconazole, nefazodone, nelfinavir, ranolazine, pravastatin, ritonavir, saquinavir, simvastatin, telithromycin, verapamil

NC/PT Obtain baseline and periodic CBC, LFTs, renal function tests. Check complete drug list; many drug interactions require dose adjustments. Monitor for pain relief. Fatal overdoses have occurred; keep out of reach of children. Pt should avoid grapefruit juice, report to all providers all drugs and herbs taken (many potentially serious drug interactions possible), ensure protection from infection and injury, obtain periodic medical exams.

colesevelam hydrochloride (WelChol)
CLASS Antihyperlipidemic, bile acid sequestrant
PREG/CONT B/NA

IND & DOSE Monotherapy for tx of hyperlipidemia. *Adult:* 3 tablets PO bid w/ meals or 6 tablets/day PO w/ meal; max, 7 tablets/day. **To lower lipid levels, w/ HMG-CoA inhibitor.** *Adult:* 3 tablets PO bid w/ meals or

6 tablets PO once a day w/ meal; max, 6 tablets/day. **To improve glycemic control in type 2 diabetes.** *Adult:* 6 tablets/day PO or 3 tablets PO bid. **Tx of familial hypercholesterolemia.** *Child 10–17 yr:* 1.8 g PO bid or 3.7 g/day PO oral suspension.

ADV EFF Constipation to fecal impaction, flatulence, increased bleeding tendencies

INTERACTIONS Fat-soluble vitamins, oral drugs, verapamil

NC/PT Used w/ diet, exercise program. Give other oral drugs 1 hr before or 4–6 hr after drug. Monitor blood lipid levels. Mix oral suspension in 4–8 oz water; do not use dry. Establish bowel program for constipation. Pt should report unusual bleeding, severe constipation.

colestipol hydrochloride (Colestid)
CLASS Antihyperlipidemic, bile acid sequestrant
PREG/CONT C/NA

IND & DOSE Adjunctive tx for primary hypercholesterolemia. *Adult:* 5–30 g/day PO suspension once a day or in divided doses bid–qid. Start w/ 5 g PO daily or bid; increase in 5-g/day increments at 1- to 2-mo intervals. For tablets, 2–16 g/day PO in one to two divided doses; initially, 2 g once or twice daily, increasing in 2-g increments at 1- to 2-mo intervals.

ADV EFF Constipation to fecal impaction, flatulence, headache, increased bleeding tendencies

INTERACTIONS Digoxin, fat-soluble vitamins, oral drugs, thiazide diuretics

NC/PT Used w/ diet, exercise program. Give other oral drugs 1 hr before or 4-6 hr after drug. Give before meals. Monitor blood lipid levels. Mix in liquids, soups, cereal, carbonated beverages; do not give dry. Establish bowel program for constipation. Pt should swallow tablets whole and not cut, crush, or chew them; report unusual bleeding, severe constipation; use analgesic for headache.

collagenase clostridium histolyticum (Xiaflex)
CLASS Proteinase enzyme
PREG/CONT B/NA

IND & DOSE Tx of pts w/ Dupuytren's contraction w/ palpable cord. *Adult:* 0.58 mg injected into palpable cord; may repeat up to three times/cord at 4-wk intervals. **Tx of pts w/ Peyronie's disease w/ penile curvature deformity of 30 degrees or more.** *Adult:* 2 injections into the collagen-containing structure followed by penile remodeling; may repeat max of eight times.
ADV EFF Injection-site reactions, pain, **severe allergic reactions, tendon rupture,** swelling in involved hand
INTERACTIONS Anticoagulants
NC/PT Be prepared for possible severe allergic reaction. Risk of bleeding if pt on anticoagulants. Tendon rupture, damage to nerves and tissue of hand possible.

corticotropin (ACTH) (H.P. Acthar Gel)
CLASS Anterior pituitary hormone, diagnostic agent
PREG/CONT C/NA

IND & DOSE Tx of allergic states, glucocorticoid-sensitive disorders, nonsuppurative thyroiditis, tuberculous meningitis, trichinosis w/ CNS and cardiac involvement; rheumatic disorders; palliative mgt of leukemias, lymphomas. *Adult:* 40–80 units IM or subcut q 24–72 hr. **Tx of acute exacerbations of MS.** *Adult:* 80–120 units/day IM for 2–3 wk.
ADV EFF Acne, amenorrhea, **anaphylactoid reactions,** depression, ecchymoses, euphoria, fluid and electrolyte disturbances, fragile skin,

hypertension, immunosuppression, impaired wound healing, infections, muscle weakness, petechiae
INTERACTIONS Anticholinesterases, antidiabetics, barbiturates, live vaccines
NC/PT Verify adrenal responsiveness before tx. Give only IM or subcut. Taper dose when discontinuing after long-term use. Give rapidly acting corticosteroid in times of stress. Pt should avoid exposure to infections, monitor blood glucose levels periodically, avoid immunizations.

cosyntropin (Cortrosyn)
CLASS Diagnostic agent
PREG/CONT C/NA

IND & DOSE Diagnostic tests of adrenal function. *Adult:* 0.25-0.75 mg IV or IM or as IV infusion at 0.04 mg/hr.
ADV EFF Anaphylactoid reactions, bradycardia, edema, hypertension, rash, **seizures,** tachycardia
INTERACTIONS Diuretics
NC/PT Plasma cortisol levels usually peak within 45–60 min of injection. Normally, expect doubling of baseline levels.

crizotinib (Xalkori)
CLASS Antineoplastic, kinase inhibitor
PREG/CONT D/NA

IND & DOSE Tx of locally advanced or metastatic non–small-cell lung cancer that is anaplastic lymphoma kinase–positive as detected by Vysis ALK Break Apart FISH Probe Kit. *Adult:* 250 mg PO bid without regard to food. Reduce to 200 mg PO bid based on pt safety.
ADV EFF Constipation, **hepatotoxicity,** n/v/d, **prolonged QT interval, serious to fatal pneumonitis,** vision changes including blurry vision, light sensitivity, floaters, flashes of light

INTERACTIONS CYP3A inducers/inhibitors, QT-prolonging drugs
NC/PT Ensure pt has been tested for appropriate sensitivity. Monitor LFTs, pulmonary function. Institute bowel program as needed; advise safety precautions with vision changes. Pt should avoid pregnancy (contraceptives advised), breast feeding; driving, operating machinery with vision changes. Pt should report difficulty breathing, color changes of urine/stool.

crofelemer (Fulyzaq)
CLASS Antidiarrheal, calcium channel stimulator
PREG/CONT C/NA

IND & DOSE Relief of noninfectious diarrhea in adults w/ HIV/AIDS on antiretroviral therapy. *Adult:* 125 mg PO bid.
ADV EFF Bronchitis, cough, flatulence, possible URI
NC/PT Ensure cause of diarrhea is not infectious and pt also taking antiretroviral. Not for use in pregnancy, breast-feeding. Monitor diarrhea. Pt should take as directed; swallow capsule whole and not cut, crush, or chew it; report cough, increased diarrhea.

cromolyn sodium (Crolom)
CLASS Antiallergy drug
PREG/CONT C/NA

IND & DOSE Prevention, tx of allergic rhinitis. *Adult, child 2 yr and older:* 1 spray in each nostril 3–6 times/day as needed. **Tx of allergic eye disorders.** *Adult:* 1 or 2 drops in each eye 4–6 times/day as needed.
ADV EFF Allergic reaction, burning or stinging, shortness of breath, wheezing
NC/PT Eyedrops not for use w/ soft contact lenses. May take several days to 2 wk for noticeable effects; pt should continue use. If pregnant or breast-feeding, consult provider.

cyanocobalamin, intranasal (Nascobal)
CLASS Synthetic vitamin
PREG/CONT C/NA

IND & DOSE Maint of pts in hematologic remission after IM vitamin B_{12} tx for pernicious anemia, inadequate secretion of intrinsic factor, dietary deficiency, malabsorption, competition by intestinal bacteria or parasites, inadequate utilization of vitamin B_{12}; inadequate therapeutic vitamin B_{12} levels in pts w/ HIV infection, AIDS, MS, Crohn's disease. *Adult:* 1 spray (500 mcg) in one nostril once/wk
ADV EFF Headache, nasal congestion, rhinitis
INTERACTIONS Alcohol, antibiotics, colchicine, methotrexate, paraaminosalicylic acid
NC/PT Confirm diagnosis before tx. Monitor serum vitamin B_{12} levels before, at 1 mo, then q 3–6 mo during tx. Do not give w/ nasal congestion, rhinitis, URI. Pt should take drug 1 hr before or after ingesting hot foods or liquids, which can cause nasal congestion.

cyclizine (Marezine)
CLASS Anticholinergic, antiemetic, antihistamine, anti–motion sickness drug
PREG/CONT B/NA

IND & DOSE Prevention, tx of nausea, vomiting, dizziness associated w/ motion sickness. *Adult:* 50 mg PO 30 min before exposure to motion. Repeat q 4–6 hr; max, 200 mg in 24 hr. *Child 6–12 yr:* 25 mg PO up to three times/day.
ADJUST DOSE Elderly pts
ADV EFF Anorexia, confusion, drowsiness, dry mouth, dysuria, nausea, urinary frequency
INTERACTIONS Alcohol, CNS depressants
NC/PT Monitor elderly pts carefully. Pt should use before motion sickness

occurs, avoid alcohol, take safety precautions w/ CNS effects.

cyclobenzaprine hydrochloride (Amrix, Flexeril)

CLASS Centrally acting skeletal muscle relaxant
PREG/CONT B/NA

IND & DOSE Relief of discomfort associated w/ acute, painful musculoskeletal conditions, as adjunct to rest, physical therapy. *Adult:* 5 mg PO tid, up to 10 mg PO tid. Do not use for longer than 2–3 wk. For ER capsules, 15 mg once/day PO.
ADJUST DOSE Elderly pts, hepatic impairment
ADV EFF Dizziness, drowsiness, dry mouth, **MI**
INTERACTIONS Alcohol, barbiturates, CNS depressants, MAOIs, TCAs, tramadol
NC/PT Give analgesics for headache. Monitor elderly pts closely. Pt should take safety precautions for CNS effects, avoid alcohol.

DANGEROUS DRUG

cyclophosphamide (generic)

CLASS Alkylating agent, antineoplastic, nitrogen mustard
PREG/CONT D/NA

IND & DOSE Tx of malignant lymphoma, multiple myeloma, leukemias, mycosis fungoides, neuroblastoma, adenocarcinoma of ovary, retinoblastoma, carcinoma of breast; used concurrently or sequentially w/ other antineoplastics. *Adult:* Induction, 40–50 mg/kg IV in divided doses over 2–5 days or 1–5 mg/kg/day PO for 2-5 days. Or, 1–5 mg/kg/day PO, 10–15 mg/kg IV q 7–10 days, or 3–5 mg/kg IV twice wkly. **Tx of minimal change nephrotic syndrome.** *Child:* 2.5–3 mg/day PO for 60–90 days.

ADJUST DOSE Renal, hepatic impairment
ADV EFF Alopecia, anorexia, **bone marrow suppression,** hematuria to potentially fatal hemorrhagic cystitis, **interstitial pulmonary fibrosis,** n/v/d, stomatitis
INTERACTIONS Allopurinol, anticoagulants, chloramphenicol, digoxin, doxorubicin, grapefruit juice, succinylcholine
NC/PT Monitor CBC; dose adjustment may be needed. Do not give full dose within 4 wk of radiation or chemotherapy. Ensure pt well hydrated. Pts should use contraceptive measures; can cause fetal abnormalities. Pt should take oral drug on empty stomach, wear protective gloves when handling drug, not drink grapefruit juice, cover head at temperature extremes (hair loss may occur).

cycloSERINE (Seromycin Pulvules)

CLASS Antibiotic, antituberculotic
PREG/CONT C/NA

IND & DOSE Tx of active pulmonary, extrapulmonary (including renal) TB not responsive to first-line antituberculotics, w/ other antituberculotics; UTIs caused by susceptible bacteria. *Adult:* 250 mg PO bid at 12-hr intervals for first 2 wk. Max, 1 g/day; maint, 500 mg–1 g/day PO in divided doses.
ADV EFF Confusion, drowsiness, headache, **HF,** somnolence, tremor, vertigo
INTERACTIONS Alcohol, high-fat meals
NC/PT Culture before tx. Use only when other drugs have failed. Use w/ other anti-TB agents. Pt should avoid alcohol, take safety precautions for CNS effects, should not take w/ high-fat meal or discontinue drug without consulting prescriber. Name confusion w/ cycloserine, cyclosporine, and cyclophosphamide; use caution.

cycloSPORINE (Gengraf, Neoral, Sandimmune)
CLASS Immunosuppressant
PREG/CONT C/NA

BBW Monitor pts for infections, malignancies; risks increase. Monitor LFTs, renal function tests before and during tx; marked decreases in function may require dose adjustment or discontinuation. Monitor BP. Heart transplant pts may need concomitant antihypertensive tx.

IND & DOSE Px and tx of organ rejection in pts w/ kidney, liver, heart transplants. *Adult:* 15 mg/kg/day PO (*Sandimmune*) initially given 4–12 hr before transplantation; continue dose postop for 1–2 wk, then taper by 5% per wk to maint level of 5–10 mg/kg/day. Or by IV infusion (*Sandimmune*) at 1/3 oral dose (ie, 5–6 mg/kg/day 4–12 hr before transplantation as slow infusion over 2–6 hr); continue this daily dose postop. Switch to oral drug as soon as possible. **Tx of rheumatoid arthritis.** *Adult:* 2.5 mg/kg/day (*Gengraf, Neoral*) PO in divided doses bid; may increase up to 4 mg/kg/ day. If no benefit after 16 wk, discontinue. **Tx of recalcitrant plaque psoriasis.** *Adult:* 2.5 mg/kg/day (*Gengraf, Neoral*) PO divided bid for 4 wk, then may increase up to 4 mg/kg/day. If response unsatisfactory after 6 wk at 4 mg/kg/day, discontinue.
ADV EFF Acne, diarrhea, gum hyperplasia, hirsutism, hyperkalemia, hypertension, hypomagnesemia, renal impairment, tremors
INTERACTIONS Amiodarone, androgens, azole antifungals, carbamazepine, colchicine, diltiazem, foscarnet, grapefruit juice, high-fat meal, HMG-CoA reductase inhibitors, hormonal contraceptives, hydantoins, macrolides, metoclopramide, nephrotoxic agents, nicardipine, orlistat, phenobarbital, rifampin, St. John's wort, SSRIs
NC/PT Mix oral sol w/ milk, chocolate milk, orange juice at room temp; do not allow to stand before drinking. Do not refrigerate. Use parenteral route only if pt cannot take oral form. Monitor LFTs, renal function, CBC, BP carefully; toxicity possible. Not for use in pregnancy (barrier contraceptives advised). Pt should avoid grapefruit juice, St John's wort, exposure to infection; should not take w/ high-fat meal or discontinue without consulting prescriber. Interacts w/ many drugs; pt should inform all caregivers he is taking drug. Name confusion w/ cyclosporine, cycloserine, and cyclophosphamide; use caution.

cyproheptadine hydrochloride (generic)
CLASS Antihistamine
PREG/CONT B/NA

IND & DOSE Relief of s&sx associated w/ perennial, seasonal allergic rhinitis; other allergic reactions; tx of cold urticaria. *Adult:* 4 mg PO tid. Maint, 4–20 mg/day in three divided doses; max, 0.5 mg/kg/day. *Child 7–14 yr:* 4 mg PO bid-tid. Max, 16 mg/day. *Child 2–6 yr:* 2 mg PO bid. Max, 12 mg/day.
ADJUST DOSE Elderly pts
ADV EFF Agranulocytosis, anaphylactic shock, bronchial secretion thickening, dizziness, drowsiness, epigastric distress, disturbed coordination, pancytopenia
INTERACTIONS Alcohol, anticholinergics, CNS depressants, fluoxetine, metyrapone, MAOIs
NC/PT Use syrup if pt cannot swallow tablets. Give w/ food. Monitor response.

DANGEROUS DRUG
cytarabine (cytosine arabinoside) (DepoCyt, Tarabine PFS)
CLASS Antimetabolite, antineoplastic
PREG/CONT D/NA

IND & DOSE AML, ALL induction, maint of remission. *Adult:* For induction, 100 mg/m^2/day by continuous IV infusion (days 1–7) or 100 mg/m^2 IV q 12 hr (days 1–7); same dose for maint. Longer rest period may be needed. *Child:* Dose based on body weight and surface area. **Tx of meningeal leukemia.** *Adult:* 5–75 mg/m^2 IV once daily for 4 days or once q 4 days. Most common dose, 30 mg/m^2 q 4 days until CSF normal, then one more tx. **Tx of lymphomatous meningitis.** *Adult:* 50 mg liposomal cytarabine intrathecal q 14 days for two doses, then q 14 days for three doses. Repeat q 28 days for four doses.

ADV EFF Alopecia, anorexia, **bone marrow depression,** fever, n/v/d, rash, stomatitis, thrombophlebitis

INTERACTIONS Digoxin

NC/PT Monitor CBC; dose adjustment based on bone marrow response. Premedicate w/ antiemetics. Do not come in contact w/ liposomal forms. Provide mouth care, comfort measures. Not for use in pregnancy. Pt should take safety measures w/ CNS effects, avoid exposure to infection, cover head at temp extremes (hair loss possible).

---

dabigatran etexilate mesylate hydrochloride
(Pradaxa)
CLASS Anticoagulant, direct thrombin inhibitor
PREG/CONT C/NA

BBW Increased risk of thrombotic events when discontinuing. Consider adding another anticoagulant if stopping drug for any reason other than pathological bleeding.

IND & DOSE To reduce risk of stroke, systemic embolism in pts w/ **nonvalvular atrial fibrillation.** *Adult:* 150 mg PO bid. Converting from warfarin: Stop warfarin and begin dabigatran when INR is under 2. Converting from parenteral anticoagulant: Start dabigatran 0–2 hr before next dose of parenteral drug would have been given, or at discontinuation of continu-

ous infusion of parenteral anticoagulant. If starting on parenteral anticoagulant, wait 12 hr (if CrCl 30 mL/min or more) or 24 hr (if CrCl under 30 mL/min) after last dose of dabigatran before starting parenteral drug.

ADJUST DOSE Renal impairment
ADV EFF Bleeding, dyspepsia, **gastric hemorrhage,** gastritis, gastritislike symptoms, **rebound increased risk of thrombotic events w/ abrupt withdrawal, serious hypersensitivity reactions**

INTERACTIONS Aspirin, NSAIDs, platelet inhibitors, rifampin, warfarin

NC/PT Contraindicated in pts with artificial heart valves. Increased risk of bleeding; use caution. Consider using another anticoagulant if stopping drug. Not for use in pregnancy, breast-feeding. Pt should take at about same time each day; swallow capsule whole and not cut, crush, or chew it; protect drug from moisture; keep in original container or blister pack; mark container and use within 60 days; pt should alert all health care providers he is taking drug; report unusual bleeding. Pt should not double-up doses; should not stop drug suddenly (risk of thrombotic events).

---

dabrafenib (Tafinlar)
CLASS Antineoplastic, kinase inhibitor
PREG/CONT D/NA

IND & DOSE Tx of unresectable or metastatic melanoma w/ BRAF V600E mutations alone or in combination w/ trametinib. *Adult:* 150 mg/day PO at least 1 hr before or 2 hr after meal.

ADV EFF Alopecia, arthralgia, **cutaneous malignancies,** fever, headache, **hemolytic anemia,** hyperglycemia, hyperkeratosis, palmar-plantar erythrodysesthesia, **tumor promotion of wild-type BRAF melanoma,** uveitis/iritis

INTERACTIONS CYP3A4/CYP2C8 inhibitors/inducers

NC/PT Ensure proper dx and appropriate BRAF mutation. Assess for other malignancies; monitor LFTs, blood glucose; have pt schedule eye exams. Pt should avoid pregnancy, breastfeeding; use analgesics for headache; monitor skin; report vision changes, rash or skin lesions, fever.

DANGEROUS DRUG

dacarbazine hydrochloride
(DTIC-Dome)

CLASS Alkylating agent, antineoplastic
PREG/CONT C/NA

BBW Arrange for lab tests (LFTs; WBC, RBC, platelet count) before and frequently during tx; serious bone marrow suppression, hepatotoxicity possible. Carcinogenic in animals; monitor accordingly.

IND & DOSE Tx of metastatic malignant melanoma. *Adult, child:* 2–4.5 mg/kg/day IV for 10 days, repeated at 4-wk intervals, or 250 mg/m²/day IV for 5 days, repeated q 3 wk. **Second line tx of Hodgkin disease.** *Adult, child:* 150 mg/m²/day IV for 5 days w/ other drugs, repeated q 4 wk, or 375 mg/m² IV on day 1 w/ other drugs, repeated q 15 days.

ADV EFF Anaphylaxis, anorexia, bone marrow suppression, hepatic necrosis, local tissue damage w/ extravasation, n/v/d, photosensitivity

NC/PT Arrange for lab tests carefully; may limit dose. Give IV only; monitor site carefully. Extravasation can cause serious local damage; apply hot packs if this occurs. Restrict fluids and food for 4–6 hr before tx; may use antiemetics. Prepare calendar of tx days. Pt should avoid exposure to infection, sun.

DANGEROUS DRUG

dactinomycin
(Cosmegen)

CLASS Antibiotic, antineoplastic
PREG/CONT D/NA

BBW Use strict handling procedures; extremely toxic to skin and eyes. If extravasation, burning, stinging occur at injection site, stop infusion immediately, apply cold compresses to area, and restart in another vein. Local infiltration w/ injectable corticosteroid and flushing w/ saline may lessen reaction.

IND & DOSE Tx of Wilms' tumor, rhabdomyosarcoma, Ewing's sarcoma, in combination therapy; testicular cancer (metastatic nonseminomatous). *Adult:* 1,000 mcg/m² IV on day 1 of combination regimen or daily for 5 days; max, 15 mcg/kg/day or 400–600 mcg/m²/day IV for 5 days. *Child:* 15 mcg/kg/day IV for 5 days; max, 15 mcg/kg/day or 400–600 mcg/m²/day IV for 5 days. **Tx of gestational trophoblastic neoplasia.** *Adult:* 12 mcg/kg/day IV for 5 days when used as monotherapy; 500 mcg IV on days 1 and 2 in combination therapy. **Palliative tx or adjunct to tumor resection via isolation-perfusion technique for solid malignancies.** *Adult:* 50 mcg/kg for lower extremity or pelvis; 35 mcg/kg for upper extremity.

ADV EFF Agranulocytosis, alopecia, anemia, aplastic anemia, bone marrow suppression, cheilitis, dysphagia, esophagitis, fatigue, fever, hepatotoxicity, lethargy, myalgia, skin eruptions, stomatitis, tissue necrosis w/ extravasation

NC/PT Use strict handling procedures; toxic to skin and eyes. Monitor CBC, LFTs carefully; may limit dose. Give IV only. Monitor site carefully; extravasation can cause serious local damage. Monitor for adverse effects, which may worsen 1–2 wk after tx. Prepare calendar of tx days. Pt should cover head at temp extremes (hair loss possible). Name confusion between dactinomycin and daptomycin; use caution.

dalfampridine (Ampyra)
CLASS Potassium channel blocker, MS drug
PREG/CONT C/NA

IND & DOSE To improve walking in pts w/ MS. *Adult:* 10 mg PO bid, 12 hr apart.
ADJUST DOSE Renal impairment, seizure disorder
ADV EFF Asthenia, back pain, balance disorder, constipation, dizziness, dyspepsia, headache, insomnia, MS relapse, nasopharyngitis, nausea, paresthesia, pharyngolaryngeal pain, UTIs
NC/PT Do not use w/ hx of seizure disorders, renal impairment. Not for use in pregnancy, breast-feeding. Pt should swallow tablet whole and not cut, crush, or chew it; use safety precautions w/ CNS effects.

dalteparin sodium (Fragmin)
CLASS Anticoagulant, low-molecular-weight heparin
PREG/CONT C/NA

BBW Carefully monitor pts w/ spinal epidural anesthesia for neurologic impairment; risk of spinal hematoma and paralysis.
IND & DOSE Tx of unstable angina. *Adult:* 120 international units/kg subcut q 12 hr w/ aspirin therapy for 5–8 days; max, 10,000 international units q 12 hr. **DVT px, abd surgery.** *Adult:* 2,500 international units subcut 1–2 hr before surgery, repeated once daily for 5–10 days after surgery. High-risk pts, 5,000 international units subcut evening before surgery, then daily for 5–10 days. **DVT px w/ hip replacement surgery.** *Adult:* 5,000 international units subcut evening before surgery

or 2,500 international units within 2 hr before surgery or 2,500 international units 4–8 hr after surgery. Then, 5,000 international units subcut each day for 5–10 days or up to 14 days. **Extended tx of venous thromboembolism.** *Adult:* Mo 1, 200 international units/kg/day subcut; max, 18,000 international units/day. Mo 2–6, 150 international units/kg/ day subcut; max, 18,000 international units/day.
ADJUST DOSE Thrombocytopenia, renal impairment
ADV EFF Bruising, chills, fever, **hemorrhage**, injection-site reaction
INTERACTIONS Antiplatelet drugs, chamomile, clopidogrel, garlic, ginger, ginkgo, ginseng, heparin, high-dose vitamin E, oral anticoagulants, salicylates, ticlopidine
NC/PT Give 1–2 hr after abd surgery. Do not give IM. Give subcut, alternating left and right abd wall. Cannot be interchanged w/ other heparin product. Do not mix w/ other injection or infusion. Have protamine sulfate on hand as antidote. Teach proper administration, disposal of needles, syringes. Pt should avoid injury, report excessive bleeding.

dantrolene sodium (Dantrium)
CLASS Direct acting skeletal muscle relaxant
PREG/CONT C/NA

BBW Monitor LFTs periodically. Arrange to discontinue at first sign of abnormality; early detection of liver abnormalities may permit reversion to normal function. Hepatotoxicity possible.
IND & DOSE Control of clinical spasticity resulting from upper motor neuron disorders. *Adult:* 25 mg PO daily. Increase to 25 mg PO tid for 7 days; then increase to 50 mg PO tid and to 100 mg PO tid if needed. *Child over 5 yr:* 0.5 mg/kg PO once daily for 7 days, then 0.5 mg/kg PO tid for

7 days, then 1 mg/kg PO tid for 7 days, then 2 mg/kg PO tid if needed. Max, 100 mg PO qid. **Preop px of malignant hyperthermia.** *Adult, child:* 4–8 mg/kg/day PO in three to four divided doses for 1–2 days before surgery; give last dose about 3–4 hr before scheduled surgery. Or, for adult, child over 5 yr, 2.5 mg/kg IV 1¼ hr before surgery infused over 1 hr. **Postcrisis follow-up.** 4–8 mg/kg/day PO in four divided doses for 1–3 days to prevent recurrence. **Tx of malignant hyperthermia.** *Adult, child over 5 yr:* Discontinue all anesthetics as soon as problem recognized. Give dantrolene by continuous rapid IV push beginning at minimum of 1 mg/kg and continuing until sx subside or maximum cumulative dose of 10 mg/kg reached.
ADV EFF Aplastic anemia, diarrhea, dizziness, drowsiness, fatigue, **hepatitis, HF,** malaise, weakness
INTERACTIONS Alcohol, verapamil
NC/PT Monitor baseline and periodic LFTs. Monitor IV site to prevent extravasation. Use all appropriate support and tx for malignant hyperthermia. Establish tx goal w/ oral drug; stop occasionally to assess spasticity. Discontinue if diarrhea is severe. Pt should take safety precautions, avoid alcohol.

dapagliflozin (Farxiga)
CLASS Antidiabetic, sodium-glucose cotransporter 2 inhibitor
PREG/CONT C/NA

IND & DOSE Adjunct to diet/exercise to improve glycemic control in type 2 diabetes. *Adult:* 5 mg/day PO in a.m.; max, 10 mg/day.
ADJUST DOSE Severe renal impairment
ADV EFF Bladder cancer, genital mycotic infections, hypoglycemia, hyponatremia, increased LDLs, renal impairment, UTI
INTERACTIONS Celery, coriander, dandelion root, digoxin, fenugreek,

garlic, ginger, juniper berries, phenobarbital, phenytoin, rifampin
NC/PT Not for use w/ type 1 diabetes. Monitor blood glucose, HbA1c, BP periodically. Not for use in pregnancy, breast-feeding. Pt should continue diet/exercise program, other antidiabetics as ordered; take safety measures w/ dehydration; monitor for UTI, genital infections.

dapsone (generic)
CLASS Leprostatic
PREG/CONT C/NA

IND & DOSE Tx of leprosy. *Adult, child:* 50–100 mg/day PO. Adults may need up to 300 mg/day; max in children, 100 mg/day PO. **Tx of dermatitis herpetiformis.** *Adult:* 50–300 mg/day PO. Smaller doses in children; max, 100 mg/day.
ADV EFF Blurred vision, headache, **hepatic impairment,** insomnia, n/v/d, photosensitivity, ringing in ears, **severe allergic reactions,** tinnitus
INTERACTIONS Probenecid, rifampin, trimethoprim
NC/PT Obtain baseline, periodic LFTs. Not for use in pregnancy, breast-feeding. Pt should complete full course of therapy, avoid sun exposure, take safety precautions w/ vision changes.

daptomycin (Cubicin)
CLASS Cyclic-lipopeptide antibiotic
PREG/CONT B/NA

IND & DOSE Tx of complicated skin, skin-structure infections caused by susceptible strains of gram-positive bacteria. *Adult:* 4 mg/kg IV over 30 min or as IV injection over 2 min in normal saline injection q 24 hr for 7–14 days. **Tx of Staphylococcus aureus bacteremia.** *Adult:* 6 mg/kg/day IV over 30 min or as IV injection over 2 min for 2–6 wk or longer.

ADJUST DOSE Renal impairment
ADV EFF Constipation, dizziness, eosinophilic pneumonia, injection-site reactions, insomnia, myopathy, n/v/d, **pseudomembranous colitis,** superinfections
INTERACTIONS HMG-CoA inhibitors, oral anticoagulants, tobramycin
NC/PT Culture before tx. Monitor CPK for myopathy. Discontinue and give support for pseudomembranous colitis. Discontinue if signs of eosinophilic pneumonia. Treat superinfections. Name confusion between dactinomycin and daptomycin; use caution.

---

darbepoetin alfa
(Aranesp)
CLASS Erythropoiesis-stimulating hormone
PREG/CONT C/NA

BBW Increased risk of death and serious CV events if Hgb target exceeds 11 g/dL. Use lowest level of drugs needed to increase Hgb to lowest level needed to avoid transfusion. Risk of DVT is higher in pts receiving erythropoietin-stimulating agents preop to decrease need for transfusion; note darbepoetin not approved for this use. Increased risk of death or tumor progression when drug used in cancer pts w/ Hgb target range exceeding 11 g/dL; monitor Hgb closely in these pts.
IND & DOSE Tx of anemia associated w/ chronic renal failure, including during dialysis. Adult: 0.45 mcg/kg IV or subcut once/wk. Target Hgb level, 12 g/dL. Tx of chemotherapy-induced anemia in pts w/ nonmyeloid malignancies. 2.25 mcg/kg subcut once/wk; adjust to maintain acceptable Hgb levels. Or 500 mcg by subcut injection once q 3 wk; adjust to maintain Hgb level no higher than 12 g/dL.
ADJUST DOSE Chronic renal failure
ADV EFF Abd pain, arthralgia, asthenia, cough, **development of anti-erythropoietin antibodies w/ subsequent pure red cell aplasia and**

extreme anemia, diarrhea, dizziness, dyspnea, edema, fatigue, headache, hypotension, hypertension, **MI,** myalgias, n/v/d, **rapid cancer growth, seizure,** stroke, URI
NC/PT Ensure correct diagnosis; not substitute for emergency transfusion. Monitor Hgb levels closely; max, 12 g/dL. Monitor preop pt for increased risk of DVTs. Do not give in sol w/ other drugs. Evaluate iron stores before and periodically during tx. Frequent blood tests will be needed. Teach pt proper administration and disposal of needles and syringes. Pt should take safety precautions for CNS effects, mark calendar for injection dates.

---

darifenacin hydrobromide (Enablex)
CLASS Urinary antispasmodic, muscarinic receptor antagonist
PREG/CONT C/NA

IND & DOSE Tx of overactive bladder. Adult: 7.5 mg/day PO w/ liquid and swallowed whole. May increase to 15 mg/day PO as early as wk 2.
ADJUST DOSE Hepatic impairment
ADV EFF Constipation, dry mouth, glaucoma, urine retention
INTERACTIONS Anticholinergics, clarithromycin, flecainide, itraconazole, ketoconazole, nefazodone, nelfinavir, ritonavir, thioridazine, TCAs
NC/PT Ensure correct diagnosis; rule out underlying medical issues. Monitor IOP. Not for use in pregnancy, breast-feeding. Pt should swallow tablet whole and not cut, crush, or chew it; use sugarless lozenges for dry mouth.

---

darunavir (Prezista)
CLASS Antiviral/protease inhibitor
PREG/CONT C/NA

IND & DOSE Tx of pts w/ HIV infection that has progressed

following standard tx. *Adult:*
600 mg PO bid w/ ritonavir 100 mg
PO bid w/ food (tx-experienced)
800 mg PO bid w/ ritonavir 100 mg
PO bid (tx-naive). *Child 3–under 18 yr,
10 kg or more:* Base dose on weight
and surface area (see
manufacturer's guidelines).
ADJUST DOSE Hepatic impairment
ADV EFF Abd pain, diabetes, headache, **hepatitis, increased bleeding
w/ hemophilia,** n/v/d, rash to **Ste-
vens Johnson syndrome,** redistribution of body fat
INTERACTIONS Alfuzosin, cisapride, dihydroergotamine, ergotamine, lovastatin, methylergonovine,
pimozide, oral midazolam, rifampin,
St. John's wort, sildenafil, simvastatin, triazolam
NC/PT Contraindicated for use w/
many other drugs; check complete
drug list before tx. Monitor LFTs
regularly; not for use w/ severe hepatic impairment. Not for use in children
under 3; fatalities have occurred.
Monitor blood glucose. Not for use in
pregnancy, breast-feeding. Pt should
report rash, changes in color of urine
or stool.

---

dasatinib (Sprycel)
CLASS Antineoplastic, kinase
inhibitor
PREG/CONT D/NA

IND & DOSE Tx of adults w/ all
stages of CML; newly diagnosed or
resistant Philadelphia chromosome–positive ALL. *Adult:* Chronic
CML, 100 mg/day PO. ALL/other
phases of CML, 140 mg/day PO.
ADV EFF Bone marrow suppression, diarrhea, dyspnea, fatigue, fluid
retention, hemorrhage, **HF,** nausea,
**pulmonary artery hypertension, QT
prolongation,** rash
INTERACTIONS Antacids; CYP3A4
inducers, inhibitors; grapefruit juice
NC/PT Obtain baseline and periodic
ECG. Monitor CBC closely; dose ad-

justment may be needed. Not for use
in pregnancy, breast-feeding. Men
should not father a child during tx. Pt
should swallow tablets whole and not
cut, crush, or chew them; avoid
grapefruit juice; avoid exposure to infection, injury; report severe swelling,
bleeding.

DAUNOrubicin citrate
(DaunoXome)
CLASS Antineoplastic
PREG/CONT D/NA

BBW Cardiac toxicity possible;
monitor ECG, enzymes (dose
adjustment may be needed). Serious
bone marrow depression possible;
monitor CBC (dose adjustment may
be needed).
IND & DOSE Tx of advanced HIV-
associated Kaposi's sarcoma. *Adult:*
400 mg/m² IV over 1hr q 2 wk.
ADJUST DOSE Renal, hepatic impairment
ADV EFF Abd pain, anorexia, **bone
marrow suppression, cancer, cardiac toxicity,** fatigue, fever, headache,
hepatotoxicity, n/v/d
INTERACTIONS Cyclophosphamide, hepatotoxic drugs, myelosup-
pressants
NC/PT Obtain baseline and periodic
ECG, enzymes. Monitor CBC closely;
dose adjustment may be needed.
Monitor injection site; extravasation
can cause serious damage. Not for use
in pregnancy, breast-feeding.

---

decitabine (Dacogen)
CLASS Antineoplastic antibiotic
PREG/CONT D/NA

IND & DOSE Tx of pts w/ myelodysplastic syndromes. *Adult:* 15 mg/m²
IV over 3 hr q 8 hr for 3 days; repeat q
6 wk.
ADJUST DOSE Renal, hepatic
impairment

ADV EFF Anemia, constipation, cough, diarrhea, fatigue, hyperglycemia, nausea, neutrophilia, petechiae, pyrexia, thrombocytopenia
NC/PT Monitor CBC closely; dose adjustment may be needed. Premedicate w/ antiemetic. Not for use in pregnancy (contraceptive use during and for 1 mo after tx), breast-feeding. Men should not father a child during and for 2 mo after tx. Pt should avoid exposure to infection, injury.

deferasirox (Exjade)
CLASS Chelate
PREG/CONT C/NA

BBW May cause potentially fatal renal, hepatic reactions; monitor closely.
IND & DOSE Tx of chronic iron overload from blood transfusions; tx of iron overload related to thalassemia in pts 10 yr and older. *Adult, child 2 yr and older (10 yr and older w/ thalassemia):* 20 mg/kg/day PO; max, 30 mg/kg/day. Adjust dose based on serum ferritin levels.
ADJUST DOSE Renal impairment
ADV EFF Abd pain; **hepatic, renal impairment;** n/v/d; rash; hearing, vision changes
INTERACTIONS Bisphosphonates, iron chelating agents
NC/PT Monitor LFTs, renal function before, wkly for 2 wk, then monthly during tx. Dose adjusted based on serum ferritin levels. Pt should take safety precautions for CNS effects.

deferoxamine mesylate (Desferal)
CLASS Chelate
PREG/CONT C/NA

IND & DOSE Tx of chronic iron overload. *Adult, child 2 yr and older:* 0.5–1 g IM qid; 2 g IV w/ each unit of blood, or 2,040 mg/day as continuous subcut infusion over 8–24 hr. IM preferred. **Tx of acute iron toxicity.**

Adult, child: 1 g IM or IV, then 0.5 g q 4 hr for two doses, then q 4–12 hr based on pt response. Max for child, 6 g/day.
ADV EFF Abd pain, hearing/vision changes, infections, injection-site reactions, n/v/d, **respiratory distress syndrome,** rash, discolored urine
NC/PT Not for use in primary hemochromatosis. Monitor hearing, vision, lung function. Caution in pregnancy, breast-feeding. Urine may be discolored. Pt should take safety measures for CNS effects.

degarelix (generic)
CLASS Antineoplastic
PREG/CONT X/NA

IND & DOSE Tx of advanced prostate cancer. *Adult:* 240 mg subcut as two 120-mg injections, then maint of 80 mg subcut q 28 days.
ADV EFF Hot flashes, injection-site reaction, loss of libido, **QT prolongation,** weight gain
INTERACTIONS QT-prolonging drugs
NC/PT Obtain baseline and periodic ECG. Monitor injection sites for reaction. Alert pt that flushing, hot flashes, changes in libido possible.

delavirdine mesylate (Rescriptor)
CLASS Antiviral, nonnucleoside reverse transcriptase inhibitor
PREG/CONT C/NA

BBW Give concurrently w/ appropriate antiretrovirals; not for monotherapy.
IND & DOSE Tx of HIV-1 infection w/ other appropriate antiretrovirals. *Adult, child over 16 yr:* 400 mg PO tid w/ appropriate antiretrovirals.
ADV EFF Diarrhea, flulike symptoms, headache, nausea, rash
INTERACTIONS Antacids, antiarrhythmics, benzodiazepines, calcium channel blockers, clarithromycin,

dapsone, ergot derivatives, indinavir, quinidine, rifabutin, saquinavir, St. John's wort, warfarin

NC/PT Must give w/ other antiretrovirals. Monitor T cells, LFTs. Monitor for opportunistic infections. Disperse 100-mg tablets in water before giving; let stand. Stir to form uniform dispersion. Have pt drink, rinse glass, and drink the rinse. Pt should use appropriate precautions (drug is not a cure); consult all health care providers (drug interacts w/ many drugs); avoid St. John's wort.

demeclocycline hydrochloride (generic)
CLASS Tetracycline
PREG/CONT D/NA

IND & DOSE Tx of infections caused by susceptible bacteria strains; when penicillin contraindicated. *Adult:* General guidelines, 150 mg PO qid or 300 mg PO bid. *Child 8 yr and older:* 3–6 mg/lb/day (6.6–13.2 mg/kg/day) PO in two to four divided doses. **Tx of gonococcal infections.** *Adult:* 600 mg PO, then 300 mg q 12 hr for 4 days to total 3 g. **Tx of streptococcal infections.** *Adult:* 150 mg PO qid for 10 days.

ADV EFF Anemia; anorexia; discoloration, inadequate calcification of fetal primary teeth if used in pregnancy; discoloration, inadequate calcification of permanent teeth if used during dental development; eosinophilia; glossitis; hemolytic thrombocytopenia; leukocytosis; leukopenia; liver failure; neutropenia; n/v/d; phototoxic reaction; rash

INTERACTIONS Antacids, dairy products, digoxin, hormonal contraceptives, iron, magnesium, penicillin

NC/PT Not for use in pregnancy (use of barrier contraceptives advised), breast-feeding. Pt should take on empty stomach w/ full glass of water, not take w/ iron or dairy products, avoid sun exposure.

denileukin diftitox (Ontak)
CLASS Biological protein
PREG/CONT D/NA

BBW Severe hypersensitivity reactions possible; have life support equipment on hand. Capillary leak syndrome possible; pt may lose visual acuity, color vision.

IND & DOSE Tx of cutaneous T-cell lymphoma in pts who express CD25 component of IL-2 receptor. *Adult:* 9 or 18 mcg/kg/day IV over 15 min for 5 consecutive days q 21 days.

ADV EFF Cough, diarrhea, dyspnea, fatigue, headache, n/v, peripheral edema, pruritus, pyrexia, rigors

NC/PT Premedicate w/ antihistamine and acetaminophen. Have emergency equipment available for hypersensitivity reactions. Warn pt of potential vision loss. Caution in pregnancy; not for use in breast-feeding. Pt should report sudden weight gain, rash, difficulty breathing, vision changes.

denosumab (Prolia, Xgeva)
CLASS RANK ligand inhibitor
PREG/CONT D (Xgeva), X (Prolia)/NA

IND & DOSE Tx of postmenopausal osteoporosis in women at high risk for fracture; tx of bone loss in breast cancer pts receiving aromatase inhibitors; tx of bone loss in prostate cancer pts receiving androgen deprivation therapy. *Adult:* 60 mg by subcut injection in upper arm, thigh, or abdomen q 6 mo (*Prolia* only). **Px of skeletal-related events in pts w/ bone metastases from solid tumors.** *Adult:* 120 mg by subcut injection q 4 wk (*Xgeva* only). **Tx of unresectable giant cell tumor of the bone (*Xgeva*).** *Adult, adolescent:* 120 mg subcut q 4 wk w/ additional 120 mg subcut on days 8, 15 of first month, w/ calcium, vitamin D.

ADJUST DOSE Renal impairment

ADV EFF Back pain, **cancer, constipation,** cystitis, hypercholesterolemia, hypocalcemia, **infection (serious to life-threatening), osteonecrosis of jaw**

NC/PT Obtain baseline serum calcium levels; repeat regularly. Give subcut into abdomen, upper thigh, or upper arm; rotate injection sites. Not for use in pregnancy, breast-feeding. Pt should take 1,000 mg/day calcium and 400 units/day vitamin D, have regular cancer screening, avoid exposure to infection, report signs of infection, get regular dental care to prevent jaw problems.

desipramine hydrochloride
(Norpramin)

CLASS Antidepressant, TCA
PREG/CONT C/NA

BBW Risk of suicidality in children, adolescents, young adults. Monitor pt; inform caregivers.

IND & DOSE Relief of depression **sx.** *Adult:* 100–200 mg/day PO as single dose or in divided doses; max, 300 mg/day.

ADJUST DOSE Adolescents, elderly pts

ADV EFF Agranulocytosis, anticholinergic effects, confusion, constipation, disturbed concentration, dry mouth, **MI,** nasal congestion, orthostatic hypotension, photosensitivity, sedation, **stroke,** urine retention, withdrawal symptoms after prolonged use

INTERACTIONS Anticholinergics, cimetidine, clonidine, fluoxetine, MAOIs, oral anticoagulants, quinolones, sympathomimetics

NC/PT Give major portion of dose at bedtime. Monitor elderly pts for increased adverse effects. Obtain CBC if fever, signs of infection occur. Pt should avoid alcohol, sun exposure;

use sugarless lozenges for dry mouth; take safety precautions w/ CNS effects; report difficulty urinating, fever, thoughts of suicide.

DANGEROUS DRUG

desirudin (Iprivask)

CLASS Anticoagulant, thrombin inhibitor
PREG/CONT C/NA

BBW Risk of epidural, spinal hematoma w/ resultant long-term or permanent paralysis. Weigh risks before using epidural or spinal anesthesia, spinal puncture.

IND & DOSE PX of DVT in pts undergoing elective hip replacement. *Adult:* 15 mg subcut q 12 hr for 9–12 days. Give initial dose 5–15 min before surgery after induction of anesthesia.

ADJUST DOSE Renal impairment

ADV EFF **Hemorrhage,** injection-site reactions

INTERACTIONS Drugs that prolong bleeding

NC/PT Give by deep subcut injection; alternate sites. Monitor blood clotting tests carefully. Protect pt from injury.

desloratadine (Clarinex, Clarinex Reditabs)

CLASS Antihistamine
PREG/CONT C/NA

IND & DOSE Relief of nasal and nonnasal sx of seasonal allergic rhinitis in pts 2 yr and older; tx of chronic idiopathic urticaria and perennial allergies caused by indoor and outdoor allergens in pts 6 mo and older. *Adult, child 12 yr and older:* 5 mg/day PO or 2 tsp (5 mg/10 mL) syrup/day PO. *Child 6–11 yr:* 1 tsp syrup (2.5 mg/5 mL)/day PO, or 2.5-mg rapidly disintegrating tablet/day PO. *Child 12 mo–5yr:* 1/2 tsp syrup/day (1.25 mg/2.5 mL) PO. *Child 6–11 mo:* 2 mL syrup/day (1 mg) PO.

ADJUST DOSE Renal, hepatic impairment
ADV EFF Dry mouth, dry throat, dizziness
NC/PT Do not use *Clarinex Reditabs* w/ phenylketonuria. Pt should use humidifier if dryness a problem, suck sugarless lozenges for dry mouth, take safety precautions if dizzy.

---

desmopressin acetate
(DDAVP, Stimate)
CLASS Hormone
PREG/CONT B/NA

IND & DOSE Tx of neurogenic diabetes insipidus. *Adult:* 0.1–0.4 mL/day intranasally as single dose or divided into two to three doses, or 0.5–1 mL/day subcut or IV divided into two doses, or 0.05 mg PO bid; adjust according to water turnover pattern (DDAVP only). *Child 3 mo–12 yr:* 0.05–0.3 mL/day intranasally as single dose or divided into two doses, or 0.05 mg PO daily; adjust according to water turnover pattern (DDAVP only). Tx of hemophilia A, von Willebrand disease (type I). *Adult:* 0.3 mcg/kg diluted in 50 mL sterile physiologic saline; infuse IV slowly over 15–30 min 30 min preop; intranasal, 1 spray/nostril 2 hr preop for total dose of 300 mcg. *Child 11 mo and older:* 1 spray/nostril (150 mcg); total dose, 300 mcg. Less than 50 kg, 150 mcg as single spray.
ADV EFF Local redness, swelling, burning at injection site; **water intoxication**
INTERACTIONS Carbamazepine, chlorpropamide, SSRIs, TCAs
NC/PT Refrigerate sol, injection. Use rhinal tube to deposit deep into nasal cavity; use air-filled syringe or blow into tube. Monitor nasal passages. Monitor for hyponatremia. Monitor pts w/ CV disorders. Individualize dose to establish diurnal water turnover patterns to allow sleep.

---

desvenlafaxine succinate (Pristiq)
CLASS Antidepressant, serotonin-norepinephrine reuptake inhibitor
PREG/CONT C/NA

BBW High risk of suicidality in children, adolescents, young adults; monitor for suicidal ideation, especially when beginning tx or changing dose. Not approved for children.
IND & DOSE Tx of major depressive disorders. *Adult:* 50 mg/day PO w/ or without food; range, 50–400 mg/day.
ADJUST DOSE Severe renal impairment
ADV EFF Constipation, decreased appetite, dizziness, dry mouth, **eosinophilic pneumonia**, fatigue, glaucoma, headache, hyperhidrosis, **interstitial lung disease**, n/v/d, **suicidal ideation**
INTERACTIONS Alcohol, aspirin, CNS depressants, MAOIs, NSAIDs, SSRIs, St. John's wort, venlafaxine, warfarin
NC/PT Limit access in suicidal pts. Do not give within 14 days of MAOIs. Taper gradually when stopping. Monitor IOP periodically. Not for use in pregnancy, breast-feeding. May take several wks to see effects. Tablet matrix may appear in stool. Pt should swallow tablet whole and not cut, crush, or chew it; report thoughts of suicide.

---

dexamethasone
(Aerosorb-Dex, DexPak TaperPak),
dexamethasone sodium phosphate (generic)
CLASS Glucocorticoid, hormone
PREG/CONT C/NA

IND & DOSE Short-term tx of various inflammatory, allergic disorders. *Adult:* 0.75–9 mg/day PO, or 0.5–9 mg/day IM or IV. *Child:* Base dose on formulas for child dosing using age, body weight. Tx of cerebral

edema. **Adult:** 10 mg IV, then 4 mg IM q 6 hr until cerebral edema sx subside. Change to oral therapy, 1–3 mg tid, as soon as possible; taper over 5–7 days. **Tx of unresponsive shock.** **Child:** 1–6 mg/kg as single IV injection (as much as 20 mg initially; repeated injections q 2–6 hr have been used). **Intra-articular or soft-tissue administration for tx of arthritis, psoriatic plaques.** **Adult:** 0.2–6 mg (depending on joint or soft-tissue injection site). **Control of bronchial asthma requiring corticosteroids.** **Adult:** 3 inhalations tid–qid; max, 12 inhalations/day. **Child:** 2 inhalations tid–qid; max, 8 inhalations/day. **Relief of seasonal or perennial rhinitis sx.** **Adult:** 2 sprays (168 mcg) into each nostril bid–tid; max, 12 sprays (1,008 mcg)/day. **Child:** 1 or 2 sprays (84–168 mcg) into each nostril bid, depending on age; max, 8 sprays (672 mcg)/day. **Tx of inflammation of eyelid, conjunctiva, cornea, globe.** **Adult, child:** Instill 1 or 2 drops into conjunctival sac q hr during day and q 2 hr during night; taper as 1 drop q 4 hr, then 1 drop tid–qid. For ointment, apply thin coating in lower conjunctival sac tid–qid; reduce dose to bid, then once daily. **Relief of inflammatory and pruritic manifestations of dermatoses.** **Adult, child:** Apply sparingly to affected area bid–qid.
ADV EFF Acne, amenorrhea, depression, euphoria, fluid/electrolyte disturbances, headache, HPA suppression, hyperglycemia, hypertension, immunosuppression, impaired wound healing, infection, insomnia, irregular menses, local irritation, muscle weakness, secondary adrenal suppression, **seizures,** vertigo
INTERACTIONS Corticotropin, live vaccines, phenobarbital, phenytoin, rifampin, salicylates
NC/PT Give daily doses before 9 a.m. to mimic normal peak corticosteroid blood levels. Taper dose w/ high doses or long-term use. Monitor serum glucose. Protect pt from exposure to infection; do not give to pt w/ active

infection. Not for use in breast-feeding. Apply topical drug sparingly to intact skin. Pt should not overuse joints after intra-articular injection.

dexchlorpheniramine maleate (generic)
CLASS Antihistamine
PREG/CONT B/NA

IND & DOSE Relief of sx associated w/ perennial, seasonal allergic rhinitis; vasomotor rhinitis; allergic conjunctivitis; mild, uncomplicated urticaria, angioedema; amelioration of allergic reactions to blood or plasma; dermatographism; adjunct tx in anaphylactic reactions. **Adult, child older than 12 yr:** 4–6 mg PO at bedtime or q 8–10 hr during day. **Child 6–12 yr:** 4 mg PO once daily at bedtime (syrup only).
ADJUST DOSE Elderly pts
ADV EFF Agranulocytosis, anaphylactic shock, disturbed coordination, dizziness, drowsiness, epigastric distress, **pancytopenia,** sedation, thickening of bronchial secretions, thrombocytopenia
INTERACTIONS Alcohol, CNS depressants
NC/PT Adjust dose to lowest possible to manage sx. Pt should swallow tablet whole and not cut, crush, or chew it; avoid alcohol; take safety precautions for CNS effects.

dexlansoprazole (Dexilant)
CLASS Antisecretory, proton pump inhibitor
PREG/CONT B/NA

IND & DOSE Healing, maint of healing of erosive esophagitis. **Adult:** 60 mg/day PO for up to 8 wk, then 30 mg/day PO. **Tx of heartburn, GERD.** **Adult:** 30 mg/day PO for up to 4 wk.
ADV EFF N/v/d, possible increase in *Clostridium difficile* diarrhea, possible loss of bone density

INTERACTIONS Ampicillin, atazanavir, digoxin, iron salts, ketoconazole, warfarin
NC/PT Not for use in breast-feeding. May be opened, contents sprinkled over 1 tbsp applesauce, and swallowed immediately. Pt should swallow capsule whole and not cut, crush, or chew it; report severe diarrhea.

DANGEROUS DRUG

dexmedetomidine hydrochloride (Precedex)
CLASS Sedative/hypnotic
PREG/CONT C/NA

IND & DOSE ICU sedation of mechanically ventilated pts. *Adult:* 1 mcg/kg IV over 10 min, then 0.2–0.7 mcg/kg/hr using IV infusion pump.
ADJUST DOSE Elderly pts
ADV EFF Agitation, bradycardia, dry mouth, hypotension, **respiratory failure**
INTERACTIONS Anesthetics, CNS depressants, opioids
NC/PT Not for use in pregnancy, breast-feeding. Monitor pt continuously during tx. Do not use for longer than 24 hr.

dexmethylphenidate hydrochloride (Focalin, Focalin XR)
CLASS CNS stimulant
PREG/CONT C/C-II

BBW Use caution w/ hx of substance dependence or alcoholism. Dependence, severe depression, psychotic reactions possible w/ withdrawal.
IND & DOSE Tx of ADHD as part of total tx program. *Adult, child 6 yr and older:* 2.5 mg PO bid; may increase as needed in 2.5- to 5-mg increments to max 10 mg PO bid. ER capsules: Initially 5 mg/day PO for children; increase in 5-mg increments to 30 mg/day. Start adults at 10 mg PO; increase in 10-mg increments to 20 mg/day. *Already on methylpheni-*

date: Start at one-half methylphenidate dose w/ max of 10 mg PO bid.
ADV EFF Abd pain, anorexia, dizziness, insomnia, nausea, nervousness, tachycardia
INTERACTIONS Alcohol, antihypertensives, dopamine, epinephrine, MAOIs, phenobarbital, phenytoin, primidone, SSRIs, TCAs, warfarin
NC/PT Ensure proper diagnosis before use; interrupt periodically to re-evaluate. Do not give within 14 days of MAOIs. Controlled substance; secure storage. May sprinkle contents on applesauce; pt should take immediately. Pt should swallow ER capsules whole and not cut, crush, or chew them; take as part of comprehensive tx program; take early in day to avoid interrupting sleep; avoid alcohol and OTC products.

dexpanthenol (Panthoderm)
CLASS Emollient, GI stimulant
PREG/CONT C/NA

IND & DOSE Prevention of postoperative adynamic ileus. *Adult:* 250–500 mg IM or IV diluted in sol; repeat in 2 hr, then q 6 hr until danger of adynamic ileus has passed. Tx of adynamic ileus. *Adult:* 500 mg IM or IV diluted in sol; repeat in 2 hr, then q 6 hr as needed. Topical tx of mild eczema, dermatosis, bee stings, diaper rash, chafing. *Adult, child:* Apply once or twice daily to affected areas.
ADV EFF Abd pain, anorexia, dizziness, insomnia, nausea, nervousness, tachycardia
INTERACTIONS Intestinal colic, n/v/d, slight hypotension
NC/PT Monitor BP w/ IV use. Intestinal colic possible.

dexrazoxane (Totect)
CLASS Lyophilizate
PREG/CONT D/NA

IND & DOSE Tx of extravasation of IV anthracycline chemotherapy.

Adult: Days 1, 2: 1,000 mg/m² IV; max, 2,000 mg IV. Day 3: 500 mg/m² IV; max, 1,000 mg infused over 2 hr.
ADJUST DOSE Renal impairment
ADV EFF Bone marrow suppression, injection-site pain, n/v/d, pyrexia
NC/PT Available in emergency kit. Monitor bone marrow. Not for use in pregnancy, breast-feeding. Use pain-relief measures for extravasation site.

---

dextran, high-molecular-weight (Dextran 70, Gentran 70, Macrodex)
CLASS Plasma volume expander
PREG/CONT C/NA

IND & DOSE Adjunct tx for shock or impending shock when blood or blood products are not available. *Adult:* 500–1,000 mL IV at 20–40 mL/min as emergency procedure; max, 20 mL/kg first 24 hr of tx. *Child:* Base dose on body weight or surface area; max, 20 mL/kg IV total dose.
ADJUST DOSE Renal impairment
ADV EFF Anaphylactoid reaction, coagulation problems, **HF,** hypervolemia, injection-site reactions, rash
NC/PT Give IV only. Use clear sols only. Monitor for hypervolemia, HF. Pt should report difficulty breathing.

---

dextran, low-molecular-weight (Dextran 40, Gentran 40, 10% LMD, Rheomacrodex)
CLASS Plasma volume expander
PREG/CONT C/NA

IND & DOSE Adjunct tx for shock or impending shock when blood or blood products are not available. *Adult, child:* Total dose of 20 mL/kg IV in first 24 hr; max, 10 mL/kg beyond 24 hr. Discontinue after 5 days. **Hemodiluent in extracorporeal circulation.** *Adult:*

10–20 mL/kg added to perfusion circuit; max, 20 mL/kg. **Px for DVT, PE in pts undergoing procedures w/ high risk of thromboembolic events.** *Adult:* 500–1,000 mL IV on day of surgery. Continue at 500 mL IV for additional 2–3 days. Thereafter, may give 500 mL q second to third day for up to 2 wk.
ADV EFF Hypotension, hypervolemia, injection-site reactions, rash
NC/PT Give IV only. Use clear sols only. Monitor for hypervolemia. Monitor urine output. Pt should report difficulty breathing.

---

dextroamphetamine sulfate (Dexedrine Spansule)
CLASS Amphetamine, CNS stimulant
PREG/CONT C/C-II

BBW High abuse potential. Avoid prolonged use; prescribe sparingly. Misuse may cause sudden death or serious CV events. Increased risk w/ heart problems or structural heart anomalies.
IND & DOSE Tx of narcolepsy. *Adult, child over 12 yr:* 10 mg/day PO in divided doses. Increase in 10-mg/day increments at wkly intervals; range, 5–60 mg/day PO in divided doses. *Child 6–12 yr:* 5 mg/day PO. Increase in 5-mg increments at wkly intervals until optimal response obtained. **Adjunct tx for abnormal behavioral syndrome (ADHD hyperkinetic syndrome).** *Adult:* 5 mg PO once or twice daily; max, 40 mg/day. *Child 6 yr and older:* 5 mg PO daily–bid. Increase in 5-mg/day increments at wkly intervals; max, 40 mg/day. *Child 3–5 yr:* 2.5 mg/day PO. Increase in 2.5-mg/day increments at wkly intervals.
ADV EFF Diarrhea, dizziness, dry mouth, hypertension, insomnia, overstimulation, palpitations, restlessness, tachycardia, unpleasant taste

INTERACTIONS Acetazolamide, antihypertensives, furazolidone, MAOIs, sodium bicarbonate, urinary acidifiers
NC/PT Baseline ECG recommended. Ensure proper diagnosis. Do not give within 14 days of MAOIs. Incorporate into comprehensive social and behavioral tx plan. Controlled substance; store securely. Give early in day. Provide periodic drug breaks. Monitor BP, growth in children. Not for use in pregnancy. Pt should swallow ER capsules whole and not cut, crush, or chew them.

dextromethorphan hydrobromide (Creo-Terpin, Delsym, DexAlone, Hold DM, etc)
CLASS Nonopioid antitussive
PREG/CONT C/NA

IND & DOSE Control of nonproductive cough. *Adult, child 12 yr and older:* Gelcaps, 30 mg PO q 6–8 hr; max, 120 mg/day. Lozenges, 5–15 mg PO q 1–4 hr; max, 120 mg/day. Liquid, syrup, strips, 10–20 mg PO q 4 hr or 30 mg q 6–8 hr; max, 120 mg/day. ER suspension, 60 mg PO q 12 hr; max, 120 mg/day. *Child 6–11 yr:* Lozenges, 5–10 mg PO q 1–4 hr; max, 60 mg/day. Liquid, syrup, strips, 15 mg PO q 6–8 hr; max, 60 mg/day. Freezer pops, 2 pops q 6–8 hr. *Child 2–6 yr:* Liquid, syrup, 7.5 mg PO q 6–8 hr; max, 30 mg/day. Freezer pops, 1 pop q 6–8 hr.
ADV EFF Respiratory depression (w/ overdose)
INTERACTIONS MAOIs
NC/PT Ensure proper use and advisability of suppressing cough. Do not use within 14 days of MAOIs. Pt should avoid OTC products w/ same ingredients, report persistent cough w/ fever.

diazepam (Diastat AcuDial, Valium)
CLASS Antiepileptic, anxiolytic, benzodiazepine
PREG/CONT D/C-IV

IND & DOSE Tx of anxiety disorders, skeletal muscle spasm, seizure disorders. *Adult:* 2–10 mg PO bid–qid, or 0.2 mg/kg rectally. Treat no more than one episode q 5 days. May give second dose in 4–12 hr. *Child 6–11 yr:* 0.3 mg/kg rectally. *Child 2–5 yr:* 0.5 mg/kg rectally. *Child over 6 mo:* 1–2.5 mg PO tid–qid initially. **Tx of anxiety.** *Adult:* 2–10 mg IM or IV; repeat in 3–4 hr if needed. **Alcohol withdrawal.** *Adult:* 10 mg IM or IV initially, then 5–10 mg in 3–4 hr if needed. **Endoscopic procedures.** *Adult:* 10 mg or less (up to 20 mg) IV just before procedure or 5–10 mg IM 30 min before procedure. **Relief of muscle spasm.** *Adult:* 5–10 mg IM or IV initially, then 5–10 mg in 3–4 hr if needed. **Status epilepticus.** *Adult:* 5–10 mg preferably by slow IV. May repeat q 5–10 min to total dose of 30 mg. May repeat in 2–4 hr. *Child 5 yr and older:* 1 mg IV q 2–5 min to max of 10 mg; may repeat in 2–4 hr. *Child over 1 mo–under 5 yr:* 0.2–0.5 mg slowly IV q 2–5 min to max of 5 mg. **Preoperative anxiety.** *Adult:* 10 mg IM. **Cardioversion.** *Adult:* 5–15 mg IV 5–10 min before procedure. **Tx of tetanus.** *Child 5 yr and older:* 5–10 mg IV q 3–4 hr. *Child over 1 mo–under 5 yr:* 1–2 mg IM or IV slowly q 3–4 hr as needed.
ADJUST DOSE Elderly pts, debilitating diseases
ADV EFF Apathy, bradycardia, confusion, constipation, **CV collapse**, depression, diarrhea, disorientation, fatigue, incontinence, lethargy, libido changes, light-headedness, paradoxical excitement, tachycardia, urine retention
INTERACTIONS Alcohol, cimetidine, disulfiram, hormonal contraceptives, omeprazole, ranitidine, theophylline

NC/PT Do not give intra-arterially; change to oral route as soon as possible. Monitor carefully w/ IV route. Keep pt in bed for 3 hr; do not allow pt to drive after injection. Taper dose after long-term use. Suggest medical alert ID. Not for use in pregnancy (barrier contraceptives advised). Pt should take safety precautions w/ CNS effects.

---

diazoxide (Proglycem)
CLASS Glucose-elevating drug
PREG/CONT C/NA

IND & DOSE Mgt of hypoglycemia due to hyperinsulinism in infants and children and to inoperable pancreatic islet cell malignancies. *Adult, child:* 3–8 mg/kg/day PO in two to three divided doses q 8–12 hr. *Infant, newborn:* 8–15 mg/kg/day PO in two to three doses q 8–12 hr.
ADJUST DOSE Renal impairment
ADV EFF Anxiety, hirsutism, hyperglycemia, hypotension, **HF,** n/v, **thrombocytopenia**
INTERACTIONS Chlorpropamide, glipizide, glyburide, hydantoins, tolazamide, tolbutamide, thiazides
NC/PT Check serum glucose, daily weight to monitor fluid retention. Protect suspension from light; have insulin on hand if hyperglycemia occurs. Excessive hair growth will end when drug stopped. Pt should report weight gain of more than 3 lb/day.

---

diclofenac epolamine (Flector, Solaraze, Voltaren), diclofenac potassium (Cambia, Cataflam, Zipsor), diclofenac sodium (Solaraze)
CLASS Analgesic
PREG/CONT C (1st, 2nd trimesters); D (3rd trimester)/NA

BBW Possible increased risk of CV events, GI bleed, renal insufficiency; monitor accordingly.

IND & DOSE Tx of pain, including dysmenorrhea. *Adult:* 50 mg PO tid or 1 transdermal patch *(Flector)* applied to most painful area bid. **Tx OF OSTEOARTHRITIS** *Adult:* 100–150 mg/day PO in divided doses *(Voltaren),* or 50 mg bid–tid PO *(Cataflam).* For upper extremities, apply 2 g gel to affected area qid; for lower extremities, apply 4 g gel to affected area qid *(Voltaren).* Tx of rheumatoid arthritis. *Adult:* 150–200 mg/day PO in divided doses *(Voltaren),* or 50 mg bid–tid PO *(Cataflam).* **Tx of ankylosing spondylitis.** *Adult:* 100–125 mg/day PO. Give as 25 mg qid, w/ extra 25-mg dose at bedtime *(Voltaren),* or 25 mg PO qid w/ additional 25 mg at bedtime if needed *(Cataflam).* **Tx of acute migraine.** *Adult:* 50-mg packet mixed in 30–60 mL water PO as single dose at onset of headache *(Cambia).* **Tx of mild to moderate pain.** *Adult:* 25 mg liquid-filled capsule PO qid *(Zipsor; not interchangeable w/ other forms of diclofenac).* **Tx of actinic keratosis.** *Adult:* Cover lesion w/ topical gel, smooth into skin; do not cover w/ dressings or cosmetics *(Solaraze).* **Relief of postop inflammation from cataract extraction.** *Adult:* 1 drop to affected eye qid starting 24 hr after surgery for 2 wk.
ADV EFF Anaphylactoid reactions to fatal anaphylactic shock, constipation, diarrhea, dizziness, **CV events,** dyspepsia, GI pain, headache, nausea
INTERACTIONS Anticoagulants, lithium
NC/PT Give w/ meals if GI upset occurs. Add packets for oral suspension to 30–60 mL water. Remove old transdermal patch before applying new one to intact, dry skin. Institute emergency procedures if overdose occurs. Pt should swallow tablets whole and not cut, crush, or chew them; avoid sun if using topical gel; take safety precautions for CNS effects.

dicyclomine hydrochloride (Bentyl)

CLASS Anticholinergic, antispasmodic, parasympatholytic
PREG/CONT B/NA

IND & DOSE Tx of functional bowel or IBS. *Adult:* 160 mg/day PO divided into four equal doses or 80 mg/day IM in four divided doses; do not give IV.
ADJUST DOSE Elderly pts
ADV EFF Altered taste perception, blurred vision, decreased sweating, dry mouth, dysphagia, irritation at injection site, n/v/d, urinary hesitancy, urine retention
INTERACTIONS Amantadine, antipsychotics, atenolol, digoxin, TCAs
NC/PT IM use is only temporary; switch to oral form as soon as possible. Ensure hydration, temp control. Pt should avoid hot environments, empty bladder before taking if urine retention occurs, perform mouth care for dry mouth.

didanosine (ddI, dideoxyinosine) (Videx, Videx EC)

CLASS Antiviral
PREG/CONT B/NA

BBW Monitor for pancreatitis (abd pain, elevated enzymes, n/v). Stop drug; resume only if pancreatitis ruled out. Monitor pts w/ hepatic impairment; decrease may be needed if toxicity occurs. Fatal liver toxicity w/ lactic acidosis possible. Noncirrhotic portal hypertension, sometimes fatal, has occurred.
IND & DOSE Tx of pts w/ HIV infection w/ other antiretrovirals. *Adult, child:* DR capsules: 60 kg or more, 400 mg/day PO; 25–60 kg, 250 mg/day PO; 20–25 kg, 200 mg/day PO. Oral sol: 60 kg or more, 200 mg PO bid or 400 mg/day PO; under 60 kg, 125 mg PO bid or 250 mg/day PO. *Child over 8 mo:* Pediatric powder, 120 mg/m² PO bid. *Child 2 wk–8 mo:* 100 mg/m² PO bid.

ADJUST DOSE Renal, hepatic impairment
ADV EFF Abd pain, headache, hemopoietic depression, **hepatotoxicity, lactic acidosis,** n/v, **pancreatitis**
INTERACTIONS Antifungals, allopurinol, fluoroquinolones, ganciclovir, methadone, tetracyclines
NC/PT Monitor CBC, pancreatic enzymes, LFTs. Give on empty stomach 1 hr before or 2 hr after meals. Pediatric sol can be made by pharmacists; refrigerate. Pt should not cut, crush, or chew ER forms.

diflunisal (generic)

CLASS Analgesic, anti-inflammatory, antipyretic, NSAIDs
PREG/CONT C/NA

BBW Possible increased risk of CV events, GI bleeding; monitor accordingly. Do not use to treat periop pain after CABG surgery.
IND & DOSE Tx of mild to moderate pain. *Adult, child over 12 yr:* 1,000 mg PO initially, then 500 mg q 8–12 hr PO. Tx of osteoarthritis, rheumatoid arthritis. *Adult, child over 12 yr:* 500–1,000 mg/day PO in two divided doses; maint, no more than 1,500 mg/day.
ADV EFF Anaphylactoid reactions to anaphylactic shock, CV event, diarrhea, dizziness, dyspepsia, GI pain, headache, insomnia, nausea, rash
INTERACTIONS Acetaminophen, antacids, aspirin
NC/PT Give w/ food if GI upset. Pt should swallow tablets whole and not cut, crush, or chew them; take safety precautions for CNS effects; report unusual bleeding.

DANGEROUS DRUG

digoxin (Lanoxin)

CLASS Cardiac glycoside
PREG/CONT C/NA

IND & DOSE Tx of HF, atrial fibrillation. *Adult:* Loading dose, 0.25 mg/day

IV or PO for pts under 70 yr w/ good renal function; 0.125 mg/day PO or IV for pts over 70 yr or w/ impaired renal function; 0.0625 mg/day PO or IV w/ marked renal impairment. Maint, 0.125–0.5 mg/day PO. *Child:* Premature, 20 mcg/kg PO or 15–25 mcg/kg IV; neonate, 30 mcg/kg PO or 20–30 mcg/kg IV; 1–24 mo, 40–50 mcg/kg PO or 30–50 mcg/kg IV; 2–10 yr, 30–40 mcg/kg PO or 25–35 mcg/kg IV; over 10 yr, 10–15 mcg/kg PO or 8–12 mcg/kg IV as loading dose. Maint, 25%–35% of loading dose in divided doses; range, 0.125–0.5 mg/day PO.
ADJUST DOSE Elderly pts, impaired renal function
ADV EFF Arrhythmias, GI upset, headache, weakness, yellow vision
INTERACTIONS Amiodarone, bleomycin, charcoal, cholestyramine, colestipol, cyclophosphamide, cyclosporine, dobutamine in sol, erythromycin, ginseng, hawthorn, licorice, loop diuretics, metoclopramide, methotrexate, oral aminoglycosides, penicillamine, psyllium, quinidine, St. John's wort, tetracyclines, thiazide diuretics, thyroid hormone, verapamil
NC/PT Monitor apical pulse; withhold if under 60 in adults, under 90 in children. Check dose carefully. Do not give IM. Give on empty stomach. Monitor for therapeutic drug levels: 0.5–2 ng/mL. Pt should have to take pulse, weigh self daily, consult prescriber before taking OTC drugs or herbs, avoid St. John's wort, report slow or irregular pulse, yellow vision.

digoxin immune fab (DigiFab)
CLASS Antidote
PREG/CONT C/NA

IND & DOSE Tx of potentially life-threatening digoxin toxicity (serum digoxin over 10 ng/mL, serum potassium over 5 mEq/L in setting of

digoxin toxicity). *Adult, child:* Dose determined by serum digoxin level or estimate of amount of digoxin ingested. If no estimate possible and serum digoxin level unavailable, use 800 mg IV (20 vials *DigiFab*) See manufacturer's details; dose varies by digoxin level.
ADV EFF Anaphylaxis, HF, low cardiac output, hypokalemia
NC/PT Ensure no sheep allergies. Monitor serum digoxin before tx. Have life-support equipment on hand. Do not redigitalize until drug has cleared (several days to a wk). Serum digoxin levels unreliable for up to 3 days after administration. Pt should report difficulty breathing.

dihydroergotamine mesylate (D.H.E. 45, Migranal)
CLASS Antimigraine, ergot
PREG/CONT X/NA

BBW Serious to life-threatening ischemia if taken w/ potent CYP3A4 inhibitors, including protease inhibitors, macrolide antibiotics; concurrent use contraindicated.
IND & DOSE Tx of migraine w/ or without aura; acute tx of cluster headaches. *Adult:* 1 mg IM, IV, or subcut at first sign of headache; may repeat at 1-hr intervals. Max, 3 mg, or 1 intranasal spray (0.5 mg) in each nostril followed in 15 min by another spray in each nostril (max, 3 mg).
ADV EFF CV events, nausea, numbness, rhinitis, tingling
INTERACTIONS CYP3A4 inhibitors, peripheral vasoconstrictors, sumatriptan
NC/PT Not for use in pregnancy, breast-feeding. May give antiemetic if nausea severe. Monitor BP; look for signs of vasospasm. Pt should to prime pump four times before use (nasal spray), report numbness or tingling, chest pain.

diltiazem hydrochloride
(Cardizem, Diltzac)
CLASS Antianginal, antihypertensive, calcium channel blocker
PREG/CONT C/NA

IND & DOSE Tx of angina pectoris. *Adult:* Initially, 30 mg PO qid before meals and at bedtime; gradually increase at 1- to 2-day intervals to 180–360 mg PO in three to four divided doses. Or, 120–360 mg/day (ER, SR forms) PO, depending on brand. Tx of essential hypertension. *Adult:* 180–240 mg PO daily *(Cardizem CD, Cartia XT).* 120–540 mg PO daily *(Cardizem LA).* 180–240 mg PO daily *(Diltia XT, Dilt-CD, Dilt-XR).* 120–240 mg PO daily *(Tiazac, Taztia XT).* Tx of supraventricular tachycardia, atrial fibrillation, atrial flutter. *Adult:* Direct IV bolus, 0.25 mg/kg over 2 min; second bolus of 0.35 mg/kg over 2 min after 15 min if response inadequate. Or, 5–10 mg/hr by continuous IV infusion w/ increases up to 15 mg/hr; may continue for up to 24 hr.
ADV EFF Asthenia, **asystole**, bradycardia, dizziness, edema, flushing, light-headedness, nausea
INTERACTIONS Beta blockers, cyclosporine, grapefruit juice
NC/PT Monitor closely while establishing dose. Pt should swallow ER/SR tablets whole and not cut, crush, or chew them; avoid grapefruit juice; report irregular heart beat, swelling.

dimenhyDRINATE
(Dimetabs, Dramamine, Dymenate)
CLASS Anticholinergic, antihistamine, anti–motion sickness drug
PREG/CONT B/NA

IND & DOSE Px, tx of n/v or vertigo of motion sickness. *Adult:* 50–100 mg PO q 4–6 hr; for px, pt should take first dose 30 min before exposure to motion. Max, 400 mg/24 hr. Or, 50 mg IM as needed, or 50 mg in 10 mL sodium chloride injection IV over 2 min. *Child 6–12 yr:* 25–50 mg PO q 6–8 hr; max, 150 mg/day.
ADJUST DOSE Elderly pts
ADV EFF Anaphylaxis, confusion, dizziness, drowsiness, heaviness/weakness of hands, lassitude, nervousness, restlessness, vertigo
INTERACTIONS Alcohol, CNS depressants
NC/PT Have epinephrine on hand during IV use. Pt should use 30 min before motion sickness–inducing event, avoid alcohol, take safety precautions w/ CNS effects.

dimercaprol (BAL in Oil)
CLASS Antidote, chelate
PREG/CONT C/NA

IND & DOSE Tx of arsenic, gold poisoning *Adult, child:* 25 mg/kg deep IM four times/day for 2 days, two times/day on third day, then once daily for 10 days. Tx of mercury poisoning. *Adult, child:* 5 mg/kg IM, then 2.5 mg/kg once daily or bid for 10 days. Tx of lead poisoning w/ edetate calcium. *Adult, child:* 4 mg/kg IM for first dose, then at 4-hr intervals w/ edetate calcium for 2–7 days.
ADJUST DOSE Hepatic impairment
ADV EFF Abd pain, burning sensation in lips/mouth, constricted feeling in throat/chest, headache, nausea, sweating
INTERACTIONS Alcohol, CNS depressants
NC/PT Use extreme caution w/ peanut allergy. Use deep IM injection. Pt should report constricted feeling in throat/chest, difficulty breathing.

dimethyl fumarate
(Tecfidera)
CLASS MS drug, nicotinic
receptor agonist
PREG/CONT C/NA

IND & DOSE Tx of relapsing MS.
Adult: 120 mg PO bid for 7 days; then
240 mg PO bid.
ADV EFF Abd pain, dizziness, dyspepsia, flushing, lymphopenia, n/v/d,
rash
NC/PT Obtain baseline and periodic
CBC, LFTs; withhold w/ serious infection. Use cautiously w/ pregnancy,
breast-feeding. Pt should swallow capsule whole and not cut, crush, or chew
it (may open and sprinkle on food);
avoid infections; dress in layers if flushing occurs; report continued n/v/d, severe rash, worsening of MS sx.

dinoprostone (Cervidil,
Prepidil, Prostin E2)
CLASS Abortifacient,
prostaglandin
PREG/CONT C/NA

IND & DOSE Termination of pregnancy 12–20 wk from first day of last
menstrual period; evacuation of
uterus in mgt of missed abortion.
Adult: 1 suppository (20 mg) high
into vagina; keep pt supine for 10 min
after insertion. May give additional
suppositories at 3- to 5-hr intervals,
based on uterine response and tolerance, for up to 2 days. **Initiation of
cervical ripening before labor induction.** *Adult:* 0.5 mg gel via provided
cervical catheter w/ pt in dorsal position and cervix visualized using spec-
ulum. May repeat dose if no response
in 6 hr. Wait 6–12 hr before beginning
oxytocin IV to initiate labor. For insert: Place 1 insert transversely in posterior fornix of vagina. Keep pt supine
for 2 hr (1 insert delivers 0.3 mg/hr
over 12 hr). Remove, using retrieval
system, at onset of active labor or
12 hr after insertion.

ADV EFF Dizziness, headache, hypotension, n/v/d, **perforated uterus**
NC/PT Store suppositories in freezer; bring to room temp before insertion. Keep pt supine after vaginal insertion. Ensure abortion complete.
Give antiemetics, antidiarrheals if
needed. Monitor for uterine tone,
bleeding. Give support, encourage-
ment for procedure/progressing labor. Name confusion among *Prostin
VR Pediatric* (alprostadil), *Prostin FZ*
(dinoprost), *Prostin E2* (dinoprosa-
tone), *Prostin 15* (carboprost in
Europe); use extreme caution.

diphenhydrAMINE
hydrochloride (Benadryl
Allergy, Diphen AF,
Diphenhist)
CLASS Antihistamine, anti–
motion sickness,
antiparkinsonian, sedative
PREG/CONT B/NA

IND & DOSE Relief of sx of various
allergic reactions, motion sickness.
Adult: 25–50 mg PO q 4–6 hr; max,
300 mg/24 hr. Or, 10–50 mg IV or
deep IM or up to 100 mg if needed;
max, 400 mg/day. *Child 6–12 yr:*
12.5–25 mg PO tid–qid, or 5 mg/kg/day
PO, or 150 mg/m²/day PO; max,
150 mg/day. Or, 5 mg/kg/day or
150 mg/m²/day IV or deep IM injection. Max, 300 mg/day divided into
four doses. **Nighttime sleep aid.**
Adult: 50 mg PO at bedtime. **Cough
suppression.** *Adult:* 25 mg PO q 4 hr;
max, 150 mg/day (syrup). *Child 6–12 yr:*
12.5 mg PO q 4 hr. Max, 75 mg/24 hr
(syrup).
ADJUST DOSE Elderly pts
ADV EFF Agranulocytosis, anaphylactic shock, bronchial secretion
thickening, disturbed coordination,
dizziness, drowsiness, epigastric distress, **hemolytic anemia, hypoplastic anemia, leukopenia, pancytopenia, thrombocytopenia**
INTERACTIONS Alcohol, CNS depressants, MAOIs

NC/PT Monitor response; use smallest dose possible. Use syrup if swallowing tablets difficult. Pt should avoid alcohol, take safety precautions w/ CNS effects.

---

dipyridamole (Persantine)

CLASS Antianginal, antiplatelet, diagnostic agent
PREG/CONT B/NA

IND & DOSE Px of thromboembolism in pts w/ artificial heart valves, w/ warfarin. *Adult:* 75–100 mg PO qid. Diagnostic aid to assess CAD in pts unable to exercise. *Adult:* 0.142 mg/kg/min IV over 4 min.

ADV EFF Abd distress, dizziness, headache

INTERACTIONS Adenosine
NC/PT Monitor continually w/ IV use. Give oral drug at least 1 hr before meals. Pt should take safety precautions for light-headedness.

---

disopyramide phosphate (Norpace, Norpace CR)

CLASS Antiarrhythmic
PREG/CONT C/NA

BBW Monitor for possible refractory arrhythmias that can be life-threatening; reserve use for life-threatening arrhythmias.

IND & DOSE Tx of life-threatening ventricular arrhythmias. *Adult, child:* 400–800 mg/day PO in divided doses q 6 hr, or q 12 hr if using CR forms. Rapid control of ventricular arrhythmias. *Adult:* 300 mg (immediate-release) PO. If no response w/in 6 hr, 200 mg PO q 6 hr; may increase to 250–300 mg q 6 hr if no response in 48 hr. For pts w/ cardiomyopathy, no loading dose; 100 mg (immediate-release) PO q 6–8 hr.

ADJUST DOSE Renal, hepatic failure

ADV EFF Blurred vision, constipation, dry nose/eye/throat, **HF**, itching,

malaise, muscle aches and pains, urinary hesitancy, urine retention

INTERACTIONS Antiarrhythmics, erythromycin, phenytoin, quinidine
NC/PT Monitor ECG carefully. Make pediatric suspension (1–10 mg/mL) by adding contents of immediate-release capsule to cherry syrup, if desired. Store in amber glass bottle; refrigerate up to 1 mo. Evaluate pt for safe, effective serum levels (2–8 mcg/mL). Pt should swallow CR forms whole and not cut, crush, or chew them; not stop taking without consulting prescriber; maintain hydration, empty bladder before taking.

---

disulfiram (Antabuse)

CLASS Antialcoholic, enzyme inhibitor
PREG/CONT C/NA

BBW Never give to intoxicated pt or without pt's knowledge. Do not give until pt has abstained from alcohol for at least 12 hr.

IND & DOSE Aid in mgt of selected chronic alcoholics who want to remain in state of enforced sobriety. *Adult:* 500 mg/day PO in single dose for 1–2 wk. If sedative effect occurs, give at bedtime or decrease dose. Maint, 125–500 mg/day PO; max, 500 mg/day.

ADV EFF Dizziness, fatigue, headache, metal- or garlic-like aftertaste, skin eruptions; if taken w/ alcohol, **arrhythmias, CV collapse, death, HF, MI**

INTERACTIONS Alcohol, caffeine, chlordiazepoxide, diazepam, metronidazole, oral anticoagulants, theophyllines
NC/PT Do not give until pt has abstained from alcohol for at least 12 hr. Monitor LFTs, CBC before and q 6 mo of tx. May crush tablets and mix w/ liquid beverages. Institute supportive measures if pt drinks alcohol during tx. Pt should abstain from all forms of alcohol (serious to fatal reactions possible if combined), wear/carry

medical ID, take safety precautions for CNS effects.

DANGEROUS DRUG

DOBUTamine hydrochloride (generic)

CLASS Beta₁-selective adrenergic agonist, sympathomimetic
PREG/CONT B/NA

IND & DOSE Short-term tx of cardiac decompensation. *Adult:* Usual rate, 2–20 mcg/kg/min IV to increase cardiac output; rarely, rates up to 40 mcg/kg/min. *Child:* 0.5–1 mcg/kg/min as continuous IV infusion. Maint, 2–20 mcg/kg/min.
ADV EFF Headache, hypertension, nausea, PVCs, tachycardia
INTERACTIONS Methyldopa, TCAs
NC/PT Monitor urine flow, cardiac output, pulmonary wedge pressure, ECG, BP closely during infusion; adjust dose, rate accordingly. Arrange to digitalize pt w/ atrial fibrillation w/ rapid ventricular rate before giving dobutamine (dobutamine facilitates AV conduction). Name confusion between dobutamine and dopamine; use caution.

DANGEROUS DRUG

docetaxel (Docefrez, Taxotere)

CLASS Antineoplastic
PREG/CONT D/NA

BBW Do not give unless blood counts are within acceptable range (neutrophils over 1,500 cells/m²). Do not give w/ hepatic impairment; increased risk of toxicity and death. Monitor LFTs carefully. Monitor for hypersensitivity reactions, possibly severe. Do not give w/ hx of hypersensitivity. Monitor carefully for fluid retention; treat accordingly.
IND & DOSE Tx of breast cancer. *Adult:* 60–100 mg/m² IV infused over 1 hr q 3 wk. **Tx of non-small-cell lung**

cancer. *Adult:* 75 mg/m² IV over 1 hr q 3 wk. **First-line tx of non-small-cell lung cancer.** *Adult:* 75 mg/m² over 1 hr, then 75 mg/m² cisplatin IV over 30–60 min q 3 wk. **Tx of androgen-independent metastatic prostate cancer.** *Adult:* 75 mg/m² IV q 3 wk as 1-hr infusion w/ 5 mg prednisone PO bid constantly throughout tx. Reduce dose to 60 mg/m² if febrile neutropenia, severe or cumulative cutaneous reactions, moderate neurosensory s&sx, or neutrophil count under 500/mm³ occurs for longer than 1 wk. Stop tx if reactions continue w/ reduced dose. **Tx of operable node-positive breast cancer.** *Adult:* 75 mg/m² IV 1 hr after doxorubicin 50 mg/m² and cyclophosphamide 500 mg/m² q 3 wk for 6 courses. **Induction for squamous cell cancer of head and neck before radiotherapy.** *Adult:* 75 mg/m² as 1-hr IV infusion, then cisplatin 75 mg/m² IV over 1 hr on day 1, then 5-FU 750 mg/m²/day IV for 5 days. Repeat q 3 wk for four cycles before radiotherapy starts. **Induction for squamous cell cancer of head and neck before chemoradiotherapy.** *Adult:* 75 mg/m² as 1-hr IV infusion, then cisplatin 100 mg/m² as 30-min–3-hr infusion, then 5-FU 1,000 mg/m²/day as continuous infusion on days 1–4. Give q 3 wk for three cycles before chemoradiotherapy starts. **Tx of advanced gastric adenocarcinoma.** *Adult:* 75 mg/m² IV as 1-hr infusion, then cisplatin 75 mg/m² IV as 1–3-hr infusion (both on day 1), then 5-FU 750 mg/m²/day IV as 24-hr infusion for 5 days. Repeat cycle q 3 wk.
ADJUST DOSE Hepatic impairment
ADV EFF Alopecia, arthralgia, asthenia, **bone marrow suppression, fluid retention,** hypersensitivity reactions, infection, myalgia, n/v/d, stomatitis
INTERACTIONS Cyclosporine, erythromycin, immunosuppressants, ketoconazole
NC/PT Handle drug carefully. Premedicate w/ oral corticosteroids to reduce fluid retention. Monitor CBC

before each dose; adjust dose as needed. Monitor LFTs; do not give w/ hepatic impairment. Monitor for fluid retention; treat accordingly. Protect from infection. Give antiemetics if needed. Pt should cover head at temp extremes (hair loss possible), mark calendar for tx days, take safety precautions for CNS effects. Name confusion between *Taxotere* (docetaxel) and *Taxol* (paclitaxel); use extreme caution.

dofetilide (Tikosyn)
CLASS Antiarrhythmic
PREG/CONT C/NA

BBW Monitor ECG before and periodically during administration. Monitor pt continually for at least 3 days. May adjust dose based on maint of sinus rhythm. Risk of induced arrhythmias.

IND & DOSE Conversion of atrial fibrillation (AF) or flutter to normal sinus rhythm; maint of sinus rhythm after conversion from AF. *Adult:* Dose based on ECG response and CrCl. CrCl over 60 mL/min, 500 mcg PO bid; CrCl 40–60 mL/min, 250 mcg PO bid; CrCl 20–under 40 mL/min, 125 mcg PO bid; CrCl under 20 mL/min, use contraindicated.

ADJUST DOSE Renal impairment
ADV EFF Fatigue, dizziness, headache, **ventricular arrhythmias**
INTERACTIONS Antihistamines, cimetidine, ketoconazole, phenothiazines, TCAs, trimethoprim, verapamil; contraindicated w/ amiodarone, disopyramide, procainamide, quinidine, sotalol

NC/PT Determine time of arrhythmia onset. Monitor ECG before and periodically during tx. Monitor serum creatinine before and q 3 mo during tx. Do not attempt cardioversion within 24 hr of starting tx. Pt should take bid at about same time each day, keep follow-up appointments, take safety precautions w/ CNS effects.

dolasetron mesylate (Anzemet)
CLASS Antiemetic, serotonin receptor blocker
PREG/CONT B/NA

IND & DOSE Px, tx of n/v associated w/ emetogenic chemotherapy (oral only). *Adult:* 100 mg PO within 1 hr before chemotherapy. *Child 2–16 yr:* 1.8 mg/kg PO tablets or injection diluted in apple or apple-grape juice within 1 hr before chemotherapy. **Px, tx of postop n/v.** *Adult:* 100 mg PO within 2 hr before surgery, or 12.5 mg IV about 15 min before stopping anesthesia for px, or 12.5 mg IV as soon as needed for tx. *Child 2–16 yr:* 1.2 mg/kg PO tablets or injection diluted in apple or apple-grape juice within 2 hr before surgery, or 0.35 mg/kg IV about 15 min before stopping anesthesia for px, or 0.35 mg/kg IV as soon as needed for tx. Max, 12.5 mg/dose.
ADV EFF Fatigue, diarrhea, dizziness, headache, prolonged QT, tachycardia
INTERACTIONS Anthracycline, QT-prolonging drugs, rifampin
NC/PT Do not use IV for chemotherapy-induced n/v. Monitor ECG before and regularly during tx. Pt should perform proper mouth care, use sugarless lozenges, use analgesics for headache, take safety precautions w/ CNS effects.

dolutegravir (Tivicay)
CLASS Antiviral, integrase inhibitor
PREG/CONT B/NA

IND & DOSE Tx of HIV-1 infection in combination w/ other antiretrovirals. *Adult, child 12 yr and older weighing at least 40 kg:* 50 mg/day PO; w/ efavirenz, fosamprenavir/ritonavir, tipranavir/ritonavir, rifampin, or suspected resistance, 50 mg PO bid.

ADV EFF Abd pain, diarrhea, fat redistribution, headache, hepatotoxicity in pts with hepatitis B or C, insomnia, nausea

INTERACTIONS Antacids, buffered drugs, calcium supplements, efavirenz, fosamprenavir/ritonavir, iron supplements, laxatives, rifampin, sucralfate, tipranavir/ritonavir

NC/PT Screen for hepatitis B or C before tx. Must be given w/ other antiretrovirals; give cation-containing drugs at least 2 hr before or 6 hr after dolutegravir. Pt should continue other HIV drugs; space antacids apart from dosing; avoid pregnancy, breast-feeding; take precautions to avoid spread; not run out of prescription; report sx of infection, difficulty breathing, changes in urine/stool color.

---

donepezil hydrochloride (Aricept, Aricept ODT)

CLASS Alzheimer drug, anticholinesterase inhibitor
PREG/CONT C/NA

IND & DOSE Tx of Alzheimer-type dementia, including severe dementia. *Adult:* 5 mg/day PO at bedtime; may increase to 10 mg daily after 4–6 wk; 10 mg PO daily for severe disease. May use 23 mg/day after 10 mg/day for at least 3 mo.

ADV EFF Abd pain, anorexia, dyspepsia, fatigue, **hepatotoxicity**, insomnia, muscle cramps, n/v/d, rash

INTERACTIONS Anticholinergics, cholinesterase inhibitors, NSAIDs, theophylline

NC/PT Monitor hepatic function. Give at bedtime. Pt should place disintegrating tablet on tongue, allow to dissolve, then drink water; take safety precautions; report severe n/v/d. Name confusion between *Aricept* (donepezil) and *Aciphex* (rabeprazole); use caution.

DOPamine hydrochloride (generic)

CLASS Dopaminergic, sympathomimetic
PREG/CONT C/NA

BBW To prevent sloughing/necrosis after extravasation, infiltrate area w/ 10–15 mL saline containing 5–10 mg phentolamine as soon as possible after extravasation.

IND & DOSE Correction of hemodynamic imbalance, low cardiac output, hypotension. *Adult:* Pts likely to respond to modest increments of cardiac contractility and renal perfusion, 2–5 mcg/kg/min IV initially. More seriously ill pts, 5 mcg/kg/min IV initially. Increase in increments of 5–10 mcg/kg/min to rate of 20–50 mcg/kg/min.

ADV EFF Angina, dyspnea, ectopic beats, hypotension, n/v, palpitations, tachycardia

INTERACTIONS MAOIs, methyldopa, phenytoin, TCAs; do not mix in IV sol w/ other drugs

NC/PT Use extreme caution in calculating doses. Base dosing on pt response. Give in large vein; avoid extravasation. Monitor urine output, cardiac output, BP during infusion. Name confusion between dopamine and dobutamine; use caution.

---

doripenem (Doribax)

CLASS Carbapenem antibiotic
PREG/CONT B/NA

IND & DOSE Tx of complicated intra-abdominal infections, UTIs caused by susceptible bacteria strains. *Adult:* 500 mg IV over 1 hr q 8 hr for 5–14 days (intra-abdominal infection) or 10 days (UTI, pyelonephritis).

ADJUST DOSE Renal impairment
ADV EFF Diarrhea including *Clostridium difficile* diarrhea, headache, nausea, phlebitis, rash

INTERACTIONS Probenecid, valproic acid
NC/PT Culture, sensitivity before tx. Monitor injection site for phlebitis. Not for use in pregnancy (barrier contraceptives advised), breast-feeding. Monitor for *C. difficile* diarrhea. Provide supportive tx for up to 2 mo after tx ends.

---

dornase alfa (Pulmozyme)
CLASS Cystic fibrosis drug
PREG/CONT B/NA

IND & DOSE Mgt of cystic fibrosis to improve pulmonary function, w/ other drugs. *Adult, child:* 2.5 mg inhaled through recommended nebulizer; bid use beneficial to some.
ADV EFF Chest pain, laryngitis, pharyngitis, rash, rhinitis
NC/PT Assess respiratory function regularly. Store in refrigerator; not stable after 24 hr at room temp. Do not mix in nebulizer w/ other drugs; review proper use of nebulizer. Pt should continue other drugs for cystic fibrosis.

---

doxapram hydrochloride (Dopram)
CLASS Analeptic, respiratory stimulant
PREG/CONT B/NA

IND & DOSE Stimulation of respiration in pts w/ drug-induced postanesthesia respiratory depression. *Adult:* Single injection of 0.5–1 mg/kg IV; max, 1.5 mg/kg as total single injection or 2 mg/kg when given as multiple injections at 5-min intervals. **Tx of COPD associated acute hypercapnia.** *Adult:* Mix 400 mg in 180 mL IV infusion; start infusion at 1–2 mg/min (0.5–1 mL/min); no longer than 2 hr. Max, 3 mg/min. **Mgt of drug-induced CNS depression.** *Adult:* 1–2 mg/kg IV; repeat in 5 min. Repeat q 1–2 hr until pt awakens. Or, priming dose of 1–2 mg/kg IV; if no response, infuse 250 mg in 250 mL dextrose or saline sol at rate of 1–3 mg/min, discontinue after 2 hr if pt awakens; repeat in 30 min–2 hr if relapse occurs. Max, 3 g/day.
ADV EFF Bronchospasm, cough, hypertension, increased reflexes, **seizures**
INTERACTIONS Aminophylline, enflurane, halothane, MAOIs, muscle relaxants, sympathomimetics, theophylline
NC/PT Give IV only. Monitor for extravasation. Continuously monitor pt until fully awake. Discontinue if sudden hypotension, deterioration occur.

---

doxazosin mesylate (Cardura, Cardura XL)
CLASS Antihypertensive, alpha-adrenergic blocker
PREG/CONT C/NA

IND & DOSE Tx of mild to moderate hypertension. *Adult:* 1 mg PO daily; maint, 2, 4, 8, or 16 mg PO daily. May increase q 2 wk. Do not use ER tablets. **Tx of BPH.** *Adult:* 1 mg PO daily; maint, 2, 4, 8 mg daily. Or, ER tablets, 4 mg PO once daily at breakfast. Max, 8 mg/day PO.
ADV EFF Diarrhea, dizziness, dyspepsia, edema, fatigue, headache, lethargy, nausea, orthostatic hypotension, palpitations, sexual dysfx, tachycardia
INTERACTIONS Alcohol, antihypertensives, nitrates, sildenafil
NC/PT Monitor pt carefully w/ first dose; chance of orthostatic hypotension, dizziness, syncope greatest w/ first dose. Monitor for edema, BPH s&sx. Pt should swallow ER tablets whole and not cut, crush, or chew them, take safety precautions.

---

doxepin hydrochloride (Prudoxin, Silenor, Sinequan, Zonalon)
CLASS Antidepressant, TCA
PREG/CONT C/NA

BBW Increased risk of suicidality in children, adolescents, young adults; monitor carefully.

IND & DOSE Tx of mild to moderate anxiety, depression. *Adult:* 25 mg PO tid. Individualize dose; range, 75–150 mg/day. **Tx of more severe anxiety, depression.** *Adult:* 50 mg PO tid; max, 300 mg/day. **Tx of mild symptoms or emotional symptoms accompanying organic disease.** *Adult:* 25–50 mg PO. **Tx of pruritus.** *Adult:* Apply cream four times/day at least 3–4 hr apart for 8 days. Do not cover dressing. **Tx of insomnia w/ difficulty in sleep maintenance (***Silenor***).** *Adult:* 3–6 mg PO 30 min before bed.

ADV EFF Anticholinergic effects, confusion, constipation, disturbed concentration, dry mouth, **MI**, orthostatic hypotension, photosensitivity, sedation, **stroke**, urine retention, withdrawal symptoms w/ prolonged use

INTERACTIONS Alcohol, anticholinergics, barbiturates, cimetidine, clonidine, disulfiram, ephedrine, epinephrine, fluoxetine, furazolidone, hormonal contraceptives, levodopa, MAOIs, methylphenidate, nicotine, norepinephrine, phenothiazines, QT-prolonging drugs, thyroid medication

NC/PT Restrict drug access in depressed, suicidal pts. Give major portion at bedtime. Dilute oral concentrate w/ approximately 120 mL water, milk, fruit juice just before administration. Pt should be aware of sedative effects (avoid driving, etc); not mix w/ other sleep-inducing drugs, alcohol; avoid prolonged exposure to sun, sunlamps; report thoughts of suicide. Name confusion between Sinequan and saquinavir; use caution.

---

doxercalciferol (Hectorol)
CLASS Vitamin D analogue
PREG/CONT B/NA

IND & DOSE To reduce parathyroid hormone in mgt of secondary hyperparathyroidism in pts undergoing chronic renal dialysis; secondary hyperparathyroidism in pts w/ stage 3, 4 chronic kidney disease without

dialysis. *Adult:* 10 mcg PO three times/wk at dialysis; max, 20 mcg three times/wk. Without dialysis, 1 mcg/day PO; max, 3.5 mcg/day.

ADV EFF Dizziness, dyspnea, edema, headache, malaise, N/V

INTERACTIONS Cholestyramine, magnesium-containing antacids, mineral oil, phenothiazines, QT-prolonging drugs, thyroid medication

NC/PT Monitor for vitamin D toxicity. Give w/ non-aluminum-containing phosphate binders. Monitor vitamin D levels predialysis.

DANGEROUS DRUG

DOXOrubicin hydrochloride (Doxil)
CLASS Antineoplastic
PREG/CONT D/NA

BBW Accidental substitution of liposomal form for conventional form has caused serious adverse reactions; check carefully before giving. Monitor for extravasation, burning, stinging. If these occur, discontinue; restart in another vein. For local subcut extravasation, local infiltration w/ corticosteroid may be ordered. Flood area w/ normal saline; apply cold compress. If ulceration, arrange consult w/ plastic surgeon. Monitor pt's response often at start of tx: serum uric acid, cardiac output (listen for S_3). CBC changes may require dose decrease; consult physician. Risk of HF, myelosuppression, liver damage. Record doses given to monitor total dosage; toxic effects often dose-related, as total dose approaches 550 mg/m².

IND & DOSE To produce regression in ALL, AML; Wilms' tumor; neuroblastoma; soft-tissue, bone sarcoma; breast, ovarian carcinoma; transitional cell bladder carcinoma; thyroid carcinoma; Hodgkin, non-Hodgkin lymphoma; bronchogenic carcinoma. *Adult:* 60–75 mg/m² as single IV injection given at 21-day intervals. Alternate schedule: 30 mg/m² IV on each of 3 successive days, repeated q 4 wk. **Tx of AIDS-related Kaposi sarcoma** (liposomal form). *Adult:* 20 mg/m² IV q 3 wk starting w/ initial rate of 1 mg/min. **Tx of ovarian cancer that has progressed or recurred after platinum-based chemotherapy.** *Adult:* 50 mg/m² IV at 1 mg/min; if no adverse effects, complete infusion in 1 hr. Repeat q 4 wk.

ADJUST DOSE Elevated bilirubin

ADV EFF Anaphylaxis, cardiac toxicity, complete but reversible alopecia, mucositis, myelosuppression, n/v, red urine

INTERACTIONS Digoxin

NC/PT Do not give IM or subcut. Monitor for extravasation. Ensure hydration. Not for use in pregnancy. Name confusion between conventional doxorubicin and liposomal doxorubicin; use caution.

---

doxycycline (Atridox, Doryx, Doxy 100, Oracea, Vibramycin)

CLASS Tetracycline
PREG/CONT D/NA

IND & DOSE *Tx of infections caused by susceptible bacteria strains; tx of infections when penicillin contraindicated. Adult, child over 8 yr, over 45 kg:* 200 mg IV in one or two infusions (each over 1–4 hr) on first tx day, then 100–200 mg/day IV, depending on infection severity. Or, 200 mg PO on day 1, then 100 mg/day PO. *Child over 8 yr, under 45 kg:*. 4.4 mg/kg IV in one or two infusions, then 2.2–4.4 mg/kg/day IV in one or two infusions. Or, 4.4 mg/kg PO in two divided doses on first tx day, then 2.2–4.4 mg/kg/day on subsequent days. **Tx of rosacea.** *Adult:* 40 mg/day PO in a.m. on empty stomach w/ full glass of water for up to 9 mo. **Tx of primary or secondary syphilis.** *Adult, child over 8 yr, over 45 kg:* 100 mg PO bid for 14 days. **Tx of acute gonococcal infection.** *Adult, child over 8 yr, over 45 kg:* 100 mg PO, then 100 mg at bedtime, then 100 mg bid for 3 days.

Or, 300 mg PO, then 300 mg in 1 hr. **Px of traveler's diarrhea.** *Adult, child over 8 yr, over 45 kg:* 100 mg/day PO. **Px of malaria.** *Adult, child over 8 yr, over 45 kg* 100 mg PO daily. *Child over 8 yr, under 45 kg:* 2 mg/kg/day PO; max, 100 mg/day. **Px of anthrax.** *Adult, child over 8 yr, over 45 kg:* 100 mg PO bid for 60 days. *Child over 8 yr, under 45 kg:* 2.2 mg/kg PO bid for 60 days. **CDC recommendations for STDs.** *Adult, child over 8 yr, over 45 kg:* 100 mg PO bid for 7–28 days depending on disease. **Periodontal disease.** *Adult, child over 8 yr, over 45 kg:* 20 mg PO bid, after scaling, root planing. **Tx of Lyme disease.** *Child over 8 yr, less than 45 kg:* 2.2 mg/kg PO bid for 60 days or 100 mg PO bid for 14–21 days.

ADJUST DOSE Elderly pts, renal impairment

ADV EFF Anorexia, bone marrow suppression, discoloring of teeth/inadequate bone calcification (of fetus when used during pregnancy, of child when used if under 8 yr), exfoliative dermatitis, glossitis, hepatic failure, n/v/d, phototoxic reactions, rash, superinfections

INTERACTIONS Alkali, antacids, barbiturates, carbamazepine, dairy foods, digoxin, iron, penicillins, phenytoins

NC/PT Culture before tx. Give w/ food if GI upset severe. Not for use in pregnancy, breast-feeding. Pt should complete full course of therapy, avoid sun exposure.

---

dronabinol (delta-9-tetrahydrocannabinol, delta-9-THC) (Marinol)

CLASS Antiemetic, appetite suppressant
PREG/CONT C/C-III

IND & DOSE *Tx of n/v associated w/ cancer chemotherapy. Adult, child:* 5 mg/m² PO 1–3 hr before chemotherapy administration. Repeat q 2–4 hr after chemotherapy, for total of four to six doses/day. If 5 mg/m² ineffective and no significant side effects, increase by 2.5–mg/m² increments to max, 15 mg/m²/dose. **Tx of anorexia associated w/ weight loss in pts w/ AIDS.** *Adult, child:* 2.5 mg PO bid before lunch and dinner. May reduce to 2.5 mg/day as single evening or bedtime dose; max, 10 mg PO bid (max not recommended for children).

ADV EFF Dependence w/ use over 30 days, depression, dry mouth, dizziness, drowsiness, hallucinations, headache, heightened awareness, impaired coordination, irritability, sluggishness, unsteadiness, visual disturbances

INTERACTIONS Alcohol, anticholinergics, antihistamines, CNS depressants, dofetilide, ritonavir, TCAs

NC/PT Store capsules in refrigerator. Supervise pt during first use to evaluate CNS effects. Discontinue if psychotic reactions; warn pt about CNS effects. Pt should avoid marijuana (drug contains same active ingredient), take safety precautions for CNS effects, avoid alcohol and OTC sleeping aids.

dronedarone (Multaq)
CLASS Antiarrhythmic
PREG/CONT X/NA

BBW Contraindicated in pts w/ symptomatic HF or recent hospitalization for HF; double risk of death. Contraindicated in pts with AF who cannot be cardioverted; double risk of death, stroke.

IND & DOSE To reduce risk of CV hospitalization in pts w/ paroxysmal or persistent AF or atrial flutter w/ recent episode of either and associated CV risk factors who are in sinus rhythm or will be cardioverted. *Adult:* 400 mg PO bid w/ a.m. and p.m. meal.

ADV EFF Asthenia, **HF**, n/v/d, QT prolongation, rash, **serious hepatotoxicity, stroke**

INTERACTIONS Antiarrhythmics, beta blockers, calcium channel blockers, CYP3A inhibitors/inducers, digoxin, grapefruit juice, sirolimus, statins, St. John's wort, tacrolimus

NC/PT Obtain baseline, periodic ECG. Do not use in pt w/ permanent AF or serious HF. Monitor LFTs during tx. Not for use in pregnancy, breastfeeding. Pt should avoid grapefruit juice, St. John's wort; keep complete list of all drugs and report use to all health care providers; comply w/ frequent ECG monitoring; not make up missed doses; report difficulty breathing, rapid weight gain, extreme fatigue.

droperidol (generic)
CLASS General anesthetic
PREG/CONT C/NA

BBW May prolong QT interval; reserve use for pts unresponsive to other tx. Monitor pt carefully.
IND & DOSE To reduce n/v associated w/ surgical procedures. *Adult:* 2.5 mg IM or IV. May use additional 1.2 mg w/ caution. *Child 2–12 yr:* 0.1 mg/kg IM or IV.
ADJUST DOSE Renal, hepatic impairment
ADV EFF Chills, drowsiness, hallucinations, hypotension, **prolonged QT w/ potentially fatal arrhythmias**, tachycardia
INTERACTIONS CNS depressants, opioids, QT-prolonging drugs
NC/PT Reserve use. Monitor ECG continually during tx and recovery. Pt should take safety precautions for CNS effects.

droxidopa (Northera)
CLASS Norepinephrine precursor
PREG/CONT C/NA

BBW Risk of supine hypertension. Raise head of bed to lessen effects; lower dose or discontinue drug if supine hypertension cannot be managed.

IND & DOSE Tx of orthostatic hypotension in adults w/ neurogenic orthostatic hypotension caused by autonomic failure. *Adult:* 100 mg PO tid; titrate in 100-mg-tid segments to max 600 mg PO tid. Effectiveness beyond 2 wk is unknown.

ADJUST DOSE Renal impairment

ADV EFF Confusion, dizziness, exacerbation of ischemic heart disease, fatigue, fever, headache, hypertension, nausea, supine hypertension

INTERACTIONS Carbidopa, levodopa

NC/PT Monitor BP carefully; raise head of bed to decrease supine hypertension. Administer last dose at least 3 hr before bedtime. Pt should avoid breast-feeding; take safety precautions w/ CNS changes; report drugs used for tx of Parkinson's disease, severe headache, chest pain, palpitations.

duloxetine hydrochloride (Cymbalta)
CLASS Antidepressant, serotonin/norepinephrine reuptake inhibitor
PREG/CONT C/NA

BBW Monitor for increased depression (agitation, irritability, increased suicidality), especially at start of tx and dose change. Most likely in children, adolescents, young adults. Provide appropriate interventions, protection. Drug not approved for children.

IND & DOSE Tx of major depressive disorder. *Adult:* 20 mg PO bid; max, 120 mg/day. Allow at least 14 days if switching from MAOI, 5 days if switching to MAOI. Tx of generalized anxiety disorder. *Adult:* 60 mg/day PO; max, 120 mg/day. Tx of diabetic neuropathic pain. *Adult:* 60 mg/day PO as single dose. Tx of fibromyalgia; chronic musculoskeletal pain. *Adult:* 30 mg/day PO for 1 wk; then increase to 60 mg/day.

ADV EFF Constipation, diarrhea, dizziness, dry mouth, fatigue, **hepatotoxicity,** sweating

INTERACTIONS Alcohol, aspirin, flecainide, fluvoxamine, linezolid, lithium, MAOIs, NSAIDs, phenothiazines, propafenone, quinidine, SSRIs, St. John's wort, tramadol, TCAs, triptans, warfarin

NC/PT Not for use in pregnancy, breast-feeding. Taper when discontinuing. Pt should swallow capsules whole and not cut, crush, or chew them; avoid alcohol, St John's wort; report thoughts of suicide; take safety precautions w/ dizziness.

dutasteride (Avodart)
CLASS BPH drug, androgen hormone inhibitor
PREG/CONT X/NA

IND & DOSE Tx of symptomatic BPH in men w/ an enlarged prostate gland *Adult:* 0.5 mg/day PO. W/ tamsulosin, 0.5 mg/day PO w/ tamsulosin 0.4. mg/day PO.

ADV EFF Decreased libido, enlarged breasts, GI upset

INTERACTIONS Cimetidine, ciprofloxacin, diltiazem, ketoconazole, ritonavir, saw palmetto, verapamil

NC/PT Assess to ensure BPH dx. Monitor prostate periodically. Pt should not father child and will not be able to donate blood during and for 6 mo after tx. Pregnant women should not handle capsule. Pt should swallow capsule whole and not cut, crush, or chew it; avoid saw palmetto.

dyphylline (Lufyllin, Lufyllin-400)
CLASS Bronchodilator, xanthine
PREG/CONT C/NA

IND & DOSE Symptomatic relief or px of bronchial asthma, reversible bronchospasm associated w/ chronic bronchitis, emphysema. *Adult:* Up to 15 mg/kg PO q 6 hr.

ADJUST DOSE Elderly, impaired pts
ADV EFF Headache, insomnia, n/v/d, seizures
INTERACTIONS Benzodiazepines, beta blockers, caffeine, halothane, mexiletine, NMJs, probenecid
NC/PT Have diazepam on hand for seizures. Give around the clock. Pt should avoid excessive intake of caffeine-containing beverages, take w/ food if GI effects severe.

---

ecallantide (Kalbitor)
CLASS Plasma kallikrein inhibitor
PREG/CONT C/NA

BBW Risk of severe anaphylaxis; have medical support on hand.
IND & DOSE Tx of acute attacks of hereditary angioedema. *Adult, child 16 yr and older:* 30 mg subcut as three 10-mg injections; may repeat once in 24 hr.
ADV EFF Anaphylaxis, fever, headache, injection-site reactions, nasopharyngitis, n/v/d
NC/PT Give only when able to provide medical support for anaphylaxis. Not for use in pregnancy, breast-feeding. Pt should report difficulty breathing.

---

eculizumab (Soliris)
CLASS Complement inhibitor, monoclonal antibody
PREG/CONT C/NA

BBW Pt must have received meningococcal vaccine at least 2 wk before tx. Drug increases risk of infection serious to fatal meningococcal infections have occurred.
IND & DOSE Tx of pts w/ paroxysmal nocturnal hemoglobinuria to reduce hemolysis. *Adult:* 600 mg IV over 35 min q 7 days for first 4 wk, then 900 mg IV as fifth dose 7 days later, then 900 mg IV q 14 days. *Child under 18 yr:* Base

dose on body weight; see manufacturer's recommendations. Tx of pts w/ atypical hemolytic uremic syndrome to inhibit complement-mediated thrombotic microangiopathy. *Adult:* 900 mg IV over 35 min for first 4 wk, then 1,200 mg IV for fifth dose 1 wk later, then 1,200 mg IV q 2 wk.
ADV EFF Back pain, headache, hemolysis, hypertension, meningococcal infections, nasopharyngitis, n/v/d, UTI
NC/PT Monitor for s&sx of meningococcal infection. Stopping drug can cause serious hemolysis. Must monitor pt for 8 wk after stopping; inform pt of risk for meningococcal infections. Not for use in pregnancy, breast-feeding. Pt should wear medical alert tag.

---

edetate calcium disodium (Calcium Disodium Versenate)
CLASS Antidote
PREG/CONT B/NA

BBW Reserve use for serious conditions requiring aggressive therapy; serious toxicity possible.
IND & DOSE Tx of acute/chronic lead poisoning, lead encephalopathy. *Adult, child:* For blood levels 20–70 mcg/dL, 1,000 mg/m²/day IV or IM for 5 days. For blood levels higher than 70 mcg/dL, combine w/ dimercaprol.
ADV EFF Electrolyte imbalance, headache, n/v/d, orthostatic hypotension
INTERACTIONS Zinc insulin
NC/PT Give IM or IV. Avoid excess fluids w/ encephalopathy. Establish urine flow by IV infusion before tx. Monitor BUN, electrolytes. Keep pt supine for short period after tx to prevent orthostatic hypotension. Pt should prepare calendar of tx days.

edrophonium chloride
(Enlon, Reversol)

CLASS Anticholinesterase, antidote, diagnostic agent, muscle stimulant
PREG/CONT C/NA

IND & DOSE Differential dx, adjunct in evaluating myasthenia gravis tx. *Adult:* Inject 10 mg IM. May retest w/ 2 mg IM after 30 min to rule out false-negative results. Or, 10 mg drawn into tuberculin syringe w/ IV needle. Inject 2 mg IV in 15–30 sec; leave needle in vein. If no reaction after 45 sec, inject remaining 8 mg. May repeat test after 30 min. *Child over 34 kg:* 2 mg IV or 5 mg IM. *Child 34 kg or less:* 1 mg or 2 mg IM. *Infants:* 0.5 mg IV. **Evaluation of myasthenia gravis tx.** *Adult:* 1–2 mg IV 1 hr after oral intake of edrophonium. Response determines effectiveness of tx. **Edrophonium test in crisis.** *Adult:* Secure controlled respiration immediately if pt apneic, then give test. If pt in cholinergic crisis, giving edrophonium will increase oropharyngeal secretions and further weaken respiratory muscles. If crisis myasthenic, giving edrophonium will improve respiration, and pt can be treated w/ longer-acting IV anticholinesterases. To give test, draw up no more than 2 mg into syringe. Give 1 mg IV initially. Carefully observe cardiac response. If after 1 min dose does not further impair pt, inject remaining 1 mg. If after 2-mg dose no clear improvement in respiration, discontinue all anticholinesterases; control ventilation by tracheostomy, assisted respiration. **Antidote for NMJ blockers.** *Adult:* 10 mg IV slowly over 30–45 sec so that onset of cholinergic reaction can be detected; repeat when necessary. Max, 40 mg.

ADV EFF Abd cramps; **anaphylaxis;** bradycardia; **cardiac arrest;** cardiac arrhythmias; dysphagia; increased lacrimation, pharyngeal/tracheobronchial secretions, salivation; miosis; urinary frequency/incontinence

INTERACTIONS Corticosteroids, succinylcholine

NC/PT Give slowly IV; have atropine sulfate on hand as antidote and antagonist to severe reaction. Testing can frighten pt; offer support, explain procedure.

efavirenz (Sustiva)

CLASS Antiviral, nonnucleoside reverse transcriptase inhibitor
PREG/CONT D/NA

IND & DOSE Tx of HIV/AIDS w/ other antiretrovirals. *Adult:* 600 mg/day PO w/ protease inhibitor or other nucleoside reverse transcriptase inhibitor. In combination w/ voriconazole 400 mg PO q 12 hr: 300 mg/day efavirenz PO. *Child 3 mo and older:* 40 kg or more, 600 mg/day PO; 32.5–under 40 kg, 400 mg/day PO; 25–under 32.5 kg, 350 mg/day PO; 20–under 25 kg, 300 mg/day PO; 15–under 20 kg, 250 mg/day PO; 10–under 15 kg, 200 mg/day PO; 5–under 10 kg, 150 mg/day PO; 3.5–under 5 kg, 100 mg/day PO.

ADV EFF Asthenia, dizziness, drowsiness, headache, n/v/d, rash

INTERACTIONS Alcohol, cisapride, ergot derivatives, hepatotoxic drugs, indinavir, methadone, midazolam, pimozide, rifabutin, rifampin, ritonavir, saquinavir, St. John's wort, triazolam, voriconazole

NC/PT Blood test needed q 2 wk. Ensure drug part of combination therapy. Give at bedtime for first 2–4 wk to minimize CNS effects. Not for use in pregnancy, breast-feeding. Not a cure; pt should use precautions. Pt should swallow tabs whole and not cut, crush, or chew them; avoid alcohol, report all drugs, herbals taken (including St. John's wort) to health care provider; seek regular medical care.

eletriptan hydrobromide (Relpax)

CLASS Antimigraine, triptan
PREG/CONT C/NA

IND & DOSE Tx of acute migraine w/ or without aura. *Adult:* 20–40 mg PO. If headache improves, then returns, may give second dose after at least 2 hr. Max, 80 mg/day.
ADV EFF Hypertonia, hypoesthesia, MI, pharyngitis, sweating, vertigo
INTERACTIONS Clarithromycin, ergots, itraconazole, ketoconazole, nefazodone, nelfinavir, ritonavir, SS-RIs, other triptans
NC/PT Tx only; not for migraine px. No more than two doses in 24 hr. Closely monitor BP w/ known CAD; discontinue if s&sx of angina. Not for use in pregnancy. Pt should take safety precautions for CNS effects, maintain usual measures for migraine relief.

elosulfase alfa (Vimizim)

CLASS Enzyme
PREG/CONT C/NA

BBW Risk of life-threatening anaphylaxis, hypersensitivity reaction. Monitor pt closely; be prepared to deal w/ anaphylaxis. Pts w/ acute respiratory illness at risk for life-threatening pulmonary complications; delay use with respiratory illness.
IND & DOSE Tx of mucopolysaccharidosis type IVA (Morquio A syndrome). *Adult, child 5 yr and over:* 2 mg/kg IV infused over 3.5–4.5 hr once a wk.
ADV EFF Abd pain, chills, fatigue, fever, headache, **hypersensitivity reaction,** vomiting
NC/PT Pretreat w/ antihistamines, antipyretic 30–60 min before infusion. Slow or stop infusion if sx of hypersensitivity reaction. Use cautiously in pregnancy, breast-feeding. Pt should report difficulty breathing, cough, rash, chest pain.

eltrombopag (Promacta)

CLASS Thrombopoietin receptor agonist
PREG/CONT C/NA

BBW Risk of severe to fatal hepatotoxicity. Monitor LFTs closely; adjust dose or discontinue as needed.
IND & DOSE Tx of chronic immune idiopathic thrombocytopenic purpura in pts unresponsive to usual tx. *Adult:* 50–75 mg/day PO. Start Eastern Asian pts at 25 mg/day.
ADJUST DOSE Moderate hepatic failure
ADV EFF Back pain, **bone marrow fibrosis,** cataracts, headache, **hepatotoxicity,** n/v/d, pharyngitis, **thrombotic events,** URI, UTI
INTERACTIONS Antacids, dairy products, oral anticoagulants, statins
NC/PT Do not give within 4 hr of antacids, dairy products. Monitor CBC, LFTs regularly for safety, dose adjustment. Not for use w/ blood cancers; worsening possible. Monitor for cataracts or vision changes. Not for use in pregnancy, breast-feeding. Pt should report chest pain, bleeding, yellowing of eyes, skin.

emtricitabine (Emtriva)

CLASS Antiviral, nucleoside reverse transcriptase inhibitor
PREG/CONT B/NA

BBW Use caution w/ current/suspected hepatitis B; serious disease resurgence possible. Withdraw drug, monitor pt w/ sx of lactic acidosis or hepatotoxicity, including hepatomegaly, steatosis.
IND & DOSE Tx of HIV-1 infection w/ other antiretrovirals. *Adult:* 200 mg/day PO or 240 mg (24 mL) oral sol/day PO. *Child 3 mo–17 yr:* 6 mg/kg/day PO to max 240 mg (24 mL) oral sol. For child over 33 kg able to swallow capsule, one 200-mg

capsule/day PO. *Child under 3 mo:* 3 mg/kg/day oral sol PO.
ADJUST DOSE Renal impairment
ADV EFF Abd pain, asthenia, cough, dizziness, headache, insomnia, **lactic acidosis,** n/v/d, rash, redistribution of body fat, rhinitis, **severe hepatomegaly w/ steatosis**
INTERACTIONS Atripla, lamivudine, Truvada; contraindicated
NC/PT HIV antibody testing before tx. Monitor LFTs, renal function regularly. Ensure use w/ other antiretrovirals. Not for use in pregnancy, breast-feeding. Not a cure; pt should use safety precautions. Pt should try to maintain nutrition, hydration (GI effects will occur).

enalapril maleate
(Epaned, Vasotec),
enalaprilat (Vasotec I.V.)
CLASS ACE inhibitor, antihypertensive
PREG/CONT D/NA

BBW Possible serious fetal injury or death if used in second, third trimesters; advise contraceptive use
IND & DOSE Tx of hypertension. *Adult:* Initially, 5 mg/day PO; range, 10–40 mg/day. Discontinue diuretics for 2–3 days before tx; if not possible, start w/ 2.5 mg/day PO or 1.25 mg IV q 6 hr; monitor pt response. If on diuretics, 0.625 mg IV over 5 min; repeat in 1 hr if needed, then 1.25 mg IV q 6 hr. *Child 1mo–16 yr:* 0.08 mg/kg PO once daily; max, 5 mg. **Tx of HF.** *Adult:* 2.5 mg PO bid or bid w/ diuretics, digitalis; max, 40 mg/day. **Tx of asymptomatic left ventricular dysfx.** *Adult:* 2.5 mg PO bid; target dose, 20 mg/day in two divided doses.
ADJUST DOSE Elderly pts, renal impairment, HF
ADV EFF Cough; decreased Hct, Hgb; diarrhea; dizziness; fatigue; **renal failure**
INTERACTIONS Indomethacin, NSAIDs, rifampin

NC/PT Adjust dose if pt also on diuretic. Peak effect may not occur for 4 hr. Monitor BP before giving second dose; monitor closely in situations that might lead to BP drop. Mark chart if surgery required; pt may need fluid support. Not for use in pregnancy (contraceptives advised). Pt should take safety precautions w/ CNS effects.

enfuvirtide (Fuzeon)
CLASS Anti-HIV drug, fusion inhibitor
PREG/CONT B/NA

IND & DOSE Tx of HIV-1 infection in tx-experienced pts w/ evidence of HIV-1 replication despite ongoing tx, w/ other antiretrovirals. *Adult:* 90 mg bid by subcut injection into upper arm, anterior thigh, or abdomen. *Child 6–16 yr:* 2 mg/kg bid by subcut injection; max, 90 mg/dose into upper arm, anterior thigh, or abdomen.
ADV EFF Dizziness, injection-site reactions, n/v/d, **pneumonia**
NC/PT Ensure pt also on other antiretrovirals; rotate injection sites (upper arm, anterior thigh, abdomen). Refrigerate reconstituted sol; use within 24 hr. Not for use in pregnancy, breast-feeding. Not a cure; pt should use safety precautions. Teach pt proper administration and disposal of syringes, needles.

DANGEROUS DRUG
enoxaparin (Lovenox)
CLASS Low-molecular-weight heparin
PREG/CONT B/NA

BBW Increased risk of spinal hematoma, neurologic damage if used w/ spinal/epidural anesthesia. If must be used, monitor pt closely.
IND & DOSE Px of DVT after hip, knee replacement surgery. *Adult:* 30 mg subcut bid, w/ initial dose 12–24 hr after surgery. Continue for

7–10 days; then may give 40 mg daily subcut for up to 3 wk. **Px of DVT after abd surgery.** Adult: 40 mg/day subcut begun within 2 hr before surgery, continued for 7–10 days; has been used up to 14 days. **Px of DVT in high-risk pts.** 40 mg/day subcut for 6–11 days; has been used up to 14 days. **Px of ischemic complications of unstable angina and non-Q-wave MI.** Adult: 1 mg/kg subcut q 12 hr for 2–8 days. **Tx of DVT.** Adult: 1 mg/kg subcut q 12 hr (for outpts); 1.5 mg/kg subcut q 12 hr or 1 mg/kg subcut q 12 hr (for inpts). **Tx of MI.** Adult: 75 yr and older, 0.75 mg/kg subcut q 12 hr (max, 75 mg for first two doses only). Under 75 yr, 30-mg IV bolus plus 1 mg/kg subcut followed by 1 mg/kg subcut q 12 hr w/ aspirin (max, 100 mg for first two doses only).

ADJUST DOSE Renal impairment

ADV EFF Bruising, chills, fever, **hemorrhage,** injection-site reactions

INTERACTIONS Aspirin, cephalosporins, chamomile, garlic, ginger, ginkgo, ginseng, high-dose vitamin E, NSAIDs, penicillins, oral anticoagulants, salicylates

NC/PT Give as soon as possible after hip surgery, within 12 hr of knee surgery, and within 2 hr preop for abd surgery. Use deep subcut injection, not IM; alternate sites. Do not mix w/ other injections or sols. Store at room temp. Have protamine sulfate on hand as antidote. Check for s&sx of bleeding; protect pt from injury. Teach pt proper administration and disposal of syringes, needles.

entacapone (Comtan)
CLASS Antiparkinsonian
PREG/CONT C/NA

IND & DOSE Adjunct w/ levodopa/carbidopa in tx of s&sx of idiopathic Parkinson's disease in pts experiencing "wearing off" of drug effects. Adult: 200 mg PO concomitantly w/ levodopa/carbidopa; max, eight times/day.

ADV EFF Confusion, disorientation, dizziness, dry mouth, dyskinesia, fever, **hallucinations,** hyperkinesia, hypotension, n/v, orthostatic hypotension, **rhabdomyolysis**

INTERACTIONS Ampicillin, apomorphine, chloramphenicol, cholestyramine, dobutamine, dopamine, epinephrine, erythromycin, isoetharine, isoproterenol, MAOIs, methyldopa, norepinephrine, rifampin

NC/PT Give only w/ levodopa/carbidopa; do not give within 14 days of MAOIs. Not for use in pregnancy (contraceptives advised), breast-feeding. Pt should use sugarless lozenges for dry mouth, take safety precautions w/ CNS effects.

entecavir (Baraclude)
CLASS Antiviral, nucleoside analogue
PREG/CONT C/NA

BBW Withdraw drug, monitor pt if s&sx of lactic acidosis or hepatotoxicity, including hepatomegaly and steatosis. Do not use in pts w/ HIV unless pt receiving highly active antiretroviral tx, because of high risk of HIV resistance. Offer HIV testing to all pts before starting entecavir. Severe, acute hepatitis B exacerbations have occurred in pts who discontinue antihepatitis tx. Monitor pts for several mo after drug cessation; restarting antihepatitis tx may be warranted.

IND & DOSE Tx of chronic hepatitis B infection in pts w/ evidence of active viral replication and active disease. Adult, child 16 yr and older w/ no previous nucleoside tx: 0.5 mg/day PO on empty stomach at least 2 hr after meal or 2 hr before next meal. Adult, child 16 yr and older w/ hx of viremia also receiving lamivudine or w/ known resistance mutations: 1 mg/day PO on empty stomach at least 2 hr after meal or 2 hr before next meal.

ADJUST DOSE Renal impairment

ADV EFF Acute exacerbation of hepatitis B when discontinuing, dizziness, fatigue, headache, nausea
INTERACTIONS Nephrotoxic drugs
NC/PT Assess renal function regularly. Give on empty stomach at least 2 hr after meal or 2 hr before next meal. Not a cure; pt should take precautions. Not for use in pregnancy, breast-feeding. Pt should not run out of or stop drug suddenly (severe hepatitis possible), should take safety precautions w/ dizziness, report unusual muscle pain.

---

enzalutamide (Xtandi)
CLASS Androgen receptor inhibitor, antineoplastic
PREG/CONT X/NA

IND & DOSE Tx of metastatic castration-resistant prostate cancer in pts previously on docetaxel. *Adult:* 160 mg/day PO once daily.
ADV EFF Arthralgia, asthenia, anxiety, back pain, diarrhea, dizziness, edema, flushing, headache, hematuria, hypertension, paresthesia, **seizures**, weakness
INTERACTIONS Midazolam, omeprazole, pioglitazone, warfarin; avoid concurrent use. Gemfibrozil
NC/PT Monitor for CNS reactions; provide safety precautions. Not for use in pregnancy. Pt should swallow capsule whole and not cut, crush, or chew it; use caution w/ CNS effects; report falls, severe headache, problems thinking clearly.

DANGEROUS DRUG

ephedrine sulfate (generic)
CLASS Bronchodilator, sympathomimetic, vasopressor
PREG/CONT C/NA

IND & DOSE Tx of hypotensive episodes, allergic disorders. *Adult:* 25–50 mg IM (fast absorption) or subcut (slower absorption), or 5–25 mg IV

slowly; may repeat in 5–10 min. *Child:* 0.5 mg/kg or 16.7 mg/m² IM or subcut q 4–6 hr. Tx of acute asthma, allergic disorders. *Adult:* 12.5–25 mg PO q 4 hr.
ADJUST DOSE Elderly pts
ADV EFF Anxiety, **CV collapse w/ hypotension**, dizziness, dysuria, fear, **hypertension resulting in intracranial hemorrhage,** pallor, **palpitations, precordial pain in pts w/ ischemic heart disease,** restlessness, **tachycardia,** tenseness
INTERACTIONS Caffeine, ephedra, guarana, ma huang, MAOIs, methyldopa, TCAs, urinary acidifiers/alkalinizers
NC/PT Protect sol from light. Give only if sol clear; discard unused portion. Monitor CV status, urine output. Avoid prolonged systemic use. Pt should avoid OTC products w/ similar action, take safety precautions w/ CNS effects.

DANGEROUS DRUG

epinephrine bitartrate (Primatene Mist), **epinephrine hydrochloride** (Adrenaclick, AsthmaNefrin, EpiPen Auto-Injector)
CLASS Antiasthmatic, cardiac stimulant, sympathomimetic, vasopressor
PREG/CONT C/NA

IND & DOSE Tx in cardiac arrest. *Adult:* 0.5–1 mg (5–10 mL of 1:10,000 sol) IV during resuscitation, 0.5 mg q 5 min. Intracardiac injection into left ventricular chamber, 0.3–0.5 mg (3–5 mL of 1:10,000 sol). **Hypersensitivity, bronchospasm.** *Adult:* 0.1–0.25 mg (1–2.5 mL of 1:10,000 sol) injected slowly IV or 0.2–1 mL of 1:1,000 sol subcut or IM, or 0.1–0.3 mL (0.5–1.5 mg) of 1:200 sol subcut. *Child:* 1:1,000 sol, 0.01 mg/kg or 0.3 mL/m² (0.01 mg/kg or 0.3 mg/m²) subcut. Repeat q 4 hr if needed; max, 0.5 mL (0.5 mg) in single dose. For neonates, 0.01 mg/kg subcut; for infants, 0.05 mg subcut as initial dose. Repeat q 20–30 min as needed. *Child 30 kg or less:* 1:10,000 sol, 0.15 mg or 0.01 mg/kg autoinjector. **Temporary relief from acute attacks of bronchial asthma, COPD.** *Adult, child 4 yr and older:* 1 inhalation, wait 1 min, then may use once more. Do not repeat for at least 3 hr. Or, place not more than 10 drops into nebulizer reservoir, place nebulizer nozzle into partially opened mouth, have pt inhale deeply while bulb is squeezed one to three times (not more than q 3 hr).

ADJUST DOSE Elderly pts

ADV EFF Anxiety, **CV collapse w/ hypotension,** dizziness, dysuria, fear, **hypertension resulting in intracranial hemorrhage,** pallor, **palpitations, precordial pain in pts w/ ischemic heart disease,** restlessness, **tachycardia,** tenseness

INTERACTIONS Beta blockers, chlorpromazine, ephedra, guarana, ma huang, methyldopa, propranolol, TCAs

NC/PT Use extreme caution when calculating doses; small margin of safety. Protect sol from light, heat. Rotate subcut injection sites. Have alpha-adrenergic blocker on hand for hypertensive crises/pulmonary edema, beta blocker on hand for cardiac arrhythmias. Do not exceed recommended dose of inhalants. Pt should take safety precautions w/ CNS effects.

DANGEROUS DRUG

epirubicin hydrochloride (Ellence)
CLASS Antineoplastic antibiotic
PREG/CONT D/NA

BBW Cardiac toxicity possible; monitor ECG closely. Severe tissue necrosis w/ extravasation. Secondary acute myelogenous leukemia possible. Reduce dose in hepatic impairment. Monitor for severe bone marrow suppression.

IND & DOSE Adjunct tx in pts w/ evidence of axillary node tumor involvement after resection of primary breast cancer. *Adult:* 100–120 mg/m² IV in repeated 3- to 4-wk cycles, all on day 1; given w/ cyclophosphamide and 5-FU.

ADJUST DOSE Elderly pts; hepatic, severe renal impairment

ADV EFF Alopecia, **bone marrow suppression, HF,** infection, **leukemia,** local injection-site toxicity/rash, n/v/d, **renal toxicity, thromboembolic events**

INTERACTIONS Cardiotoxic drugs, cimetidine, live vaccines

NC/PT Monitor baseline and periodic ECG to evaluate for toxicity. Premedicate w/ antiemetic. Monitor injection site carefully. Monitor CBC regularly; dose adjustment may be needed. Not for use in pregnancy, breast-feeding. Pt should mark calendar of tx dates.

---

eplerenone (Inspra)
CLASS Aldosterone receptor blocker, antihypertensive
PREG/CONT B/NA

IND & DOSE Tx of hypertension. *Adult:* 50 mg/day PO as single dose; may increase to 50 mg PO bid after minimum 4-wk trial period. Max, 100 mg/day. **Tx of HF post-MI.** *Adult:* Initially, 25 mg/day PO; titrate to 50 mg/day over 4 wk. If serum potassium lower than 5, increase dose; if 5–5.4, no adjustment needed; if 5.5–5.9, decrease dose; if 6 or higher, withhold dose.

ADV EFF Dizziness, gynecomastia, headache, **hyperkalemia, MI**

INTERACTIONS ACE inhibitors, amiloride, ARBs, NSAIDs, spironolactone, triamterene; serious reactions w/ erythromycin, fluconazole, itraconazole, ketoconazole, lithium, saquinavir, verapamil

NC/PT Monitor potassium, renal function; suggest limiting potassium-rich foods. Not for use in pregnancy, breast-feeding. Pt should avoid OTC drugs that might interact, weigh self daily, report changes of 3 lb or more/day.

epoetin alfa (EPO, erythropoietin) (Epogen, Procrit)

CLASS Recombinant human erythropoietin
PREG/CONT C/NA

BBW Increased risk of death, serious CV events if Hgb target is over 11 g/dL. Use lowest levels of drug needed to increase Hgb to lowest level needed to avoid transfusion. Incidence of DVT higher in pts receiving erythropoietin-stimulating agents preop to reduce need for transfusion; consider antithrombotic px if used for this purpose. Pts w/ cancer at risk for more rapid tumor progression, shortened survival, death when Hgb target is over 12 g/dL. Increased risk of death in cancer pts not receiving radiation or chemotherapy.

IND & DOSE Tx of anemia of chronic renal failure. *Adult:* 50–100 units/kg three times/wk IV for dialysis pts, IV or subcut for nondialysis pts. Maint, 75–100 units/kg three times/wk. If on dialysis, median dose is 75 units/kg three times/wk. Target Hgb range, 10–11 g/dL. *Child 1 mo–16 yr:* 50 units/kg IV or subcut three times/wk. Tx of anemia in HIV-infected pts on AZT therapy. *Adult:* For pts receiving AZT dose of 4,200 mg/wk or less w/ serum erythropoietin levels of 500 milliunits/mL or less, 100 units/kg IV or subcut three times/wk for 8 wk. Tx of anemia in cancer pts on chemotherapy (*Procrit* only). *Adult:* 150 units/kg subcut three times/wk or 40,000 units subcut wkly. After 8 wk, can increase to 300 units/kg or 60,000 units subcut wkly. *Child 1 mo–16 yr:* 600 units/kg IV; max, 60,000 units/dose in child 5 yr and older. To reduce allogenic blood transfusions in surgery.

Adult: 300 units/kg/day subcut for 10 days before surgery, on day of surgery, and 4 days after surgery. Or, 600 units/kg/day subcut 21, 14, and 7 days before surgery and on day of surgery. Tx of anemia of prematurity. *Child:* 25–100 units/kg/dose IV three times/wk.

ADV EFF Arthralgia, asthenia, chest pain, **development of anti-erythropoietin antibodies,** dizziness, edema, fatigue, headache, hypertension, n/v/d, **seizures, stroke, tumor progression/shortened survival (w/ cancers)**

NC/PT Confirm nature of anemia. Do not give in sol w/ other drugs. Monitor access lines for clotting. Monitor Hgb (target range, 10–11 g/dL; max, 11 g/dL). Evaluate iron stores before and periodically during tx; supplemental iron may be needed. Monitor for sudden loss of response and severe anemia w/ low reticulocyte count; withhold drug and check for anti-erythropoietin antibodies. Must give subcut three times/wk. Pt should keep blood test appointments to monitor response to drug, report difficulty breathing, chest pain, severe headache.

epoprostenol sodium (Flolan, Veletri)

CLASS Prostaglandin
PREG/CONT B/NA

IND & DOSE Tx of primary pulmonary hypertension in pts unresponsive to standard tx. *Adult:* 2 ng/kg/min IV w/ increases of 2 ng/kg as tolerated through infusion pump using central line; 20–40 ng/kg/min common range after 6 mo

ADV EFF Anxiety, agitation, chest pain, flushing, headache, hypotension, muscle aches, n/v/d, pain; **rebound pulmonary hypertension (w/ sudden stopping)**

INTERACTIONS Antihypertensives, diuretics, vasodilators

NC/PT Must deliver through continuous infusion pump. Use caution in pregnancy, breast-feeding. Teach pt, significant other maint and use of pump. Do not stop suddenly; taper if discontinuing. Pt should use analgesics for headache, muscle aches.

eprosartan mesylate
(Teveten)
CLASS Antihypertensive, ARB
PREG/CONT D/NA

BBW Rule out pregnancy before starting tx. Suggest barrier birth control; fetal injury, deaths have occurred. If pregnancy detected, discontinue as soon as possible.
IND & DOSE Tx of hypertension. *Adult:* 600 mg PO daily. Can give in divided doses bid w/ target dose of 400–800 mg/day.
ADJUST DOSE Renal impairment
ADV EFF Abd pain, diarrhea, dizziness, headache, URI symptoms
INTERACTIONS Potassium-elevating drugs
NC/PT If BP not controlled, may add other antihypertensives. Monitor fluid intake. Use caution if pt goes to surgery; volume depletion possible. Not for use in pregnancy (barrier contraception advised), breast-feeding. Pt should use care in situations that could lead to volume depletion.

DANGEROUS DRUG

eptifibatide (Integrelin)
CLASS Antiplatelet, glycoprotein IIb/IIIa receptor agonist
PREG/CONT B/NA

IND & DOSE Tx of acute coronary syndrome. *Adult:* 180 mcg/kg IV (max, 22.6 mg) over 1–2 min as soon as possible after dx, then 2 mcg/kg/min (max, 15 mg/hr) by continuous IV infusion for up to 72 hr. If pt is to undergo percutaneous coronary intervention (PCI), continue for 18–24 hr after procedure, up to 96 hr of tx. Px of ischemia w/ PCI. 180 mcg/kg IV as

bolus immediately before PCI, then 2 mcg/kg/min by continuous IV infusion for 18–24 hr. May give second bolus of 180 mcg/kg 10 min.
ADJUST DOSE Renal impairment
ADV EFF Bleeding, dizziness, headache, hypotension, rash
INTERACTIONS Anticoagulants, clopidogrel, dipyridamole, NSAIDs, thrombolytics, ticlopidine
NC/PT Used w/ aspirin, heparin. Arrange for baseline and periodic CBC, PT, aPTT, active clotting time; maintain aPTT of 50–70 sec and active clotting time of 300–350 sec. Avoid invasive procedures. Ensure compression of sites. Pt should use analgesics for headache, take safety precautions for dizziness.

ergotamine tartrate
(Ergomar)
CLASS Antimigraine, ergot
PREG/CONT X/NA

IND & DOSE Px, tx of vascular headaches. *Adult:* 2 mg under tongue at first sign of headache. May repeat at 30-min intervals; max, 6 mg/day or 10 mg/wk.
ADV EFF Cyanosis, gangrene, headache, hypertension, ischemia, itching, n/v, pulmonary fibrosis, tachycardia
INTERACTIONS Beta blockers, epinephrine, macrolide antibiotics, nicotine, protease inhibitors, sympathomimetics
NC/PT Not for use in pregnancy, breast-feeding. Pt should take at first sign of headache; not take more than 3 tablets in 24 hr; report difficulty breathing, numbness or tingling, chest pain.

eribulin mesylate
(Halaven)
CLASS Antineoplastic, microtubular inhibitor
PREG/CONT D/NA

IND & DOSE Tx of metastatic breast cancer in pts previously treated w/ at least two chemotherapeutic regimens. *Adult:* 1.4 mg/m²

IV over 2–5 min on days 1 and 8 of 21-day cycle.
ADJUST DOSE Hepatic, renal impairment
ADV EFF Alopecia, asthenia, **bone marrow suppression,** constipation, nausea, **QT prolongation, peripheral neuropathy**
INTERACTIONS Dextrose-containing solutions, QT-prolonging drugs
NC/PT Obtain baseline ECG; monitor QT interval. Monitor for bone marrow suppression, (adjust dose accordingly), peripheral neuropathy (dose adjustment may be needed). Not for use in pregnancy, breast-feeding. Protect from infection. Hair loss possible. Pt should cover head at extremes of temp; report fever, chills, cough, burning on urination.

erlotinib (Tarceva)
CLASS Antineoplastic, monoclonal antibody
PREG/CONT D/NA

IND & DOSE Tx of locally advanced or metastatic non-small-cell lung cancer after failure of other chemotherapy. *Adult:* 150 mg/day PO on empty stomach. **Tx of locally advanced, unresectable or metastatic pancreatic cancer, w/ gemcitabine.** *Adult:* 100 mg/day PO w/ IV gemcitabine.
ADJUST DOSE Hepatic, renal impairment; lung dysfx
ADV EFF Abd pain, anorexia, **bleeding, corneal ulcerations,** cough, dyspnea, **exfoliative skin disorders,** fatigue, **GI perforation, hepatic failure, hemolytic anemia, interstitial pulmonary disease, MI,** n/v/d, rash, **renal failure**
INTERACTIONS Antacids, cigarette smoking, CYP3A4 inducers/inhibitors, midazolam
NC/PT Monitor LFTs, renal function regularly. Monitor pulmonary status. Assess cornea before and periodically during tx. Provide skin care, including sunscreen, alcohol-free emollient

cream. Not for use in pregnancy, breast-feeding. Pt should report severe diarrhea, difficulty breathing, worsening rash, vision changes.

ertapenem (Invanz)
CLASS Carbapenem antibiotic
PREG/CONT B/NA

IND & DOSE Tx of community-acquired pneumonia; skin, skin-structure infections, including diabetic foot infections; complicated GU, intra-abdominal infections; acute pelvic infections caused by susceptible bacteria strains; px of surgical-site infection after colorectal surgery. *Adult, child 13 yr and older:* 1 g IM or IV each day. Length of tx varies w/ infection: intra-abdominal, 5–14 days; urinary tract, 10–14 days; skin, skin-structure, 7–14 days; community-acquired pneumonia, 10–14 days; acute pelvic, 3–10 days. *Child 3 mo–12 yr:* 15 mg/kg IV or IM bid for 3–14 days; max, 1 g/day.
ADJUST DOSE Renal impairment
ADV EFF Anaphylaxis, headache, hypersensitivity reaction, local pain/phlebitis at injection site; n/v/d, **pseudomembranous colitis.**
NC/PT Culture before tx. Give by deep IM injection; have emergency equipment on hand for hypersensitivity reactions. Monitor injection site for reaction. Treat superinfections. Pt should report severe or bloody diarrhea, pain at injection site. Name confusion between *Avinza* (ER morphine) and *Invanz* (ertapenem); use extreme caution.

erythromycin salts (Eryderm, Eryped, Erythrocin)
CLASS Macrolide antibiotic
PREG/CONT B/NA

IND & DOSE Tx of infections caused by susceptible bacteria. *Adult:* General guidelines, 15–20 mg/kg/day by continuous IV infusion or up to 4 g/day in divided doses q 6 hr; or 250 mg (400 mg ethylsuccinate) PO q 6 hr or 500 mg PO q 12 hr or 333 mg PO q 8 hr, up to 4 g/day, depending on infection severity. *Child:* General guidelines, 30–50 mg/kg/day PO in divided doses. Specific dose determined by infection severity, age, weight. **Tx of streptococcal infections.** *Adult:* 250 mg PO q 6 hr or 500 mg PO q 12 hr (for group A beta-hemolytic streptococcal infections, continue tx for at least 10 days). **Tx of Legionnaires' disease.** *Adult:* 1–4 g/day PO or IV in divided doses for 10–21 days. **Tx of dysenteric amebiasis.** *Adult:* 250 mg PO q 6 hr or 333 mg PO q 8 hr for 10–14 days. *Child:* 30–50 mg/kg/day PO in divided doses for 10–14 days. **Tx of acute PID** *(Neisseria gonorrhoeae). Adult:* 500 mg IV q 6 hr for 3 days, then 250 mg PO q 6 hr or 333 mg PO q 8 hr or 500 mg PO q 12 hr for 7 days. **Tx of chlamydial infections.** *Adult:* Urogenital infections during pregnancy, 500 mg PO qid or 666 mg PO q 8 hr for at least 7 days; ½ this dose q 8 hr for at least 14 days if intolerant to first regimen. Urethritis in males, 800 mg ethylsuccinate PO tid for 7 days. *Child:* 50 mg/kg/day PO in divided doses, for at least 2 (conjunctivitis of newborn) or 3 (pneumonia of infancy) wk. **Tx of primary syphilis.** *Adult:* 30–40 g PO in divided doses over 10–15 days. **CDC recommendations for STDs.** *Adult:* 500 mg PO qid for 7–30 days, depending on infection. **Tx of pertussis.** *Child:* 40–50 mg/kg/day PO in divided doses for 14 days. **Tx of superficial ocular infections caused by susceptible strains.** *Adult, child:* ½-inch ribbon instilled into conjunctival sac of affected eye two to six times/day, depending on infection severity. **Tx of acne** (dermatologic sol). *Adult, child:* Apply to affected areas a.m. and p.m. **Tx of skin infections caused by susceptible bacteria.** *Adult, child:* Apply

flexible hydroactive dressings and granules; keep in place for 1–7 days.
ADV EFF Abd pain, **anaphylaxis,** anorexia, local irritation w/ topical use; n/v/d, **pseudomembranous colitis,** superinfections
INTERACTIONS Calcium channel blockers, carbamazepine, corticosteroids, cyclosporine, digoxin, disopyramide, ergots, grapefruit juice, midazolam, oral anticoagulants, proton pump inhibitors, quinidine, statins, theophylline
NC/PT Culture before tx. Give oral drug on empty stomach round the clock for best results. Monitor LFTs w/ long-term use. Keep topical form to clean, dry area. Pt should avoid grapefruit juice, report severe or bloody diarrhea.

escitalopram oxalate (Lexapro)
CLASS Antidepressant, SSRI
PREG/CONT C/NA

BBW Monitor for suicidality, especially when starting tx or altering dose. Increased risk in children, adolescents, young adults.
IND & DOSE Tx of major depressive disorder. *Adult:* 10 mg/day PO as single dose; may increase to 20 mg/day after minimum of 1-wk trial period. Maint, 10–20 mg/day PO. *Child 12–17 yr:* 10 mg/day PO as single dose; max, 20 mg/day. **Tx of generalized anxiety disorder.** *Adult:* 10 mg/day PO; may increase to 20 mg/day after 1 wk if needed.
ADJUST DOSE Elderly pts, hepatic impairment
ADV EFF Anaphylaxis, angioedema, dizziness, ejaculatory disorders, nausea, somnolence, suicidality
INTERACTIONS Alcohol, carbamazepine, citalopram, lithium, MAOIs, SSRIs, St. John's wort
NC/PT Limit supply in suicidal pts. Do not use within 14 days of MAOIs. Taper after long-term use. Not for use in pregnancy, breast-feeding. Use

safety precautions. May need 4 wk to see effects. Pt should not stop drug suddenly; avoid alcohol, St John's wort; report thoughts of suicide. Name confusion between escitalopram and citalopram and *Lexapro* (escitalopram) and *Loxitane* (loxapine); use caution.

eslicarbazepine acetate
(Aptiom)

CLASS Antiepileptic, sodium channel blocker

PREG/CONT C/NA

IND & DOSE Adjunct tx for partial-onset seizures. *Adult:* 400 mg/day PO; after 1 wk, increase to 800 mg/day PO. Max, 1,200 mg/day.

ADJUST DOSE Severe renal impairment (not recommended)

ADV EFF Anaphylaxis, dizziness, double vision, drowsiness, fatigue, headache, hyponatremia, liver damage, n/v, suicidality

INTERACTIONS Carbamazepine, hormonal contraceptives, phenobarbital, phenytoin, primidone

NC/PT Ensure proper dx. Monitor LFTs, serum electrolytes; ensure safety precautions w/ CNS effects. Pt should avoid pregnancy, breastfeeding; take safety precautions w/ CNS effects; report thoughts of suicide, difficulty breathing, changes in color of urine/stool.

DANGEROUS DRUG

esmolol hydrochloride
(Brevibloc)

CLASS Antiarrhythmic, beta-selective adrenergic blocker

PREG/CONT C/NA

IND & DOSE Tx of supraventricular tachycardia; noncompensatory tachycardia; intraop, postop tachycardia and hypertension. *Adult:* Initial loading dose, 500 mcg/kg/min IV for 1 min, then maint of 50 mcg/kg/min for 4 min. If response inadequate after

5 min, repeat loading dose and follow w/ maint infusion of 100 mcg/kg/min. Repeat titration as needed, increasing rate of maint dose in 50-mcg/kg/min increments. As desired heart rate or safe endpoint is approached, omit loading infusion and decrease incremental dose in maint infusion to 25 mcg/kg/min (or less), or increase interval between titration steps from 5 to 10 min. Usual range, 50–200 mcg/kg/min. Up to 24-hr infusions have been used; up to 48 hr may be well tolerated. Individualize dose based on pt response; max, 300 mcg/kg/min.

ADV EFF Hypotension, inflammation at injection site, light-headedness, midscapular pain, rigors, weakness

INTERACTIONS Ibuprofen, indomethacin, piroxicam, verapamil

NC/PT Do not give undiluted. Do not mix in sol w/ sodium bicarbonate, diazepam, furosemide, thiopental. Not for long-term use. Closely monitor BP, ECG.

esomeprazole magnesium (Nexium)

CLASS Antisecretory, proton pump inhibitor

PREG/CONT B/NA

IND & DOSE Healing of erosive esophagitis. *Adult:* 20–40 mg PO daily for 4–8 wk. Maint, 20 mg PO daily. *Child 1–11 yr:* 20 kg or more, 10–20 mg/day PO for up to 8 wk; under 20 kg, 10 mg/day PO for up to 8 wk. Tx of symptomatic GERD. *Adult:* 20 mg PO daily for 4 wk. Can use additional 4-wk course. *Child 12–17 yr:* 20–40 mg/day PO daily for 8 wk. *Child 1–11 yr:* 10 mg/day PO for up to 8 wk. Tx of duodenal ulcer. *Adult:* 40 mg/day PO for 10 days w/ 1,000 mg PO bid amoxicillin and 500 mg PO bid clarithromycin. Reduction of risk of gastric ulcers w/ NSAID use. *Adult:* 20–40 mg PO daily for 6 mo. Short-term tx of GERD when oral therapy not possible.

Adult, child 1 mo–17 yr: 20–40 mg IV by injection over at least 3 min or IV infusion over 10–30 min.

ADJUST DOSE Severe hepatic impairment

ADV EFF Abd pain, **bone loss w/ long-term use,** *Clostridium difficile* diarrhea, dizziness, headache, hypomagnesemia, n/v/d, pneumonia, sinusitis, URI

INTERACTIONS Atazanavir, benzodiazepines, digoxin, iron salts, ketoconazole

NC/PT Give at least 1 hr before meals; may give through NG tube. Monitor LFTs periodically. Limit IV use to max 10 days. Pt should swallow capsules whole and not cut, crush, or chew them; take safety precautions w/ CNS effects.; report diarrhea, difficulty breathing. Name confusion between esomeprazole and omeprazole, *Nexium* (esomeprazole) and *Nexavar* (sorafenib); use caution.

---

estazolam (generic)

CLASS Benzodiazepine, sedative-hypnotic
PREG/CONT X/C-IV

IND & DOSE Tx of insomnia, recurring insomnia, acute or chronic medical conditions requiring restful sleep. *Adult:* 1 mg PO before bedtime; may need up to 2 mg.

ADJUST DOSE Elderly pts, debilitating disease,

ADV EFF Anaphylaxis, angioedema, apathy, bradycardia, constipation, **CV collapse**, depression, diarrhea, disorientation, drowsiness, drug dependence w/ withdrawal syndrome, dyspepsia, lethargy, light-headedness, tachycardia, urine retention

INTERACTIONS Alcohol, aminophylline, barbiturates, opioids, phenothiazines, rifampin, TCAs, theophylline

NC/PT Monitor LFTs, renal function. Taper after long-term use. Pt should avoid alcohol, use only as needed

(can be habit-forming), take safety precautions w/ CNS effects.

---

estradiol, estradiol acetate, estradiol cypionate, estradiol hemihydrate, estradiol valerate (Delestrogen, Estrace, Estring, Evamist, Femring, Vagifem)

CLASS Estrogen
PREG/CONT X/NA

BBW Arrange for pretreatment and periodic (at least annual) hx and physical; should include BP, breasts, abdomen, pelvic organs, Pap test. May increase risk of endometrial cancer. Do not use to prevent CV events, dementia; may increase risks, including thrombophlebitis, PE, stroke, MI. Caution pt of risks of estrogen use. Stress need for pregnancy prevention during tx, frequent medical follow-up, periodic rests from tx.

IND & DOSE Relief of moderate to severe vasomotor symptoms, atrophic vaginitis, kraurosis vulvae associated w/ menopause. *Adult:* 1–2 mg/day PO. Adjust dose to control symptoms. For gel, 0.25 g 0.1% gel applied to right or left upper thigh on alternating days; may increase to 0.5 or 1 g/day to control symptoms. For topical spray (*Evamist*), 1 spray once daily to forearm; may increase to 2–3 sprays daily. Cyclic therapy (3 wk on/1 wk off) recommended, especially in women w/ no hysterectomy. 1–5 mg estradiol cypionate in oil IM q 3–4 wk. 10–20 mg estradiol valerate in oil IM q 4 wk. 0.014- to 0.05-mg system applied to skin wkly or twice wkly. If oral estrogens have been used, start transdermal system 1 wk after withdrawal of oral form. Given on cyclic schedule (3 wk on/1 wk off). Attempt to taper or discontinue q 3–6 mo. Vaginal cream: 2–4 g intravaginally daily for 1–2 wk, then reduce to ½ dose for similar period followed by maint of 1 g one to three times/wk thereafter. Discontinue or taper at 3- to 6-mo intervals. Vaginal ring: Insert one ring high into vagina. Replace q 90 days. Vaginal tablet: 1 tablet inserted vaginally daily for 2 wk, then twice wkly. Emulsion: Apply lotion to legs, thighs, or calves once daily. Apply gel to one arm once daily. **Tx of female hypogonadism, female castration, primary ovarian failure.** *Adult:* 1–2 mg/day PO. Adjust to control symptoms. Cyclic therapy (3 wk on/1 wk off) recommended. 1.5–2 mg estradiol cypionate in oil IM at monthly intervals. 10–20 mg estradiol valerate in oil IM q 4 wk. 0.05-mg system applied to skin twice wkly as above. **Tx of prostate cancer** (inoperable). *Adult:* 1–2 mg PO tid; give long-term. 30 mg or more estradiol valerate in oil IM q 1–2 wk. **Tx of breast cancer** (inoperable, progressing). *Adult:* 10 mg tid PO for at least 3 mo. **Prevention of postpartum breast engorgement.** *Adult:* 10–25 mg estradiol valerate in oil IM as single injection at end of first stage of labor. **Px of osteoporosis.** *Adult:* 0.5 mg/day PO cyclically (23 days on, 5 days rest) starting as soon after menopause as possible.

ADV EFF Acute pancreatitis, abd cramps, bloating, **cancer**, chloasma, **cholestatic jaundice, colitis**, dysmenorrhea, edema, **hepatic adenoma**, menstrual flow changes, n/v/d, pain at injection site, photosensitivity, premenstrual syndrome, **thrombotic events**

INTERACTIONS Barbiturates, carbamazepine, corticosteroids, phenytoins, rifampin

NC/PT Give cyclically for short-term use. Give w/ progestin for women w/ intact uterus. Provide proper administration for each drug type. Potentially serious adverse effects. Not for use in pregnancy, breast-feeding. Pt should get regular pelvic exams, avoid sun exposure, report pain in calves/chest, lumps in breast, vision or speech changes.

estrogens, conjugated
(Cenestin, Enjuvia, Premarin)

CLASS Estrogen
PREG/CONT X/NA

BBW Arrange for pretreatment and periodic (at least annual) hx and physical; should include BP, breasts, abdomen, pelvic organs, Pap test. May increase risk of endometrial cancer. Do not use for dementia; may increase risks, including thrombophlebitis, PE, stroke, MI. Caution pt of risks of estrogen use. Stress need for pregnancy prevention during tx, frequent medical follow-up, periodic rests from tx.

IND & DOSE Relief of moderate to severe vasomotor symptoms associated w/ menopause. *Adult:* 0.3–0.625 mg/day PO. **Tx of atrophic vaginitis, kraurosis vulvae associated w/ menopause.** *Adult:* 0.5–2 g vaginal cream daily intravaginally or topically, depending on severity. Taper or discontinue at 3- to 6-mo intervals. Or, 0.3 mg/day PO continually. **Tx of female hypogonadism.** *Adult:* 0.3–0.625 mg/day PO for 3 wk, then 1 wk rest. **Tx of female castration, primary ovarian failure.** *Adult:* 1.25 mg/day PO. **Tx of prostate cancer** (inoperable). *Adult:* 1.25–2.5 mg PO tid. **Tx of osteoporosis.** *Adult:* 0.3 mg/day PO continuously or cyclically (25 days on/5 days off). **Breast cancer** (inoperable, progressing). *Adult:* 10 mg PO tid for at least 3 mo. **Abnormal uterine bleeding due to hormonal imbalance.** 25 mg IV or IM. Repeat in 6–12 hr as needed. More rapid response w/ IV route.

ADV EFF Acute pancreatitis, abd cramps, bloating, **cancer**, chloasma, **cholestatic jaundice, colitis**, dysmenorrhea, edema, headache, **hepatic adenoma**, menstrual flow changes, n/v/d, pain at injection site, photosensitivity, premenstrual syndrome, **thrombotic events**

INTERACTIONS Barbiturates, carbamazepine, corticosteroids, phenytoins, rifampin

NC/PT Give cyclically for short-term use. Give w/ progestin for women w/ intact uterus. Review proper administration for each drug type. Potentially serious adverse effects. Not for use in pregnancy, breast-feeding. Pt should get regular pelvic exams, avoid sun exposure, report pain in calves/chest, lumps in breast, vision or speech changes.

estrogens, esterified (Menest)

CLASS Estrogen
PREG/CONT X/NA

BBW Arrange for pretreatment and periodic (at least annual) hx and physical; should include BP, breasts, abdomen, pelvic organs, Pap test. May increase risk of endometrial cancer. Do not use to prevent CV events or dementia; may increase risks, including thrombophlebitis, PE, stroke, MI. Caution pt of risks of estrogen use. Stress need for pregnancy prevention during tx, frequent medical follow-up, periodic rests from drug tx. Give cyclically for short-term only when treating postmenopausal conditions because of endometrial neoplasm risk. Taper to lowest effective dose; provide drug-free wk each mo.

IND & DOSE Relief of moderate to severe vasomotor symptoms, atrophic vaginitis, kraurosis vulvae associated w/ menopause. *Adult:* 0.3–1.25 mg/day PO given cyclically (3 wk on/1 wk off). Use lowest possible dose. Tx of female hypogonadism. *Adult:* 2.5–7.5 mg/day PO in divided doses for 20 days on/10 days off. Female castration, primary ovarian failure. *Adult:* 1.25 mg/day PO given cyclically. Prostate cancer (inoperable). *Adult:* 1.25–2.5 mg PO tid. Inoperable, progressing breast cancer. *Adult:* 10 mg PO tid for at least 3 mo.

ADV EFF Acute pancreatitis, abd cramps, bloating, **cancer**, chloasma, **cholestatic jaundice**, colitis, dysmenorrhea, edema, headache, **hepatic adenoma**, menstrual flow changes, n/v/d, pain at injection site, photosensitivity, premenstrual syndrome, **thrombotic events**

INTERACTIONS Barbiturates, carbamazepine, corticosteroids, phenytoins, rifampin

NC/PT Give cyclically for short-term use. Give w/ progestin for women w/ intact uterus. Review proper administration for each drug type. Potentially serious adverse effects. Not for use in pregnancy, breast-feeding. Pt should get regular pelvic exams, avoid sun exposure, report pain in calves/chest, lumps in breast, vision or speech changes.

estropipate (generic)

CLASS Estrogen
PREG/CONT X/NA

BBW Arrange for pretreatment and periodic (at least annual) hx and physical; should include BP, breasts, abdomen, pelvic organs, Pap test. May increase risk of endometrial cancer. Do not use to prevent CV events or dementia; may increase risks, including thrombophlebitis, PE, stroke, MI. Caution pt of risks of estrogen use. Stress need for pregnancy prevention during tx, frequent medical follow-up, periodic rests from drug tx. Give cyclically for short term only when treating postmenopausal conditions because of endometrial neoplasm risk. Taper to lowest effective dose; provide drug-free wk each mo.

IND & DOSE Relief of moderate to severe vasomotor sx, atrophic vaginitis, kraurosis vulvae associated w/ menopause. *Adult:* 0.75–6 mg/day PO given cyclically (3 wk on/1 wk off). Use lowest possible dose. Tx of female hypogonadism, female castration, primary ovarian failure. *Adult:* 1.5–9 mg/day PO for first

3 wk, then rest period of 8–10 days. Repeat if no bleeding at end of rest period. **Px of osteoporosis.** *Adult:* 0.75 mg/day PO for 25 days of 31-day cycle/mo.

ADV EFF Acute pancreatitis, abd cramps, bloating, **cancer,** chloasma, **cholestatic jaundice, colitis,** dysmenorrhea, edema, headache, **hepatic adenoma,** menstrual flow changes, n/v/d, pain at injection site, photosensitivity, premenstrual syndrome, **thrombotic events**

INTERACTIONS Barbiturates, carbamazepine, corticosteroids, phenytoins, rifampin

NC/PT Give cyclically for short-term use. Give w/ progestin for women w/ intact uterus. Review proper administration for each drug type. Potentially serious adverse effects. Not for use in pregnancy, breast-feeding. Pt should get regular pelvic exams, avoid sun exposure, report pain in calves/chest, lumps in breast, vision or speech changes.

eszopiclone (Lunesta)
CLASS Nonbenzodiazepine hypnotic, sedative-hypnotic
PREG/CONT C/C-IV

IND & DOSE Tx of insomnia. *Adult:* 2 mg PO immediately before bedtime. May increase to 3 mg PO.

ADJUST DOSE CYP3A4 inhibitor use, elderly pts, severe hepatic impairment

ADV EFF Anaphylaxis, angioedema, dizziness, headache, nervousness, somnolence, **suicidality**

INTERACTIONS Alcohol, clarithromycin, itraconazole, ketoconazole, nefazodone, nelfinavir, rifampin, ritonavir

NC/PT Not for use in pregnancy, breast-feeding. Pt should swallow tablet whole and not cut, crush, or chew it; take only if in bed and able to stay in bed for 8 hr; avoid alcohol; not take w/ high-fat meal; report thoughts of suicide.

etanercept (Enbrel)
CLASS Antiarthritic, disease-modifying antirheumatic drug
PREG/CONT B/NA

BBW Monitor for infection s&sx; discontinue if infection occurs. Risk of serious infections (including TB), death. Increased risk of lymphoma, other cancers in children taking for juvenile rheumatoid arthritis, Crohn's disease, other inflammatory conditions; monitor accordingly.

IND & DOSE To reduce s&sx of ankylosing spondylitis, rheumatoid arthritis, psoriatic arthritis. *Adult:* 50 mg/wk subcut. *Child 2–17 yr:* 0.8 mg/kg/wk subcut; max, 50 mg/wk. **To reduce s&sx of plaque psoriasis.** *Adult:* 50 mg/dose subcut twice wkly 3 or 4 days apart for 3 mo; maint, 50 mg/wk subcut.

ADV EFF Bone marrow suppression, demyelinating disorders (MS, myelitis, optic neuritis), cancers, increased risk of serious infections, dizziness, headache, irritation at injection site, URIs

INTERACTIONS Immunosuppressants, vaccines

NC/PT Obtain baseline and periodic CBC, neurologic function tests. Rotate injection sites (abdomen, thigh, upper arm). Monitor for infection. Do regular cancer screening. Teach proper administration, disposal of syringes, needles. Pt should avoid exposure to infection, maintain other tx for rheumatoid disorder (drug not a cure).

ethacrynic acid (Edecrin)
CLASS Loop diuretic
PREG/CONT B/NA

IND & DOSE To reduce edema associated w/ systemic diseases. *Adult:* 50–200 mg/day PO; may give IV as 50 mg slowly to max, 100 mg. *Child:* 25 mg/day PO; adjust in 25-mg/day increments if needed.

ADV EFF Abd pain, **agranulocytosis**, dehydration, dysphagia, fatigue, headache, hepatic impairment, hypokalemia, n/v/d, vertigo, weakness
INTERACTIONS Diuretics
NC/PT Switch to oral form as soon as possible. Give w/ food if GI upset. Monitor potassium; supplement as needed. Not for use in breast-feeding. Pt should weigh self daily; report changes of 3 lb/day or more.

ethambutol hydrochloride
(Myambutol)
CLASS Antituberculotic
PREG/CONT C/NA

IND & DOSE Tx of pulmonary TB w/ at least one other antituberculotic. *Adult, child 13 yr and older:* 15 mg/kg/day PO as single oral dose. Continue until bacteriologic conversion permanent and max clinical improvement has occurred. Retreatment: 25 mg/kg/day as single oral dose. After 60 days, reduce to 15 mg/kg/day as single dose.
ADV EFF Anorexia, fever, headache, malaise, n/v/d, optic neuritis, **toxic epidermal necrolysis, thrombocytopenia**
INTERACTIONS Aluminum salts
NC/PT Ensure use w/ other antituberculotics. Give w/ food. Monitor CBC, LFTs, renal function, ophthalmic exam. Pt should not stop suddenly; have regular medical checkups; report changes in vision, color perception; take safety precautions w/ CNS effects.

ethionamide (Trecator)
CLASS Antituberculotic
PREG/CONT C/NA

IND & DOSE Tx of pulmonary TB unresponsive to first-line tx, w/ at least one other antituberculotic. *Adult:* 15–20 mg/kg/day PO to max 1 g/day. *Child:* 10–20 mg/kg/day PO in two or

three divided doses after meals (max, 1 g/day), or 15 mg/kg/24 hr as single dose.
ADV EFF Alopecia, asthenia, depression, drowsiness, **hepatitis**, metallic taste, n/v/d, orthostatic hypotension, peripheral neuritis
NC/PT Ensure use w/ other antituberculotics. Concomitant use of pyridoxine recommended to prevent or minimize s&sx of peripheral neuritis. Give w/ food. Monitor LFTs before tx and q 2–4 wk during tx. Not for use in pregnancy. Pt should not stop suddenly, have regular medical checkups, take safety precautions w/ CNS effects.

ethosuximide (Zarontin)
CLASS Antiepileptic, succinimide
PREG/CONT C/NA

IND & DOSE Control of absence (petit mal) seizures. *Adult, child 6 yr and older:* 500 mg/day PO. Increase by small increments to maint level; increase by 250 mg q 4–7 days until control achieved. *Child 3–6 yr:* 250 mg/day PO. Increase in small increments until optimal 20 mg/kg/day in one dose or two divided doses.
ADV EFF Abd pain, **agranulocytosis, aplastic anemia**, ataxia, blurred vision, constipation, cramps, dizziness, drowsiness, **eosinophilia, generalized tonic-clonic seizures, granulocytopenia**, irritability, **leukopenia, monocytosis**, nervousness, n/v/d, **pancytopenia, Stevens-Johnson syndrome**
INTERACTIONS Alcohol, CNS depressants, primidone
NC/PT Reduce dose, discontinue, or substitute other antiepileptic gradually. Taper when discontinuing. Monitor CBC. Stop drug at signs of rash. Evaluate for therapeutic serum level (40–100 mcg/mL). Not for use in pregnancy (contraceptives advised). Pt should avoid alcohol, wear medical ID, avoid exposure to infection, take safety precautions w/ CNS effects.

ethotoin (Peganone)
CLASS Antiepileptic, hydantoin
PREG/CONT D/NA

IND & DOSE Control of tonic-clonic, complex partial (psychomotor) seizures. *Adult:* 1 g/day PO in four to six divided doses; increase gradually over several days. Usual maint dose, 2–3 g/day PO in four to six divided doses. *Child 1 yr and older:* 750 mg/day PO in four to six divided doses; maint range, 500 mg/day to 1 g/day PO in four to six divided doses.
ADV EFF Abd pain, **agranulocytosis, aplastic anemia,** ataxia, blurred vision, confusion, constipation, cramps, dizziness, drowsiness, **eosinophilia, epidermal necrolysis,** fatigue, **granulocytopenia, hepatotoxicity,** irritability, leukopenia, **lymphoma, monocytosis,** nervousness, n/v/d, nystagmus, **pancytopenia, pulmonary fibrosis, Stevens-Johnson syndrome**
INTERACTIONS Acetaminophen, amiodarone, antineoplastics, carbamazepine, chloramphenicol, cimetidine, corticosteroids, cyclosporine, diazoxide, disopyramide, disulfiram, doxycycline, estrogens, fluconazole, folic acid, hormonal contraceptives, isoniazid, levodopa, methadone, metyrapone, mexiletine, phenacemide, phenylbutazone, primidone, rifampin, sulfonamides, theophyllines, trimethoprim, valproic acid
NC/PT May use w/ other antiepileptics. Reduce dosage, discontinue, or substitute other antiepileptic gradually. Taper when discontinuing. Monitor CBC. Stop drug at signs of rash. Monitor LFTs. Give w/ food to enhance absorption. Evaluate for therapeutic serum levels (15–50 mcg/mL). Not for use in pregnancy (contraceptives advised). Evaluate lymph node enlargement during tx. Frequent medical follow-up needed. Pt should avoid alcohol, wear medical ID, avoid exposure to infection, take safety precautions w/ CNS effects, use good dental care to limit gum hyperplasia.

etidronate disodium (Didronel)
CLASS Bisphosphonate, calcium regulator
PREG/CONT C/NA

IND & DOSE Tx of Paget's disease. *Adult:* 5–10 mg/kg/day PO for up to 6 mo; or 11–20 mg/kg/day PO for up to 3 mo. If retreatment needed, wait at least 90 days between tx regimens. **Tx of heterotopic ossification.** *Adult:* 20 mg/kg/day PO for 2 wk, then 10 mg/kg/day PO for 10 wk (after spinal cord injury); 20 mg/kg/day PO for 1 mo preop (after total hip replacement), then 20 mg/kg/day PO for 3 mo postop.
ADJUST DOSE Renal impairment
ADV EFF Bone pain, headache, n/v/d
INTERACTIONS Antacids, aspirin, food
NC/PT For Paget's disease, ensure 3 mo rest periods between tx. Monitor serum calcium level. Pt should take w/ full glass of water 2 hr before meals, take calcium and vitamin D as needed, report muscle twitching.

etodolac (generic)
CLASS Analgesic, NSAID
PREG/CONT C/NA

BBW Increased risk of CV events, GI bleeding; monitor accordingly.
IND & DOSE Mgt of s&sx of osteoarthritis, rheumatoid arthritis. *Adult:* 600–1,000 mg/day PO in divided doses. Maint range, 600–1,200 mg/day in divided doses; max, 1,200 mg/day (20 mg/kg for pts under 60 kg). ER, 400–1,000 mg/day PO; max, 1,200 mg/day. **Mgt of s&sx of juvenile rheumatoid arthritis** (ER tablets). *Child 6–16 yr:* Over 60 kg, 1,000 mg/day PO as 500 mg PO bid; 46–60 kg, 800 mg/day PO as 400 mg

PO bid; 31–45 kg, 600 mg/day PO; 20–30 kg, 400 mg/day PO. **Analgesia, acute pain.** *Adult:* 200–400 mg PO q 6–8 hr; max, 1,200 mg/day.
ADV EFF Anaphylactoid reactions, **bleeding,** blurred vision, constipation, **CV events,** diarrhea, dizziness, dyspepsia, GI pain, **hepatic failure, renal impairment**
INTERACTIONS Anticoagulants, antihypertensives, antiplatelets
NC/PT Pt should take w/ meals, use safety precautions w/ CNS effects.

DANGEROUS DRUG

etoposide (VP-16)
(Etopophos, Toposar)
CLASS Antineoplastic, mitotic inhibitor
PREG/CONT D/NA

BBW Obtain platelet count, Hgb, Hct, WBC count w/ differential before tx and each dose. If severe response, discontinue; consult physician. Severe myelosuppression possible. Monitor for severe hypersensitivity reaction; arrange supportive care.
IND & DOSE Tx of testicular cancer. *Adult:* 50–100 mg/m²/day IV on days 1 to 5, or 100 mg/m²/day IV on days 1, 3, 5 q 3–4 wk w/ other chemotherapeutics. **Tx of small-cell lung cancer.** *Adult:* 35 mg/m²/day IV for 4 days to 50 mg/m²/day for 5 days; repeat q 3–4 wk after recovery from toxicity or switch to oral form (two times IV dose rounded to nearest 50 mg).
ADJUST DOSE Renal impairment
ADV EFF Alopecia, **anaphylactoid reactions,** anorexia, fatigue, hypotension, **myelotoxicity,** n/v/d, somnolence
INTERACTIONS Anticoagulants, antihypertensives, antiplatelets
NC/PT Avoid skin contact; use rubber gloves. If contact occurs, immediately wash w/ soap, water. Do not give IM, subcut. Monitor BP during infusion. Give antiemetic if nausea severe. Not for use in pregnancy (contraceptives advised). Pt should cover head at temp extremes (hair loss possible), mark

calendar of tx days, avoid exposure to infection, have blood tests regularly.

etravirine (Intelence)
CLASS Antiviral, nonnucleoside reverse transcriptase inhibitor
PREG/CONT B/NA

IND & DOSE Tx of HIV-1 infection in tx-experienced pts w/ evidence of viral replication and HIV-1 strains resistant to nonnucleoside reverse transcriptase inhibitors and other antiretrovirals, w/ other drugs. *Adult:* 200 mg PO bid after meal. *Child 6–under 18 yr:* 30 kg or more, 200 mg PO bid; 25 to under 30 kg, 150 mg PO bid; 20 to under 25 mg, 125 mg PO bid; 16–under 20 kg, 100 mg PO bid.
ADV EFF Altered fat distribution, diarrhea, fatigue, headache, **severe hypersensitivity reactions**
INTERACTIONS Antiarrhythmics, atazanavir, azole, carbamazepine, clarithromycin, clopidogrel, delavirdine, fosamprenavir, indinavir, maraviroc, nelfinavir, nevirapine, phenobarbital, phenytoin, rifabutin, rifampin, rifapentine, ritonavir, St. John's wort, tipranavir, warfarin
NC/PT Always give w/ other antivirals. Stop at first sign of severe skin reaction. Pt should swallow tablets whole and not cut, crush, or chew them. If it cannot swallow, put tablets in glass of water, stir; when water is milky, have pt drink whole glass, rinse several times, and drink rinse each time to get full dose. Not for use in breast-feeding. Pt should not use w/ St. John's wort, take precautions to prevent transmission (drug not a cure), have blood tests regularly.

everolimus (Afinitor, Zortress)
CLASS Antineoplastic, kinase inhibitor
PREG/CONT D/NA

BBW Zortress only: Risk of serious infections, cancer development; risk

of venous thrombosis, kidney loss; risk of nephrotoxicity w/ cyclosporine. Increased mortality if used w/ heart transplant; not approved for this use.
IND & DOSE Tx of advanced renal carcinoma after failure w/ sunitinib, sorafenib; tx of subependymal giant-cell astrocytoma in pts not candidates for surgery. *Adult:* 5–10 mg/day PO w/ food. Tx of pts 1 yr and older with tuberous sclerosis complex who have developed brain tumor. *Adult, child:* 4.5 mg/m² PO once/day with food. Px of organ rejection in adult at low to moderate risk receiving kidney transplant (*Zortress*). *Adult:* 0.75 mg PO bid w/ cyclosporine starting as soon as possible after transplant.
ADJUST DOSE Hepatic impairment
ADV EFF Elevated blood glucose, lipids, serum creatinine; oral ulcerations, pneumonitis, serious to fatal infections, stomatitis
INTERACTIONS Live vaccines, strong CYP3A4 inducers (increase everolimus dose to 20 mg/day), CYP3A4 inhibitors
NC/PT Give w/ food. Provide oral care. Monitor respiratory status; protect from infections. Not for use in pregnancy, breast-feeding. Pt should report difficulty breathing, fever.

exemestane (Aromasin)
CLASS Antineoplastic
PREG/CONT X/NA

IND & DOSE Tx of advanced breast cancer in postmenopausal women whose disease has progressed after tamoxifen; adjunct tx of postmenopausal women w/ estrogen receptor–positive early breast cancer who have received 2–3 yr of tamoxifen; switch to exemestane to finish 5-yr course. *Adult:* 25 mg/day PO w/ meal.
ADV EFF Anxiety, decreased bone marrow density, depression, GI upset, headache, hot flashes, nausea, sweating
INTERACTIONS CYP3A4 inducers/inhibitors, estrogens, St. John's wort

NC/PT Monitor LFTs, renal function. Give supportive therapy for adverse effects. Not for use in pregnancy, breast-feeding. Pt should not use St. John's wort.

exenatide (Bydureon, Byetta)
CLASS Antidiabetic, incretin mimetic drug
PREG/CONT C/NA

BBW ER form increases risk of thyroid C-cell tumors; contraindicated w/ personal/family hx of medullary thyroid cancer and in pts w/ multiple endocrine neoplasia syndrome.
IND & DOSE Adjunct to diet, exercise for tx of type 2 diabetes; as add-on tx w/ insulin glargine, metformin to improve glycemic control in type 2 diabetes. *Adult:* 5–10 mcg by subcut injection bid at any time within 60 min before a.m. and p.m. meals or two main meals of day, approximately 6 hr apart. ER form, 2 mg by subcut injection once q 7 days.
ADJUST DOSE Renal impairment
ADV EFF Dizziness, **hypoglycemia**, injection-site reaction, **hemorrhagic or necrotizing pancreatitis**, nausea
INTERACTIONS Alcohol, antibiotics, oral contraceptives, warfarin
NC/PT Maintain diet, exercise. Monitor serum glucose. Monitor for pancreatitis. Rotate injection sites (thigh, abdomen, upper arm). Give within 1 hr of meal; if pt not going to eat, do not give. Use caution w/ pregnancy, breast-feeding. Review hypoglycemia s&sx.

ezetimibe (Zetia)
CLASS Cholesterol-absorption inhibitor, cholesterol-lowering drug
PREG/CONT C/NA

IND & DOSE Adjunct to diet, exercise to lower cholesterol. *Adult, child over 10 yr:* 10 mg/day PO

without regard to food. May give at same time as HMG-CoA reductase inhibitor, fenofibrate. If combined w/ bile acid sequestrant, give at least 2 hr before or 4 hr after bile acid sequestrant.
ADV EFF Abd pain, diarrhea, dizziness, headache, URI
INTERACTIONS Cholestyramine, cyclosporine, fenofibrate, gemfibrozil
NC/PT Ensure use of diet, exercise program. Monitor serum lipid profile. Not for use in pregnancy, breast-feeding. Frequent blood tests needed. Pt should use safety precautions w/ CNS effects, continue other lipid-lowering drugs if prescribed.

ezogabine (Potiga)
CLASS Antiepileptic, neuronal potassium channel opener
PREG/CONT C/NA

BBW Risk of suicidal ideation/suicidality; monitor accordingly.
IND & DOSE Adjunct to tx of partial seizures when other measures have failed. *Adult:* 100 mg PO tid for 1 wk; maint, 200–400 mg PO tid, w/ other antiepileptics.
ADV EFF Abnormal coordination, aphasia, asthenia, blurred vision, confused state, dizziness, fatigue, prolonged QT, somnolence, tremor, urine retention, suicidal ideation, vertigo
INTERACTIONS Alcohol, carbamazepine, digoxin, phenytoin
NC/PT Obtain baseline ECG; review QT interval periodically. Taper slowly when withdrawing. Not for use in pregnancy, breast-feeding. Pt should empty bladder before taking, continue other tx for seizures as prescribed, avoid alcohol, use safety precautions w/ CNS effects, report thoughts of suicide.

factor IX concentrates
(AlphaNine SD, Bebulin VH, BeneFix, Mononine)
CLASS Antihemophilic
PREG/CONT C/NA

IND & DOSE Control of bleeding w/ factor IX deficiency (hemophilia B, Christmas disease). *Adult:* Base dose on factor IX levels. Guidelines: *BeneFix,* 1.3 units/kg × body weight (kg) × desired increase (% of normal) IV daily to bid for up to 7 days; *Bebulin VH,* body weight (kg) × desired increase (% of normal) × 1.2 units/kg IV daily to bid for up to 10 days. *Others:* 1 international unit/kg × body weight (kg) × desired increase (% of normal) IV daily to bid. **Px of factor IX deficiency.** *Adult, child:* 20–30 units/kg IV once or twice/wk; increase if surgery planned.
ADV EFF AIDS, Creutzfeldt-Jakob disease, headache, infusion reaction, nausea, **thrombotic events**
NC/PT Must give IV; infuse slowly. Monitor for infusion reaction; slow infusion. Regular blood tests of clotting factors needed. Review s&sx of thrombotic events. Pt should wear medical ID.

factor XIII concentrate
(human) (Corifact)
CLASS Clotting factor
PREG/CONT C/NA

IND & DOSE Routine px of congenital factor XIII deficiency. *Adult, child:* 40 units/kg IV over not less than 4 mL/min, then base dose on pt response. Repeat q 28 days, maintaining trough activity level of 5%–20%.
ADV EFF Anaphylaxis, arthralgia, **blood-transferred diseases**, chills, factor XIII antibody formation, fever, headache, hepatic impairment, **thrombotic events**
NC/PT Alert pt to risk of blood-related disease. Teach pt s&sx of thrombotic events, allergic reaction,

immune reaction (break-through bleeding).

famciclovir sodium
(Famvir)
CLASS Antiviral
PREG/CONT B/NA

IND & DOSE Mgt of herpes zoster. *Adult:* 500 mg PO q 8 hr for 7 days. **Tx of genital herpes, first episode in immunocompetent pts.** *Adult:* 250 mg PO tid for 7–10 days. **Tx of recurrent genital herpes.** *Adult:* 125 mg PO bid for 5 days, or 1,000 mg PO bid for 1 day. **Chronic suppression of recurrent genital herpes.** *Adult:* 250 mg PO bid for up to 1 yr. **Tx of recurrent orolabial or genital herpes simplex infection in HIV-infected pts.** *Adult:* 500 mg PO q 12 hr for 7 days. **Tx of recurrent herpes labialis.** *Adult:* 1,500 mg PO as single dose.
ADJUST DOSE Renal impairment
ADV EFF Cancer, diarrhea, fever, granulocytopenia, headache, rash, thrombocytopenia
INTERACTIONS Cimetidine, digoxin
NC/PT Monitor CBC before, q 2 days during, at least wkly after tx. Pt should continue precautions to prevent transmission (drug not a cure), avoid exposure to infection, take analgesics for headache.

famotidine (Pepcid)
CLASS Histamine-2 receptor antagonist
PREG/CONT B/NA

IND & DOSE Acute tx of active duodenal ulcer. *Adult:* 40 mg PO or IV at bedtime, or 20 mg PO or IV bid; discontinue after 6–8 wk. *Child 1–12 yr:* 0.5 mg/kg/day PO at bedtime or divided into two doses (up to 40 mg/day), or 0.25 mg/kg IV q 12 hr (up to 40 mg/day) if unable to take orally. **Maint tx of duodenal ulcer.** *Adult:*

20 mg PO at bedtime. **Benign gastric ulcer.** *Adult:* 40 mg PO daily at bedtime. **Tx of hypersecretory syndrome.** *Adult:* Initially, 20 mg PO q 6 hr. Taper; up to 160 mg PO q 6 hr has been used. Or, 20 mg IV q 12 hr in pts unable to take orally. *Children 1–12 yr:* 0.25 mg/kg IV q 12 hr (up to 40 mg/day) if unable to take orally. **Tx of GERD.** *Adult:* 20 mg PO bid for up to 6 wk. For GERD w/ esophagitis, 20–40 mg PO bid for up to 12 wk. *Child 1–12 yr:* 1 mg/kg/day PO divided into two doses (up to 40 mg bid). *Child 3 mo–1 yr:* 0.5 mg/kg PO bid for up to 8 wk. *Under 3 mo:* 0.5 mg/kg/dose oral suspension once daily for up to 8 wk. **Px, relief of heartburn, acid indigestion.** *Adult:* 10–20 mg PO for relief; 10–20 mg PO 15–60 min before eating for prevention. Max, 20 mg/24 hr.
ADJUST DOSE Renal impairment
ADV EFF Constipation, diarrhea, headache
NC/PT Reserve IV use for pts unable to take orally; switch to oral as soon as possible. Give at bedtime. May use concurrent antacid to relieve pain. Pt should place rapidly disintegrating tablet on tongue; swallow w/ or without water.

fat emulsion, intravenous (Intralipid, Liposyn)
CLASS Caloric drug, nutritional drug
PREG/CONT C/NA

BBW Give to preterm infants only if benefit clearly outweighs risk; deaths have occurred.
IND & DOSE Parenteral nutrition. *Adult:* Should not constitute more than 60% of total calorie intake. *10%:* Infuse IV at 1 mL/min for first 15–30 min; may increase to 2 mL/min. Infuse only 500 mL first day; increase following day. Max, 2.5 g/kg/day. *20%:* Infuse at 0.5 mL/min for first 15–30 min. Infuse only 250 mL

Liposyn II or 500 mL *Intralipid* first day; increase following day. Max, 3 g/kg/day. *30%:* Infuse at 1 mL/min (0.1 g fat/min) for first 15–30 min; max, 2.5 g/kg/day. *Child:* Should not constitute more than 60% of total calorie intake. *10%:* Initial IV infusion rate, 0.1 mL/min for first 10–15 min. *20%:* Initial infusion rate, 0.05 mL/min for first 10–15 min. If no untoward reactions, increase rate to 4 g/kg in 4 hr; max, 4 g/kg/day. *30%:* Initial infusion rate, 0.1 mL/min (0.01 g fat/min) for first 10–15 min; max, 3 g/kg/day. **Tx of essential fatty acid deficiency.** Supply 8%–10% of caloric intake by IV fat emulsion.
ADV EFF Headache, leukopenia, nausea, **sepsis, thrombocytopenia,** thrombophlebitis
NC/PT Supplied in single-dose containers. Do not store partially used bottles or resterilize for later use. Do not use w/ filters. Do not use bottle in which there appears to be separation from emulsion. Monitor closely for fluid, fat overload. Monitor lipid profile, nitrogen balance closely; monitor for thrombotic events, sepsis. Pt should report pain at injection site.

febuxostat (Uloric)
CLASS Antigout drug, xanthine oxidase inhibitor
PREG/CONT C/NA

IND & DOSE Long-term mgt of hyperuricemia in pts w/ gout. *Adult:* 40 mg/day PO; if serum uric acid level not under 6 mg/dL in 2 wk, may increase to 80 mg/day.
ADJUST DOSE Hepatic, renal impairment
ADV EFF Gout flares, **MI,** nausea, stroke
INTERACTIONS Azathioprine, mercaptopurine theophyllines (use contraindicated)
NC/PT Obtain baseline, periodic uric acid levels. May use w/ antacids, other drugs to control gout. Store at room temp, protected from light. Use cau-

tion in pregnancy, breast-feeding. Pt should report chest pain, numbness, tingling.

felodipine (Plendil)
CLASS Antihypertensive, calcium channel blocker
PREG/CONT C/NA

IND & DOSE Tx of essential hypertension. *Adult:* 5 mg/day PO; range, 2.5–10 mg/day PO.
ADJUST DOSE Elderly pts, hepatic impairment
ADV EFF Dizziness, fatigue, flushing, headache, lethargy, light-headedness, nausea, peripheral edema
INTERACTIONS Antifungals, barbiturates, carbamazepine, cimetidine, grapefruit juice, hydantoins, ranitidine
NC/PT Monitor cardiac rhythm, BP carefully during dose adjustment. Pt should swallow tablet whole and not cut, crush, or chew it; avoid grapefruit juice; report swelling in hands, feet.

fenofibrate (Antara, Fenoglide, Lofibra, Lipofen, TriCor, Triglide, Trilipix)
CLASS Antihyperlipidemic
PREG/CONT C/NA

IND & DOSE Adjunct to diet, exercise for tx of hypertriglyceridemia. *Adult:* 48–145 mg (*TriCor*) PO, or 67–200 mg (*Lofibra*) PO w/ meal, or 50–160 mg/day (*Triglide*) PO daily, or 43–130 mg/day PO (*Antara*), or 50–150 mg/day PO (*Lipofen*), or 40–120 mg/day PO (*Fenoglide*), or 45–135 mg/day PO (*Trilipix*). **Adjunct to diet, exercise for tx of primary hypercholesterolemia, mixed dyslipidemia.** *Adult:* 145 mg/day PO (*TriCor*), or 200 mg/day (*Lofibra*) PO w/ meal, or 160 mg/day (*Triglide*), or 130 mg/day PO (*Antara*), or 150 mg/day PO (*Lipofen*), or 120 mg/day PO (*Fenoglide*), or 135 mg/day PO (*Trilipix*); if combined w/ statin, 135 mg/day PO (*Trilipix*).

ADJUST DOSE Elderly pts, renal impairment
ADV EFF Decreased libido, ED, flu-like symptoms, myalgia, nausea, **pancreatitis**, rash
INTERACTIONS Anticoagulants, bile acid sequestrants, immunosuppressants, nephrotoxic drugs, statins
NC/PT Obtain baseline, periodic lipid profile, LFTs, CBC w/ long-term therapy. Differentiate between brand names; doses vary. Balance timing of administration if used w/ other lipid-lowering drugs. Use caution in pregnancy; not for use in breast-feeding. Pt should swallow DR capsules whole and not cut, crush, or chew them; continue exercise, diet programs; report muscle weakness, aches.

---

fenoprofen calcium
(Nalfon)

CLASS Analgesic, NSAID
PREG/CONT B (1st, 2nd trimesters); D (3rd trimester)/NA

BBW Increased risk of CV events, GI bleeding; monitor accordingly.
IND & DOSE Tx of rheumatoid arthritis, osteoarthritis. *Adult:* 400–600 mg PO tid or qid. May need 2–3 wk before improvement seen. **Tx of mild to moderate pain.** *Adult:* 200 mg PO q 4–6 hr as needed.
ADJUST DOSE Renal impairment
ADV EFF Agranulocytosis, anaphylactoid reactions to fatal anaphylactic shock, aplastic anemia, dizziness, dyspepsia, **eosinophilia**, GI pain, granulocytopenia, headache, impaired vision, insomnia, **leukemia**, nausea, neutropenia, pancytopenia, rash, somnolence, **thrombocytopenia**
INTERACTIONS ACE inhibitors, anticoagulants, antiplatelets, aspirin, phenobarbital
NC/PT Not for use in pregnancy (contraceptives advised). Pt should take w/ meals, use safety precautions

w/ CNS effects, report bleeding, tarry stools, vision changes.

---

fentanyl (Abstral, Actiq, Duragesic, Fentora, Lazanda, Onsolis, SUBSYS)

CLASS Opioid agonist analgesic
PREG/CONT C/C-II

BBW Ensure appropriate use because drug potentially dangerous; respiratory depression, death possible. Have opioid antagonist, facilities for assisted or controlled respiration on hand during parenteral administration. Use caution when switching between forms; doses vary. Transdermal, nasal forms not for use in opioid–nontolerant pts. Not for acute or postop use. Do not substitute for other fentanyl product. Keep out of children's reach; can be fatal. Potentiation of effects possible when given w/ macrolide antibiotics, ketoconazole, itraconazole, protease inhibitors; potentially fatal respiratory depression possible.
IND & DOSE Analgesic adjunct for anesthesia. *Adult:* Premedication, 50–100 mcg IM 30–60 min before surgery. Adjunct to general anesthesia, initially, 2–20 mcg/kg; maint, 2–50 mcg IV or IM. 25–100 mcg IV or IM when vital sign changes indicate surgical stress, lightening of analgesia. W/ oxygen for anesthesia, total high dose, 50–100 mcg/kg IV. Adjunct to regional anesthesia, 50–100 mcg IM or slowly IV over 1–2 min. *Child 2–12 yr:* 2–3 mcg/kg IV as vital signs indicate. **Control of postop pain, tachypnea, emergence delirium.** *Adult:* 50–100 mcg IM; repeat in 1–2 hr if needed. **Mgt of chronic pain in pts requiring continuous opioid analgesia over extended period.** *Adult:* 25 mcg/hr transdermal system; may need replacement in 72 hr if pain has not subsided. Do not use torn, damaged systems; serious overdose possible. *Children 2–12 yr:*

25 mcg/hr transdermal system; pts should be opioid-tolerant and receiving at least 60 mg oral morphine equivalents/day. **Tx of breakthrough pain in cancer pts treated w/ and tolerant to opioids.** *Adult:* Place unit (*Actiq*) in mouth between cheek, lower gum. Start w/ 200 mcg; may start redosing 15 min after previous lozenge completed. No more than two lozenges/breakthrough pain episode. For buccal tablets, initially 100-mcg tablet between cheek, gum for 14–25 min; may repeat in 30 min. For buccal soluble film, remove film, place inside cheek; will dissolve within 5–30 min. For sublingual tablets, initially 100 mcg sublingually; wait at least 2 hr between doses. For nasal spray, 100 mcg as single spray in one nostril. Max, 800 mcg as single spray in one nostril or single spray in each nostril/episode. Wait at least 2 hr before treating new episode. No more than four doses in 24 hr.

ADV EFF **Apnea, cardiac arrest,** clamminess, confusion, constipation, dizziness, floating feeling, headache, lethargy, light-headedness, local irritation, n/v, sedation, **shock,** sweating, vertigo
INTERACTIONS Alcohol, barbiturates, CNS depressants, grapefruit juice, itraconazole, ketoconazole, macrolide antibiotics, MAOIs, protease inhibitors
NC/PT Adjust dose as needed, tolerated for pain relief. Apply transdermal system to nonirritated, nonirradiated skin on flat surface of upper torso. Clip, do not shave, hair. May need 12 hr for full effect. Do not use torn, damaged transdermal systems; serious overdose possible. Give to breast-feeding women 4–6 hr before next scheduled feeding. Buccal soluble film, nasal spray only available through restricted access program. Pt should avoid grapefruit juice, remove old transdermal patch before applying new one, take safety precautions w/ CNS effects, report difficulty breathing. Name confusion between fentanyl and sufentanil; use extreme caution.

ferrous salts (ferrous aspartate, ferrous fumarate, ferrous gluconate, ferrous sulfate, ferrous sulfate exsiccated) (Femiron, Feosol, Fer-In-Sol, Ferro-Sequels, Slow Fe, Slow Release Iron)
CLASS Iron preparation
PREG/CONT A/NA

BBW Warn pt to keep out of reach of children; leading cause of fatal poisoning in child under 6 yr.
IND & DOSE **Dietary iron supplement.** *Adult:* Men, 8–11 mg/day PO; women, 8–18 mg/day PO. Pregnant, breast-feeding women, 9–27 mg/day PO. *Child:* 7–11 mg/day PO. **Px, tx of iron deficiency anemia.** *Adult:* 150–300 mg/day (6 mg/kg/day) PO for approximately 6–10 mo. *Child:* 3–6 mg/kg/day PO.
ADV EFF Anorexia, **coma, death w/ overdose;** constipation; GI upset; n/v
INTERACTIONS Antacids, chloramphenicol, cimetidine, ciprofloxacin, coffee, eggs, levodopa, levothyroxine, milk, norfloxacin, ofloxacin, tea, tetracycline
NC/PT Establish correct diagnosis. Regularly monitor Hct, Hgb. Use straw for liquid forms (may stain teeth). Give w/ food if GI upset severe. Stool may be green to black; tx may take several mo. Laxative may be needed. Pt should avoid eggs, milk, coffee, tea; keep out of reach of children (serious to fatal toxicity possible).

ferumoxytol (Feraheme)
CLASS Iron preparation
PREG/CONT C/NA

IND & DOSE **Tx of iron deficiency anemia in pts w/ chronic renal failure.** *Adult:* 510 mg IV as undiluted sol at 30 mg/sec, then 510 mg IV in 3–8 days.
ADV EFF Constipation, diarrhea, dizziness, **hypersensitivity**

reactions, hypotension, iron overload, nausea, peripheral edema
NC/PT Alters MRI results for up to 3 mo after use; will not alter CT scans or X-rays. Do not give if iron overload. Monitor for hypersensitivity reaction up to 30 min after infusion; have life support available. Monitor BP during and for 30 min after administration. Use caution in pregnancy; not for use in breast-feeding. Pt should take safety precautions w/ CNS effects, report difficulty breathing, itching, swelling.

fesoterodine fumarate (Toviaz)
CLASS Antimuscarinic
PREG/CONT C/NA

IND & DOSE Tx of overactive bladder. *Adult:* 4 mg/day PO; may increase to max 8 mg/day.
ADJUST DOSE Renal impairment; hepatic impairment (not recommended)
ADV EFF Blurred vision, constipation, decreased sweating, dry eyes, dry mouth, increased IOP, urine retention
INTERACTIONS Alcohol, clarithromycin, itraconazole, ketoconazole
NC/PT Monitor IOP before, periodically during tx. Pt should swallow tablet whole and not cut, crush, or chew it; use sugarless lozenges, mouth care for dry mouth; take safety precautions for vision changes; stay hydrated in heat conditions (decreased ability to sweat); avoid alcohol.

fexofenadine hydrochloride (Allegra)
CLASS Antihistamine
PREG/CONT C/NA

IND & DOSE Symptomatic relief of sx associated w/ seasonal allergic rhinitis. *Adult, child 12 yr and older:* 60 mg PO bid or 180 mg PO once daily; or 10 mL suspension PO bid. *Child 6–12 yr:* 30 mg orally disintegrating

tablet (ODT) PO bid, or 5 mL suspension PO bid. *Child 2–12 yr:* 5 mL suspension PO bid. **Chronic idiopathic urticaria.** *Adult, child 12 yr and older:* 60 mg PO bid or 180 mg PO once daily. *Child 6–12 yr:* 30 mg ODT PO bid, or 5 mL suspension PO bid. *Child 2–12 yr:* 5 mL suspension PO bid..
ADJUST DOSE Elderly pts, renal impairment
ADV EFF Drowsiness, fatigue, nausea
INTERACTIONS Antacids, erythromycin, itraconazole ketoconazole
NC/PT Arrange for humidifier if nasal dryness, thickened secretions a problem; encourage hydration. Pt should use in a.m. before exposure to allergens, take safety precautions w/ CNS effects.

fibrinogen concentrate, human (RiaSTAP)
CLASS Coagulation factor
PREG/CONT C/NA

IND & DOSE Tx of acute bleeding episodes in pts w/ congenital fibrinogen deficiency. *Adult, child:* 70 mg/kg by slow IV injection not over 5 mL/min; adjust dose to target fibrinogen level of 100 mg/dL.
ADJUST DOSE Elderly pts, renal impairment
ADV EFF Anaphylactic reactions, arterial thrombosis, blood-transmitted diseases, chills, **DVT,** fever, **MI,** n/v, **PE,** rash
NC/PT Made from human blood; risk of blood-transmitted diseases. Risk of thromboembolic events, severe hypersensitivity reactions. Pt should report chest/leg pain, chest tightness, difficulty breathing, continued fever.

fidaxomicin (Dificid)
CLASS Macrolide antibiotic
PREG/CONT B/NA

IND & DOSE Tx of *Clostridium difficile* diarrhea. *Adult:* 200 mg PO bid for 10 days.

ADV EFF Abd pain, dyspepsia, **gastric hemorrhage,** n/v
NC/PT Culture stool before tx. Not for systemic infections; specific to *C. difficile* diarrhea. Pt should complete full course of tx, report severe vomiting, bloody diarrhea.

filgrastim (Neupogen)
CLASS Colony-stimulating factor
PREG/CONT C/NA

IND & DOSE To decrease incidence of infection in pts w/ nonmyeloid malignancies receiving myelosuppressive anticancer drugs; to reduce time to neutrophil recovery, duration of fever after induction or consolidation chemotherapy tx of acute myeloid leukemia. *Adult:* 5 mcg/kg/day subcut or IV as single daily injection. May increase in increments of 5 mcg/kg for each chemotherapy cycle; range, 4–8 mcg/kg/day. **To reduce duration of neutropenia after bone marrow transplant.** *Adult:* 10 mcg/kg/day IV or continuous subcut infusion. **Tx of severe chronic neutropenia.** *Adult:* 6 mcg/kg subcut bid (congenital neutropenia); 5 mcg/kg/day subcut as single injection (idiopathic, cyclic neutropenia). **To mobilize hematopoietic progenitor cells into blood for leukapheresis collection.** *Adult:* 10 mcg/kg/day subcut at least 4 days before first leukapheresis; continue to last leukapheresis.
ADV EFF Alopecia, bone pain, n/v/d
NC/PT Obtain CBC, platelet count before and twice wkly during tx. Do not give within 24 hr of chemotherapy. Give daily for up to 2 wk or neutrophils are 10,000/mm³. Store in refrigerator. Do not shake vial; do not reuse vial, needles, syringes. Teach pt proper administration, disposal of needles, syringes. Pt should avoid exposure to infection, cover head at temp extremes (hair loss possible).

finasteride (Propecia, Proscar)
CLASS Androgen hormone inhibitor
PREG/CONT X/NA

IND & DOSE Tx of symptomatic BPH. *Adult:* 5 mg daily PO w/ or without meal; may take 6–12 mo for response (*Proscar*). **Px of male-pattern baldness.** *Adult:* 1 mg/day PO for 3 mo or more before benefit seen (*Propecia*).
ADV EFF Decreased libido, ED, gynecomastia
NC/PT Confirm dx of BPH. Protect from light. Pregnant women should not touch tablet. Pt may not donate blood during and for 6 mo after tx. Pt should monitor urine flow for improvement; may experience loss of libido

fingolimod (Gilenya)
CLASS MS drug
PREG/CONT C/NA

IND & DOSE Tx of relapsing forms of MS. *Adult:* 0.5 mg/day PO.
ADV EFF Back pain, bradycardia, cough, decreased lung capacity, depression, diarrhea, dyspnea, headache, increased liver enzymes, infections, macular edema
INTERACTIONS Amiodarone, antineoplastics, beta blockers, calcium channel blockers, immunomodulators, immunosuppressants, ketoconazole, live vaccines. procainamide, quinidine, sotalol
NC/PT Use caution w/ hypertension or hx of CAD. Obtain baseline, periodic ophthalmic evaluation because of macular edema risk. Monitor for bradycardia for at least 6 hr after first dose. Obtain spirometry studies if dyspnea occurs. Not for use in pregnancy (contraceptives advised during and for 2 mo after tx), breast-feeding. Pt should avoid exposure to infection, take safety

precautions w/ CNS effects, report difficulty breathing.

flavoxate hydrochloride (generic)

CLASS Parasympathetic blocker, urinary antispasmodic
PREG/CONT B/NA

IND & DOSE Symptomatic relief of dysuria, urgency, nocturia, suprapubic pain, frequency/incontinence due to cystitis, prostatitis, urethritis, urethrocystitis, urethrotrigonitis. *Adult, child 12 yr and older:* 100–200 mg PO tid or qid. Reduce dose when symptoms improve. Use max 1,200 mg/day in severe urinary urgency after pelvic radiotherapy.
ADV EFF Blurred vision, drowsiness, dry mouth, eosinophilia, headache, leukopenia, nervousness, n/v, vertigo
INTERACTIONS Anticholinergics, cholinergics
NC/PT Treat for underlying problem leading to s&sx. Obtain eye exam before, during tx. Pt should use sugarless lozenges for dry mouth, report blurred vision.

flecainide acetate (Tambocor)

CLASS Antiarrhythmic
PREG/CONT C/NA

BBW Increased risk of nonfatal cardiac arrest, death in pts w/ recent MI, chronic atrial fibrillation. Monitor cardiac rhythm carefully; risk of potentially fatal proarrhythmias.
IND & DOSE Px, tx of life-threatening ventricular arrhythmias. *Adult:* 100 mg PO q 12 hr. Increase in 50-mg increments bid q fourth day until efficacy achieved; max, 400 mg/day. Px of paroxysmal atrial fibrillation/flutter associated w/ symptoms and paroxysmal supraventricular tachycardias. *Adult:* 50 mg PO q 12 hr; may increase in 50-mg increments bid q 4 days until efficacy achieved; max,

300 mg/day. **Transfer to flecainide.** Allow at least 2–4 plasma half-lives to elapse after other antiarrhythmics discontinued before starting flecainide.
ADJUST DOSE Elderly pts; renal, hepatic impairment
ADV EFF Abd pain, arrhythmias, chest pain, constipation, dizziness, drowsiness, dyspnea, fatigue, headache, leukopenia, n/v, visual changes
INTERACTIONS Amiodarone, cimetidine, disopyramide (avoid marked drop in cardiac output), propranolol
NC/PT Check serum potassium before starting tx; evaluate for therapeutic serum levels (0.2–1 mcg/mL). Monitor response closely; have life support equipment on hand. Pt should take q 12 hr (arrange timing to avoid interrupting sleep), use safety precautions w/ CNS effects, report chest pain, palpitations.

floxuridine (FUDR)

CLASS Antimetabolite, antineoplastic
PREG/CONT D/NA

IND & DOSE Palliative mgt of GI adenocarcinoma metastatic to liver. *Adult:* 0.1–0.6 mg/kg/day via intra-arterial infusion.
ADV EFF Bone marrow suppression, infections, gastric ulceration, glossitis, hepatic impairment, n/v/d, renal impairment, stomatitis
INTERACTIONS Immunosuppressants, live vaccines
NC/PT Obtain baseline, periodic CBC. Check for mouth ulcerations, dental infections; mouth care essential. Protect from exposure to infections. Not for use in pregnancy, breast-feeding. Pt should report severe GI pain, bloody diarrhea.

fluconazole (Diflucan)

CLASS Antifungal
PREG/CONT D/NA

IND & DOSE Tx of oropharyngeal candidiasis: *Adult:* 200 mg PO or IV on first day, then 100 mg/day for at least 2 wk. **Tx of esophageal candidiasis.** *Adult:* 200 mg PO or IV on first day, then 100 mg/day, up to 400 mg/day for minimum of 3 wk, at least 2 wk after resolution. *Child:* 6 mg/kg PO or IV on first day, then 3 mg/kg/day for 3 wk, at least 2 wk after resolution. **Tx of vaginal candidiasis.** *Adult:* 150 mg PO as single dose. **Tx of systemic candidiasis.** *Adult:* 400 mg PO or IV daily. *Child:* 6–12 mg/kg PO or IV. **Tx of candidal UTI/peritonitis.** *Adult:* 50–200 mg/day PO or IV. **Tx of cryptococcal meningitis.** *Adult:* 400 mg PO or IV on first day, then 200 mg/day up to 400 mg/day for 10–12 wk after cultures of CSF become negative. *Child:* 12 mg/kg PO or IV on first day, then 6 mg/kg/day for 10–12 wk after cultures of CSF become negative. **Suppression of cryptococcal meningitis in AIDS pts.** *Adult:* 200 mg PO or IV daily. *Child:* 6 mg/kg PO or IV daily. **Px of candidiasis in bone marrow transplants.** *Adult:* 400 mg PO daily for several days before onset of neutropenia and for 7 days after neutrophil count above 1,000/mm³.

ADJUST DOSE Renal impairment
ADV EFF Abd pain, headache, n/v/d, **renal toxicity**
INTERACTIONS Benzodiazepines, cimetidine, cyclosporine, oral hypoglycemics, phenytoin, rifampin, warfarin anticoagulants, zidovudine
NC/PT Culture before tx. For IV, oral use only. Monitor renal function wkly. Frequent medical follow-up needed. Pt should take hygiene measures to prevent infection spread, use analgesics for headache.

---

flucytosine (Ancobon)
CLASS Antifungal
PREG/CONT C/NA

BBW Monitor serum flucytosine levels in pts w/ renal impairment (levels over 100 mcg/mL associated w/ toxicity).

IND & DOSE Tx of serious infections caused by susceptible *Candida, Cryptococcus* strains. *Adult:* 50–150 mg/kg/ day PO at 6-hr intervals.
ADJUST DOSE Renal impairment
ADV EFF Anemia, **cardiac arrest,** confusion, dizziness, **leukopenia,** n/v/d, **rash, respiratory arrest, thrombocytopenia**
NC/PT Give capsules few at a time over 15-min to decrease GI upset, diarrhea. Monitor LFTs, renal/hematologic function periodically during tx. Pt should take safety precautions w/ CNS effects; report fever, difficulty breathing.

DANGEROUS DRUG

fludarabine phosphate (generic)
CLASS Antimetabolite, antineoplastic
PREG/CONT D/NA

BBW Stop tx if s&sx of toxicity (CNS complaints, stomatitis, esophagopharyngitis, rapidly falling WBC count, intractable vomiting, diarrhea, GI ulceration/bleeding, thrombocytopenia, hemorrhage, hemolytic anemia); serious to life-threatening infections possible. Consult physician.
IND & DOSE Chronic lymphocytic leukemia (CLL); unresponsive B-cell CLL. *Adult:* 40 mg/m² PO or 25 mg/m² IV over 30 min for 5 consecutive days. Begin each 5-day course q 28 days.
ADJUST DOSE Renal impairment
ADV EFF Anorexia, autoimmune hemolytic anemia, bone marrow toxicity, chills, **CNS toxicity (including blindness, coma, death),** cough, dyspnea, edema, fatigue, fever, headache, infection, n/v/d, pneumonia, pruritus, **pulmonary toxicity,** stomatitis, **tumor lysis syndrome,** visual disturbances, weakness
INTERACTIONS Pentostatin
NC/PT Obtain CBC before tx, each dose. Monitor pulmonary function regularly. Not for use in pregnancy

(contraceptives advised). Pt should not crush tablets; avoid contact w/ skin, mucous membranes; mark calendar of tx days; take safety precautions for CNS effects; avoid exposure to infections; report bruising, excess bleeding, black stools, difficulty breathing.

fludrocortisone acetate
(Florinef Acetate)

CLASS Corticosteroid
PREG/CONT C/NA

IND & DOSE Partial replacement tx in adrenocortical insufficiency. *Adult:* 0.05–0.1 mg/day PO. **Tx of salt-losing adrenogenital syndrome.** *Adult:* 0.1–0.2 mg/day PO.
ADJUST DOSE Elderly pts; hepatic, renal impairment
ADV EFF Anxiety, cardiac enlargement, depression, edema, HF, hypertension, hypokalemic acidosis, infection, weakness
INTERACTIONS Amphotericin B, anabolic steroids, antidiabetics, aspirin, barbiturates, digitalis, diuretics, hormonal contraceptives, phenytoin, rifampin, warfarin
NC/PT Monitor BP, serum electrolytes, blood glucose before, periodically during tx. Protect from infection. Frequent medical follow-up, blood tests needed. Use caution in pregnancy, breast-feeding. Pt should wear medical ID, report all drugs used to health care provider (many drug interactions possible).

flumazenil (Romazicon)

CLASS Antidote, benzodiazepine receptor antagonist
PREG/CONT C/NA

BBW Possible increased risk of seizures, especially in pts on long-term benzodiazepine tx and pts w/ serious cyclic antidepressant overdose; take appropriate precautions.

IND & DOSE Reversal of conscious sedation or in general anesthesia. *Adult:* 0.2 mg (2 mL) IV over 15 sec, wait 45 sec; if ineffectual, repeat at 60-sec intervals. Max cumulative dose, 1 mg (10 mL). *Children over 1 yr:* 0.01 mg/kg (up to 0.2 mg) IV over 15 sec; wait 45 sec. Repeat at 60-sec intervals. Max cumulative dose, 0.05 mg/kg or 1 mg, whichever lowest. **Mgt of suspected benzodiazepine overdose.** *Adult:* 0.2 mg IV over 30 sec; repeat w/ 0.3 mg IV q 30 sec. May give further doses of 0.5 mg over 30 sec at 1-min intervals. Max cumulative dose, 3 mg.
ADV EFF Amnesia, dizziness, increased sweating, n/v, pain at injection site, **seizures**, vertigo
INTERACTIONS Alcohol, CNS depressants, food
NC/PT IV use only, into running IV in large vein. Have emergency equipment on hand; continually monitor response. Provide safety measures for CNS effects for at least 18–24 hr after use. Give pt written information (amnesia may be prolonged). Pt should avoid alcohol for 18–24 hr after administration.

flunisolide (Aerospan HFA)

CLASS Corticosteroid
PREG/CONT C/NA

BBW Taper systemic steroids carefully during transfer to inhalational steroids; deaths from adrenal insufficiency have occurred.

IND & DOSE Intranasal relief/mgt of nasal sx of seasonal, perennial allergic rhinitis. *Adult:* 2 sprays (50 mcg) in each nostril bid; may increase to 2 sprays in each nostril tid (total dose, 300 mcg/day). Max, 400 mcg/day. *Child 6–14 yr:* 1 spray in each nostril tid or 2 sprays in each nostril bid (total dose, 150–200 mcg/day). Max, 200 mcg/day. **Inhalation maint tx of asthma.** *Adult:* 2 inhalations by mouth bid. Max, 640 mcg/day.

Child 12 yr and older: Adult dosage. *Child 6–11 yr:* 1 inhalation bid. Max, 160 mcg bid.

ADV EFF Epistaxis, fungal infection, headache, nasal irritation, rebound congestion

NC/PT May use decongestant drops to facilitate penetration if needed. Not for acute asthma attack. Pt should not stop suddenly, rinse mouth after each use of inhaler.

DANGEROUS DRUG

fluorouracil (Adrucil, Carac, Efudex, Fluoroplex)

CLASS Antimetabolite, antineoplastic
PREG/CONT D/NA

BBW Stop tx at s&sx of toxicity (stomatitis, esophagopharyngitis, rapidly falling WBC count, intractable vomiting, diarrhea, GI ulceration/bleeding, thrombocytopenia, hemorrhage); serious to life-threatening reactions have occurred. Consult physician.

IND & DOSE Palliative mgt of carcinoma of colon, rectum, breast, stomach, pancreas in selected pts considered incurable by surgery or other means. *Adult:* 12 mg/kg/day IV for 4 successive days, infused slowly over 24 hr; max, 800 mg/day. If no toxicity, 6 mg/kg/day IV on days 6, 8, 10, 12, w/ no drug tx on days 5, 7, 9, 11. Stop tx at end of day 12. If no toxicity, repeat q 30 days. If toxicity, 10–15 mg/kg/wk IV as single dose after s&sx of toxicity subside; max, 1 g/wk. Adjust dose based on response; tx may be prolonged (12–60 mo). **Tx of actinic or solar keratoses.** *Adult:* Apply bid to cover lesions. 0.5% and 1% used on head, neck, chest; 2% and 5% used on hands. Continue until inflammatory response reaches erosion, necrosis, and ulceration stage, then stop. Usual tx course, 2–4 wk. Complete healing may not occur for 1–2 mo after tx stops. **Tx of superficial basal cell carcinoma.** *Adult:* 5% strength bid in amount sufficient to

cover lesions, for at least 3–6 wk. Tx may be needed for 10–12 wk.

ADJUST DOSE Poor risk, undernourished pts

ADV EFF Alopecia, anorexia, cramps, dermatitis, duodenal ulcer, duodenitis, enteritis, gastritis, glossitis, lethargy, **leukopenia**, local irritation w/ topical use, malaise, n/v/d, photosensitivity, rash, stomatitis, **thrombocytopenia**

NC/PT Obtain CBC before and regularly during tx. Ensure dx of topical lesions. Thoroughly wash hands after applying topical form; avoid occlusive dressings w/ topical form. Stop tx at s&sx of toxicity. Frequent medical follow-up needed. Pt should mark calendar for tx days; cover head at temp extremes (hair loss possible); avoid exposure to sun, infections; report black tarry stools, unusual bleeding or bruising.

---

fluoxetine hydrochloride (Prozac, Sarafem)

CLASS Antidepressant, SSRI
PREG/CONT C/NA

BBW Establish suicide precautions for severely depressed pts. Limit quantity dispensed; high risk of suicidality in children, adolescents, young adults.

IND & DOSE Tx of depression. *Adult:* 20 mg/day PO in a.m.; max, 80 mg/day. Once stabilized, may switch to 90-mg DR capsules PO once/wk. *Child 8–18 yr:* 10 mg/day PO; may increase to 20 mg/day after 1 wk or after several wk for lowweight children. **Tx of depressive episodes of bipolar I disorder.** *Adult:* 20 mg/day PO w/ 5 mg olanzapine. **Tx of tx-resistant depression.** *Adult:* 20–50 mg/day PO w/ 5–20 mg olanzapine. **Tx of OCD.** *Adult:* 20 mg/day PO; range, 20–60 mg/day PO. May need up to 5 wk for effectiveness. Max, 80 mg/day. *Adolescent, higher-weight child:* 10 mg/day PO; range,

20–60 mg/day PO. *Adolescent, lower-weight child:* 10 mg/day PO; range, 20–30 mg/day. **Tx of bulimia.** *Adult:* 60 mg/day PO in a.m. **Tx of panic disorder.** *Adult:* 10 mg/day PO for first wk; max, 60 mg/day. **Tx of PMDD (Sarafem).** *Adult:* 20 mg/day PO. Or 20 mg/day PO starting 14 days before anticipated beginning of menses, continuing through first full day of menses; then no drug until 3 days before next menses. Max, 80 mg/day.

ADJUST DOSE Elderly pts, hepatic impairment

ADV EFF Anorexia, anxiety, asthenia, constipation, dizziness, drowsiness, dry mouth, dyspepsia, fever, headache, insomnia, light-headedness, nervousness, n/v/d, painful menstruation, pharyngitis, pruritus, rash, **seizures**, sexual dysfx, sweating, URI, urinary frequency, weight changes

INTERACTIONS Alcohol, benzodiazepines, ER drugs, linezolid, lithium, MAOIs, opioids, serotoninergic drugs, St. John's wort, TCAs, thioridazine

NC/PT Do not use within 14 days of MAOIs. Give in a.m. Full antidepressant effect may not occur for up to 4–6 wk. Taper when stopping. Not for use in pregnancy. Pt should avoid alcohol, St. John's wort; take safety precautions w/ CNS effects; report thoughts of suicide. Name confusion between Sarafem (fluoxetine) and Serophene (clomiphene); use caution.

fluphenazine decanoate, fluphenazine hydrochloride (generic)

CLASS Antipsychotic, dopaminergic blocker, phenothiazine
PREG/CONT C/NA

BBW Establish suicide precautions for severely depressed pts. Limit quantity dispensed; high risk of suicidality in children, adolescents, young adults.

IND & DOSE Mgt of manifestations of psychotic disorders. *Adult:* 2.5–10 mg/day PO in divided doses q 6–8 hr; usual maint dose, 1–5 mg/day. Or, 1.25 mg/day IM (range, 2.5–10 mg) divided and given q 6–8 hr; parenteral dose is ⅓ to ½ oral dose (fluphenazine hydrochloride). **Long-term or parenteral neuroleptic therapy.** *Adult:* 12.5–25 mg IM or subcut; max, 100 mg/dose (fluphenazine decanoate).

ADJUST DOSE Elderly pts

ADV EFF Akathisia, anemia, aplastic anemia, autonomic disturbances, bronchospasm, cardiac arrest, dystonias, eosinophilia, hemolytic anemia, hyperthermia, hypoglycemia, laryngospasm, leukocytosis, leukopenia, **NMS**, photosensitivity, pseudoparkinsonism, refractory arrhythmias, seizures, sudden death related to asphyxia; tardive dyskinesia, thrombocytopenic or nonthrombocytopenic purpura

INTERACTIONS Alcohol, anticholinergics, barbiturates, CNS depressants, metrizamide

NC/PT Dilute oral concentrate in 60 mL suitable diluent not containing caffeine, tannic acid (tea), pectinates (apple juice). Monitor CBC, renal function, LFTs; adjust dose accordingly. Pt should take safety precautions w/ CNS effects; avoid exposure to sun, infection; maintain hydration; report unusual bleeding.

flurazepam hydrochloride (generic)

CLASS Benzodiazepine, sedative-hypnotic
PREG/CONT X/C-IV

IND & DOSE Tx of insomnia. *Adult:* 15–30 mg PO at bedtime.

ADJUST DOSE Elderly pts, debilitating disease

ADV EFF Anaphylaxis, angioedema, apathy, bradycardia, confusion, constipation, **CV collapse**, depression, diarrhea, disorientation, drowsiness, drug dependence w/ withdrawal, fatigue, gynecomastia, lethargy, light-headedness, restlessness, tachycardia, urine retention

INTERACTIONS Alcohol, aminophylline, barbiturates, cimetidine, disulfiram, hormonal contraceptives, opioids, phenothiazines, rifampin, SSRIs, theophylline, TCAs

NC/PT Monitor LFTs, renal function. Taper gradually after long-term use. Not for use in pregnancy (barrier contraceptives advised). Pt should take safety precautions w/ CNS effects, report worsening depression, difficulty breathing, edema.

flurbiprofen (Ansaid, Ocufen)

CLASS Analgesic, NSAID
PREG/CONT B (oral); C (ophthalmic)/NA

BBW Increased risk of CV events, GI bleeding; monitor accordingly. Contraindicated for tx of periop CABG pain.

IND & DOSE Acute or long-term tx of s&sx of rheumatoid arthritis, osteoarthritis; relief of moderate to mild pain. *Adult:* 200–300 mg PO in divided doses bid, tid, or qid. Max, 100 mg/dose. *Inhibition of intraop miosis. Adult:* 1 drop ophthalmic sol approximately q 30 min, starting 2 hr before surgery (total, 4 drops).

ADV EFF Agranulocytosis, aplastic anemia, bleeding, bone marrow depression, bronchospasm, dizziness, dyspepsia, **eosinophilia**, **fatal anaphylactic shock**, fatigue, **gastric ulcer**, GI pain, **granulocytopenia**, headache, insomnia, **leukopenia**, nausea, neutropenia, **pancytopenia**, **renal impairment**, somnolence, **thrombocytopenia**, transient local stinging/ burning w/ ophthalmic sol

NC/PT Give w/ food if GI upset severe. Not for use in pregnancy (barrier contraceptives advised). Pt should take safety precautions w/ CNS effects; report fever, rash, black stools, swelling in ankles/fingers.

DANGEROUS DRUG

flutamide (generic)

CLASS Antiandrogen, antineoplastic
PREG/CONT D/NA

BBW Arrange for periodic monitoring of LFTs during long-term tx; severe hepatotoxicity possible.

IND & DOSE Tx of locally advanced, metastatic prostatic carcinoma. *Adult:* 250 mg PO tid. Begin tx at same time as initiation of LH-RH analogue.

ADV EFF Anemia, dizziness, drowsiness, ED, GI disturbances, gynecomastia, **hepatic necrosis, hepatitis**, hot flashes, leukopenia, loss of libido, n/v/d, photosensitivity, rash

NC/PT Give w/ other drugs used for medical castration. Monitor LFTs regularly. Periodic blood tests will be needed. Pt should take safety precautions w/ CNS effects, avoid exposure to sunlight.

fluvastatin sodium (Lescol)

CLASS Antihyperlipidemic, statin
PREG/CONT X/NA

IND & DOSE Adjunct to diet, exercise to lower cholesterol, LDL; to slow progression of CAD, reduce risk of need for revascularization w/ CAD. *Adult:* 40 mg/day PO. Maint, 20–80 mg/day PO; give 80 mg/day as two 40-mg doses, or use 80-mg ER form. *Tx of heterozygous familial hypercholesterolemia. Child 9–16 yr:* 20 mg/day PO. Adjust q 6 wk to max 40 mg bid or 80 mg ER form PO once/day.

ADV EFF Abd pain, blurred vision, cataracts, constipation, cramps, flatulence, headache, **rhabdomyolysis**

INTERACTIONS Azole antifungals, cyclosporine, erythromycin, gemfibrozil, grapefruit juice, niacin, other statins, phenytoin, warfarin

NC/PT Give in evening. Periodic ophthalmic exams will be needed. Not for use in pregnancy (barrier contraceptives advised). Pt should swallow ER form whole and not cut, crush, or chew it; continue diet, exercise program; avoid grapefruit juice; report muscle pain w/ fever, changes in vision.

fluvoxamine maleate
(Luvox)
CLASS Antidepressant, SSRI
PREG/CONT C/NA

BBW Establish suicide precautions for severely depressed pts. Limit quantity dispensed. Increased risk of suicidal ideation, behavior in children, adolescents, young adults.
IND & DOSE Tx of OCD, social anxiety disorders. *Adult:* 50 mg PO at bedtime; range, 100–300 mg/day. Or, 100–300 mg/day CR capsules PO. *Child 8–17 yr:* 25 mg PO at bedtime. Divide doses over 50 mg/day; give larger dose at bedtime. Max for child up to 11 yr, 200 mg/day.
ADJUST DOSE Elderly pts, hepatic impairment
ADV EFF Anorexia, anxiety, asthenia, constipation, dizziness, drowsiness, dry mouth, dyspepsia, fever, headache, insomnia, light-headedness, nervousness, n/v/d, painful menstruation, pharyngitis, pruritus, rash, **seizures**, sexual dysfx, sweating, URI, urinary frequency, weight changes
INTERACTIONS Alprazolam, beta blockers, carbamazepine, cigarette smoking, clozapine, diltiazem, MAO-Is, methadone, quetiapine, statins, St. John's wort, TCAs, theophylline, triazolam, warfarin
NC/PT Give in evening. Monitor for serotonin syndrome. Taper when stopping. Pt should swallow CR capsule whole and not cut, crush, or chew it; take safety precautions w/ CNS effects; report thoughts of suicide.

folic acid (Folvite)
CLASS Folic acid, vitamin supplement
PREG/CONT A/NA

IND & DOSE Tx of megaloblastic anemias due to sprue, nutritional deficiency, pregnancy; anemias of infancy, childhood. *Adult:* 1 mg/day PO, IM, IV, subcut; maint, 0.4 mg/day. In pregnancy/breast-feeding, 0.8 mg/day PO. *Child (maint):* Over 4 yr, 0.4 mg/day PO; under 4 yr, up to 0.3 mg/day PO; infants, 0.1 mg/day
ADV EFF Pain, discomfort at injection site
INTERACTIONS Aminosalicylic acid, phenytoin, sulfasalazine
NC/PT Ensure correct anemia dx. Give orally if possible. Monitor for hypersensitivity reactions. Pt should report pain at injection site, difficulty breathing.

follitropin alfa (Gonal-F)
CLASS Fertility drug
PREG/CONT X/NA

IND & DOSE Induction of ovulation. *Adult:* 75 international units/day subcut. Increase by 37.5 international units/day after 14 days; may increase again after 7 days. Do not use for longer than 35 days. Stimulation of multiple follicles for in vitro fertilization. *Adult:* 150 international units/day subcut on days 2, 3 of cycle; continue for 10 days. Adjust based on response. Max, 450 international units subcut; then 5,000–10,000 international units HCG. Promotion of spermatogenesis. *Adult:* 150–300 international units subcut two to three times/wk w/ HCG. May use for up to 18 mo.
ADV EFF Multiple births, nausea, ovarian cyst, **ovarian hyperstimulation, pulmonary/vascular complications,** URI
NC/PT Ensure uterine health. Monitor regularly; monitor for thrombotic

events. Alert pt to risk of multiple births. Teach proper administration, disposal of needles, syringes.

follitropin beta (Follistim AQ)

CLASS Fertility drug
PREG/CONT X/NA

IND & DOSE Induction of ovulation.
Adult: 75 international units/day subcut. Increase by 37.5 international units/day after 14 days; may increase again after 7 days. Do not use for longer than 35 days. **Stimulation of multiple follicles for in vitro fertilization.** *Adult:* 150–225 international units/day subcut or IM for at least 4 days; adjust based on response. Follow w/ HCG.
ADV EFF Multiple births, nausea, ovarian cyst, **ovarian hyperstimulation, pulmonary/vascular complications,** URI
NC/PT Ensure uterine health. Give subcut in navel or abdomen. Monitor regularly; monitor for thrombotic events. Alert pt to risk of multiple births. Teach proper administration, disposal of needles, syringes.

fomepizole (Antizol)

CLASS Antidote
PREG/CONT C/NA

IND & DOSE Antidote for antifreeze, methanol poisoning. *Adult:* 15 mg/kg loading dose IV, then 10 mg/kg IV q 12 hr for 12 doses by slow IV infusion over 30 min.
ADV EFF Acidosis, bradycardia, dizziness, electrolyte disturbances, headache, hypotension, injection-site reaction, lymphangitis, **multiorgan failure,** nausea, nystagmus, phlebitis, **seizures, shock**
INTERACTIONS Alcohol
NC/PT Monitor ECG, electrolytes, renal function, LFTs, BP. Monitor injection site. May be used w/hemodialysis if needed to clear toxins.

Give q 4 hr during dialysis. Pt should take safety precautions w/ CNS effects.

DANGEROUS DRUG
fondaparinux (Arixtra)

CLASS Antithrombotic, low-molecular-weight heparin
PREG/CONT C/NA

BBW Carefully monitor pts receiving spinal/epidural anesthesia; risk of spinal hematoma, neurologic damage.
IND & DOSE Px of venous thrombotic events in pts undergoing surgery for hip fracture, hip or knee replacement; in pts undergoing abd surgery; extended px of DVT that may lead to PE after hip surgery. *Adult:* 2.5 mg/day subcut starting 6–8 hr after surgical closure and continuing for 5–9 days. May add 24 days after initial course for pts undergoing hip fracture surgery. **Tx of DVT, acute PE, w/ warfarin.** *Adult:* Over 100 kg, 10 mg/day subcut for 5–9 days; begin warfarin within 72 hr. 50–100 kg, 7.5 mg/day subcut for 5–9 days. Under 50 kg, 5 mg/day subcut for 5–9 days.
ADJUST DOSE Elderly pts, renal impairment
ADV EFF Anemia, bruising, fever, **hemorrhage,** local reaction at injection site, nausea
INTERACTIONS Cephalosporins, garlic, ginkgo, NSAIDs, oral anticoagulants, penicillins, salicylates, vitamin E
NC/PT Give drug 6–8 hr after surgical closure. Give by deep subcut injections; do not give IM. Store at room temp. Do not mix w/ other sols or massage injection site. Rotate injection sites. Provide safety measures to prevent bleeding. Teach proper technique for injection, disposal of needles/syringes. Pt should avoid NSAIDs, report bleeding, black tarry stools, severe headache.

formoterol fumarate
(Foradil Aerolizer,
Perforomist)

CLASS Antiasthmatic, beta
agonist
PREG/CONT C/NA

BBW Long-acting beta agonists may
increase risk of asthma-related
deaths; use only if clearly warranted.
Use without concomitant inhaled corticosteroid contraindicated.

IND & DOSE Maintenance tx of
COPD. *Adult:* Oral inhalation of contents of 1 capsule (12 mcg) using *Aerolizer* inhaler q 12 hr; max, 24 mcg
daily. Or, one 20-mcg/2 mL vial by
oral inhalation using jet nebulizer connected to air compressor bid (a.m.
and p.m.); max, 40 mcg/day. **Prevention of exercise-induced bronchospasm.** *Adult, child 12 yr and older:*
Oral inhalation of contents of 1 capsule (12 mcg) using *Aerolizer* inhaler
15 min before exercise. **Maintenance
tx of asthma.** *Adult, child 5 yr and older:* Oral inhalation of contents of
1 capsule (12 mcg) using *Aerolizer* inhaler q 12 hr; max, 1 capsule q 12 hr.
ADV EFF Headache, nervousness,
prolonged QT interval, throat/mouth
irritation, tremors, viral infections
INTERACTIONS Beta blockers,
QT-prolonging drugs
NC/PT Teach proper use of inhaler,
nebulizer; periodically monitor use.
Provide safety information for tremors, analgesics for headache. Ensure
continued use of other drugs for
COPD, bronchospasm. Pt should use
15 min before activity if used for exercise-induced asthma. Name confusion
between *Foradil* (formoterol) and *Toradol* (ketorolac); use extreme caution.

fosamprenavir (Lexiva)
CLASS Antiviral, protease inhibitor
PREG/CONT C/NA

IND & DOSE Tx of HIV infection w/
other antiretrovirals. *Adult:*
1,400 mg PO bid. W/ ritonavir:
1,400 mg PO plus ritonavir
100 mg/day PO, or 1,400 mg/day PO
plus ritonavir 200 mg/day PO, or
700 mg PO bid w/ ritonavir 100 mg
PO bid. In protease-experienced pts:
700 mg PO bid w/ ritonavir 100 mg
PO bid. *Child 2–5 yr (tx-naïve):*
30 mg/kg oral suspension PO bid;
max, 1,400 mg bid. *Child 6 yr and older (tx-naïve):* 30 mg/kg oral suspension PO bid; max, 1,400 mg bid. Or,
18 mg/kg oral suspension PO w/ ritonavir 3 mg/kg PO bid; max, 700 mg
fosamprenavir plus 100 mg ritonavir
bid. *Child 6 yr and older (tx-experienced):* 18 mg/kg oral suspension w/
3 mg/kg ritonavir PO bid; max,
700 mg fosamprenavir w/ 100 mg
ritonavir bid.
ADJUST DOSE Hepatic impairment
ADV EFF Depression, headache, hyperglycemia, **MI**, n/v/d, redistribution
of body fat, **Stevens-Johnson
syndrome**
INTERACTIONS Dihydroergotamine, ergotamine, flecainide, lovastatin, methylergonovine, midazolam,
pimozide, piroxicam, propafenone, rifabutin, simvastatin, triazolam—do
not use w/ any of preceding drugs.
Amiodarone, amitriptyline, amlodipine, carbamazepine, cyclosporine,
delavirdine, diltiazem, efavirenz, felodipine, hormonal contraceptives,
imipramine, isradipine, itraconazole,
ketoconazole, lidocaine, lopinavir/
ritonavir, nevirapine, nicardipine,
nifedipine, nimodipine, nisoldipine,
phenobarbital, phenytoin, quinidine,
rifampin, saquinavir, sildenafil,
St. John's wort, tacrolimus, vardenafil,
verapamil
NC/PT Carefully check other drugs
being used; interacts w/ many drugs.
Give w/ other antiretrovirals. Monitor
LFTs, blood glucose. Monitor for
rash. Not for use in pregnancy (barrier contraceptives advised). Pt should
monitor glucose carefully if diabetic;
avoid St. John's wort; tell all health
care providers about all drugs, herbs
being taken; report rash, chest pain.

fosfomycin tromethamine (Monurol)

CLASS Antibacterial, urinary tract anti-infective
PREG/CONT B/NA

IND & DOSE Tx of uncomplicated UTIs in women caused by susceptible strains. *Adult, child 12 yr and older:* 1 packet dissolved in water PO as single dose.

ADV EFF Dizziness, headache, nausea, rash

INTERACTIONS Metoclopramide
NC/PT Culture before tx. Do not give dry. Mix in 90–120 mL water (not hot); stir to dissolve. Pt should contact prescriber if no improvement, take safety precautions if dizziness occurs.

fosinopril sodium (Monopril)

CLASS ACE inhibitor, antihypertensive
PREG/CONT D/NA

BBW Pt should avoid pregnancy (suggest contraceptive); fetal damage possible if used in second, third trimesters. Switch to different drug if pregnancy occurs.

IND & DOSE Tx of hypertension. *Adult:* 10 mg/day PO. Range, 20–40 mg/day PO; max, 80 mg. **Adjunct tx of HF.** *Adult:* 10 mg/day PO; observe for 2 hr for hypotension. For pt w/ moderate to severe renal failure, 5 mg/day PO; max, 40 mg/day.

ADV EFF Angioedema, cough, nausea, orthostatic hypotension, rash
INTERACTIONS Antacids, indomethacin, lithium, NSAIDs, potassium-sparing diuretics
NC/PT Alert surgeon about use; postop fluid replacement may be needed. Not for use in pregnancy (barrier methods advised). Pt should use care in situations that might lead to BP drop, change positions slowly if light-headedness occurs. Name confusion between fosinopril and lisinopril; use caution.

fosphenytoin sodium (Cerebyx)

CLASS Antiepileptic, hydantoin
PREG/CONT D/NA

BBW Pt should avoid pregnancy; fetal damage possible. Suggest use of contraceptive.

IND & DOSE Short-term control of status epilepticus. *Adult:* Loading dose, 15–20 mg PE/kg at 100–150 mg PE/min IV. **Px, of seizures during or after neurosurgery.** *Adult:* Loading dose, 10–20 mg PE/kg IM or IV; maint, 4–6 mg PE/kg/day. **Substitution for oral phenytoin therapy.** *Adult:* Substitute IM or IV at same total daily dose as phenytoin; for short-term use only.

ADJUST DOSE Hepatic, renal impairment

ADV EFF Ataxia, dizziness, drowsiness, hypotension, nausea, pruritus, twitching

INTERACTIONS Acetaminophen, amiodarone, antineoplastics, carbamazepine, chloramphenicol, cimetidine, corticosteroids, cyclosporine, diazoxide, disopyramide, disulfiram, doxycycline, estrogens, fluconazole, folic acid, hormonal contraceptives, isoniazid, levodopa, methadone, metyrapone, mexiletine, phenacemide, phenylbutazone, primidone, rifampin, sulfonamides, theophyllines, trimethoprim, valproic acid
NC/PT Give IV slowly to prevent severe hypotension. Monitor infusion site carefully; sols are very alkaline, irritating. For short-term use only (up to 5 days); switch to oral phenytoin as soon as possible. Not for use in pregnancy (contraceptives advised). Pt should take safety precautions w/ CNS effects. Name confusion w/ *Cerebyx* (fosphenytoin), *Celebrex* (celecoxib), *Celexa*

(citalopram), and *Xanax* (alprazolam); use caution.

frovatriptan succinate
(Frova)
CLASS Antimigraine, triptan
PREG/CONT C/NA

IND & DOSE Tx of acute migraine w/ or without aura. *Adult:* 2.5 mg PO as single dose at first sign of migraine; may repeat after 2 hr. Max, 3 doses/24 hr.
ADV EFF Cerebrovascular events, dizziness, headache, **MI**, n/v, tingling, **ventricular arrhythmias**
INTERACTIONS Ergots, SSRIs
NC/PT Ensure proper dx of migraine. For tx, not px. Ensure no ergots taken within 24 hr. Ensure 2 hr between doses, no more than three doses/day. Monitor BP. Not for use in migraine. Pt should take safety precautions w/ CNS effects, report chest pain/pressure.

DANGEROUS DRUG

fulvestrant (Faslodex)
CLASS Antineoplastic, estrogen receptor antagonist
PREG/CONT D/NA

IND & DOSE Tx of hormone receptor–positive breast cancer in postmenopausal women w/ disease progression after antiestrogen tx. *Adult:* 500 mg IM on days 1, 15, 29, then monthly as two concomitant 5-mL injections, one in each buttock.
ADJUST DOSE Hepatic impairment
ADV EFF Abd pain, anemia, arthritis, asthenia, back pain, bone pain, dizziness, dyspnea, hot flashes, increased cough/sweating, n/v/d, pelvic pain
INTERACTIONS Oral anticoagulants
NC/PT Rule out pregnancy; suggest contraceptives. Handle cautiously. Give by slow IM injection

over 1–2 min. Hot flashes possible. Teach proper administration, disposal of syringes, needles. Pt should mark calendar of tx days, take safety precautions w/ CNS effects.

furosemide (Lasix)
CLASS Loop diuretic
PREG/CONT C/NA

BBW Profound diuresis w/ water, electrolyte depletion possible; careful medical supervision needed.
IND & DOSE Edema associated w/ systemic disease. *Adult:* 20–80 mg/day PO as single dose; max, 600 mg/day. Or, 20–40 mg IM or IV (slow IV injection over 1–2 min); max, 4 mg/min. *Child:* 2 mg/kg/day PO; max, 6 mg/kg/day (1 mg/kg/day in preterm infants). Tx of acute pulmonary edema. *Adult:* 40 mg IV over 1–2 min. May increase to 80 mg IV over 1–2 min if response unsatisfactory after 1 hr. *Child:* 1 mg/kg IV or IM. May increase by 1 mg/kg in 2 hr until desired effect achieved. Max, 6 mg/kg. Tx of hypertension. *Adult:* 40 mg bid PO.
ADJUST DOSE Renal impairment
ADV EFF Anemia, anorexia, dizziness, hypokalemia, leukopenia, muscle cramps, n/v, orthostatic hypotension, paresthesia, photosensitivity, pruritus, thrombocytopenia, urticaria, xanthopsia
INTERACTIONS Aminoglycosides, charcoal, cisplatin, digitalis, ibuprofen, indomethacin, NSAIDs, oral antidiabetics, phenytoin
NC/PT Give early in day so diuresis will not affect sleep. Do not expose to light. Record weight daily. Arrange for potassium replacement or potassium-rich diet. Pt should avoid sun exposure, report loss or gain of more than 3 lb/day, take safety precautions w/ CNS effects. Name confusion between furosemide and torsemide; use caution.

gabapentin (Neurontin, Gralise, Horizant)

CLASS Antiepileptic
PREG/CONT C/NA

IND & DOSE *Adjunct tx of partial seizures.* *Adult:* 300 mg PO tid. Maint, 900–1,800 mg/day PO tid in divided doses; max of 2,400–3,600 mg/day has been used. Max interval between doses, 12 hr. *Child 3–12 yr:* 10–15 mg/kg/day PO in three divided doses. Range, 25–35 mg/kg/day in three divided doses (child 5 yr and older) and up to 40 mg/kg/day in three divided doses (child 3–4 yr). *Tx of postherpetic neuralgia.* *Adult:* 300 mg/day PO; 300 mg PO bid on day 2; 300 mg PO tid on day 3. Or, 1,800 mg/day PO w/ evening meal *(Gralise).* *Tx of moderate to severe restless legs syndrome.* *Adult:* 600–800 mg/day PO w/ food around 5 p.m.; max, 2,400 mg/day *(Horizant).*
ADJUST DOSE Elderly pts, renal impairment
ADV EFF Ataxia, dizziness, insomnia, suicidal ideation, tremor, weight gain
INTERACTIONS Antacids
NC/PT *Gralise* not interchangeable w/ other forms of gabapentin. Do not cut, crush, or allow pt to chew ER forms. Taper ER forms after long-term use. Pt may be at increased risk for suicidality; monitor. Suggest medical ID. Pt should take safety precautions for CNS effects.

gadobutrol (Gadavist)

CLASS Contrast agent
PREG/CONT C/NA

BBW Risk of nephrogenic systemic fibrosis, more common w/ higher-than-normal dosing or repeated dosing; monitor total dose.
IND & DOSE *Detection, visualization of areas w/ disrupted blood-brain barrier and/or abnormal CNS vascularity.*

Adult, child 2 yr and older: Dosage based on body weight: 0.1 mL/kg, given as IV bolus at 2 mL/sec; flush line w/ NSS after injection.
ADV EFF Dysgeusia, feeling hot, headache, **hypersensitivity reaction,** injection-site reaction, nausea, **nephrogenic systemic fibrosis**
NC/PT Evaluate GFR before starting tx. Monitor total dose exposure; monitor for nephrogenic systemic fibrosis. Not for use in pregnancy. Pt should report all exposure to contrast agents, itching, swelling or tightening, red or dark patches on skin, joint stiffness, muscle weakness, bone pain.

galantamine hydrobromide (Razadyne)

CLASS Alzheimer drug, cholinesterase inhibitor
PREG/CONT B/NA

IND & DOSE *Tx of mild to moderate dementia of Alzheimer type.* *Adult:* 4 mg PO bid; after 4 wk, increase to 8 mg PO bid; after 4 more wk, increase to 12 mg PO bid. Range, 16–32 mg/day in two divided doses. ER capsules, 8 mg/day PO; titrate to 16–24 mg/day PO.
ADJUST DOSE Hepatic, renal impairment
ADV EFF Abd pain, anorexia, diarrhea, dizziness, dyspepsia, n/v/d, insomnia, weight loss
INTERACTIONS Bethanechol, cimetidine, erythromycin, ketoconazole, paroxetine, potent CYP2D6/CYP3A4 inhibitors, succinylcholine
NC/PT Does not cure disease; may slow degeneration. Establish baseline functional profile. Mix sol w/ water, fruit juice, or soda. Do not cut, crush, or allow pt to chew ER form; have pt swallow whole. Antiemetics may be helpful for GI upset. Pt should take safety measures for CNS effects. Because of name confusion, manufacturer has changed name from *Reminyl* to *Razadyne.*

galsulfase (Naglazyme)

CLASS Enzyme
PREG/CONT B/NA

IND & DOSE Tx of pts w/ mucopolysaccharidosis VI to improve walking and stair climbing capacity. *Adult:* 1 mg/kg/wk by IV infusion, diluted and infused over 4 hr.

ADJUST DOSE Hepatic, renal impairment

ADV EFF Abd pain, anaphylaxis and allergic reactions, cardiorespiratory failure, chills, dyspnea, fever, headache, **immune reactions, infusion reactions,** n/v, pruritus, rash, urticaria

NC/PT Establish baseline activity. Pretreat w/ antihistamines and antipyretics; consider adding corticosteroids. Monitor continually during infusion; consider lowering dose or discontinuing if severe reactions.

ganciclovir sodium (Cytovene, Vitrasert, Zirgan)

CLASS Antiviral
PREG/CONT C/NA

BBW Obtain CBC before tx, q 2 days during daily dosing, and at least wkly thereafter. Consult physician and arrange for reduced dose if WBC or platelet counts falls. IV therapy is *only* for tx of CMV retinitis in immunocompromised pts and for px of CMV disease in transplant pts at risk for CMV.

IND & DOSE Tx of CMV retinitis. *Adult:* 5 mg/kg IV at constant rate over 1 hr q 12 hr for 14–21 days; maint, 5 mg/kg by IV infusion over 1 hr once daily 7 days/wk or 6 mg/kg once daily 5 days/wk. Or 1,000 mg PO tid w/ food or 500 mg PO six times/day q 3 hr w/ food while awake. Implant surgically placed in affected eye q 5–8 mo. *Child 2 yr and older:* Ophthalmic gel, 1 drop in affected eye(s) five times daily (approximately q 3 hr while awake) until ulcer heals. Maint, 1 drop three times daily for 7 days. **Prevention of CMV disease in transplant recipients:** *Adult:* 5 mg/kg IV over 1 hr q 12 hr for 7–14 days; then 5 mg/kg by IV infusion over 1 hr once daily 7 days/wk, or 6 mg/kg/day once daily for 5 days/wk. Prophylactic oral dose is 1,000 mg tid. **Prevention of CMV disease w/ advanced AIDS:** *Adult:* 1,000 mg PO tid.

ADJUST DOSE Renal impairment

ADV EFF Anemia, bone marrow suppression, cancer, fever, granulocytopenia, hepatic changes, inflammation at injection site, pain, rash, thrombocytopenia

INTERACTIONS Bone marrow suppressants, imipenem-cilastatin, probenecid, zidovudine

NC/PT Avoid contact w/ sol; proper disposal necessary. Do not give IM or subcut; give oral drug w/ food. Monitor CBC before and periodically during tx. Not for use in pregnancy (contraceptives for men and women advised). Tell pt surgical implant will need to be replaced q 5–8 mo; periodic eye exams, frequent blood tests will be needed.

ganirelix acetate (Antagon)

CLASS Fertility drug
PREG/CONT X/NA

IND & DOSE Inhibition of premature LH surges in women in fertility programs. *Adult:* 250 mcg/day subcut starting on day 2 or 3 of cycle.

ADV EFF Abd pain, headache, injection-site reaction, n/v, **ovarian hyperstimulation,** vaginal bleeding

NC/PT Drug part of comprehensive fertility program. Show pt proper administration technique and proper disposal of needles and syringes. Pt should report swelling, shortness of breath, severe n/v, low urine output.

DANGEROUS DRUG

gemcitabine hydrochloride (Gemzar)

CLASS Antimetabolite, antineoplastic
PREG/CONT D/NA

IND & DOSE Tx of pancreatic cancer after 5-FU tx. *Adult:* 1,000 mg/m² IV over 30 min once wkly for up to 7 wk. Subsequent cycles of once wkly for 3 out of 4 consecutive wk can be given after 1-wk rest fro tx. **First-line tx of inoperable, locally advanced or metastatic non-small-cell lung cancer:** *Adult:* 1,000 mg/m² IV over 30 min, days 1, 8, and 15 of each 28-day cycle, w/ 100 mg/m² cisplatin on day 1 after gemcitabine infusion, or 1,250 mg/m² IV over 30 min, days 1 and 8 of each 21-day cycle, w/ 100 mg/m² cisplatin on day 1 after gemcitabine infusion. **First-line therapy for metastatic breast cancer after failure of other adjuvant chemotherapy.** *Adult:* 1,250 mg/m² IV over 30 min, days 1 and 8 of each 21-day cycle, w/ 175 mg/m² paclitaxel IV as 3-hr infusion before gemcitabine on day 1 of cycle. **Tx of advanced ovarian cancer that has relapsed at least 6 mo after completion of platinum-based therapy.** *Adult:* 1,000 mg/m² IV over 30 min, days 1 and 8 of each 21-day cycle. Carboplatin given on day 1 after gemcitabine.
ADV EFF Alopecia, **bone marrow depression**, edema, fever, flulike symptoms, **interstitial pneumonitis**, n/v, pain, rash
NC/PT Monitor CBC, renal function, LFTS carefully; dose adjustment may be needed. Infuse over 30 min; longer infusions cause increased half-life/ greater toxicity. Premedicate for n/v. Pt should avoid exposure to infection, protect head in temp extremes (hair loss possible).

gemfibrozil (Lopid)

CLASS Antihyperlipidemic
PREG/CONT C/NA

IND & DOSE Adjunct to diet, exercise for tx of hypertriglyceridemia in pts w/ very high triglycerides; reduction of CAD in pts unresponsive to traditional therapies. *Adult:* 1,200 mg/day PO in two divided doses 30 min before morning and evening meals.
ADJUST DOSE Hepatic, renal impairment
ADV EFF Abd pain, blurred vision, cataract development, dizziness, dyspepsia, eczema, epigastric pain, **eosinophilia**, fatigue, headache, **leukopenia**, n/v/d, **rhabdomyolysis**
INTERACTIONS Anticoagulants, repaglinide, statins, sulfonylureas
NC/PT Use only if strongly indicated and lipid studies show a definite response; hepatic tumorigenicity occurs in lab animals. Pt should take w/ meals; continue diet, exercise program; take safety precautions w/ CNS effects; report muscle pain w/ fever.

gemifloxacin mesylate (Factive)

CLASS Fluoroquinolone antibiotic
PREG/CONT C/NA

BBW Risk of tendinitis and tendon rupture. Risk increases in pts over 60 yr, w/ concurrent corticosteroid use, and w/ kidney, heart, or lung transplant; monitor these pts accordingly. Risk of exacerbation of muscle weakness and potential crisis in pts w/ myasthenia gravis; contraindicated for use in pts w/ hx of myasthenia gravis.
IND & DOSE Tx of acute bacterial exacerbations of chronic bronchitis caused by susceptible strains. *Adult:* 320 mg/day PO for 5 days. **Tx of community-acquired pneumonia**

caused by susceptible strains.
Adult: 320 mg/day PO for 5 days;
7 days for resistant strains.
ADJUST DOSE Renal impairment
ADV EFF Abd pain, blurred vision,
dizziness, n/v/d, photosensitivity,
**prolonged QT interval, ulcerative
colitis,** sulfonylureas
INTERACTIONS Aluminum- or
potassium-containing antacids,
amiodarone, antidepressants,
antipsychotics, calcium, didanosine,
erythromycin, iron, procainamide,
quinidine, sotalol, sucralfate
NC/PT Culture before tx. Not for use
in breast-feeding. Pt should take 3 hr
before or 2 hr after taking antacids;
swallow tablet whole and not cut,
crush, or chew it; drink plenty of fluids; report acute pain or tenderness in
muscle or tendon, bloody diarrhea,
palpitations, fainting.

---

gentamicin sulfate
(Gentak, Pediatric
Gentamicin Sulfate)
CLASS Fluoroquinolone
antibiotic
PREG/CONT D (systemic); C
(ophthalmic)/NA

BBW Monitor hearing w/ long-term
tx; ototoxicity possible. Monitor renal
function, CBC, serum drug levels during long-term tx; carefully monitor pt
if combined w/ other neurotoxic or
nephrotoxic drugs.

IND & DOSE Tx of serious infections caused by susceptible bacteria strains or when causative organisms not known. **Adult:** 320 mg/day
PO for 5 days. **Tx of community-
acquired pneumonia caused by susceptible strains. Adult:** 3 mg/kg/day
IM or IV in three equal doses q 8 hr.
Up to 5 mg/kg/day in three to four
equal doses in severe infections, usually for 7–10 days. For IV use, may infuse loading dose of 1–2 mg/kg over
30–60 min. **Child:** 2–2.5 mg/kg IM or
IV q 8 hr. **Infants, neonates:** 2.5 mg/kg
IM or IV q 8 hr. **Preterm, full-term neo-**

nates 1 wk or younger: 2.5 mg/kg IM
or IV q 12 hr. **Preterm neonates under
32 wk gestational age:** 2.5 mg/kg IM
or IV q 18 hr or 3 mg/kg q 24 hr.
Tx of PID. Adult: 2 mg/kg IV, then
1.5 mg/kg IV tid plus clindamycin
600 mg IV qid. Continue for at least
4 days and at least 48 hr after pt improves, then continue clindamycin
450 mg PO qid for 10–14 days total
tx. **Tx of superficial ocular infections
due to susceptible microorganism
strains. Adult, child:** 1–2 drops in
affected eye(s) q 4 hr; use up to 2
drops hrly in severe infections or
apply ointment ½" ointment to affected
eye bid–tid. **Infection px in minor
skin abrasions, tx of superficial
skin infections. Adult, child:** Apply
tid–qid. May cover w/ sterile bandage.
ADJUST DOSE Elderly pts, renal
failure
ADV EFF Anorexia, **apnea,** arach-
noiditis at IM injection sites, **bone
marrow suppression,** dizziness, local
irritation, n/v/d, **nephrotoxicity, neuromuscular blockade,** ototoxicity,
pain, purpura, rash, **seizures,** superinfections, tinnitus
INTERACTIONS Aminoglycosides,
anesthetics, beta-lactam–type antibiotics, carbenicillin, cephalosporins,
citrate-anticoagulated blood, diuretics (potent), enflurane, methoxyflu-
rane, nondepolarizing NMJ blockers,
penicillins, succinylcholine, ticarcillin,
vancomycin
NC/PT Culture before tx. Give by
deep IM injection if possible. Avoid
long-term use. Monitor serum levels. Max peak levels, 12 mcg/mL
(6–8 mcg/mL usually adequate for
most infections); max trough levels,
2 mcg/mL. Monitor CBC, renal function, hearing. Teach proper administration of ophthalmic and topical
preparations. Pt should take safety
precautions w/ CNS effects; avoid
exposure to infection; report severe
headache, loss of hearing, difficult
breathing.

glatiramer acetate
(Copaxone)

CLASS MS drug
PREG/CONT B/NA

IND & DOSE To reduce frequency of relapses in pts w/ relapsing-re-mitting MS, including pts who have experienced a first clinical episode and have MRI features consistent w/ MS. *Adult:* 20 mg/day subcut.

ADV EFF Anxiety, asthenia, back pain, chest pain, infections, injection-site reactions (including lipoatrophy, skin necrosis), nausea, post-injection reaction, rash

NC/PT Rotate injection sites; do not use same site within a wk. Teach proper administration handling and disposal of needles and syringes. Monitor for infections. Pt should report severe injection-site reactions, chest pain w/ sweating, trouble breathing.

DANGEROUS DRUG

glimepiride (Amaryl)

CLASS Antidiabetic, sulfonylurea
PREG/CONT C/NA

IND & DOSE Adjunct to diet to lower blood glucose in pts w/ type 2 diabetes mellitus. *Adult:* 1–2 mg PO once daily w/ breakfast or first meal of day. Range, 1–4 mg PO once daily; max, 8 mg/day. **W/ met-formin or insulin to better control glucose as adjunct to diet, exercise in pts w/ type 2 diabetes mellitus.** *Adult:* 8 mg PO daily w/ first meal of day w/ low-dose insulin or metformin.

ADJUST DOSE Adrenal or pituitary insufficiency; debilitated, elderly, malnourished pts; hepatic, renal impairment

ADV EFF Allergic skin reactions, anorexia, **CV mortality**, diarrhea, epigastric distress, **eosinophilia, hypoglycemia**

INTERACTIONS Alcohol, androgens, anticoagulants, azole antifungals, beta blockers, calcium channel blockers, celery, cholestyramine, chloramphenicol, clofibrate, coriander, corticosteroids, dandelion root, diazoxide, estrogens, fenugreek, fluconazole, garlic, gemfibrozil, ginseng, histamine-2 blockers, hormonal contraceptives, hydantoins, isoniazid, juniper berries, magnesium salts, MAOIs, methyldopa, nicotinic acid, phenothiazines, probenecid, rifampin, salicylates, sulfinpyrazone, sulfonamides, sympathomimetics, TCAs, thiazides, thyroid drugs, urinary acidifiers/alkalinizers

NC/PT Monitor blood glucose. Transfer to insulin temporarily in times of stress. Ensure diet, exercise program. Arrange for complete diabetic teaching program. Not for use in pregnancy. Pt should avoid alcohol.

DANGEROUS DRUG

glipiZIDE (Glucotrol)

CLASS Antidiabetic, sulfonylurea
PREG/CONT C/NA

IND & DOSE Adjunct to diet to lower blood glucose in pts w/ type 2 diabetes mellitus. *Adult:* 5 mg PO before breakfast. Adjust dose in increments of 2.5–5 mg as determined by blood glucose response; max, 15 mg/dose. ER tablets, 5 mg/day PO; may increase to 10 mg/day after 3 mo.

ADJUST DOSE Elderly pts

ADV EFF Allergic skin reactions, anorexia, **bone marrow suppression, CV mortality**, diarrhea, epigastric distress, **eosinophilia, hypoglycemia**

INTERACTIONS Alcohol, beta blockers, chloramphenicol, clofibrate, coriander, dandelion root, diazoxide, fenugreek, garlic, gemfibrozil, ginseng, juniper berries, phenothiazines, rifampin, salicylates, sulfonamides

NC/PT Monitor blood glucose. Transfer to insulin temporarily in times of stress. Give 30 min before breakfast. Ensure diet, exercise program. Arrange for complete diabetic teaching program. Not for use in pregnancy. Pt should swallow ER tablets whole and not cut, crush, or chew them; avoid alcohol.

glucagon (GlucaGen Diagnostic Kit, GlucaGen HypoKit, Glucagon Emergency Kit)

CLASS Diagnostic agent, glucose-elevating drug
PREG/CONT B/NA

IND & DOSE Tx of hypoglycemia. *Adult, child over 20 kg:* 0.5–1 mg IV, IM, or subcut; severe hypoglycemia, 1 mL IV, IM, or subcut. Use IV if possible. *Child under 20 kg:* 0.5 mg IM, IV, or subcut, or dose equivalent to 20–30 mcg/kg. Diagnostic aid in radiologic examination of stomach, duodenum, small bowel, colon. *Adult, child over 20 kg:* Usual dose, 0.25–2 mg IV or 1–2 mg IM.
ADV EFF Hypokalemia, hypotension, n/v, **respiratory distress**
INTERACTIONS Oral anticoagulants
NC/PT Arouse pt as soon as possible. Provide supplemental carbohydrates. Evaluate insulin dose in pts w/ insulin overdose. Teach pt and significant other proper administration and disposal of needles and syringes.

glucarpidase (Voraxaze)

CLASS Carboxypeptidase enzyme
PREG/CONT C/NA

IND & DOSE Tx of pts w/ toxic plasma methotrexate concentrations w/ delayed methotrexate clearance due to impaired renal function. *Adult, child:* 50 units/kg as single IV injection.

ADV EFF Flushing, headache, hypotension, n/v, paresthesia, **serious allergic reactions**
INTERACTIONS Folate, folate antimetabolites, leucovorin
NC/PT Continue hydration, alkalinization of urine. Do not administer within 2 hr of leucovorin. Monitor closely for allergic reaction during and directly after injection. Tell pt blood levels will be monitored repeatedly during tx. Pt should report fever, chills, rash, difficulty breathing, numbness/tingling, headache.

DANGEROUS DRUG

glyBURIDE (DiaBeta, Glynase)

CLASS Antidiabetic, sulfonylurea
PREG/CONT B (Glynase); C (DiaBeta)/NA

IND & DOSE Adjunct to diet to lower blood glucose in pts w/ type 2 diabetes mellitus. *Adult:* 2.5–5 mg PO w/ breakfast (DiaBeta); 1.5–3 mg/day PO (Glynase); maint, 1.25–20 mg/day PO.
ADJUST DOSE Debilitated, elderly, malnourished pts
ADV EFF Allergic skin reactions, anorexia, blurred vision, **bone marrow suppression, CV mortality,** diarrhea, epigastric distress, **hypoglycemia**
INTERACTIONS Alcohol, beta blockers, chloramphenicol, clofibrate, coriander, dandelion root, diazoxide, fenugreek, garlic, gemfibrozil, ginseng, juniper berries, phenothiazines, rifampin, salicylates, sulfonamides
NC/PT Note dosage difference between two forms; use w/ care. Monitor blood glucose. Transfer to insulin temporarily in times of stress. Give before breakfast. Ensure diet, exercise program. Arrange for complete diabetic teaching program. Not for use in pregnancy. Pt should avoid alcohol. Name confusion between *Dia-Beta* (glyburide) and *Zebeta* (bisoprolol); use caution.

glycerol phenylbutyrate
(Ravicti)

CLASS Nitrogen-binding agent
PREG/CONT C/NA

IND & DOSE Long-term mgt of urea cycle disorders not managed by dietary/amino acid supplementation. *Adult, child 2 yr and older:* 4.5–11.2 mL/m²/day PO divided into three equal doses, rounded to nearest 0.5 mL, w/ food; max, 17.5 mL/day.
ADJUST DOSE Hepatic impairment
ADV EFF Diarrhea, flatulence, headache, **neurotoxicity**
INTERACTIONS Corticosteroids, haloperidol, probenecid, valproic acid
NC/PT Must give w/ protein-restricted diet; monitor ammonia levels; adjust dose as needed. Not for use in pregnancy, breast-feeding. Pt should take w/ food, report disorientation, confusion, impaired memory.

glycopyrrolate (Cuvposa, Robinul)

CLASS Anticholinergic, antispasmodic, parasympatholytic
PREG/CONT B/NA

IND & DOSE Adjunct tx for peptic ulcer. *Adult:* 1 mg PO tid or 2 mg bid–tid. Maint: 1 mg bid; max, 8 mg/day. Tx of chronic, severe drooling caused by neurologic disorders. *Child: 3–16 yr:* 0.02 mg/kg PO tid; titrate in 0.02-mg increments q 5–7 days. Max, 0.1 mg/kg PO tid; do not exceed 1.5–3 mg/dose. Tx of peptic ulcer. *Adult:* 0.1–0.2 mg IM or IV tid–qid. Preanesthetic medication. *Adult:* 0.004 mg/kg IM 30–60 min before anesthesia. *Child 2 yr–under 12 yr:* 0.004 mg/kg IM 30 min–1 hr before anesthesia. *Child 1 mo–2 yr:* Up to 0.009 mg/kg IM may be needed. Intraop to decrease vagal traction reflexes. *Adult:* 0.1 mg IV; repeat as needed at 2- to 3-min intervals. *Child over 1 mo:* 0.004 mg/kg IV, not to exceed 0.1 mg in single dose. May repeat at 2- to 3-min intervals. Reversal of neuromuscular blockade. *Adult, child over 1 mo:* W/ neostigmine, pyridostigmine, 0.2 mg IV for each 1 mg neostigmine or 5 mg pyridostigmine; give IV simultaneously.
ADV EFF Altered taste perception, blurred vision, decreased sweating, dry mouth, dysphagia, irritation at injection site, n/v, photosensitivity, urinary hesitancy, urine retention
INTERACTIONS Amantadine, anticholinergics, digitalis, haloperidol, phenothiazines
NC/PT Check dose carefully. Ensure adequate hydration. Pt should empty bladder before each dose, avoid hot environments (may be subject to heat stroke) and sun exposure, suck sugarless lozenges, perform mouth care for dry mouth.

gold sodium thiomalate
(Aurolate)

CLASS Antirheumatic, gold compound
PREG/CONT C/NA

BBW Monitor lung, renal function; obtain CBC regularly. Discontinue at first sign of toxicity; can cause serious to fatal bone marrow suppression and renal toxicity.
IND & DOSE Tx of selected, early cases of adult and juvenile rheumatoid arthritis. *Adult:* 10 mg IM wk 1; 25 mg IM wk 2 and 3; then 25–50 mg IM to total dose of 1 g. Maint, 25–50 mg IM q other wk for 2–30 wk. *Child:* 10 mg IM as test dose, then 1 mg/kg/wk IM; max, 50 mg/dose.
ADV EFF Abd pain, **bone marrow suppression**, diarrhea, fainting, fever, grey-blue skin, hair loss, headache, infection, injection-site reactions, photosensitivity, rash, **seizures**, stomatitis
INTERACTIONS ACE inhibitors, chloroquine immunosuppressants, phenylbutazone, phenytoin, primaquine

NC/PT Monitor closely. Rotate injection sites; local reactions common. May use corticosteroids for severe reactions. Give analgesics as needed. Use cautiously in pregnancy. Pt should avoid exposure to infection and sunlight.

golimumab (Simponi)

CLASS Monoclonal antibody, TNF inhibitor
PREG/CONT B/NA

BBW Serious infections possible, including TB, sepsis, invasive fungal infections. Discontinue if infection or sepsis develops. Perform TB test before tx. If TB present, start TB tx and monitor pt carefully throughout tx. Increased risk of lymphoma and other cancers in children and adolescents; monitor accordingly.
IND & DOSE Tx of active rheumatoid arthritis, active psoriatic arthritis, ankylosing spondylitis. *Adult:* 50 mg/mo subcut or 2 mg/kg IV over 30 min wk 0, 4, then q 8 wk.
ADV EFF Dizziness, **increased risk of demyelinating disorders, infections,** injection-site reactions, nasopharyngitis
INTERACTIONS Abatacept, anakinra, adalimumab, certolizumab, etanercept, infliximab, live vaccines, rituximab
NC/PT TB test before tx. Store in refrigerator; bring to room temp before use. Rotate injection sites. For IV, use inline filter; do not infuse w/ other drugs. Monitor for CNS changes, infection. Not for use in breast-feeding. Teach proper administration and disposal of needles and syringes. Pt should avoid live vaccines, take safety precautions for dizziness, have regular medical follow-up; report fever, numbness and tingling, worsening of arthritis.

---

goserelin acetate (Zoladex)

CLASS Antineoplastic, hormone
PREG/CONT X; D (w/ breast cancer)/NA

IND & DOSE Palliative tx of advanced prostate or breast cancer. *Adult:* 3.6 mg q 28 days subcut (long-term use). **Mgt of endometriosis.** *Adult:* 3.6 mg subcut q 28 days for 6 mo. **Endometrial thinning before ablation.** *Adult:* One to two 3.6-mg subcut depots 4 wk apart; surgery should be done 4 wk after first dose (within 2–4 wk after second dose if two are used). **Tx of stage B₂–C prostate cancer.** *Adult:* Start tx 8 wk before start of radiation therapy and continue during radiation therapy; 3.6-mg depot 8 wk before radiation, then one 10.8-mg depot 28 days later. Or, four injections of 3.6-mg depot at 28-day intervals, two depots preceding and two during radiotherapy.
ADV EFF Cancer, decreased erections, dizziness, dysmenorrhea, edema, gynecomastia, hot flashes, lower urinary tract symptoms, sexual dysfunction, vaginitis
NC/PT Implant in upper abdomen q 28 days or q 3 mo. Mark calendar for injection dates. Not for use in pregnancy (contraceptives advised), breast-feeding. Pt should report pain at injection site, discuss sexual dysfx w/ health care provider.

granisetron hydrochloride (Kytril, Sancuso)

CLASS Antiemetic, 5-HT₃ receptor antagonist
PREG/CONT B/NA

IND & DOSE Tx, px of chemotherapy-induced n/v. *Adult, child over 2 yr:* 10 mcg/kg IV over 5 min starting within 30 min of chemotherapy, only on days of chemotherapy. Or 1 mg PO bid or 2 mg/day PO as 1 dose, beginning up to 1 hr before chemotherapy and second dose 12 hr after chemotherapy, only on days of chemotherapy. Or, for adults, apply 1 patch to clean, dry skin on upper, outer arm 24–48 hr before chemotherapy. Keep patch in place minimum of 24 hr after completion of chemotherapy, then remove; may be left in place for up to 7 days. **Tx, px of radiation induced n/v.** *Adult, child over 2 yr:* 2 mg PO once daily 1 hr before radiation. **Px, tx of postop n/v.** *Adult, child over 2 yr:* 1 mg IV over 30 sec before induction or reversal of anesthesia.

ADV EFF Asthenia, chills, decreased appetite, fever, headache

NC/PT Use only as directed. Apply transdermal patch to clean, dry skin; leave in place up to 7 days. Pt should perform mouth care, use sugarless lozenges to help relieve nausea, report sever headache.

guaifenesin (Altarussin, Diabetic Tussin, Mucinex, Siltussin)
CLASS Expectorant
PREG/CONT C/NA

IND & DOSE **Symptomatic relief of respiratory conditions characterized by dry, nonproductive cough; mucus in respiratory tract.** *Adult, child over 12 yr:* 200–400 mg PO q 4 hr; max, 2.4 g/day. Or 1–2 tablets PO (600-mg ER tablets) q 12 hr; max, 2.4 g/day. *Child 6–12 yr:* 100–200 mg PO q 4 hr; max, 1.2 g/day or 600 mg (ER) PO q 12 hr. *Child 2–6 yr:* 50–100 mg PO q 4 hr; max, 600 mg/day.

ADV EFF Dizziness, headache, n/v
NC/PT Pt should swallow ER tablet whole and not cut, crush, or chew it, use for no longer than 1 wk, consult prescriber if cough persists, take safety precautions for dizziness. Name confusion between *Mucinex* (guaifenesin) and *Mucomyst* (acetyl-cysteine); use caution.

guanfacine hydrochloride (Intuniv, Tenex)
CLASS Antihypertensive, sympatholytic
PREG/CONT B/NA

IND & DOSE **Mgt of hypertension.** *Adult, child over 12 yr:* 1 mg/day PO at bedtime. **Tx of ADHD.** *Adult, child 6 yr and older:* 1 mg/day PO; titrate at increments of 1 mg/wk to range of 1–4 mg/day *(Intuniv).*

ADJUST DOSE Elderly pts; hepatic, renal impairment

ADV EFF Constipation, dizziness, dry mouth, ED, sedation, weakness

NC/PT Taper when stopping; decrease by no more than 1 mg q 3–7 days. Pt should swallow ER form whole and not cut, crush, or chew it, take immediate-release form at bedtime, continue tx program for ADHD, take safety precautions for CNS effects, use sugarless lozenges for dry mouth.

haloperidol, haloperidol decanoate, haloperidol lactate (Haldol)
CLASS Antipsychotic, dopaminergic blocker
PREG/CONT C/NA

BBW Increased risk of death in elderly pts w/ dementia-related psychosis; drug not approved for this use.

IND & DOSE **Tx of psychiatric disorders, Tourette syndrome.** *Adult:* 0.5–2 mg PO bid–tid w/ moderate symptoms; 3–5 mg PO bid–tid for more resistant pts. Or IM dose 10–15 times daily oral dose in elderly pts stabilized on 10 mg/day or less; 20 times daily oral dose in pts stabilized on high doses and tolerant to oral haloperidol. Max, 3 mL/injection site; repeat at 4-wk intervals. **Prompt control of acutely agitated pts w/ severe symptoms.** *Adult:* 2–5 mg (up to 10–30 mg) q 60 min or q 4–8 hr IM as necessary. **Tx of psychiatric disorders.** *Child 3–12 yr or 15–40 kg:* 0.5 mg/day (25–50 mcg/kg/day) PO; may increase in increments of 0.5 mg q 5–7 days as needed in general, then 0.05–0.15 kg/day PO bid–tid. **Nonpsychotic and Tourette syndromes, behavioral disorders, hyperactivity.** *Child 3–12 yr or 15–40 kg:* 0.05–0.075 mg/day PO bid–tid.

ADJUST DOSE Elderly pts

ADV EFF Akathisia, anemia, **aplastic anemia**, autonomic disturbances, bronchospasm, **cardiac arrest**, dry mouth, dystonia, **eosinophilia**, **hemolytic anemia**, hyperthermia, **hypoglycemia**, **laryngospasm**, leukocytosis, **leukopenia**, **NMS**, photosensitivity, pseudoparkinsonism, **refractory arrhythmias**, **seizures**, **sudden death related to asphyxia**, tardive dyskinesia, **thrombocytopenic or nonthrombocytopenic purpura**

INTERACTIONS Anticholinergics, carbamazepine, ginkgo, lithium

NC/PT Do not use IM in children. Do not give IV. Gradually withdraw after maint tx. Monitor for renal toxicity. Urine may be pink to brown. Pt should take safety precautions for CNS effects, avoid sun exposure, maintain fluid intake, use sugarless lozenges for dry mouth.

DANGEROUS DRUG

heparin sodium (generic)
CLASS Anticoagulant
PREG/CONT C/NA

IND & DOSE *Px, tx of venous thrombotic events.* *Adult:* IV loading dose, 5,000 units; then 10,000–20,000 units subcut followed by 8,000–10,000 units subcut q 8 hr or 15,000–20,000 units q 12 hr. Or initial dose, 10,000 units IV, then 5,000–10,000 units IV q 4–6 hr. Or loading dose, 5,000 units IV, then 20,000–40,000 units/day by IV infusion. *Child:* IV bolus of 50 units/kg, then 100 units/kg IV q 4 hr, or 20,000 units/m²/24 hr by continuous IV infu-

sion. **Px of postop thromboembolism.** *Adult:* 5,000 units by deep subcut injection 2 hr before surgery and q 8–12 hr thereafter for 7 days or until pt fully ambulatory. **Surgery of heart and blood vessels for pts undergoing total body perfusion.** *Adult:* Not less than 150 units/kg IV. IV often-used guideline: 300 units/kg for procedures less than 60 min, 400 units/kg for longer procedures. Add 400–600 units to 100 mL whole blood. **Clot prevention in blood samples.** *Adult:* 70–150 units/ 10–20 mL whole blood.

ADV EFF Bleeding, bruising, chills, fever, **hemorrhage**, injection-site reactions, hair loss, liver enzyme changes, **white clot syndrome**

INTERACTIONS Aspirin, cephalosporins, chamomile, garlic, ginger, ginkgo, ginseng, high-dose vitamin E, NSAIDs, penicillins, oral anticoagulants, salicylates

NC/PT Adjust dose based on coagulation tests; target aPTT, 1.5–2.5 times control. Incompatible in sol w/ many drugs; check before combining. Give by deep subcut injection; do not give IM. Apply pressure to all injection sites; check for signs of bleeding. Have protamine sulfate on hand as antidote. Pt should protect from injury, report bleeding gums, black or tarry stools, severe headache.

hetastarch (Hespan, Voluven)
CLASS Plasma expander
PREG/CONT C/NA

IND & DOSE *Adjunct tx for plasma volume expansion in shock due to hemorrhage, burns, surgery, sepsis, trauma.* *Adult:* 500–1,000 mL IV; max, 1,500 mL/day. In acute hemorrhagic shock, rates approaching 20 mL/kg/hr IV often needed (*Hespan*); up to 50 mL/kg/day IV *Voluven* injection. *Adjunct tx in leukapheresis to improve harvesting, increase yield of granulocytes.* *Adult:* 250–700 mL

infused at constant fixed ratio of 1:8 to 1:13 to venous whole blood. Safety of up to two procedures/wk and total of seven to ten procedures using hetastarch have been established.
ADV EFF Bleeding, chills, headache, itching, mild influenza-like reactions, submaxillary and parotid gland enlargement, n/v
NC/PT Do not mix in sol w/ other drugs. Have emergency support on hand. Pt should report difficulty breathing, severe headache.

histrelin implant (Vantas)

CLASS Antineoplastic, GNRH
PREG/CONT X/NA

IND & DOSE Palliative tx of advanced prostate cancer. *Adult:* 1 implant inserted subcut and left for 12 mo. May be removed after 12 mo and new implant inserted.
ADV EFF Diabetes, fatigue, hot flashes, hyperglycemia, injection-site reactions **MI, renal impairment, spinal cord compression, stroke,** testicular atrophy
NC/PT Monitor serum glucose, renal function, injection site. Pt should report chest pain, numbness or tingling, injection-site reactions.

hyaluronic acid derivatives (Euflexxa, Hyalgan, Synvisc)

CLASS Glucosamine polysaccharide
PREG/CONT C/NA

IND & DOSE Tx of pain in osteoarthritis of knee in pts unresponsive to traditional therapy. *Adult:* 2 mL/wk by intra-articular injection in knee for total of three to five injections.
ADV EFF Headache, joint swelling, pain at injection site
NC/PT Avoid strenuous exercise and prolonged weight bearing for 48 hr after injection. Headache may occur.

hyaluronidase (Amphadase, Hylenex, Vitrase)

CLASS Enzyme
PREG/CONT C/NA

IND & DOSE To increase absorption of injected drugs. *Adult, child:* Add 150 units to injection sol. **Hypodermoclysis.** *Adult:* 150 units injected under skin close to clysis. *Child under 3 yr:* Limit total dose to 200 mL/clysis. *Premature infants:* Max, 25 mL/kg at rate of no more than 2 mL/min. **Adjunct to subcut urography.** *Adult:* 75 units subcut over each scapula followed by injection of contrast media at same sites.
ADV EFF Chills, dizziness, edema, hypotension, injection-site reactions, n/v
INTERACTIONS Benzodiazepines, furosemide, phenytoin
NC/PT Do not use w/ dopamine or alpha-adrenergic drugs or in inflamed or infected areas. Do not apply to cornea or use for insect bites or stings; monitor injection site.

hydrALAZINE hydrochloride (Apresoline)

CLASS Antihypertensive, vasodilator
PREG/CONT C/NA

IND & DOSE Tx of essential hypertension. *Adult:* 10 mg PO qid for first 2–4 days; increase to 25 mg PO qid for first wk. Second and subsequent wks: 50 mg PO qid. Or 20–40 mg IM or IV, repeated as necessary if unable to take orally. *Child:* 0.75 mg/kg/day PO in divided doses q 6 hr (max, 7.5 mg/kg/day PO in four divided doses, or 200 mg/day PO). Or 1.7–3.5 mg/kg IM or IV divided into four to six doses if unable to take orally.

Tx of eclampsia. **Adult:** 5–10 mg q 20 min by IV bolus. If no response after 20 mg, try another drug.
ADV EFF Angina, anorexia, **blood dyscrasias,** dizziness, headache, n/v/d, orthostatic hypotension, palpitations, peripheral neuritis, rash, tachycardia
INTERACTIONS Adrenergic blockers
NC/PT Use parenteral drug immediately after opening ampule. Withdraw drug gradually, especially in pts who have experienced marked BP reduction. Pt should take safety precautions w/ orthostatic hypotension, CNS effects; take w/ food; report chest pain, numbness or tingling, fever.

hydrochlorothiazide
(HydroDIURIL, Hydro-Par, Microzide Capsules)
CLASS Thiazide diuretic
PREG/CONT B/NA

IND & DOSE Adjunct tx of edema from systemic disease. **Adult:** 25–100 mg PO daily until dry weight attained. Then, 25–100 mg/day PO or intermittently, up to 200 mg/day. **Child:** 1–2 mg/kg/day PO in one or two doses. Max, 100 mg/day in two doses (2–12 yr), 37.5 mg/day in two doses (6 mo–2 yr), up to 3 mg/kg/day in two doses (under 6 mo). **Tx of hypertension.** **Adult:** 12.5–50 mg PO; max, 50 mg/day.
ADJUST DOSE Elderly pts
ADV EFF Anorexia, dizziness, drowsiness, dry mouth, muscle cramps, n/v, nocturia, photosensitivity, polyuria, vertigo
INTERACTIONS Amphotericin B, antidiabetics, cholestyramine, colestipol, corticosteroids, lithium, loop diuretics, NMJ blockers
NC/PT Monitor BP; reduced dose of other antihypertensives may be needed. Give w/ food. Mark calendar for intermittent therapy. Pt should measure weight daily, take early in day so sleep not interrupted, use safety precautions for CNS effects, avoid sun exposure, report weight changes of 3 lb/day.

hydrocodone bitartrate
(Zohydro ER)
CLASS Opioid agonist analgesic
PREG/CONT C/C-II

BBW Risks of addiction, severe to fatal respiratory depression, death w/ accidental consumption by children, life-threatening neonatal withdrawal if used in pregnancy, fatal plasma levels if combined w/ alcohol.
IND & DOSE Mgt of pain requiring continuous analgesic for prolonged period. **Adult:** Initially, 10 mg PO q 12 hr for opioid-naïve or opioid-nontolerant pts; increase as needed in 10-mg increments q 12 hr q 3–7 days.
ADJUST DOSE Elderly, impaired pts; severe renal, hepatic impairment
ADV EFF Abd pain, back pain, confusion, constipation, dizziness, dry mouth, fatigue, headache, n/v/d, pruritus, respiratory depression
INTERACTIONS Alcohol, anticholinergics, barbiturate anesthetics, CNS depressants, CYP3A4 inhibitors, MAOIs, other opioids, protease inhibitors
NC/PT Monitor pt carefully; ensure appropriate use of drug. Ensure opioid antagonist and emergency equipment readily available. Safety issues w/ CNS changes. Taper when discontinuing. Pt should swallow capsule whole, not cut, crush, or chew it; discontinue slowly; avoid pregnancy, breast-feeding, alcohol; take safety precautions w/ CNS changes; report difficulty breathing, severe constipation, pain unrelieved by drug.

hydrocortisone salts
(Cortaid, Pandel, Solu-Cortef, Westcort)
CLASS Corticosteroid
PREG/CONT C/NA

IND & DOSE Replacement tx in adrenal cortical insufficiency, allergic states, inflammatory disorders, hematologic disorders, trichinosis, ulcerative colitis, MS. *Adult, child:* 5–200 mg/day PO based on severity and pt response, or 100–500 mg IM or IV q 2, 4, or 6 hr. Retention enema for tx of ulcerative colitis, proctitis. *Adult, child:* 100 mg nightly for 21 days. **Anorectal cream, suppositories to relieve discomfort of hemorrhoids, perianal itching or irritation.** *Adult, child:* 1 applicator daily or bid for 2 or 3 wk and q second day thereafter. **Dermatologic preparations to relieve inflammatory and pruritic manifestations of dermatoses.** *Adult, child:* Apply sparingly to affected area bid–qid. **Tx of acute/chronic ophthalmic inflammatory conditions.** *Adult, child:* 1–2 drops per eye one to two times/day.

ADV EFF Anaphylactoid reactions, amenorrhea, ecchymoses, fluid retention, headache, **HF,** hypokalemia, hypotension, immunosuppression, infection, irregular menses, local pain or irritation at application site, muscle weakness, pancreatitis, peptic ulcer, striae, vertigo

INTERACTIONS Anticoagulants, anticholinesterases, cholestyramine, estrogen, hormonal contraceptives, ketoconazole, live vaccines, phenobarbital, phenytoin, rifampin, salicylates

NC/PT Give daily before 9 a.m. to mimic normal peak diurnal corticosteroid levels and minimize HPA suppression. Rotate IM injection sites. Use minimal doses for minimal duration to minimize adverse effects. Taper doses when discontinuing high-dose or long-term tx; arrange for increased dose when pt is subject to unusual stress. W/ topical use, use caution w/ occlusive dressings; tight or plastic diapers over affected area can increase systemic absorption. Suggest medical ID. Pt should protect from infection; report swelling, difficulty breathing.

DANGEROUS DRUG

hydromorphone hydrochloride (Dilaudid, Dilaudid-HP, Exalgo)

CLASS Opioid agonist analgesic
PREG/CONT C; D (Labor & delivery)/C-II

BBW Monitor dose and intended use; vary w/ form. Serious effects, abuse, misuse possible. Extended-release form for opioid-tolerant pts only; fatal respiratory depression possible. Extended-release form not for use w/ acute or postop pain or as an as-needed drug. Pt must swallow extended-release tablets whole; broken, chewed, or crushed tablets allow rapid release of drug and could cause fatal overdose.

IND & DOSE Relief of moderate to severe pain; acute and chronic pain. *Adult:* 2–4 mg PO q 4–6 hr. Liquid, 2.5–10 mg PO q 3–6 hr. ER tablets, 8–64 mg/day PO. Or 1–2 mg IM/subcut q 4–6 hr as needed, or by slow IV injection over 2–3 min, or 3 mg rectally q 6–8 hr.

ADJUST DOSE Elderly pts; hepatic, renal impairment

ADV EFF Apnea, cardiac arrest, circulatory depression, constipation, dizziness, flushing, light-headedness, n/v, respiratory arrest, respiratory depression, sedation, shock, sweating, visual disturbances

INTERACTIONS Alcohol, anticholinergics, antihistamines, barbiturate anesthetics, MAOIs, opioid agonist/antagonists

NC/PT Ensure opioid antagonist and facilities for assisted or controlled respiration are readily available during parenteral administration. Breastfeeding pts should take 4–6 hr before scheduled feeding. Refrigerate rectal suppositories. Pt should swallow ER tablets whole, and not cut, crush, or chew them; avoid alcohol, antihistamines; take laxative for constipation; use safety precautions for CNS effects; report chest pain, difficulty breathing.

hydroxocobalamin
(Cyanokit)

CLASS Antidote
PREG/CONT C/NA

IND & DOSE Tx of known or suspected cyanide poisoning. *Adult:* 5 g by IV infusion over 15 min; may give second dose over 15–120 min by IV infusion.
ADV EFF Anaphylaxis, chest tightness, dyspnea, edema, **hypertension**, injection-site reactions, nausea, photosensitivity, rash, red skin and mucous membranes (up to 2 wk), red urine (up to 5 wk)
NC/PT Support pt during acute poisoning. Run in separate IV line; do not mix w/ other drugs. Monitor BP. Not for use in pregnancy, breast-feeding. Tell pt urine may be red for up to 5 wk, skin and mucous membranes may be red for 2 wk. Pt should avoid exposure to sunlight during that period, report difficulty breathing.

hydroxyprogesterone caproate (Makena)

CLASS Progestin
PREG/CONT B/NA

IND & DOSE To reduce risk of preterm birth in women w/ singleton pregnancy and hx of singleton spontaneous preterm birth. *Adult:* 250 mg IM once wkly, beginning between 16 wk, 0 days' and 20 wk, 6 days' gestation. Continue wkly injections until wk 37 of gestation, or until delivery, whichever comes first.
ADV EFF Depression, fluid retention, glucose intolerance, injection-site reactions, nausea, pruritus, **thromboembolic events**, urticaria
NC/PT IM injection into upper outer area of buttocks once/wk. Vial stable for 5 wk at room temp; protect from light. Monitor injection sites; periodically check serum glucose. Mark calendar for injection days. Pt should report leg, chest pain.

hydroxyurea (Droxia, Hydrea)

CLASS Antineoplastic
PREG/CONT D/NA

IND & DOSE Tx of melanoma; recurrent, metastatic, or inoperable ovarian cancer. *Adult:* 80 mg/kg PO as single dose q third day or 20–30 mg/kg PO as single daily dose (*Hydrea*).
Concomitant therapy w/ irradiation for primary squamous cell carcinoma of head and neck. *Adult:* 80 mg/kg PO as single daily dose q third day. Begin 7 days before irradiation; continue during and for a prolonged period after radiation therapy (*Hydrea*).
Tx of resistant chronic myelocytic leukemia. *Adult:* 20–30 mg/kg PO as single daily dose (*Hydrea*). **To reduce sickle cell anemia crises** (*Droxia*). *Adult:* 15 mg/kg/day PO as single dose; may increase by 5 mg/kg/day q 12 wk until max of 35 mg/kg/day reached. If blood levels become toxic, stop drug and resume at 2.5 mg/kg/day less than dose that resulted in toxicity when blood levels return to normal; increase q 12 wk in 2.5-mg/kg/day intervals if blood levels remain acceptable.
ADJUST DOSE Renal impairment
ADV EFF Anorexia, bone marrow depression, cancer, dizziness, headache, n/v, stomatitis
INTERACTIONS Uricosuric agents
NC/PT Handle w/ extreme care; may cause cancer. Use gloves when handling capsule. Monitor CBC before and q 2 wk during tx. Capsule should not be cut, crushed, or chewed; have pt swallow whole. If pt unable to swallow capsule, may empty into glass of water; pt should swallow immediately. Not for use in pregnancy (barrier contraceptives advised). Pt should drink 10–12 glasses of fluid each day, take safety precautions for CNS effects, protect from exposure to infections, report unusual bleeding.

hydrOXYzine hydrochloride, hydrOXYzine pamoate (Vistaril)

CLASS Antiemetic, antihistamine, anxiolytic
PREG/CONT C/NA

IND & DOSE Symptomatic relief of anxiety. *Adult, child over 6 yr:* 50–100 mg PO qid. *Child under 6 yr:* 50 mg/day PO in divided doses. **Mgt of pruritus.** *Adult:* 25 mg PO tid–qid. *Child:* 50–100 mg PO ul IM. **Sedation, antiemetic (preop/postop).** *Adult:* 25 mg PO or IM tid–qid. *Child:* 0.6 mg/kg PO or IM. **Psychiatric and emotional emergencies.** 50–100 mg IM immediately and q 4–6 hr as needed.
ADV EFF Constipation, dizziness, drowsiness, dry mouth, hypersensitivity reactions, sedation, tremors, urine retention
INTERACTIONS Alcohol, barbiturates, CNS depressants, opioids
NC/PT Do not give parenteral sol subcut, IV, or intra-arterially; tissue necrosis has occurred. Give IM injections deep into upper outer quadrant of buttocks or midlateral thigh (adults) or midlateral thigh muscles (children). Pt should take safety precautions w/ CNS effects, use sugarless lozenges for dry mouth, avoid alcohol.

hyoscyamine sulfate (IB-Stat, Levbid, Levsin/SL, Symax)

CLASS Anticholinergic, antispasmodic, belladonna alkaloid
PREG/CONT C/NA

IND & DOSE Adjunct tx in IBS, peptic ulcer, spastic or functional GI disorders, cystitis, neurogenic bladder or bowel disorders, parkinsonism, biliary or renal colic, rhinitis. *Adult:* 0.125–0.25 mg PO q 4 hr or as needed. Or 1–2 mL oral sol q 4 hr as needed (max, 12 mL/day). Or 1–2 oral sprays q 4 hr as needed (max, 12 sprays/day). Or ½–1 orally disintegrating tablet 3–4 times/day 30 min–1 hr before meals and at bedtime. Or 1–2 tsp elixir PO q 4 hr as needed (max, 12 tsp/day). Or 0.375–0.75 mg ER tablet PO q 12 hr; may give q 8 hr if needed (max, 4 capsules/day). Or 0.25–0.5 mg subcut, IM, or IV 2–4 times/day at 4-hr intervals as needed. *Child 12 yr and older:* 1–2 tablets PO q 4 hr as needed (max, 12 tablets in 24 hr). Or ½–1 orally disintegrating tablets PO tid–qid 30 min–1 hr before meals and at bedtime. Or 1–2 mL oral sol PO q 4 hr or as needed (max, 12 mL in 24 hr). Or 1–2 ER capsules PO q 12 hr; adjust to 1 capsule q 8 hr if needed (max, 4 capsules in 24 hr). Or 1–2 tsp elixir PO q 4 hr or as needed (max, 12 tsp in 24 hr). Or 1–2 oral sprays q 4 hr as needed. *Child 2 yr–under 12 yr:* ½–1 tablet PO q 4 hr as needed (max, 6 tablets in 24 hr). Or 0.25–1 mL oral sol PO q 4 hr or as needed (max, 6 mL in 24 hr). Or may give elixir, dose based on weight. **To reduce secretions preanesthesia.** *Adult:* 0.005 mg/kg IV or IM 30–60 min before induction. *Child over 2 yr:* 5 mcg/kg IV 30–60 min before anesthesia. **Tx of drug-induced bradycardia.** *Adult, child over 2 yr:* 0.125 mg (0.25 mL) IV. Repeat as needed. **Reversal of neuromuscular blockade.** *Adult, child over 2 yr:* 0.2 mg IV, IM, or subcut for q 1 mg neostigmine.
ADV EFF Anaphylaxis, decreased sweating, dizziness, drowsiness, dry mouth, fever, nausea, palpitations, urinary hesitancy, urticaria
INTERACTIONS Antacids, amantadine, anticholinergics, antihistamines, haloperidol, MAOIs, phenothiazines, TCAs
NC/PT Ensure adequate hydration. Pt should empty bladder before each dose, swallow whole (not cut, crush, or chew ER forms), take safety precautions for CNS effects, use sugarless lozenges for dry mouth, take 30–60 min before meals; report difficulty breathing, fainting, palpitations.

ibandronate sodium
(Boniva)

CLASS Bisphosphonate, calcium regulator
PREG/CONT C/NA

IND & DOSE Tx, px of osteoporosis in postmenopausal women. *Adult:* 2.5 mg/day PO, or 150-mg tablet PO once/mo, or 3 mg IV over 15–30 sec q 3 mo.
ADJUST DOSE Renal impairment
ADV EFF Abd/back pain, bronchitis, diarrhea, dizziness, dyspepsia, headache, hypertension, **jaw osteonecrosis,** myalgia, pneumonia
INTERACTIONS Aluminum, iron, magnesium antacids; food, milk
NC/PT Monitor serum calcium levels. Ensure adequate intake of vitamin D/calcium. Use caution in pregnancy; not for use in breast-feeding. Obtain periodic bone density exams. Pt should take in a.m. w/ full glass of water at least 60 min before first beverage, food, or medication of day; stay upright for 60 min after taking to avoid potentially serious esophageal erosion; mark calendar for once/mo or q-3-mo tx; report difficulty swallowing, pain/burning in esophagus.

DANGEROUS DRUG

ibritumomab (Zevalin)

CLASS Antineoplastic, monoclonal antibody
PREG/CONT D/NA

BBW Risk of serious to fatal infusion reactions, prolonged bone marrow suppression, cutaneous/mucocutaneous reactions; monitor, support pt accordingly.
IND & DOSE Tx of relapsed or refractory low-grade follicular transformed B-cell non-Hodgkin lymphoma; previously treated follicular non-Hodgkin lymphoma w/ relapse

after first-line tx. *Adult:* 250 mg/m²
IV rituximab, then 5 mCi/kg as 10-min IV push. Repeat in 7–9 days.
ADV EFF Abd pain, asthenia, cough, fatigue, fever, **infusion reactions, leukemia,** nasopharyngitis, n/v/d, **prolonged bone marrow suppression, severe cutaneous/mucocutaneous reactions**
INTERACTIONS Live vaccines, platelet inhibitors
NC/PT Premedicate w/ acetaminophen, diphenhydramine before each infusion. Monitor for extravasation; move to other limb if this occurs. Not for use in pregnancy (barrier contraceptives advised), breast-feeding. Pt should avoid exposure to infection; report bleeding, fever or s&sx of infection, rash, mouth sores.

ibrutinib (Imbruvica)

CLASS Antineoplastic, kinase inhibitor
PREG/CONT PREG/CONT D/NA

IND & DOSE Tx of mantle cell lymphoma when at least one other tx has been tried. *Adult:* 560 mg PO once daily.
ADJUST DOSE Hepatic impairment (contraindicated)
ADV EFF Abd pain, anemia, **bone marrow suppression,** bruising, constipation, dyspnea, edema, fatigue, n/v/d, renal toxicity, **secondary malignancies,** URI
INTERACTIONS CYP3A inducers/inhibitors
NC/PT Ensure proper dx. Monitor renal function; screen for secondary malignancies. Not for use in pregnancy (contraceptive use advised), breast-feeding. Pt must swallow capsule whole, not cut, crush, or chew it. Pt should avoid exposure to infection; report color changes in urine/stool, severe diarrhea, fever, bleeding, sx of infection.

ibuprofen (Advil, Caldolor, Motrin)

CLASS Analgesic, NSAID
PREG/CONT B (1st, 2nd trimesters); D (3rd trimester)/NA

BBW Increased risk of CV events, GI bleeding; monitor accordingly. Contraindicated for tx of periop pain after CABG.

IND & DOSE Tx of mild to moderate pain, fever, migraine headache, primary dysmenorrhea. *Adult, child 12 yr and older:* 400 mg PO q 4–6 hr; max, 3,200/day. Or, 400–800 mg IV over 30 min q 6 hr for pain. Or, 400 mg IV over 30 min for fever; may follow with 400 mg IV q 4–6 hr or 100–200 mg IV q 4 hr to control fever. *Child 6 mo–11 yr:* Base dose on weight, given q 6–8 hr. 32–42 kg, 300 mg PO; 27–31 kg, 250 mg PO; 22–26 kg, 200 mg PO; 16–21 kg, 150 mg PO; 11–15 kg, 100 mg PO; 8–10 kg, 75 mg PO; 5–7 kg, 50 mg. Oral drops: 9–11 kg or 12–23 mo, 1.875 mL (75 mg) PO; 5–8 kg or 6–11 mo, 1.25 mL (50 mg) PO. Tx of osteoarthritis, rheumatoid arthritis. *Adult:* 1,200–3,200 mg/day PO (300 mg qid or 400, 600, 800 mg tid or qid; individualize dose). Tx of juvenile arthritis. *Child 6 mo–11 yr:* 30–50 mg/kg/day PO in three to four divided doses; 20 mg/kg/day for milder disease.

ADV EFF Agranulocytosis, anaphylactoid reactions to anaphylactic shock, bronchospasm, dizziness, dyspepsia, edema, eye changes, headache, GI bleeding, GI pain, HF, insomnia, nausea, pancytopenia, rash, somnolence, stomatitis

INTERACTIONS ACE inhibitors, anticoagulants, beta blockers, bisphosphonates, bumetanide, ethacrynic acid, furosemide, ginkgo, lithium

NC/PT Ensure hydration w/ IV use. Stop if eye changes, renal or hepatic impairment. Give w/ food if GI upset. Pt should avoid OTC products that may contain ibuprofen, take safety precautions w/ CNS effects, report ankle swelling, black tarry stool, vision changes.

DANGEROUS DRUG

ibutilide fumarate (Corvert)

CLASS Antiarrhythmic
PREG/CONT C/NA

BBW Have emergency equipment on hand during and for at least 4 hr after administration; can cause potentially life-threatening arrhythmias. Use caution when selecting pts for tx.

IND & DOSE Rapid conversion of atrial fibrillation (AF)/flutter of recent onset to sinus rhythm. *Adult:* 60 kg or more, 1 vial (1 mg) IV over 10 min; may repeat after 10 min if arrhythmia not terminated; under 60 kg, 0.1 mL/kg (0.01 mg/kg) IV over 10 min; may repeat after 10 min if arrhythmia not terminated.

ADV EFF Dizziness, headache, nausea, numbness/tingling in arms, ventricular arrhythmias

INTERACTIONS Amiodarone, antihistamines, digoxin, disopyramide, quinidine, phenothiazines, procainamide, sotalol, TCAs

NC/PT Determine time of arrhythmia onset; most effective if less than 90 days. Ensure pt anticoagulated for at least 2 wk if AF lasts more than 2 days. Have emergency equipment on hand. Provide follow-up for medical evaluation. Pt should report chest pain, difficulty breathing.

---

icatibant (Firazyr)

CLASS Bradykinin receptor antagonist
PREG/CONT C/NA

IND & DOSE Tx of acute attacks of hereditary angioedema. *Adult:* 30 mg subcut in abdomen; may repeat after at least 6 hr. Max, 3 injections/day.

ADV EFF Dizziness, drowsiness, fever, injection-site reaction.
INTERACTIONS ACE inhibitors
NC/PT Teach proper administration, disposal of needles, syringes. Rotate injection sites; do not inject into scars, inflamed/infected areas. Use caution in pregnancy, breast-feeding. Pt should take safety precautions w/ CNS effects, go to emergency department after injecting if laryngeal attack occurs.

icosapent ethyl (Vascepa)
CLASS Antihypertriglyceridemic, ethyl ester
PREG/CONT C/NA

IND & DOSE Adjunct to diet to reduce triglyceride levels in adults with severe (500 mg/dL or higher) hypertriglyceridemia. *Adult:* 2 g PO bid w/ food.
ADV EFF Arthralgia, bleeding, **hepatic impairment,** hypersensitivity reaction
INTERACTIONS Anticoagulants, platelet inhibitors
NC/PT Monitor LFTs carefully; use caution w/ known fish/shellfish allergy. Pt should swallow capsule whole and not cut, crush, or chew it; continue diet/exercise program.

DANGEROUS DRUG

idarubicin hydrochloride (Idamycin PFS)
CLASS Antineoplastic antibiotic
PREG/CONT D/NA

BBW Do not give IM, subcut because of severe local reaction, tissue necrosis; give IV only. Risk of myocardial toxicity; monitor accordingly. Monitor response to tx frequently at start of tx. Monitor serum uric acid level, CBC, cardiac output (listen for S_3), LFTs. Changes in uric acid levels may need dose decrease; consult physician.

IND & DOSE Tx of AML w/ other drugs. *Adult:* 12 mg/m²/day for 3 days by slow IV injection (10–15 min) w/ cytarabine. May give cytarabine as 100 mg/m²/day by continuous IV infusion for 7 days or as 25-mg/m² IV bolus, then 200 mg/m²/day IV for 5 days by continuous infusion. May give second course when toxicity has subsided, if needed, at 25% dose reduction.
ADJUST DOSE Hepatic, renal impairment
ADV EFF Alopecia, **anaphylaxis,** anorexia, **cancer, cardiac toxicity,** headache, **HF,** injection-site reactions, **myelosuppression, mucositis,** n/v
NC/PT Monitor injection site for extravasation. Monitor CBC, LFTs, renal function, cardiac output frequently during tx. Ensure adequate hydration. Not for use in pregnancy (barrier contraceptives advised). Pt should cover head at temp extremes (hair loss possible), get regular medical follow-up, report swelling, chest pain, difficulty breathing.

idursulfase (Elaprase)
CLASS Enzyme
PREG/CONT C/NA

BBW Risk of severe to life-threatening anaphylactic reactions during infusion; have emergency equipment on hand. Monitor closely.
IND & DOSE Tx of Hunter's syndrome. *Adult, child over 5 yr:* 0.5 mg/kg IV infused over 1–3 hr q wk.
ADV EFF **Anaphylaxis,** fever, hypertension, rash, respiratory impairment
NC/PT Start first infusion slowly to monitor for infusion reaction (8 mL/min for first 15 min, then increase by 8 mL/min at 15-min intervals; max, 100 mL/hr). Do not infuse w/ other products in same line. Use caution in pregnancy, breast-feeding. Pt should report difficulty breathing, rash.

DANGEROUS DRUG

ifosfamide (Ifex)

CLASS Alkylating agent, antineoplastic, nitrogen mustard
PREG/CONT D/NA

BBW Arrange for blood tests to evaluate hematopoietic function before starting tx and wkly during tx; serious hemorrhagic toxicities have occurred. Provide extensive hydration consisting of at least 2 L oral or IV fluid/day to prevent bladder toxicity. Arrange to give protector, such as mesna, to prevent hemorrhagic cystitis.

IND & DOSE Third-line chemotherapy of germ-cell testicular cancer w/ other drugs; third-line tx of bone, soft-tissue sarcomas. *Adult:* 1.2 g/m²/day IV over at least 30 min for 5 consecutive days; repeat q 3 wk, or after recovery from hematologic toxicity. For px of bladder toxicity, give more than 2 L fluid/day IV or PO. Use mesna IV to prevent hemorrhagic cystitis.

ADJUST DOSE Renal impairment
ADV EFF Alopecia, anorexia, confusion, hallucinations, immunosuppression, leukopenia, n/v, **potentially fatal hemorrhagic cystitis,** somnolence
INTERACTIONS Grapefruit juice
NC/PT For px of bladder toxicity, give more than 2 L fluid/day IV or PO. Use mesna IV to prevent hemorrhagic cystitis. Maintain hydration (at least 10–12 glasses fluid/day). Can cause fetal harm; contraceptives advised (for men/women) during and for few wks after tx. Pt should avoid grapefruit juice, cover head at temp extremes (hair loss possible), report painful urination, blood in urine.

iloperidone (Fanapt)

CLASS Atypical antipsychotic
PREG/CONT C/NA

BBW Increased risk of death if used in elderly pts w/ dementia-related psychosis. Do not use for these pts; not approved for this use.

IND & DOSE Acute tx of schizophrenia. *Adult:* Range, 12–24 mg/day PO; titrate based on orthostatic hypotension tolerance. Initially, 1 mg PO bid; then 2, 4, 6, 8, 10, 12 mg PO bid on days 2, 3, 4, 5, 6, 7 respectively.

ADJUST DOSE Hepatic impairment
ADV EFF Dizziness, fatigue, hyperglycemia, nausea, **NMS,** orthostatic hypotension, **QT prolongation,** weight gain
INTERACTIONS Alcohol, antihypertensives, CNS depressants, fluoxetine, itraconazole, ketoconazole, other QT-prolonging drugs, paroxetine, St. John's wort
NC/PT Obtain baseline ECG; periodically monitor QT interval. Titrate over first wk to decrease orthostatic hypotension. Monitor serum glucose. Use caution in pregnancy; not for use in breast-feeding. Pt should take safety measures w/ CNS effects, avoid alcohol/St. John's wort; change positions carefully, report fever, thoughts of suicide, fainting.

iloprost (Ventavis)

CLASS Vasodilator
PREG/CONT C/NA

IND & DOSE Tx of pulmonary artery hypertension in pts w/ NY Heart Association Class II to IV symptoms. *Adult:* 2.5–5 mcg inhaled 6–9 times/day while awake; max, 45 mcg/day.
ADV EFF Back pain, **bronchospasm,** cough, dizziness, headache, **hypotension,** insomnia, light-headedness, muscle cramps, n/v, palpitations, **pulmonary hypotension,** syncope
INTERACTIONS Anticoagulants, antihypertensives, vasodilators
NC/PT Review proper use of inhaler. Use caution in pregnancy; not for use in breast-feeding. Pt should take safety measures w/ CNS effects, report difficulty breathing, fainting.

DANGEROUS DRUG
imatinib mesylate
(Gleevec)

CLASS Antineoplastic, protein tyrosine kinase inhibitor
PREG/CONT D/NA

IND & DOSE Tx of chronic phase CML. *Adult:* 400 mg/day PO as once-a-day dose; may consider 600 mg/day. *Child over 2 yr:* 260 mg/m²/day PO as one dose, or divided a.m. and p.m. **Tx of accelerated phase or blast crisis CML.** *Adult:* 600 mg/day PO as single dose; may consider 400 mg PO bid. **Tx of newly diagnosed CML.** *Child over 2 yr:* 340 mg/m² PO; max, 600 mg/day. **Tx of ALL.** *Adult:* 600 mg/day PO. **Tx of aggressive systemic mastocytosis (ASM), hypereosinophilic syndrome/chronic eosinophilic leukemia, myelodysplastic/myeloproliferative diseases, metastatic malignant GI stromal tumors; adjunct tx after surgical resection of Kit-positive GI stromal tumors.** *Adult:* 400 mg/day PO. **Tx of ASM w/ eosinophilia.** *Adult:* 100 mg/day PO. **Tx of unresectable, recurrent, or metastatic dermatofibrosarcoma protuberans.** *Adult:* 800 mg/day PO.
ADJUST DOSE Hepatic, renal impairment
ADV EFF Bone marrow suppression, fluid retention, headache, **left ventricular dysfx**, n/v/d, rash, **severe HF**
INTERACTIONS Azithromycin, carbamazepine, clarithromycin, cyclosporine, dexamethasone, grapefruit juice, itraconazole, ketoconazole, levothyroxine, pimozide, phenobarbital, phenytoin, rifampin, simvastatin, St. John's wort, warfarin
NC/PT Monitor CBC. Not for use in pregnancy (barrier contraceptives advised). Monitor child for growth retardation. Give w/ meals. May disperse in glass of water or apple juice; give immediately using 50 mL for 10-mg tablet, 200 mL for 400-mg tablet. Pt should not cut or crush tablet, take analgesics for headache, avoid grapefruit juice/St. John's wort, report sudden fluid retention.

imipramine hydrochloride, imipramine pamoate
(Tofranil)

CLASS Antidepressant, TCA
PREG/CONT C/NA

BBW Limit drug access for depressed, potentially suicidal pts. Increased risk of suicidality, especially in children, adolescents, young adults; monitor accordingly.

IND & DOSE Tx of depression. *Adult:* Hospitalized pts, 100–150 mg/day PO in divided doses; may increase to 200 mg/day. After 2 wk, may increase to 250–300 mg/day. Outpts, 75 mg/day PO, increasing to 150 mg/day. Max, 200 mg/day; range, 50–150 mg/day. *Adolescent:* 30–40 mg/day PO. **Tx of childhood enuresis.** *Child 6 yr and older:* 25 mg/day PO 1 hr before bedtime. May increase to 75 mg PO nightly in child over 12 yr, 50 mg PO nightly in child under 12 yr. Max, 2.5 mg/kg/day.
ADJUST DOSE Elderly pts
ADV EFF Anticholinergic effects, arrhythmias, **bone marrow depression**, confusion, constipation, disturbed concentration, dry mouth, **MI**, nervousness, orthostatic hypotension, photosensitivity, sedation, **stroke**, urine retention, withdrawal symptoms after prolonged use
INTERACTIONS Anticholinergics, clonidine, MAOIs, oral anticoagulants, St. John's wort, sympathomimetics
NC/PT Give major portion at bedtime. Consider dose change w/ adverse effects. Not for use in pregnancy, breast-feeding. Pt should avoid sun exposure, take safety measures w/ CNS effects, report thoughts of suicide, excessive sedation.

indacaterol (Arcapta Neohaler)

CLASS Bronchodilator, long-acting beta agonist
PREG/CONT C/NA

BBW Increased risk of asthma-related deaths; not indicated for tx of asthma.

IND & DOSE Long-term maint bronchodilator tx for pts w/ COPD: *Adult:* 75 mcg/day inhaled w/ *Arcapta Neohaler.*

ADV EFF Arrhythmias, asthma-related deaths, **bronchospasm**, cough, headache, **hypertension**, nausea, nasopharyngitis, pharyngeal pain, **seizures**
INTERACTIONS Adrenergic drugs, beta blockers, corticosteroids, diuretics, MAOIs, QT-prolonging drugs, TCAs, xanthines
NC/PT Not for acute or deteriorating situations. Do not exceed recommended dose. Should be used with inhaled corticosteroid. Review proper use of inhaler. Pt should report worsening of condition, chest pain, severe difficulty breathing.

indapamide (generic)

CLASS Thiazide-like diuretic
PREG/CONT B/NA

IND & DOSE Tx of edema associated w/ HF. *Adult:* 2.5–5 mg/day PO. Tx of hypertension. *Adult:* 1.25–2.5 mg/day PO. Consider adding another drug if control not achieved.
ADV EFF Agranulocytosis, anorexia, **aplastic anemia**, dizziness, dry mouth, hypotension, n/v, photosensitivity, vertigo
INTERACTIONS Antidiabetics, cholestyramine, colestipol, lithium, thiazide diuretics
NC/PT Give w/ food if GI upset occurs. Give early in a.m. Pt should weigh self daily and record, report weight change of 3 lb/day, take safety precautions w/ CNS effects, use sugarless lozenges for dry mouth, avoid sun exposure.

indinavir sulfate (Crixivan)

CLASS Antiviral, protease inhibitor
PREG/CONT C/NA

IND & DOSE Tx of HIV infection w/ other drugs. *Adult, child 12 yr and older:* 800 mg PO q 8 hr. W/ delavirdine, 600 mg PO q 8 hr; w/ delavirdine, 400 mg PO tid; w/ didanosine, give more than 1 hr apart on empty stomach; w/ itraconazole, 600 mg PO q 8 hr; w/ itraconazole, 200 mg PO bid; w/ ketoconazole, 600 mg PO q 8 hr; w/ rifabutin, 1,000 mg PO q 8 hr (reduce rifabutin by 50%).
ADJUST DOSE Hepatic impairment
ADV EFF Dry skin, flulike symptoms, headache, hyperbilirubinemia, n/v/d
INTERACTIONS Ergots, midazolam, pimozide, triazolam; do not use w/ preceding drugs. Atazanavir, azole antifungals, benzodiazepines, carbamazepine, delavirdine, efavirenz, fentanyl, grapefruit juice, interleukins, nelfinavir, nevirapine, phenobarbital, phenytoin, rifabutin, rifampin, rifamycin, ritonavir, sildenafil, St. John's wort, venlafaxine
NC/PT Protect capsules from moisture; store in container provided and keep desiccant in bottle. Give drug q 8 hr around clock. Maintain hydration. Check all drugs pt taking; many interactions possible. Not a cure for disease; advise pt to use precautions. Pt should avoid grapefruit juice, St. John's wort; continue other HIV drugs; drink at least 1.5 L of water/day; report severe diarrhea.

indomethacin, indomethacin sodium trihydrate (Indocin)

CLASS NSAID
PREG/CONT B (1st, 2nd trimesters); D (3rd trimester)/NA

BBW Increased risk of CV events, GI bleeding; monitor accordingly.

Adverse reactions dose-related; use lowest effective dose.

IND & DOSE Relief of s&sx of osteoarthritis, rheumatoid arthritis, ankylosing spondylitis. *Adult:* 25 mg PO bid or tid; may use total daily dose of 150–200 mg/day PO. **Tx of acute painful shoulder.** *Adult:* 75–150 mg/day PO in three or four divided doses for 7–14 days. **Tx of acute gouty arthritis.** *Adult:* 50 mg PO tid until pain tolerable; then decrease until not needed (within 3–5 days). Do not use SR form. **Closure of hemodynamically significant patent ductus arteriosus in preterm infants 500–1,750 g.** *Infant:* 3 IV doses at 12- to 24-hr intervals. 2–7 days old: 0.2 mg/kg IV for all three doses. Under 48 hr old: 0.2 mg/kg IV, then 0.1 mg/kg, then 0.1 mg/kg.

ADV EFF Anaphylactoid reactions to anaphylactic shock. aplastic anemia, apnea w/ IV use, bleeding ulcer, bone marrow suppression, dizziness, drowsiness, eye changes, headache, insomnia, n/v, **pulmonary hemorrhage w/ IV use**, rash

INTERACTIONS ACE inhibitors, adrenergic blockers, ARBs, bisphosphonates, lithium, loop diuretics, potassium-sparing diuretics

NC/PT Do not use SR form for gouty arthritic. Give w/ food. Monitor eyes w/ long-term therapy. Monitor LFTs, renal function. Pt should avoid OTC drugs without first checking w/ prescriber. Take safety precautions w/ CNS effects, report black or tarry stools, bleeding.

infliximab (Remicade)
CLASS Monoclonal antibody
PREG/CONT B/NA

BBW Risk of serious to life-threatening infections, activation of TB, malignancies, including fatal hepatosplenic T-cell lymphoma. Monitor pt; reserve for approved uses.

IND & DOSE Tx of Crohn's disease, ulcerative colitis, ankylosing spondylitis, psoriatic arthritis, plaque psoriasis. *Adult, child:* 5 mg IV at 0, 2, 6 wk; maint, 5 mg/kg IV q 8 wk (q 6 wk for ankylosing spondylitis). **Tx of rheumatoid arthritis.** *Adult:* 3 mg IV at 0, 2, 6 wk; maint, 3 mg/kg IV q 8 wk.

ADV EFF Abd pain, bone marrow suppression, cancer, demyelinating diseases, headache, hepatitis B reactivation, hepatotoxicity, HF, infusion reactions, **serious to fatal infections**

INTERACTIONS TNF blockers, tocilizumab, methotrexate, immunosuppressants

NC/PT Obtain TB test before starting tx. Monitor CBC before each dose; adjustment may be needed. Monitor LFTs. Assess for s&sx of infection. Pt should get routine cancer screening, report edema, chest pain, fever, signs of infection.

insoluble Prussian blue (Radiogardase)
CLASS Ferric hexacyanoferrate
PREG/CONT C/NA

IND & DOSE Tx of pts w/ known or suspected internal contamination w/ radioactive cesium and/or radioactive or nonradioactive thallium. *Adult:* 3 g PO tid. *Child 2–12 yr:* 1 g PO tid.

ADV EFF Constipation

NC/PT Monitor radioactivity levels. Take appropriate precautions to avoid exposure. Treat for constipation if indicated. Excreted in urine, feces; pt should flush toilet several times, clean up spilled urine, feces.

DANGEROUS DRUG

insulin, insulin lispro (Humalog), insulin aspart (Novolog), insulin detemir (Levemir), insulin glargine (Lantus), insulin glulisine (Apidra), isophane insulin

CLASS Hormone
PREG/CONT B; C (aspart, glargine, glulisine)/NA

IND & DOSE Tx of type 1 diabetes, severe ketoacidosis, diabetic coma; short-course tx when glucose control needed. *Adult, child:* 0.5–1 unit/kg/day subcut. Base adjustment on serum glucose levels, pt response. Can give regular and glulisine IV. **Tx of type 2 diabetes when glucose control cannot be maintained.** *Adult:* 10 mg/day subcut; range, 2–100 units/day *(Lantus)* or 0.1–0.2 units/kg subcut or 10 units/day or bid subcut *(Levemir).* See *Insulin pharmacokinetics.*
ADV EFF Anaphylaxis or angioedema, hypoglycemia, injection-site reactions, ketoacidosis, rash

INTERACTIONS Alcohol, atypical antipsychotics, beta blockers, celery, coriander, corticosteroids, dandelion root, diuretics, fenugreek, garlic, ginseng, juniper berries, MAOIs, salicylates
NC/PT Double-check doses for child. Use caution when mixing two types of insulin; always draw regular insulin into syringe first. If mixing w/ lispro, draw lispro first. Use mixtures of regular and NPH or regular and lente within 5–15 min of combining. Do not mix *Lantus* (glargine), *Levemir* (detemir) in sol w/ other drugs, including other insulins. Usage based on onset, peak, duration; varies among insulins. Do not freeze; protect from heat extremes. Monitor serum glucose frequently. Monitor, rotate injections sites. Ensure total diabetic teaching, including diet, exercise, hygiene measures, recognition of hypo-, hyperglycemia. Pt should avoid alcohol; if using herbs, check w/ prescriber for insulin dose adjustment; wear medical ID; always eat when using insulin; report uncontrolled serum glucose.

INSULIN PHARMACOKINETICS

Type	Onset	Peak	Duration
Regular	30–60 min	2–3 hr	6–12 hr
NPH	1–1.5 hr	4–12 hr	24 hr
Lente	1–2.5 hr	7–15 hr	24 hr
Ultralente	4–8 hr	10–30 hr	>36 hr
Lispro	<15 min	30–90 min	2–5 hr
Aspart	10–20 min	1–3 hr	3–5 hr
Detemir	Slow	3–6 hr	6–23 hr
Glargine	60 min	None	24 hr
Glulisine	2–5 min	30–90 min	1–2 hr
Combination insulins	30–60 min, then 1–2 hr	2–4 hr, then 6–12 hr	6–8 hr, then 18–24 hr

---

DANGEROUS DRUG

interferon alfa-2b
(Intron-A)
CLASS Antineoplastic
PREG/CONT C/NA

BBW Risk of serious to life-threatening reactions. Monitor for severe reactions (including hypersensitivity reactions), neuropsychiatric, autoimmune, ischemic, infectious disorders. Notify physician immediately if these occur; dose reduction/discontinuation may be needed.

IND & DOSE *Tx of hairy cell leukemia. Adult:* 2 million international units/m² subcut or IM three times/wk for up to 6 mo. *Tx of condylomata acuminata. Adult:* 1 million international units/lesion intralesionally three times/wk for 3 wk; can treat up to five lesions at one time. May repeat in 12–16 wk. *Tx of chronic hepatitis C. Adult:* 3 million international units subcut or IM three times/wk for 18–24 mo. *Tx of AIDS-related Kaposi sarcoma. Adult:* 30 million international units/m² subcut or IM three times/wk. *Tx of chronic hepatitis B. Adult:* 30–35 million international units/wk subcut or IM either as 5 million international units daily or 10 million international units three times/wk for 16 wk. *Child:* 3 million international units/m² subcut three times/wk for first wk, then 6 million international units/m² subcut three times/wk for total of 16–24 wk (max, 10 million international units three times/wk). *Tx of follicular lymphoma. Adult:* 5 million international units subcut three times/wk for 18 mo w/ other chemotherapy. *Tx of malignant melanoma. Adult:* 20 million international units/m² IV over 20 min on 5 consecutive days/wk for 4 wk; maint, 10 million international units/m² IV three times/wk for 48 wk.

ADV EFF Anorexia, **bone marrow suppression,** confusion, dizziness, flulike symptoms, n/v, rash

NC/PT Obtain baseline, periodic CBC, LFTs. Do not give IV. Pt should mark calendar of tx days, get blood tests regularly, take safety precautions w/ CNS effects, report bleeding, signs of infection.

DANGEROUS DRUG

interferon alfacon-1
(Infergen)
CLASS Immunomodulator
PREG/CONT C/NA

BBW Severe to life-threatening neuropsychiatric, autoimmune, ischemic, infectious disorders possible; monitor pt accordingly.

IND & DOSE *Tx of chronic hepatitis C in pts w/ compensated liver disease and anti–hepatitis C antibodies. Adult:* 9 mcg subcut three times/wk for 24 wk; at least 48 hr between doses. If used w/ ribavirin, 15 mcg daily as single subcut injection w/ weight-based ribavirin at 1,200 mg (75 kg and over), 1,000 mg (under 75 kg) PO in two divided doses for up to 48 wk.

ADJUST DOSE Hepatic, renal impairment

ADV EFF Abd pain, arthralgia, back/body pain, **bone marrow suppression,** fatigue, fever, flulike symptoms, **hepatic failure,** myalgia, nausea, **neuropsychiatric disorders,** neutropenia, ophthalmic disorders, **pancreatitis, peripheral neuropathy, pulmonary failure, renal failure,** rigor

INTERACTIONS Bone marrow suppressants

NC/PT Obtain baseline, periodic CBC, LFTs, renal function tests. Monitor for eye changes. Not for use in pregnancy (barrier contraceptives advised), breast-feeding. Give antiemetics if needed. Teach learn proper pt administration, disposal of needles, syringes. Pt should use precautions to prevent disease spread (drug not a cure), report personality changes, thoughts of suicide, signs of infection, unusual bleeding, difficulty breathing.

interferon beta-1a
(Avonex, Rebif)

CLASS Immunomodulator, MS drug
PREG/CONT C/NA

IND & DOSE Tx of relapsing forms of MS to slow accumulation of physical disability, decrease frequency of clinical exacerbations. *Adult:* 30 mcg IM once/wk *(Avonex).* Or, 22–44 mcg subcut three times per wk *(Rebif);* start w/ 8.8 mcg three times/wk; titrate up over 5 wk to full dose of 22–44 mcg.
ADV EFF Anorexia, **bone marrow suppression,** confusion, depression, dizziness, flulike symptoms, nausea, photosensitivity
NC/PT Obtain baseline, periodic CBC, LFTs. Rotate injection sites. Teach proper administration, disposal of needles, syringes. Maintain hydration. Pt should mark calendar of tx days; avoid exposure to infections, sun; report infection, unusual bleeding, thoughts of suicide.

interferon beta-1b
(Betaseron, Extavia)

CLASS Immunomodulator, MS drug
PREG/CONT C/NA

IND & DOSE Tx of relapsing forms of MS to slow accumulation of physical disability, decrease frequency of clinical exacerbations. *Adult:* 0.25 mg subcut q other day (target); discontinue if disease unremitting for more than 6 mo. Initially, 0.0625 mg subcut q other day, wks 1–2; then 0.125 mg subcut q other day, wks 3–4; then 0.1875 mg subcut q other day, wks 5–6; target 0.25 mg subcut q other day by wk 7.
ADV EFF Anorexia, **bone marrow suppression,** confusion, depression, dizziness, flulike symptoms, nausea, photosensitivity
NC/PT Obtain baseline, periodic CBC, LFTs. Rotate injection sites. Not

for use in pregnancy (barrier contraceptives advised). Maintain hydration. Teach proper administration, disposal of needles, syringes. Pt should mark calendar of tx day; avoid exposure to infection, sun; report infection, unusual bleeding, thoughts of suicide.

interferon gamma-1b
(Actimmune)

CLASS Immunomodulator
PREG/CONT C/NA

IND & DOSE To reduce frequency/severity of serious infections associated w/ chronic granulomatous disease; to delay time to disease progression in pts w/ severe, malignant osteopetrosis; tx of renal cell carcinoma. *Adult:* 50 mcg/m² (1 million international units/m²) subcut three times/wk in pts w/ body surface area (BSA) over 0.5 m²; 1.5 mcg/kg/dose in pts w/ BSA of 0.5 m² or less subcut three times/wk. For severe reactions, withhold or reduce dose by 50%.
ADV EFF Anorexia, confusion, depression, dizziness, flulike symptoms, nausea
NC/PT Obtain baseline, periodic CBC, LFTs. Store in refrigerator. Give at night if flulike symptoms a problem. Rotate injection sites. Teach proper administration, disposal of needles, syringes. Not for use in pregnancy (barrier contraceptives advised). Maintain hydration. Pt should mark calendar of tx day; avoid exposure to infection, sun; report infection, unusual bleeding, thoughts of suicide.

iodine thyroid products
(Iosat, Lugol's Solution, Pima, SSKI, Strong Iodine Solution, ThyroSafe, ThyroShield)

CLASS Thyroid suppressant
PREG/CONT D/NA

IND & DOSE Tx of hyperthyroidism in preparation for surgery; thyrotoxic

crisis: Adult, child over 1 yr: RDA, 150 mcg/day PO. Tx, 0.3 mL PO tid (*Strong Iodine Solution, Lugol's Solution*); range, 0.1–0.9 mL/day PO. **Thyroid blocking in radiation emergency.** Adult, child over 12 yr, 68 kg or more: 130 mg PO q 24 hr (*Iosat, ThyroSafe, ThyroShield*). Child 3–18 yr, under 68 kg: 65 mg/day PO. Child 1 mo–3 yr: 32.5 mg/day PO. Child birth–1 mo: 16.25 mg/day PO.
ADV EFF Iodism, rash, swelling of salivary glands
INTERACTIONS Lithium
NC/PT Dilute strong iodine sol w/ fruit juice/water to improve taste. Crush tablets for small child. Discontinue if iodine toxicity.

---

iodoquinol (Yodoxin)
CLASS Amebicide
PREG/CONT C/NA

IND & DOSE Tx of acute, chronic intestinal amebiasis. Adult: 650 mg PO tid after meals for 20 days. Child: 10–13.3 mg/kg/day PO in three divided doses for 20 days; max, 650 mg/dose (do not exceed 1.95 g in 24 hr for 20 days).
ADV EFF Blurred vision, n/v/d, rash
INTERACTIONS Lithium
NC/PT Give after meals. Maintain nutrition. Pt should report severe GI upset, unusual fatigue.

---

ipilimumab (Yervoy)
CLASS Cytotoxic T-cell antigen 4–blocking antibody
PREG/CONT C/NA

BBW Severe to fatal immune-mediated reactions involving many organs possible; may occur during tx or wks to mos after tx ends. Permanently stop drug, treat w/ high-dose systemic corticosteroids if s&sx of immune reactions appear.
IND & DOSE Tx of unresectable or metastatic melanoma. Adult: 3 mg/kg IV over 90 min q 3 wk; total, four doses.

ADV EFF Colitis, diarrhea, endocrinopathies, fatigue, hepatitis, pruritus, rash
NC/PT Establish baseline LFTs, thyroid/endocrine/GI function, skin condition; assess regularly for changes. Not for use in pregnancy, breast-feeding. Pt should mark calendar for tx days, report severe diarrhea, increased thirst, unusual fatigue.

---

ipratropium bromide (Atrovent)
CLASS Anticholinergic, bronchodilator
PREG/CONT B/NA

IND & DOSE Maint tx of bronchospasm associated w/ COPD (sol, aerosol), chronic bronchitis, emphysema. Adult, child 12 yr and older: 500 mcg tid–qid via nebulizer, w/ doses 6–8 hr apart. Symptomatic relief of rhinorrhea associated w/ common cold. Adult, child 12 yr and older: 2 sprays 0.06%/nostril tid–qid. Child 5–11 yr: 2 sprays 0.06%/nostril tid. Symptomatic relief of rhinitis. Adult, child 6 yr and older: 2 sprays 0.03%/nostril bid-tid. Relief of rhinorrhea in seasonal allergic rhinitis. Adult, child over 5 yr: 2 sprays 0.06%/nostril qid for 3 wk.
ADV EFF Cough, dizziness, dry mouth, headache, nervousness, nausea, urine retention
NC/PT Do not use w/ peanut, soy allergies. Protect sol from light. May mix in nebulizer w/ albuterol for up to 1 hr. Review proper use of nebulizer. Ensure hydration. Pt should empty bladder before using, take safety precautions w/ CNS effects, report vision changes, rash.

---

irbesartan (Avapro)
CLASS Antihypertensive, ARB
PREG/CONT D/NA

BBW Rule out pregnancy before beginning tx. Suggest barrier contraceptives during tx; fetal injury, deaths have occurred.

IND & DOSE Tx of hypertension. *Adult, child 13–16 yr:* 150 mg/day PO; max, 300 mg/day. *Child 6–12 yr:* 75 mg/day PO; max, 150 mg/day. **To slow progression of nephropathy in pts w/ hypertension, type 2 diabetes.** *Adult:* 300 mg/day PO.
ADJUST DOSE Volume or salt depletion
ADV EFF Abd pain, **angioedema**, cough, dizziness, fatigue, headache, n/v/d, URI
INTERACTIONS CYP2C9-metabolized drugs
NC/PT Use caution w/ surgery; volume expansion may be needed. Monitor closely when decreased BP secondary to fluid volume loss possible. May give w/ meals. Not for use in pregnancy (barrier contraceptives advised), breastfeeding. Pt should take safety precautions w/ CNS effects; report fever, chills.

---

irinotecan hydrochloride
(Camptosar)
CLASS Antineoplastic, DNA topoisomerase inhibitor
PREG/CONT D/NA

BBW Obtain CBC before each infusion. Do not give when baseline neutrophil count under 1,500 /mm². Severe bone marrow suppression possible; consult physician for dose reduction or withholding if bone marrow depression evident. Monitor for diarrhea; assess hydration. Arrange to reduce dose if 4–6 stools/day; omit dose if 7–9 stools/day. If 10 or more stools/day, consult physician. May prevent or ameliorate early diarrhea w/ atropine 0.25–1 mg IV or subcut. Treat late diarrhea lasting more than 24 hr w/ loperamide; late diarrhea can be severe to life-threatening.
IND & DOSE First-line tx w/ 5-FU, leucovorin tx w/ metastatic colon, rectal carcinomas. *Adult:* 125 mg/m² IV over 90 min days 1, 8, 15, 22 w/ leucovorin 20 mg/m² IV bolus days 1, 8, 15, 22 and 5-FU

500 mg/m² IV days 1, 8, 15, 22. Restart cycle on day 43. Or, 180 mg/m² IV over 90 min days 1, 15, 29 w/ leucovorin 200 mg/m² IV over 2 hr days 1, 2, 15, 16, 29, 30 and 5-FU 400 mg/m² as IV bolus days 1, 2, 15, 16, 29, 30 followed by 5-FU 600 mg/m² IV infusion over 22 hr on days 1, 2, 15, 16, 29, 30. Restart cycle on day 43. **Tx of pts w/ metastatic colon, rectal cancer whose disease has recurred or progressed after 5-FU therapy.** *Adult:* 125 mg/m² IV over 90 min once wkly for 4 wk, then 2-wk rest; repeat 6-wk regimen, or 350 mg/m² IV over 90 min once q 3 wk.
ADV EFF Alopecia, anorexia, **bone marrow suppression**, dizziness, dyspnea, fatigue, mucositis, n/v/d
INTERACTIONS Diuretics, ketoconazole, other antineoplastics, St. John's wort
NC/PT Monitor CBC; dose adjustment based on bone marrow response. Monitor IV site for extravasation. Not for use in pregnancy (barrier contraceptives advised). Pt should mark calendar for tx days, cover head at temp extremes (hair loss possible), avoid exposure to infections, report pain at injection site, signs of infection, severe/bloody diarrhea.

---

iron dextran (Dexferrum, INFeD)
CLASS Iron preparation
PREG/CONT C/NA

BBW Monitor for hypersensitivity reactions; test dose highly recommended. Have epinephrine on hand for severe hypersensitivity reaction.
IND & DOSE Tx of iron deficiency anemia only when PO route not possible. *Adult, child:* 0.5 mL IM or IV test dose before tx; base dose on hematologic response w/ frequent Hgb determinations. Over 25 kg: Dose (mL) = [0.0442 (desired Hgb−observed Hgb) × LBW] + (0.26 × LBW), where Hgb = Hgb in g/dL and LBW = lean body weight, IV or IM.

Child over 4 mo, 5–15 kg: Dose (mL) = 0.0442 (desired Hgb−observed Hgb) × W + (0.26 × W), where W = actual weight in kg, IV or IM. **Iron replacement for blood loss.** *Adult, child:* Replacement iron (in mg) = blood loss (in mL) × Hct.
ADV EFF Anaphylaxis, arthritic reactivation, **cardiac arrest**, discoloration/pain at injection site, local phlebitis, lymphadenopathy, n/v
INTERACTIONS Chloramphenicol
NC/PT Ensure actual iron deficiency. Perform test dose at least 5 min before tx. Inject IM only into upper outer quadrant of buttocks using Z-track technique. Monitor serum ferritin. Pt should avoid oral iron or vitamins w/ iron added, report pain at injection site, difficulty breathing.

iron sucrose (Venofer)
CLASS Iron preparation
PREG/CONT B/NA

IND & DOSE Tx of iron deficiency anemia in chronic kidney disease. *Adult:* On dialysis, 100 mg IV injection over 2–5 min or 100 mg diluted IV infusion over at least 15 min. Not on dialysis, 200 mg IV injection over 2–5 min. Peritoneal dialysis, 300 mg over 1.5 hr on two occasions 14 days apart, then single infusion of 400 mg over 2.5 hr.
ADV EFF Anaphylaxis, arthralgia, chest pain, dizziness, headache, **hypotension**, injection-site reactions, **iron overload**, muscle cramps, n/v/d
NC/PT Ensure actual iron deficiency. Pt should avoid oral iron or vitamins w/ iron added, take safety precautions w/ CNS effects, report pain at injection site, difficulty breathing.

isocarboxazid (Marplan)
CLASS MAOI
PREG/CONT C/NA

BBW Increased risk of suicidality in children, adolescents, young adults; monitor accordingly.

IND & DOSE Tx of depression (not a first choice). *Adult:* Up to 40 mg/day PO.
ADJUST DOSE Hepatic, severe renal impairment
ADV EFF Constipation, **CV events**, drowsiness, dry mouth
INTERACTIONS Anesthetics, antihypertensives, buspirone, caffeine, CNS depressants, dextromethorphan, meperidine, SSRIs, sympathomimetics, TCAs, tyramine-containing foods
NC/PT Do not use w/ known cerebrovascular disorders, pheochromocytoma. Check complete drug list before giving; many interactions. Pt should avoid foods high in tyramine, use sugarless lozenges for dry mouth, report thoughts of suicide.

isoniazid (Nydrazid)
CLASS Antituberculotic
PREG/CONT C/NA

BBW Risk of serious to fatal hepatitis; monitor liver enzymes monthly.
IND & DOSE Tx of active TB. *Adult:* 5 mg/kg/day (max, 300 mg) PO or IM in single dose w/ other effective drugs. Or, 15 mg/kg (max, 900 mg) PO or IM two or three times/wk. *Child:* 10–15 mg/kg/day (max, 300 mg) PO or IM in single dose w/ other effective drugs. Or, 20–40 mg/kg (max, 900 mg/day) two or three times/wk. **Px for TB.** *Adult:* 300 mg/day PO in single dose. *Child:* 10 mg/kg/day (max, 300 mg) PO in single dose.
ADV EFF Epigastric distress, fever, gynecomastia, **hepatitis**, injection-site reactions, peripheral neuropathy, **thrombocytopenia**
INTERACTIONS Acetaminophen, alcohol, carbamazepine, enflurane, phenytoin, rifampin, tyramine-containing foods
NC/PT Concomitant administration of 10–50 mg/day pyridoxine recommended for pts who are malnourished or predisposed to neuropathy (alcoholics, diabetics). Pt should take on empty stomach; avoid alcohol, foods high in

tyramine; get regular medical checkups; take safety precautions to avoid injury (loss of sensation possible).

---

isoproterenol hydrochloride (Isuprel)

CLASS Antiasthmatic, beta agonist, bronchodilator, vasopressor

PREG/CONT C/NA

IND & DOSE Mgt of bronchospasm during anesthesia. *Adult:* 0.01–0.02 mg (0.5–1 mL diluted sol) by IV bolus; repeat when needed. *Child 7–19 yr:* 0.05–0.1 mcg/kg/min by IV bolus. Max, 1.3–2.7 mcg/kg/min. Vasopressor as adjunct tx of shock. *Adult:* 0.5–5 mcg/min; infuse IV at adjusted rate based on hr, CVP, systemic BP, urine flow. Tx of cardiac standstill, arrhythmias. *Adult:* 0.02–0.06 mg IV injection using diluted sol. Or, 5 mcg/min IV infusion using diluted sol.

ADJUST DOSE Elderly pts

ADV EFF Anxiety, apprehension, bronchospasm, cardiac arrhythmias, cough, dyspnea, fear, pallor, palpitations, **pulmonary edema**, respiratory difficulties, sweating

INTERACTIONS Antiarrhythmics, ergots, halogenated hydrocarbon anesthetics, oxytocics, TCAs

NC/PT Protect from light. Give smallest dose for minimum period. Have beta blocker on hand to reverse effects. Pt should report chest pain, tremor.

---

isosorbide dinitrate (Dilatrate SR, Isochron, Isordil Titradose), isosorbide mononitrate (Imdur, ISMO, Monoket)

CLASS Antianginal, nitrate

PREG/CONT C; B (*Imdur, Monoket*)/NA

IND & DOSE Tx of angina (dinitrate). *Adult:* 2.5–5 mg sublingual or

5- to 20-mg oral tablets; maint, 10–40 mg PO q 6 hr or tid (oral tablets/capsules). SR or ER: Initially, 40 mg, then 40–80 mg PO q 8–12 hr. Px of angina (mononitrate). *Adult:* 20 mg PO bid 7 hr apart. ER tablets: 30–60 mg/day PO; may increase to 120 mg/day. Acute px of angina (dinitrate). *Adult:* 2.5–5 mg sublingual q 2–3 hr. Give 15 min before activity that may cause angina.

ADV EFF Apprehension, collapse, dizziness, headache, hypotension, orthostatic hypotension, rebound hypertension, restlessness, tachycardia, weakness

INTERACTIONS Ergots

NC/PT Reduce dose gradually when stopping. Headache possible. Pt should place sublingual form under tongue or in buccal pouch, try not to swallow; take orally on empty stomach; take safety precautions w/ CNS effects, orthostatic hypotension; report blurred vision, severe headache, more frequent anginal attacks. Name confusion Isordil (isosorbide) and Plendil (felodipine); use caution.

---

isotretinoin (Amnesteem, Claravis, Sotret)

CLASS Acne product, retinoid

PREG/CONT X/NA

BBW Ensure pt reads, signs consent form; place form in pt's permanent record. Rule out pregnancy before tx; test for pregnancy within 2 wk of starting tx. Advise use of two forms of contraception starting 1 mo before tx until 1 mo after tx ends. Pharmacists must register pts in iPLEDGE program before dispensing drug. Pt may obtain no more than 30-day supply.

IND & DOSE Tx of severe recalcitrant nodular acne unresponsive to conventional tx. *Adult, child 12 yr and older:* 0.5–1 mg/kg/day PO; range, 0.5–2 mg/kg/day divided into two doses for 15–20 wk. Max daily dose, 2 mg/kg. If second course needed, allow rest period of at least 8 wk between courses.

ADV EFF Abd pain, bronchospasm, cheilitis, conjunctivitis, dizziness, dry nose/skin, epistaxis, eye irritation, fatigue, headache, hematuria, insomnia, lethargy, lipid changes, n/v, papilledema, skin irritation, **suicidality**, visual changes

INTERACTIONS Corticosteroids, phenytoin, tetracycline, vitamin A
NC/PT Ensure pt has read, signed consent form. Rule out pregnancy; ensure pt using contraception. Allow 8 wk between tx cycles. Only 1 mo prescription can be given. Pt may be unable to wear contact lenses. Give w/ food to improve absorption. Pt should swallow capsules whole and not cut, crush, or chew them; avoid donating blood; avoid vitamin supplements; take safety precautions w/ CNS effects; report visual changes, thoughts of suicide.

isradipine (DynaCirc CR)
CLASS Antihypertensive, calcium channel blocker
PREG/CONT C/NA

IND & DOSE Mgt of hypertension. *Adult:* 2.5 mg PO bid; max, 20 mg/day. CR, 5–10 mg/day PO.

ADJUST DOSE Elderly pts; hepatic, renal impairment

ADV EFF Dizziness, edema, headache, hypotension, nausea

INTERACTIONS Antifungals, atracurium, beta blockers, calcium, carbamazepine, digoxin, fentanyl, H₂ antagonists, pancuronium, prazosin, quinidine, rifampin, tubocurarine, vecuronium

NC/PT Monitor BP; other antihypertensives may be added as needed. Monitor BP, cardiac rhythm closely when determining dose. Pt should swallow CR tablet whole and not cut, crush, or chew it; take safety precautions w/ CNS effects; treat for headache; report swelling, palpitations.

itraconazole (Sporanox)
CLASS Antifungal
PREG/CONT C/NA

BBW Risk of severe HF; do not give if evidence of cardiac dysfunction, HF. Potential for serious CV events (including ventricular tachycardia, death) w/ lovastatin, simvastatin, triazolam, midazolam, pimozide, dofetilide, quinidine due to significant CYP450 inhibition; avoid these combinations.

IND & DOSE Tx of empiric febrile neutropenia. *Adult:* 200 mg PO bid until clinically significant neutropenia resolves. Tx of candidiasis. *Adult:* 200 mg/day PO (oral sol only) for 1–2 wk (oropharyngeal); 100 mg/day PO for at least 3 wk (esophageal); 200 mg/day PO in AIDS/neutropenic pts. Tx of blastomycosis, chronic histoplasmosis. *Adult:* 200 mg/day PO for at least 3 mo; max, 400 mg/day. Tx of systemic mycoses. *Adult:* 100–200 mg/day PO for 3–6 mo. Tx of dermatophytoses. *Adult:* 100–200 mg/day PO to bid for 7–28 days. Tx of fingernail onychomycosis. *Adult:* 200 mg bid PO for 1 wk, then 3-wk rest period; repeat. Tx of toenail onychomycosis. *Adult:* 200 mg/day PO for 12 wk. Tx of aspergillosis. *Adult:* 200–400 mg/day PO.

ADJUST DOSE Renal impairment
ADV EFF Abd pain, edema, headache, **HF, hepatotoxicity**, n/v/d, rash
INTERACTIONS Antacids, benzodiazepines, buspirone, carbamazepine, colas, cyclosporine, digoxin, grapefruit juice, histamine₂ antagonists, isoniazid, lovastatin, macrolide antibiotics, nevirapine, oral hypoglycemics, phenobarbital, phenytoin, protease inhibitors, proton pump inhibitors, rifampin, warfarin anticoagulants

NC/PT Culture before tx. Monitor LFTs; stop if s&sx of active liver disease. Check all drugs being used; many interactions possible. Not for use in pregnancy (contraceptives advised). Give capsules w/ food. For oral sol, give 100–200 mg (10–20 mL), have pt rinse and hold, then swallow sol daily for 1–3 wk. Pt should avoid grapefruit juice, colas; report difficulty breathing, stool/urine changes.

ivacaftor (Kalydeco)
CLASS Cystic fibrosis transmembrane conductance regulator potentiator
PREG/CONT B/NA

IND & DOSE Tx of cystic fibrosis (CF) in pts 6 yr and older w/ G551D mutation of CF gene. *Adult, child 6 yr and older:* 150 mg PO q 12 hr w/ fat-containing food.
ADJUST DOSE Moderate to severe hepatic impairment
ADV EFF Abd pain, congestion, dizziness, headache, hepatic impairment, nasopharyngitis, n/v, rash, URI
INTERACTIONS Grapefruit juice, moderate to strong CYP3A inhibitors, St. John's wort
NC/PT Monitor LFTs before and q 3 mo during first yr, then yearly. Give w/ fat-containing food; use safety precautions if dizziness occurs. Pt should take q 12 hr w/ fat-containing food; use caution w/ dizziness; avoid grapefruit juice, St. John's wort; report yellowing of eyes or skin, urine/stool color changes.

ivermectin (Stromectol)
CLASS Anthelmintic
PREG/CONT C/NA

IND & DOSE Tx of intestinal strongyloidiasis. *Adult:* 200 mcg/kg PO as single dose. Tx of onchocerciasis. *Adult:* 150 mcg/kg PO as single dose; may repeat in 3–12 mo.
ADV EFF Abd pain, dizziness, nausea, rash
NC/PT Culture before tx. Not for use in breast-feeding. Pt should take on empty stomach w/ water; will need repeat stool cultures; may need repeat tx.

ixabepilone (Ixempra)
CLASS Antineoplastic, microtubular inhibitor
PREG/CONT D/NA

BBW Risk of severe liver failure, severe bone marrow suppression, neurotoxicities, cardiotoxicities; select pt carefully, monitor closely.
IND & DOSE Tx of metastatic or locally advanced breast cancer in pts who have failed on anthracycline, taxane. *Adult:* 40 mg/m² IV over 3 hr q 3 wk; may combine w/ capecitabine.
ADV EFF Alopecia, anorexia, asthenia, bone marrow suppression, fatigue, n/v/d, peripheral neuropathy, severe hypersensitivity reactions, stomatitis
INTERACTIONS CYP3A4 inducers/inhibitors
NC/PT Follow CBC, LFTs closely. Premedicate w/ corticosteroids. Not for use in pregnancy (barrier contraceptives advised). Pt should mark calendar for tx days; cover head at temp extremes (hair loss possible); avoid exposure to infections; perform mouth care (for stomatitis); take safety precautions (for neuropathies); report chest pain, palpitations, difficulty breathing, numbness/tingling.

DANGEROUS DRUG

ketamine (Ketalar)
CLASS Nonbarbiturate anesthetic
PREG/CONT B/C-III

BBW Emergence reaction (confusion, hallucinations, delirium) possible; lessened with smallest effective dose and use of tactile, verbal, or visual stimuli. Severe cases require small dose of short-acting barbiturate.
IND & DOSE Induction of anesthesia. *Adult:* 1–4.5 mg/kg IV slowly or

1–2 mg/kg IV at 0.5 mg/kg/min, or 6.5–13 mg/kg IM (10 mg/kg IM produces 12–25 min anesthesia). **Induction of anesthesia in cardiac surgery.** *Adult:* 0.5–1.5 mg/kg IV at 20 mg q 10 sec. **Maintenance of general anesthesia.** *Adult:* Repeat dose in increments of ½ to full induction dose.

ADV EFF Anorexia, confusion, diplopia, dreamlike state, emergence reaction, hallucinations, hypertension, nausea, pain at injection site, vomiting
INTERACTIONS Halothane, NMJ blockers, other sedative/hypnotics, thyroid hormones
NC/PT Administered by anesthesia specialist. Ensure oxygen, oximetry, cardiac monitoring; have emergency equipment nearby. Warn pt about sedative effect: Pt should avoid driving after receiving drug, tasks requiring mental alertness/coordination, making important decisions. Pt should report difficulty breathing, pain at injection site, changes in thinking.

ketoconazole (Extina, Nizoral A-D, Xolegel)
CLASS Antifungal
PREG/CONT C/NA

BBW Risk of serious to fatal hepatotoxicity; monitor closely.

IND & DOSE Tx of susceptible, systemic fungal infections; recalcitrant dermatophytosis. *Adult:* 200 mg PO daily; for severe infections, 400 mg/day PO for 1 wk–6 mo. *Child over 2 yr:* 3.3–6.6 mg/kg PO as single dose. **To reduce scaling due to dandruff.** *Adult, child:* Moisten hair, scalp thoroughly w/ water; apply sufficient shampoo to produce lather; leave on for 5 min. Shampoo twice/wk for 4 wk with at least 3 days between shampooing. **Topical tx of tinea pedis, corporis, cruris; cutaneous candidiasis.** *Adult, child over 12 yr:* Apply thin film of gel, foam, cream once daily to affected area for 2 wk; do not

wash area for 3 hr after applying. Wait 20 min before applying makeup, sunscreen. May need 6 wk of tx. **Tx of seborrheic dermatitis.** *Adult, child over 12 yr:* Apply foam bid for 4 wk.
ADV EFF Anaphylaxis, dizziness, hepatotoxicity, local stinging on application, n/v, pruritus
INTERACTIONS Antacids, corticosteroids, cyclosporine, histamine₂ blockers, proton pump inhibitors, rifampin, tacrolimus, warfarin
NC/PT Culture before tx. Have epinephrine on hand for anaphylaxis. Monitor LFTs closely. Review proper administration. Pt may need long-term tx. Pt should use proper hygiene to prevent infection spread, avoid drugs that alter stomach acid level (if needed, pt should take ketoconazole at least 2 hr after these drugs), take safety precautions w/ CNS effects, report stool/urine changes, unusual bleeding.

ketoprofen (generic)
CLASS NSAID
PREG/CONT C (1st, 2nd trimesters); D (3rd trimester)/NA

BBW Increased risk of CV events, GI bleeding; monitor accordingly. Contraindicated for tx of perioperative pain after CABG surgery; serious adverse effects have occurred.

IND & DOSE Relief of pain from rheumatoid arthritis, osteoarthritis. *Adult:* 75 mg PO tid or 50 mg PO qid. Maint. 150–300 mg PO in three or four divided doses; max, 300 mg/day. ER form, 200 mg/day PO; or max, 200 mg/day ER. **Tx of mild to moderate pain, primary dysmenorrhea:** *Adult:* 25–50 mg PO q 6–8 hr as needed.
ADJUST DOSE Elderly pts; hepatic, renal impairment
ADV EFF Anaphylaxis, dizziness, dyspepsia, edema, **gastric/duodenal ulcer,** GI pain, headache, insomnia, nausea, **renal impairment**

INTERACTIONS Aminoglycosides, aspirin, cyclosporine, diuretics, warfarin
NC/PT Monitor renal function. Give w/ food. Not for use in pregnancy. Pt should avoid OTC products that might contain NSAIDs, report swelling, difficulty breathing, black tarry stools.

ketorolac tromethamine (Acular LS, Acuvail, Sprix)
CLASS Antipyretic, NSAID
PREG/CONT C (1st, 2nd trimesters); D (3rd trimester)/NA

BBW Increased risk of CV events, GI bleeding; monitor accordingly. Do not use during labor/delivery or in breastfeeding; serious adverse effects in fetus/baby possible. May increase risk of bleeding; do not use w/ high risk of bleeding or as px before surgery. Increased risk of severe hypersensitivity with known hypersensitivity to aspirin, NSAIDs.
IND & DOSE Short-term pain mgt (up to 5 days). *Adult:* 60 mg IM or 30 mg IV as single dose, or 30 mg IM or IV q 6 hr to max 120 mg/day. Or, 1 spray in one nostril q 6–8 hr; max, 63 mg/day (over 65 yr); 1 spray (15.75 mg) in each nostril q 6–8 hr; max, 126 mg/day (under 65 yr). *Transfer to oral:* 20 mg PO as first dose for pts who received 60 mg IM or 30 mg IV as single dose or 30-mg multiple dose, then 10 mg PO q 4–6 hr; max, 40 mg/24 hr. *Child 2–16 yr:* 1 mg/kg IM to max 30 mg, or 0.5 mg/kg IV to max 15 mg as single dose. **Relief of itching of allergic conjunctivitis.** *Adult:* 1 drop in affected eye(s) qid. **Relief of cataract postop pain, inflammation.** *Adult:* Dose varies by product; check manufacturer info.
ADJUST DOSE Elderly pts, renal impairment, weight under 50 kg
ADV EFF Anaphylaxis, dizziness, dyspepsia, edema, **gastric/duodenal ulcer,** GI pain, headache, insomnia, nausea, **renal impairment**
INTERACTIONS Aminoglycosides, aspirin, cyclosporine, diuretics, NSAIDs, warfarin

NC/PT Protect vials from light. Monitor renal function. Give to maintain serum levels, control pain. Not for use in pregnancy. Do not use ophthalmic drops w/ contact lenses. Pt should take w/ food, use safety precautions w/ CNS effects, avoid OTC products that might contain NSAIDs, report swelling, difficulty breathing, black tarry stools.

DANGEROUS DRUG

labetalol hydrochloride (Trandate)
CLASS Antihypertensive, sympathetic blocker
PREG/CONT C/NA

IND & DOSE Tx of hypertension. *Adult:* 100 mg PO bid; maint, 200–400 mg bid PO; up to 2,400 mg/day has been used. **Tx of severe hypertension.** *Adult:* 20 mg (0.25 mg/kg) IV injection slowly over 2 min; can give additional doses of 40 or 80 mg at 10-min intervals until desired BP achieved or 300-mg dose has been injected. Transfer to oral therapy as soon as possible.
ADJUST DOSE Elderly pts
ADV EFF Bronchospasm, constipation, cough, dizziness, dyspnea, ED, flatulence, gastric pain, **HF,** n/v/d, **stroke,** vertigo
INTERACTIONS Calcium channel blockers, enflurane, isoflurane, nitroglycerin
NC/PT Taper after long-term tx. Keep pt supine during infusion. Pt should not stop taking suddenly, take w/ meals, use safety precautions w/ CNS effects, report difficulty breathing, swelling.

lacosamide (Vimpat)
CLASS Antiepileptic
PREG/CONT C/NA

BBW Increased risk of suicidal ideation in children, adolescents, young adults; monitor accordingly.

IND & DOSE Adjunct tx for partial-onset seizures. *Adult, child 17 yr and older:* 50 mg PO bid; range, 200–400 mg/day PO. IV dosing is same as oral; for short-term use if oral not possible.
ADJUST DOSE Hepatic, renal impairment
ADV EFF Ataxia, prolonged PR interval, diplopia, dizziness, n/v
INTERACTIONS Other PR-prolonging drugs
NC/PT Taper after long-term tx. Not for use in pregnancy (barrier contraceptives advised), breast-feeding. Pt should not stop taking suddenly, take safety precautions w/ CNS effects, report thoughts of suicide, personality changes.

lactulose (Cephulac, Chronulac, Constilac, Enulose)
CLASS Ammonia-reducing drug, laxative
PREG/CONT B/NA

IND & DOSE Tx of portal-systemic encephalopathy. 30–45 mL (20–30 g) PO tid or qid. Adjust q 1–2 days to produce two or three soft stools/day. May use 30–45 mL/hr PO if needed. Or, 300 mL (20 g) lactulose mixed w/ 700 mL water or physiologic saline as retention enema retained for 30–60 min; may repeat q 4–6 hr. *Child:* 2.5–10 mL/day PO in divided dose for small child or 40–90 mL/day for older child suggested. Goal: Two or three soft stools daily. **Laxative.** *Adult:* 15–30 mL/day (10–20 g) PO; up to 60 mL/day has been used.
ADV EFF Belching, distention, intestinal cramping, transient flatulence
NC/PT Give laxative syrup orally w/ fruit juice, water, milk to increase palatability. Monitor serum ammonia levels. Monitor for electrolyte imbalance w/ long-term tx. Pt should not use other laxatives, not use as laxative for longer than 1 wk unless pre-

scribed, have ready access to bathroom facilities, report diarrhea.

lamivudine (Epivir, Epivir-HBV)
CLASS Antiviral, reverse transcriptase inhibitor
PREG/CONT C/NA

BBW Monitor hematologic indices, LFTs q 2 wk during tx; severe hepatomegaly w/ steatosis, lactic acidosis possible. Counsel, periodically test pts receiving *Epivir-HBV*; severe, acute hepatitis B virus (HBV) exacerbations have occurred in pts w/ both HIV and HBV infection who stop taking lamivudine.
IND & DOSE Tx of chronic hepatitis B. *Adult:* 100 mg PO daily. *Child 2–17 yr:* 3 mg/kg PO daily; max, 100 mg daily. Tx of HIV w/ other drugs. *Adult, child 16 yr and older:* 150 mg PO bid or 300 mg/day PO as single dose. *Child 3 mo–16 yr:* 4 mg/kg PO bid; max, 150 mg bid. *Over 30 kg:* 150 mg PO bid. *Over 21 kg but under 30 kg:* 75 mg PO in am and 150 mg PO in pm. *14–21 kg:* 75 mg PO bid.
ADJUST DOSE Renal impairment
ADV EFF Agranulocytosis, asthenia, diarrhea, GI pain, headache, **hepatomegaly w/ lactic acidosis**, nasal s&sx, nausea, **pancreatitis, steatosis**
INTERACTIONS Trimethoprim-sulfamethoxazole, zalcitabine
NC/PT Give w/ other antiretrovirals for HIV. Monitor for s&sx of pancreatitis; stop immediately if evident. Monitor for opportunistic infections. Not for use in pregnancy. Pt should use protection to prevent transmission (drug not a cure), get frequent blood tests, report severe headache, severe n/v.

lamotrigine (Lamictal)
CLASS Antiepileptic
PREG/CONT C/NA

BBW Risk of serious, life-threatening rash; monitor accordingly. Stop immediately if rash appears; have appropriate life support on hand.

IND & DOSE Tx of partial-onset seizures, primary generalized tonic-clonic seizures, Lennox-Gastaut syndrome. *Adult taking enzyme-inducing antiepileptics (ie, carbamazepine, phenobarbital, phenytoin) but not valproic acid:* 50 mg PO daily for 2 wk, then 100 mg PO daily in two divided doses for 2 wk. Then may increase by 100 mg/day q wk to maint of 300–500 mg/day PO in two divided doses. ER form: wk 1–2, 50 mg/day PO; wk 3–4, 100 mg/day PO; wk 5, 200 mg/day PO; wk 6, 300 mg/day PO; wk 7, 400 mg/day PO. Range, 400–600 mg/day. *Adult, child over 12 yr taking enzyme-inducing antiepileptics and valproic acid:* 25 mg PO q other day for 2 wk, then 25 mg daily for 2 wk. Then may increase by 25–50 mg q 1–2 wk to maint 100–400 mg/day PO in two divided doses. *Child 2–12 yr taking non-enzyme-inducing antiepileptics and valproic acid:* 0.15 mg/kg/day PO in one to two divided doses for 2 wk. Then 0.3 mg/kg/day PO in one to two divided doses, rounded down to nearest 5 mg for 2 wk. Maint, 1–5 mg/kg/day in one to two divided doses to max of 200 mg/day. *Child 2–12 yr taking single enzyme-inducing antiepileptic without valproic acid:* 0.6 mg/kg/day PO in two divided doses for 2 wk, then 1.2 mg/kg/day PO in two divided doses for 2 wk. Maint, 5–15 mg/kg/day in two divided doses to max 400 mg/day. **Tx of bipolar I disorder.** *Adult taking valproic acid:* 25 mg PO q other day for 2 wk, then 25 mg PO once daily for 2 wk. After 4 wk, may double dose at wkly intervals to target 100 mg/day. *Adult taking enzyme-inducing antiepileptics but not valproic acid:* 50 mg/day PO for 2 wk; then 100 mg PO daily in two divided doses for 2 wk. After 4 wk, may increase dose in 100-mg increments at wkly intervals to target maint of 400 mg/day PO in two divided doses. *Adult taking neither enzyme-inducing antiepileptics nor valproic*

acid: 25 mg/day PO for 2 wk, then 50 mg PO daily for 2 wk. After 4 wk, may double dose at wkly intervals to maint of 200 mg/day.

ADV EFF Aseptic meningitis, ataxia, dizziness, **hepatotoxicity**, nausea, **rash, Stevens-Johnson syndrome, toxic epidermal necrosis w/ multiorgan failure**

INTERACTIONS Carbamazepine, phenobarbital, phenytoin, primidone, valproic acid

NC/PT Monitor LFTs, renal function closely. Monitor for aseptic meningitis. Monitor for rash; stop if rash evident. Taper slowly over 2 wk when stopping. Ensure pt swallows ER tablets whole and does not cut, crush, or chew them. Pt should wear medical ID, take safety precautions w/ CNS effects, report rash, stool/urine changes. Name confusion between Lamictal (lamotrigine) and Lamisil (terbinafine); use caution.

---

lanreotide acetate
(Somatuline Depot)
CLASS Growth hormone (GH) inhibitor
PREG/CONT C/NA

IND & DOSE Long-term tx of acromegaly in pts unresponsive to other tx. *Adult:* 60–120 mcg subcut q 4 wk for 3 mo.

ADJUST DOSE Hepatic, renal impairment

ADV EFF Abd pain, cholelithiasis, diarrhea, flatulence, hyperglycemia, hypoglycemia, injection-site reactions, sinus bradycardia, thyroid dysfx

INTERACTIONS Antidiabetics, beta blockers, cyclosporine, insulin

NC/PT Drug injected into buttocks, alternating left and right; monitor for injection-site reactions. Monitor GH, insulin growth factor-1. Monitor serum glucose, thyroid function; intervene as indicated. Monitor for bradycardia. Monitor for use in breast-feeding. Pt should mark calendar of tx days, keep frequent follow-up appointments.

lansoprazole (Prevacid, Prevacid 24 hr)
CLASS Proton pump inhibitor
PREG/CONT B/NA

IND & DOSE Tx of active duodenal ulcer. *Adult:* 15 mg PO daily for 4 wk; maint, 15 mg/day PO. Tx of gastric ulcer. *Adult:* 30 mg/day PO for up to 8 wk. To reduce risk of gastric ulcer w/ NSAIDs. *Adult:* 15 mg/day PO for up to 12 wk. Tx of duodenal ulcers associated w/ *Helicobacter pylori*. *Adult:* 30 mg lansoprazole, 500 mg clarithromycin, 1 g amoxicillin, all PO bid for 10–14 days; or 30 mg lansoprazole, 1 g amoxicillin PO tid for 14 days. GERD. *Adult, child 12–17 yr:* 15 mg/day PO for up to 8 wk. *Child 1–11 yr:* Over 30 kg, 30 mg/day PO for up to 12 wk. 30 kg or less, 15 mg/day PO for up to 12 wk. Tx of erosive esophagitis, poorly responsive GERD. *Adult, child 12–17 yr:* 30 mg/day PO daily for up to 8 wk. Additional 8-wk course may be helpful for pts not healed after 8-wk tx. Maint, 15 mg/day PO. Tx of pathological hypersecretory conditions. *Adult:* 60 mg/day PO; up to 90 mg bid have been used. Short-term tx of erosive esophagitis (all grades). *Adult:* 30 mg/day IV over 30 min for up to 7 days; switch to oral form as soon as possible for total of 8 wk. Tx of heartburn. *Adult:* 1 capsule *Prevacid 24 hr* PO w/ full glass of water in a.m. before eating for 14 days; may repeat 14-day course q 4 mo.
ADJUST DOSE Hepatic impairment
ADV EFF Abd pain, bone loss, dizziness, headache, n/v/d, rash, URI
INTERACTIONS Ketoconazole, sucralfate, theophylline
NC/PT Give w/ meals. May open capsule, sprinkle on applesauce, *Ensure*, yogurt, cottage cheese, strained pears. For NG tube, place 15- or 30-mg tablet in syringe, draw up 4 or

10 mL water; shake gently for quick dispersal. After dispersal, inject through NG tube into stomach within 15 min. If using capsules w/ NG tube, mix granules from capsule w/ 40 mL apple juice, inject through tube, then flush tube w/ more apple juice. For orally disintegrating tablet, place on tongue, follow w/ water after it dissolves. For IV, switch to oral form for further evaluation if no symptom improvement. Arrange for further evaluation if no symptom improvement. Pt should swallow capsule whole and not cut, crush, or chew it; take safety precautions w/ CNS effects; report severe diarrhea.

lanthanum carbonate (Fosrenol)
CLASS Phosphate binder
PREG/CONT C/NA

IND & DOSE To reduce serum phosphate level in pts w/ end-stage renal disease. *Adult:* 1,500–3,000 mg/day PO w/ meals; base dose on serum phosphate level.
ADJUST DOSE Hepatic impairment
ADV EFF Allergic skin reactions, dyspepsia, GI obstruction, n/v/d, tooth injury
INTERACTIONS Antacids, levothyroxine, quinolone antibiotics
NC/PT Monitor serum phosphate level (target, 6 mg/dL or lower). Pt should chew or crush tablets, not swallow whole; take w/ meals; separate from other oral drugs by 2 hr; report severe abd pain, constipation.

DANGEROUS DRUG
lapatinib (Tykerb)
CLASS Antineoplastic, kinase inhibitor
PREG/CONT D/NA

BBW Severe to fatal hepatotoxicity has occurred; monitor LFTs closely.
IND & DOSE Tx of advanced/metastatic breast cancer w/ tumors that overexpress HER2 in women who

have received other tx. *Adult:* 1,250 mg/day PO on days 1–21 w/ capecitabine 2,000 mg/m²/day PO on days 1–14, given 12 hr apart. Repeat 21-day cycle. **Tx of HER2-positive metastatic breast cancer.** *Adult:* 1,500 mg/day PO w/ letrozole 2.5 mg/day PO.

ADJUST DOSE Cardiotoxicities, concomitant CYP3A4 inducers/inhibitors, hepatic impairment

ADV EFF Anaphylaxis, decreased left ventricular function, diarrhea, fatigue, **hepatotoxicity, interstitial pneumonitis**, n/v, **prolonged QT interval**

INTERACTIONS Antacids, carbamazepine, digoxin, grapefruit juice, ketoconazole, midazolam, paclitaxel, QT-prolonging drugs, St. John's wort

NC/PT Monitor LFTs before and regularly during tx. Monitor cardiac/respiratory function; evaluate lungs for pneumonitis. Not for use in pregnancy (contraceptives advised). Pt should take 1 hr before or after meals; avoid grapefruit juice, St. John's wort, antacids; report difficulty breathing, swelling, dizziness, color change of urine/stool.

laronidase (Aldurazyme)
CLASS Enzyme
PREG/CONT C/NA

BBW Life-threatening anaphylaxis has occurred; have medical support on hand.

IND & DOSE Tx of pts w/ Hurler, Hurler-Scheie forms of mucopolysaccharidosis 1; Scheie forms w/ moderate to severe symptoms. *Adult, child 6 yr and older:* 0.58 mg/kg IV infused over 3–4 hr once/wk.

ADV EFF Anaphylaxis, fever, hyperreflexia, hypertension, injection- site reactions, paresthesia, tachycardia, UTI

NC/PT Pretreat w/ antipyretics, antihistamines; monitor continually during infusion. Have emergency equipment on hand. Pt should mark

calendar of tx days; report injection-site pain/swelling, difficulty breathing.

leflunomide (Arava)
CLASS Antiarthritic, pyrimidine, synthesis inhibitor
PREG/CONT X/NA

BBW Advise women of childbearing age of risks of pregnancy; provide counseling for appropriate contraceptive use during tx. If pt decides to become pregnant, withdrawal program to rid body of leflunomide recommended. May use cholestyramine to rapidly decrease serum level if unplanned pregnancy suspected. Risk of severe liver injury; monitor LFTs before, periodically during tx. Not recommended w/ preexisting liver disease or liver enzymes over two times upper limit of normal (ULN). Use caution w/ other drugs that cause liver injury; start cholestyramine washout if ALT increases to three times ULN.

IND & DOSE Tx of active rheumatoid arthritis (RA); to relieve s&sx, improve functioning. *Adult:* Loading dose, 100 mg/day PO for 3 days; maint, 20 mg/day PO. May reduce to 10 mg/day PO.

ADJUST DOSE Hepatic impairment
ADV EFF Alopecia, drowsiness, diarrhea, erythematous rashes, headache, **hepatotoxicity**

INTERACTIONS Charcoal, cholestyramine, hepatotoxic drugs, rifampin

NC/PT Monitor LFTs. If ALT rise between two and three times ULN, monitor closely if continued tx desired. If ALT three times or more ULN, cholestyramine may decrease absorption; consider stopping. Not for use in pregnancy (barrier contraceptives advised). Pt should continue other RA tx, get regular medical follow-up, cover head at temp extremes (hair loss possible), take safety precautions w/ CNS effects.

lenalidomide (Revlimid)

CLASS Antianemic, immunomodulator
PREG/CONT X/NA

BBW Thalidomide derivative associated w/ birth defects; rule out pregnancy before tx. Available under limited access program. Can cause significant bone marrow suppression. Increased risk of DVT, PE.

IND & DOSE Tx of multiple myeloma, w/ dexamethasone. *Adult:* 25 mg/day PO days 1–21 of repeated 28-day cycle. *Tx of transfusion-dependent anemia due to low or intermediate risk myelodysplastic syndromes. Adult:* 10 mg/day PO. *Tx of mantle cell lymphoma in pts who progress after two prior therapies. Adult:* 25 mg/day PO on days 1–21 of repeated 28-day cycle.

ADJUST DOSE Renal impairment
ADV EFF Anemia, back pain, **bone marrow suppression, cancer,** constipation, diarrhea, dizziness, dyspnea, edema, fatigue, fever, nausea, rash, thrombocytopenia, tumor lysis syndrome, URI
INTERACTIONS Digoxin, erythropoietin-stimulating tx, estrogens
NC/PT Monitor CBC; adjust dose as needed. Rule out pregnancy; ensure contraceptive use. Not for use in breast-feeding. Pt should take safety precautions w/ CNS effects; avoid exposure to infection; get cancer screening; report s&sx of infection, unusual bleeding, muscle pain, difficulty breathing.

lepirudin (Refludan)

CLASS Anticoagulant
PREG/CONT B/NA

IND & DOSE Tx of heparin-induced thrombocytopenia associated w/ thromboembolic disease. *Adult:* 0.4 mg/kg IV bolus, then 0.15 mg/kg IV for 2–10 days.
ADJUST DOSE Renal impairment

ADV EFF Allergic skin reactions, **bleeding,** fever, injection-site reactions, liver changes, pneumonia
INTERACTIONS Other anticoagulants, thrombolytics
NC/PT Monitor aPTT ratio (target, 1.5–2.5). Monitor for signs of bleeding. Not for use in pregnancy, breastfeeding. Pt should report pain at injection site, bleeding.

letrozole (Femara)

CLASS Antiestrogen, antineoplastic, aromatase inhibitor
PREG/CONT D/NA

IND & DOSE Tx of advanced breast cancer in postmenopausal women progressing after antiestrogen tx; adjuvant tx of early receptor-positive breast cancer; extended adjuvant tx of breast cancer in postmenopausal women who have had 5 yr of tamoxifen. *Adult:* 2.5 mg/day PO; continue until tumor progression evident.
ADJUST DOSE Hepatic impairment
ADV EFF GI upset, headache, hot flashes, nausea, **thromboembolic events**
NC/PT Not for use in pregnancy (contraceptives advised). Give comfort measures for adverse effects. Pt should report urine/stool color changes.

leucovorin calcium (generic)

CLASS Folic acid derivative
PREG/CONT C/NA

IND & DOSE Leucovorin rescue, after high-dose methotrexate. *Adult:* Start within 24 hr of methotrexate dose; 10 mg/m² PO q 6 hr for 10 doses or until methotrexate level less than 0.05 micromolar. If serum creatinine is 100% greater than pretreatment level 24 hr after methotrexate dose, or based on methotrexate levels, increase leucovorin to 150 mg IV q 3 hr until serum methotrexate less than 1.0 micromolar; then 15 mg IV q 3 hr until methotrexate is under 0.05 micromolar. *Tx of megaloblastic anemia. Adult:* 1 mg/day IM; max, 1 mg/day. *Palliative tx of metastatic colon cancer. Adult:* 200 mg/m² by slow IV injection over 4 hr daily w/ 5-FU 370 mg/m² IV. Or, 20 mg/m² IV, then 5-FU 425 mg/m² IV. Repeat daily for 5 days; may repeat at 4-wk intervals.

ADV EFF Hypersensitivity reactions, pain/discomfort at injection site
INTERACTIONS 5-FU
NC/PT Give orally if possible. Monitor for hypersensitivity reactions; have emergency support on hand. Do not use intrathecally. Pt should report rash, difficulty breathing. Name confusion between *Leukeran* (chlorambucil) and leucovorin; use care.

---

leuprolide acetate
(Eligard, Lupron)
CLASS GnRH analogue
PREG/CONT X/NA

IND & DOSE *Tx of advanced prostate cancer. Adult:* 1 mg/day subcut, or depot 7.5 mg IM monthly (q 28–33 days), or 22.5 mg depot IM or subcut q 3 mo (84 days), or 30 mg depot IM or subcut q 4 mo, or 45 mg depot subcut q 6 mo. *Tx of endometriosis. Adult:* 3.75 mg as single monthly IM injection, or 11.25 mg IM q 3 mo. Continue for 6 mo. *Tx of uterine leiomyomata. Adult:* 3.75 mg as single monthly injection for 3 mo, or 11.25 mg IM once; give w/ concomitant iron tx. *Tx of central precocious puberty. Child:* 50 mcg/kg/day subcut; may increase by 10-mcg/kg/day increments. Or, 0.3 mg/kg IM depot q 4 wk. Round to nearest depot size; minimum, 7.5 mg.

ADV EFF Anorexia, constipation, dizziness, headache, hematuria, hot flashes, injection-site reactions, **MI**, n/v, peripheral edema, sweating

NC/PT Give only w/ syringe provided. Give depot injections deep into muscle. Obtain periodic tests of testosterone, PSA. Not for use in pregnancy (contraceptives advised). Stop if precocious puberty before 11 yr (girls), 12 yr (boys). Teach proper administration, disposal of needles, syringes. Pt should take safety precautions w/ CNS effects, report injection-site reaction, chest pain.

---

levalbuterol hydrochloride (Xopenex), levalbuterol tartrate (Xopenex HFA)
CLASS Antiasthmatic, beta agonist, bronchodilator
PREG/CONT C/NA

IND & DOSE *Tx, px of bronchospasm. Adult, child 12 yr and older (Xopenex):* 0.63 mg tid, q 6–8 hr by nebulization; may increase up to 1.25 mg tid by nebulization. *Child 6–11 yr (Xopenex):* 0.31 mg tid by nebulization; max, 0.63 mg tid.: *Adult, child 4 yr and older (Xopenex HFA):* 2 inhalations (90 mcg) repeated q 4–6 hr; some pts may respond to 1 inhalation (45 mcg) q 4 hr.

ADV EFF Anxiety, apprehension, BP changes, **bronchospasm**, CNS stimulation, fear, headache, nausea
INTERACTIONS Aminophylline, beta blockers, MAOIs, sympathomimetics, theophylline
NC/PT Keep unopened drug in foil pouch until ready to use; protect from heat, light. Once foil pouch open, use vial within 2 wk, protected from heat, light. Once vial is removed from pouch, use immediately. If not used, protect from light, use within 1 wk. Discard vial if sol not colorless. Teach proper use of inhaler/nebulizer. Pt should take safety precautions w/ CNS effects, not exceed recommended dose, report chest pain, difficulty breathing, worsening of condition.

levetiracetam (Keppra)
CLASS Antiepileptic
PREG/CONT C/NA

IND & DOSE Tx of partial-onset seizures. *Adult, child over 16 yr:* 500 mg PO or IV bid; max, 3,000 mg/day. ER tablets: 1,000 mg/day PO; max, 3,000 mg/day. *Child 4–16 yr:* 10 mg/kg PO bid (500–1,000 mg/day); may increase q 2 wk in 20-mg/kg increments to 30 mg/kg bid (1,500–3,000 mg/day). Daily dose of oral sol: total dose (mL/day) = daily dose (mg/kg/day) × pt weight (kg) ÷ 100 mg/mL PO. Tx of generalized tonic-clonic seizures. *Adult, child over 16 yr:* 500 mg PO bid; increase by 1,000 mg/day q 2 wk to recommended 3,000 mg/day. *Child 6–15 yr:* 10 mg/kg PO bid; increase q 2 wk by 20-mg/kg increments to recommended 60 mg/kg/day given as 30 mg/kg bid. Tx of myoclonic seizures. *Adult, child 12 yr and older:* 500 mg PO bid; slowly increase to recommended max, 3,000 mg/day.
ADJUST DOSE Renal impairment
ADV EFF Dizziness, dyspepsia, headache, **suicidality**, vertigo, vision changes
NC/PT Taper when stopping. Give w/ food. Not for use in pregnancy (barrier contraceptives advised). Pt should swallow ER tablet whole and not cut, crush, or chew it; take safety precautions w/ CNS effects; wear medical ID; report severe headache, thoughts of suicide. Name confusion between *Keppra* (levetiracetam) and *Kaletra* (lopinavir/ritonavir); use caution.

levocetirizine dihydrochloride (Xyzal)
CLASS Antihistamine
PREG/CONT B/NA

IND & DOSE Symptom relief of seasonal, perennial allergic rhinitis in pts 6 mo and older; tx of uncomplicat-ed skin effects in chronic idiopathic urticaria in pts 2 yr and older. *Adult, child 12 yr and older:* 5 mg/day PO in evening. *Child 6–11 yr:* 2.5 mg/day PO in evening. *Child 6 mo–5 yr:* 1.25 mg (½ tsp oral sol) PO once daily in evening.
ADJUST DOSE Renal impairment
ADV EFF Dry mouth, fatigue, mental alertness changes, nasopharyngitis, somnolence
INTERACTIONS Alcohol, CNS depressants
NC/PT Encourage humidifiers, adequate fluid intake to help prevent severe dryness of mucous membranes; skin care for urticaria. Not for use in pregnancy, breast-feeding. Pt should take in evening, use safety precautions w/ CNS effects.

levodopa (generic)
CLASS Antiparkinsonism
PREG/CONT C/NA

IND & DOSE Tx of parkinsonism. *Adult:* 1 g/day PO in two or more doses w/ food; increase gradually in increments not exceeding 0.75 g/day q 3–7 days as tolerated. Max, 8 g/day. Only available in combination products.
ADV EFF Abd pain, adventitious movements, anorexia, ataxia, dizziness, drowsiness, dry mouth, n/v, numbness, **suicidality**, weakness
INTERACTIONS Benzodiazepines, MAOIs, papaverine, phenytoin, pyridoxine, TCAs
NC/PT Ensure 14 days free of MAOIs before use. Give w/ meals. Decreased dose needed if tx interrupted. Observe for suicidal tendencies. Limit vitamin B_6 intake; check multivitamin use. Pt should take safety precautions w/ CNS effects, use sugarless lozenges for dry mouth, report uncontrollable movements, difficulty urinating.

levofloxacin (Levaquin)

CLASS Fluoroquinolone antibiotic

PREG/CONT C/NA

BBW Risk of tendinitis, tendon rupture. Risk increased in pts older than 60 yr, w/ concurrent corticosteroids use, and w/ kidney, heart, lung transplant. Risk of exacerbation of myasthenia gravis w/ serious muscle weakness; do not use w/ hx of myasthenia gravis.

IND & DOSE *Tx of community-acquired pneumonia.* *Adults:* 500 mg/day PO or IV for 7–14 days. *Tx of sinusitis.* *Adult:* 500 mg/day PO or IV for 10–14 days, or 750 mg/day PO or IV for 5 days. *Tx of chronic bronchitis.* *Adult:* 500 mg/day PO or IV for 7 days. *Tx of skin infection.* *Adult:* 500–750 mg/day PO or IV for 7–14 days. *Tx of UTIs, pyelonephritis.* *Adults:* 250 mg daily PO or IV for 3–10 days; complicated, 750 mg/day PO or IV for 5 days. *Tx of nosocomial pneumonia.* *Adult:* 750 mg/day PO or IV for 7–14 days. *Tx of chronic prostatitis.* *Adults:* 500 mg/day PO for 28 days, or 500 mg/day by slow IV infusion over 60 min for 28 days. *Post-exposure anthrax.* *Adult:* 500 mg/day PO or IV for 60 days. *Child 6 mo or older over 50 kg:* 500 mg/day PO for 60 days. *Child 6 mo or older under 50 kg:* 8 mg/kg q 12 hr PO for 60 days. Max, 250 mg/dose. *Tx, px of plague due to Yersinia pestis.* *Adult, child over 50 kg:* 500 mg/day PO for 10–14 days. *Child 6 mo and older but less than 50 kg:* 8 mg/kg PO q 12 hr for 10–14 days; max, 250 mg.

ADJUST DOSE Renal impairment

ADV EFF Diarrhea, dizziness, headache, insomnia, muscle/joint tenderness, photosensitivity, **prolonged QT interval**, rash, renal impairment, **tendon rupture**

INTERACTIONS Antacids, iron salts, magnesium, NSAIDs, QT-prolonging drugs, St. John's wort, sucralfate, zinc

NC/PT Culture before starting tx. Ensure hydration. Stop if hypersensitivity reaction. Separate from antacids by at least 2 hr. Pt should avoid sun exposure, avoid St John's wort, take safety precautions w/ CNS effects, report muscle/tendon pain, weakness.

levoleucovorin (Fusilev)

CLASS Folate analogue

PREG/CONT C/NA

IND & DOSE *Rescue after high-dose methotrexate; to diminish toxicity from impaired methotrexate elimination.* *Adult:* 7.5 mg IV q 6 hr for 10 doses, starting 24 hr after start of methotrexate infusion. *Palliative tx of advanced metastatic colorectal cancer, w/ 5-FU.* *Adult:* 100 mg/m² by IV injection over at least 3 min, then 5-FU 370 mg/m² by IV injection. Or, or 10 mg/m² by IV injection, then 5-FU 425 mg/m² by IV injection.

ADV EFF N/v/d, stomatitis

INTERACTIONS 5-FU, phenobarbital, phenytoin, primidone, trimethoprim-sulfamethoxazole

NC/PT Inject slowly IV, no faster than 160 mg/min because of high calcium content. Give antiemetics if needed, mouth care for stomatitis.

levomilnacipran (Fetzima)

CLASS Antidepressant, serotonin/norepinephrine reuptake inhibitor

PREG/CONT C/NA

BBW Increased risk of suicidality in children, adolescents, young adults; monitor closely.

IND & DOSE *Tx of major depressive disorder.* *Adult:* 20 mg/day PO for 2 days; then 40 mg/day PO. May increase in increments of 40 mg/day every 2 days as needed. Max, 120 mg/day.

ADJUST DOSE Severe renal impairment

ADV EFF Activation of mania, bradycardia, constipation, discontinuation syndrome, ED, hyponatremia, hypertension, n/v, palpitations, serotonin syndrome, sweating, urinary retention

INTERACTIONS Azole antifungals, buspirone, clarithromycin, diuretics, fentanyl, linezolid, lithium, methylene blue (IV), NSAIDs, St. John's wort, tramadol, tryptophan

NC/PT Monitor for hypomania, BP periodically, IOP in pts w/ glaucoma, serotonin syndrome, discontinuation syndrome. Not for use in pregnancy, breast-feeding. Pt should swallow capsule whole, not cut, crush, or chew it. Pt should avoid St. John's wort; empty bladder before taking drug; take safety precautions w/ CNS effects; report thoughts of suicide, hallucinations, continued rapid heart rate, hallucinations.

DANGEROUS DRUG

levorphanol tartrate
(generic)
CLASS Opioid agonist analgesic
PREG/CONT C/C-II

IND & DOSE Relief of moderate to severe pain. *Adult:* 2 mg PO q 3–6 hr; range, 8–16 mg/day.

ADJUST DOSE Elderly pts, impaired adults

ADV EFF Bronchospasm, **cardiac arrest,** constipation, dizziness, drowsiness, **laryngospasm,** lightheadedness, n/v, **respiratory arrest, shock,** sweating

INTERACTIONS Alcohol, antihistamines, barbiturate anesthetics, CNS depressants

NC/PT Monitor closely w/ first dose. Pt should take safety precautions w/ CNS effects, use laxative for constipation, take 4–6 hr before next feeding if breast-feeding, report difficulty breathing.

levothyroxine sodium
(Levothroid, Levoxine, Levoxyl, Synthroid, Thyro-Tabs)
CLASS Thyroid hormone
PREG/CONT A/NA

BBW Do not use for weight loss; possible serious adverse effects w/ large doses.

IND & DOSE Replacement tx in hypothyroidism. *Adult:* 12.5–25 mcg PO, w/ increasing increments of 25 mcg PO q 2–4 wk; maint, up to 200 mcg/day. Can substitute IV or IM injection for oral form when oral route not possible. Usual IV dose is 50% of oral dose. Start at 25 mcg/day or less in pts w/ long-standing hypothyroidism, known cardiac disease. Usual replacement, 1.7 mcg/kg/day. **Tx of myxedema coma without severe heart disease.** *Adult:* Initially, 200–500 mcg IV. May give additional 100–300 mcg or more second day if needed. **Thyroid suppression tx.** *Adult:* 2.6 mcg/kg/day PO for 7–10 days. **TSH suppression in thyroid cancer, nodules, euthyroid goiters.** Individualize dose based on specific disease and pt; larger amounts than used for normal suppression. **Tx of congenital hypothyroidism.** *Child:* Over 12 yr, 2–3 mcg/kg/day PO; 6–12 yr, 4–5 mcg/kg/day PO; 1–5 yr, 5–6 mcg/kg/day PO; 6–12 mo, 6–8 mcg/kg/day PO; 3–6 mo, 8–10 mcg/kg/day PO; 0–3 mo, 10–15 mcg/kg/day PO.

ADJUST DOSE Elderly pts

ADV EFF Cardiac arrest, esophageal atresia, n/v/d, tremors

INTERACTIONS Aluminum- and magnesium-containing antacids, cholestyramine, colestipol, digoxin, iron, sucralfate, theophylline, warfarin

NC/PT Monitor thyroid function. Do not add IV form to other IV fluids. Replaces normal hormone; adverse effects should not occur. Pt should swallow whole w/ full glass of water, wear medical ID, report chest pain, unusual sweating.

DANGEROUS DRUG

lidocaine hydrochloride
(Anestacon, Numby Stuff, Otocaine, Xylocaine)

CLASS Antiarrhythmic, local anesthetic
PREG/CONT B/NA

IND & DOSE Tx of ventricular arrhythmias. *Adult:* Use 10% sol for IM injection: 300 mg in deltoid or thigh muscle; may repeat in 60–90 min. Switch to IV or oral form as soon as possible. Or, 1–4 mg/min (20–50 mcg/kg/min) IV; decrease as soon as cardiac rhythm stabilizes. *Child:* Safety/efficacy not established. AHA recommends bolus of 0.5–1 mg/kg IV, then 30 mcg/kg/min w/ caution. **Local anesthetic.** *Adult, child:* Conc, diluent should be appropriate to particular local anesthetic use: 5% sol w/ glucose for spinal anesthesia, 1.5% sol w/ dextrose for low spinal or saddle block anesthesia. Dose varies w/ area to be anesthetized and reason for anesthesia; use lowest dose needed to achieve results. **Topical analgesia.** *Adult, child:* Up to 3 transdermal patches to one area of pain for up to 12 hr within 24-hr period, or apply cream, ointment, gel, sol, oral patch, spray as directed 1–3 times/day.
ADJUST DOSE Elderly, debilitated pts; HF; hepatic, renal impairment
ADV EFF Anaphylactoid reactions, back pain, **cardiac arrest**, cardiac arrhythmias, dizziness, drowsiness, fatigue, headache, hypotension, lightheadedness, **respiratory arrest**, **seizures**, urine retention
INTERACTIONS Beta blockers, cimetidine, succinylcholine
NC/PT Have life support equipment on hand; continually monitor pt response. Check conc carefully; varies by product. Monitor for safe, effective serum conc (antiarrhythmic: 1–5 mcg/ mL); conc of 6 or

more mcg/mL usually toxic. Pt should take safety precautions w/ CNS effects, report difficulty speaking/ breathing, numbness, pain at injection site.

linaclotide (Linzess)
CLASS Guanylate cyclase-C agonist, IBS drug
PREG/CONT C/NA

BBW Contraindicated in child up to 6 yr; avoid use in child 6–17 yr; caused deaths in juvenile mice.
IND & DOSE Tx of IBS w/ constipation. *Adult:* 290 mcg/day PO. **Tx of chronic idiopathic constipation.** *Adult:* 145 mcg/day PO.
ADV EFF Abd pain, diarrhea, distention, flatulence, **severe diarrhea**
NC/PT Ensure constipation is main complaint. Give on empty stomach. Have pt swallow capsule whole and not cut, crush, or chew it. Ensure pt is not under 6 yr. Pt should swallow capsule whole and not cut, crush, or chew it; take on empty stomach; store in original container protected from moisture; not give to child under 17 yr; report severe diarrhea, severe abd pain.

linagliptin (Tradjenta)
CLASS Antidiabetic, DPP-4 inhibitor
PREG/CONT B/NA

IND & DOSE Adjunct to diet, exercise to improve glycemic control in pts w/ type 2 diabetes; tx of type 2 diabetes in pts w/ severe renal impairment w/ insulin; add on tx to insulin, diet, exercise to achieve glycemic control in pts w/ type 2 diabetes. *Adult:* 5 mg PO once/day.
ADV EFF Hypoglycemia, nasopharyngitis, pancreatitis
INTERACTIONS Celery, coriander, dandelion root, fenugreek, garlic, ginger, juniper berries, potent CYP3A inhibitors

NC/PT Monitor blood glucose, HbA1c before, periodically during tx. Ensure pt continues diet, exercise, other drugs for diabetes control. Use caution in pregnancy, breast-feeding. Arrange for thorough diabetic teaching program. Report OTC/herbal use that could alter blood glucose, s&sx of infection, uncontrolled glucose level.

lincomycin hydrochloride (Lincocin)
CLASS Lincosamide antibiotic
PREG/CONT C/NA

BBW Risk of *Clostridium difficile* diarrhea, pseudomembranous colitis; monitor closely.

IND & DOSE Tx of serious infections caused by susceptible bacteria strains. *Adult:* 500 mg/day PO q 6–8 hr, or 600 mg IM q 12–24 hr, or 600 mg–1 g IV q 8–12 hr. *Child:* 30–60 mg/kg/day PO, or 10 mg/kg IM q 12–24 hr, or 10–20 mg/kg/day IV in divided doses.

ADJUST DOSE Renal impairment
ADV EFF Abd pain, **agranulocytosis, anaphylactic reactions,** anorexia, **cardiac arrest,** contact dermatitis, esophagitis, n/v/d, pain after injection, **pseudomembranous colitis,** rash
INTERACTIONS Aluminum salts, kaolin, NMJ blockers
NC/PT Culture before tx. Give orally w/ full glass of water or food. Do not give IM injection of more than 600 mg; inject deeply into muscle. Monitor LFTs, renal function. Pt should report severe, watery diarrhea.

linezolid (Zyvox)
CLASS Oxazolidinone antibiotic
PREG/CONT C/NA

IND & DOSE Tx of VREF, MRSA, pneumonia, complicated skin/skin-structure infections, including diabetic foot ulcers without osteomyelitis. *Adult, child 12 yr and older:* 600 mg IV or PO q 12 hr for 10–28 days. *Child 11 yr and under:* 10 mg/kg IV or PO q 8 hr for 10–14 days. Tx of uncomplicated skin/skin-structure infections. *Adult, child 12 yr and older:* 400 mg PO q 12 hr for 10–14 days. *Child 5–11 yr:* 10 mg/kg PO q 12 hr for 10–14 days.
ADV EFF Diarrhea, dizziness, insomnia, nausea, **pseudomembranous colitis,** rash
INTERACTIONS Aspirin, dipyridamole, MAOIs, NSAIDs, pseudoephedrine, SSRIs, St. John's wort, sympathomimetics, tyramine-containing foods
NC/PT Culture before tx. Do not mix IV solution with other solutions. Monitor platelets, BP w/ long-term use. Pt should complete full course; avoid foods high in tyramine; report all OTC and herbal use; report severe GI problems, bloody diarrhea. Name confusion between Zyvox (linezolid) and Zovirax (acyclovir); use caution.

liothyronine (Cytomel, Triostat)
CLASS Thyroid hormone
PREG/CONT A/NA

BBW Do not use for weight loss; serious adverse effects w/ large doses possible.

IND & DOSE Replacement tx in hypothyroidism. *Adult:* 25 mcg PO; maint, 25–75 mcg/day. Tx of myxedema. *Adult:* 5 mcg/day PO; maint, 50–100 mcg/day. Tx of myxedema coma, precoma. *Adult:* 25–50 mcg IV q 4–12 hr; do not give IM or subcut. Start at 10–20 mcg IV w/ heart disease. Max, 100 mcg/24 hr. Tx of simple goiter. *Adult:* 5 mcg/day PO; maint, 75 mcg/day. Thyroid suppression tx. *Adult:* 75–100 mcg/day PO for 7 days. Repeat I¹³¹ uptake test; unaffected w/ hyperthyroidism, decreased by 50% w/ euthyroidism. Tx of congenital hypothyroidism.

Child: Birth, 5 mcg/day PO. Usual maint, 20 mcg/day up to 1 yr; 50 mcg/day PO for 1–3 yr, adult dose over 3 yr.
ADJUST DOSE Elderly pts
ADV EFF Cardiac arrest, esophageal atresia, hyperthyroidism, n/v/d, tremors
INTERACTIONS Aluminum-, magnesium-containing antacids, cholestyramine, colestipol, digoxin, iron, sucralfate, theophylline, warfarin
NC/PT Monitor thyroid function. Do not add IV form to other IV fluids. Replaces normal hormone; adverse effects should not occur. Pt should swallow whole w/ full glass of water, wear medical ID, report chest pain, unusual sweating.

liotrix (Thyrolar)
CLASS Thyroid hormone
PREG/CONT A/NA

BBW Do not use for weight loss; serious adverse effects w/ large doses possible.
IND & DOSE Replacement tx in hypothyroidism. *Adult:* 30 mg/day PO; Maint, 60–120 mg/day PO (thyroid equivalent). Mgt of goiter, thyroid cancer. Use larger doses than needed for replacement surgery. Dx of thyroid function. 1.56 mcg/kg/day PO for 7–10 days. Tx of congenital hypothyroidism. *Child:* Over 12 yr, 90 mg/day PO; 6–12 yr, 60–90 mg/day PO; 1–5 yr, 45–60 mg/day PO; 6–12 mo, 30–45 mg/day PO; 0–6 mo, 15–30 mg/day PO.
ADV EFF Cardiac arrest, esophageal atresia, hyperthyroidism, n/v/d, tremors
INTERACTIONS Aluminum-, magnesium-containing antacids, cholestyramine, colestipol, digoxin, iron, sucralfate, theophylline, warfarin
NC/PT Monitor thyroid function. Replaces normal hormone; adverse effects should not occur. Pt should swallow whole w/ full glass of water, wear medical ID, report chest pain, unusual sweating.

liraglutide (Victoza)
CLASS Antidiabetic, glucagon-like peptide receptor agonist
PREG/CONT C/NA

BBW Causes thyroid medullary cancer in rodents. Not for use w/ personal, family hx of thyroid medullary cancer, multiple endocrine neoplasia syndrome type 2; monitor closely.
IND & DOSE Adjunct to diet, exercise to improve glycemic control in type 2 diabetes. *Adults:* 0.6 mg/day by subcut injection; max, 1.8 mg/day.
ADV EFF Dizziness, headache, n/v/d, **pancreatitis, papillary thyroid carcinoma**
INTERACTIONS Antidiabetic secretagogues, celery, coriander, dandelion root, drugs that delay GI emptying, garlic, ginseng, fenugreek, juniper berries
NC/PT Monitor blood glucose, HbA1c before, periodically during tx. Ensure pt continues diet, exercise, other drugs for diabetes. Provide complete diabetic teaching program. Teach proper administration, disposal of needles, syringes. Use caution in pregnancy, breast-feeding. Pt should report OTC/herbal use, difficulty swallowing, lump in throat, severe abd pain radiating to back.

lisdexamfetamine dimesylate (Vyvanse)
CLASS Amphetamine, CNS stimulant
PREG/CONT C/C-II

BBW High risk of abuse; could lead to drug dependence. Amphetamine misuse has caused serious CV events, sudden death.
IND & DOSE Tx of ADHD as part of integrated tx plan. *Adult, child 6 yr and older:* 30 mg/day PO in a.m.; may increase at wkly intervals in increments of 10–20 mg/day. Max, 70 mg/day.

ADV EFF Abd pain, **cardiac events,** decreased appetite, fever, headache, insomnia, irritability, n/v/d, **sudden death,** weight loss
INTERACTIONS Chlorpromazine, haloperidol, MAOIs, meperidine, methenamine, norepinephrine, sympathomimetics, TCAs, urine acidifiers
NC/PT Ensure proper dx. Part of comprehensive tx plan. Monitor growth in child. If pt cannot swallow whole, empty contents into glass of water, have pt drink right away. Stop periodically to validate use. Pt should avoid MAOI use within 14 days, take in a.m. to prevent insomnia, store in dry place, secure drug (controlled substance), report vision changes, manic symptoms, marked weight loss.

lisinopril (Prinivil, Zestril)
CLASS ACE inhibitor, antihypertensive
PREG/CONT D/NA

BBW Contraceptives advised. If pregnancy occurs, stop drug as soon as possible; fetal injury/death possible.
IND & DOSE Tx of hypertension. **Adults:** 10 mg/day PO; range, 20–40 mg/day. If also taking diuretic, start at 5 mg/day; monitor BP. **Child 6 yr and older:** 0.07 mg/kg/day PO; max, 5 mg/day. **Adjunct Tx of HF. Adults:** 5 mg/day PO w/ diuretics, digitalis. Effective range, 5–20 mg/day (Prinivil), 5–40 mg/day (Zestril). **To improve survival post-MI. Adults:** Start within 24 hr of MI; 5 mg PO, then 5 mg PO in 24 hr; 10 mg PO after 48 hr; then 10 mg/day PO for 6 wk.
ADJUST DOSE Elderly pts, renal impairment
ADV EFF Airway obstruction, angioedema, cough, dizziness, fatigue, gastric irritation, headache, insomnia, n/v/d, orthostatic hypotension, **pancytopenia**
INTERACTIONS Capsaicin, NSAIDs

NC/PT Mark chart if surgery scheduled; fluid replacement may be needed postop. Monitor BP; use care in situations that may lead to decreased BP. Maintain hydration. Not for use in pregnancy (contraceptives advised). Pt should take safety precautions w/ CNS effects, report swelling, difficulty breathing. Name confusion between lisinopril and fosinopril; use caution.

lithium carbonate, lithium citrate (Lithobid, Lithonate, Lithotabs)
CLASS Antimanic drug
PREG/CONT D/NA

BBW Monitor clinical status closely, especially during initial tx stages. Monitor for therapeutic serum level (0.6–1.2 mEq/L); toxicity closely related to serum level.
IND & DOSE Tx of manic episodes of bipolar disorder. **Adults:** 600 mg PO tid or 900 mg SR form PO bid to produce effective serum level between 1 and 1.5 mEq/L. Maint, 300 mg PO tid–qid to produce serum level of 0.6–1.2 mEq/L. Determine serum level at least q 2 mo in samples drawn immediately before dose (at least 8–12 hr after previous dose).
ADJUST DOSE Elderly pts, renal impairment
ADV EFF Related to serum levels: **Death,** lethargy, muscle weakness, **pulmonary complications,** slurred speech, tremor progressing to **CV collapse.** Other: Dizziness, drowsiness, GI upset, thirst, tremor
INTERACTIONS Antacids, carbamazepine, dandelion root, diuretics, haloperidol, indomethacin, iodide salts, juniper, NSAIDs, SSRIs, tromethamine, urinary alkalinizers
NC/PT Monitor serum level regularly; therapeutic range, 0.6–1.2 mEq/L. Maintain salt, fluid intake. Not for use in pregnancy (contraceptives advised). Teach toxicity warning signs.

Pt should take w/ food, milk; take safety precautions w/ CNS effects; report diarrhea, unsteady walking, slurred speech.

DANGEROUS DRUG

lomitapide (Juxtapid)
CLASS Antitriglyceride
PREG/CONT X/NA

BBW Increased transaminase elevations; monitor LFTs closely. Stop drug at s&sx of hepatotoxicity; risk of hepatic steatosis, cirrhosis.
IND & DOSE Adjunct to low-fat diet, other lipid-lowering tx to reduce LDL, total cholesterol, apolipoprotein B, non-HDL cholesterol in pts w/ homozygous familial hypercholesterolemia. *Adult:* Initially 5 mg/day PO, then at 2 wk to 10 mg/day PO, then at 4-wk intervals to 20, 40, and 60 mg/day PO.
ADJUST DOSE Hepatic, renal impairment
ADV EFF Abd pain, dyspepsia, **hepatotoxicity**, n/v/d
INTERACTIONS Bile acid sequestrants, lovastatin, simvastatin, strong or moderate CYP3A4 inhibitors, warfarin
NC/PT Available only through restricted access program. Ensure negative pregnancy test before tx and continued use of low-fat diet other lipid-lowering agents. Monitor LFTs regularly. Consider supplemental vitamin E, and fatty acids, tx for severe GI effects. Not for use in pregnancy (barrier contraceptives advised), breast-feeding. Pt should take as prescribed (dosage will be slowly increased); take w/ water (not food) in evening; swallow capsule whole and not cut, crush, or chew it; continue low-fat diet, other lipid-lowering drugs; take vitamin E, fatty acids if prescribed; report severe GI complaints, urine/stool color changes, extreme fatigue.

DANGEROUS DRUG

lomustine (CeeNU)
CLASS Alkylating agent, antineoplastic
PREG/CONT D/NA

BBW Arrange for blood tests to evaluate hematopoietic function before tx, then wkly for at least 6 wk; severe bone marrow suppression possible. Delayed suppression at or beyond 6 wk also possible.
IND & DOSE Tx of primary/metastatic brain tumors, secondary tx of Hodgkin disease in pts who relapse after primary tx w/ other drugs.
Adult, child: 130 mg/m^2 PO as single dose q 6 wk. Must make adjustments w/ bone marrow suppression: Initially, reduce to 100 mg/m^2 PO q 6 wk; do not give repeat dose until platelets over 100,000/mm^2 and leukocytes over 4,000/mm^2.
ADV EFF Alopecia, ataxia, **bone marrow suppression**, n/v, **pulmonary fibrosis**, renal toxicity
NC/PT Monitor CBC, respiratory function. Do not give full dose within 2–3 wk of radiation therapy. Not for use in pregnancy (barrier contraceptives advised). Antiemetics may be ordered. Pt should avoid exposure to infection, report unusual bleeding, difficulty breathing, s&sx of infection.

---

loperamide hydrochloride (Imodium, Pepto Diarrhea Control)
CLASS Antidiarrheal
PREG/CONT B/NA

IND & DOSE Tx of acute/chronic diarrhea, traveler's diarrhea. *Adult:* 4 mg PO, then 2 mg after each unformed stool; max, 16 mg/day. *Child:* 8–12 yr (over 30 kg): 2 mg PO tid; 6–8 yr (20–30 kg): 2 mg PO bid; 2–5 yr (13–20 kg): 1 mg PO tid. For traveler's diarrhea, 6–11 yr (22–43 kg): 2 mg PO after loose stool, then 1 mg w/ each subsequent stool; max, 4 mg/day PO

(6–8 yr) or 6 mg/day PO (9–11 yr) for 2 days.

ADV EFF Abd pain, constipation, distention, dry mouth, nausea, **pulmonary infiltrates, toxic megacolon**

NC/PT Pt should take drug after each stool; stop if no response in 48 hr; drink clear fluids to prevent dehydration; report fever, continued diarrhea, abd pain and distention.

lopinavir (lopinavir/ ritonavir) (Kaletra)

CLASS Antiviral, protease inhibitor

PREG/CONT C/NA

IND & DOSE *Note:* Doses for child under 12 yr based on weight. See manufacturer's details for specific doses. **Tx of HIV infection w/ other antiretrovirals in tx-naive pts.** *Adult, child 12 yr and older, over 40 kg:* 800 mg lopinavir, 200 mg ritonavir (four tablets or 10 mL)/day PO. *Children 6 mo–12 yr:* over 40 kg, adult dose; 15–under 40 kg, 10 mg/kg PO bid; 7–under 15 kg, 12 mg/kg PO bid. *Child 6 mo–12 yr using oral solution:* over 40 kg, adult dose; over 35–40 kg, 4.75 mL PO bid; over 30–35 kg, 4 mL PO bid; over 25–30 kg, 3.5 mL PO bid; over 20–25 kg, 2.75 mL PO bid; 15–20 kg, 2.25 mL PO bid; over 10–15 kg, 1.75 mL PO bid; 7–10 kg, 1.2 mL PO bid. **Tx of HIV infection w/ other antiretrovirals in tx-experienced pts.** *Adult, child 12 yr and older, over 40 kg:* 400 mg lopinavir, 100 mg ritonavir (two tablets or 5 mL) PO bid. **Tx of HIV infection w/ efavirenz, nevirapine, fosamprenavir without ritonavir, or nelfinavir.** *Adult, child 12 yr and older, over 40 kg:* 600 mg lopinavir, 150 mg ritonavir (three tablets) PO bid for tx-experienced pts. No adjustment needed for tx-naive pts. *Child 6 mo–12 yr:* 7–15 kg, 13 mg/kg PO bid; 15–40 kg, 11 mg/kg PO bid; over 45 kg, adult dose. **Tx of HIV infection using oral sol w/ efavirenz, nevirapine, amprenavir, or nelfinavir.** *Adult, child 12 yr*

and older, over 40 kg: Adjust dose to 533 mg lopinavir, 133 mg ritonavir (6.5 mL) bid PO w/ food. *Child 6 mo–12 yr:* over 45 kg, adult dose; over 40–45 kg, 5.75 mL bid PO; over 35–40 kg, 5 mL PO bid; over 30–35 kg, 4.5 mL PO bid; over 25–30 kg, 4 mL PO bid; over 25–30 kg, 3.25 mL PO bid; over 20–25 kg, 2.5 mL PO bid; 15–20 kg, 2.5 mL PO bid; over 10–15 kg, 2 mL PO bid; 7–10 kg, 1.5 mL PO bid.

ADV EFF Abd pain, anorexia, asthenia, lipid abnormalities, n/v/d, paresthesia, rash

INTERACTIONS Hormonal contraceptives, sildenafil, St. John's wort, tadalafil, vardenafil. Fatal reactions possible: do not give w/ amiodarone, bepridil, bupropion, clozapine, encainide, flecainide, meperidine, piroxicam, propafenone, quinidine, rifabutin. Extreme sedation/respiratory depression possible; do not give w/ alprazolam, clonazepam, diazepam, estazolam, flurazepam, midazolam, triazolam, zolpidem.

NC/PT Obtain baseline lipid profile. Store sol in refrigerator; protect from light, heat. Do not use in preterm infants. Give didanosine 1 hr before or 2 hr after lopinavir sol. May make hormonal contraceptives ineffective (barrier contraceptives advised). Pt should swallow tablet whole and not cut, crush, or chew it; use precautions to prevent spread (drug not a cure); avoid other prescription drugs, OTC/herbs until checking w/ prescriber; avoid St John's wort; report severe abd pain, numbness/tingling. Name confusion between Kaletra (lopinavir/ritonavir) and Keppra (levetiracetam).

loratadine (Alavert, Claritin)

CLASS Antihistamine

PREG/CONT B/NA

IND & DOSE Symptomatic relief of allergic rhinitis; tx of rhinitis, urticaria. *Adult, child 6 yr and over:*

10 mg/day PO. *Child 2–5 yr:* 5 mg PO daily (syrup, chewable tablets).
ADJUST DOSE Elderly pts; hepatic, renal impairment
ADV EFF Bronchospasm, dizziness, headache, increased appetite, nervousness, thickened bronchial secretions, weight gain
INTERACTIONS Alcohol, CNS depressants
NC/PT Pt should place orally disintegrating tablet on tongue, swallow after it dissolves; avoid alcohol; use humidifier for dry mucous membranes; take safety precautions w/ CNS effects.

lorazepam (Ativan)
CLASS Anxiolytic, benzodiazepine, sedative-hypnotic
PREG/CONT D/C-IV

IND & DOSE Mgt of anxiety disorders; short-term relief of anxiety symptoms. *Adults:* 2–6 mg/day PO; range, 1–10 mg/day in divided doses w/ largest dose at bedtime. **Insomnia due to transient stress.** *Adult:* 2–4 mg PO at bedtime. **Preanesthetic sedation, anxiolytic.** *Adult:* 0.05 mg/kg IM; max, 4 mg at least 2 hr before procedure. Or, 2 mg total IV or 0.044 mg/kg, whichever smaller; may give doses as high as 0.05 mg/kg to total of 4 mg 15–20 min before procedure. **Tx of status epilepticus.** *Adult:* 4 mg slowly IV at 2 mg/min. May give another 4 mg IV after 10–15 min if needed.
ADJUST DOSE Hepatic, renal impairment
ADV EFF Apathy, confusion, depression, disorientation, drowsiness, dry mouth, **CV collapse,** gynecomastia, hostility, light-headedness, nausea, restlessness
INTERACTIONS Alcohol, CNS depressants, kava, probenecid, theophyllines
NC/PT Do not give intra-arterially. Give IM injection deep into muscle.

Protect sol from light. May mix oral sol w/ water, juice, soda, applesauce, pudding. Taper gradually after long-term tx. Pt should take safety precautions w/ CNS effects; report vision changes, chest pain, fainting. Name confusion between lorazepam and alprazolam; use caution.

lorcaserin hydrochloride (Belviq)
CLASS Serotonin receptor agonist, weight-loss drug
PREG/CONT X/NA

IND & DOSE Adjunct to diet, exercise for long-term weight management in adults w/ initial body mass index of 30 kg/m^2 or more or 27 kg/m^2 or more w/ at least one weight-related condition. *Adult:* 10 mg PO bid.
ADV EFF Back pain, cognitive changes, constipation, dizziness, dry mouth, fatigue, headache, hypoglycemia, **NMS, pulmonary hypertension, suicidality, valvular heart disease**
INTERACTIONS Bupropion, dextromethorphan, linezolid, lithium, MAO-Is, selected serotonin norepinephrine reuptake inhibitors, SSRIs, St. John's wort, TCAs, tramadol, tryptophan; avoid these combinations
NC/PT Ensure appropriate use of drug; if 5% of body weight is not lost within 12 wk, stop drug. Be aware of risk of cognitive changes, suicidality; monitor for s&sx of valvular heart disease, NMS. Not for use in pregnancy, breast-feeding. Pt should take drug bid, and not change dosage; continue diet, exercise program; avoid combining w/ other weight-loss drugs; avoid St. John's wort; use safety precautions w/ dizziness, sugarless candy for dry mouth; watch for slowed thinking, sleepiness; report thoughts of suicide, changes in heart rate, mental status.

losartan potassium
(Cozaar)

CLASS Antihypertensive, ARB
PREG/CONT D/NA

BBW Rule out pregnancy before starting tx. Suggest barrier contraceptives during tx; fetal injury/death have occurred.

IND & DOSE Tx of hypertension. *Adult:* 50 mg/day PO; range, 25–100 mg/day PO once or bid. *Child 6 yr and over:* 0.7 mg/kg/day PO; max, 50 mg/day. **Tx of diabetic nephropathy.** *Adult:* 50 mg/day PO; may increase to 100 mg/day based on BP response. **Tx of hypertension w/ left ventricular hypertrophy.** *Adult:* 50–100 mg/day PO w/ 12.5–25 mg/day hydrochlorothiazide.

ADV EFF Abd pain, cough, diarrhea, dizziness, drowsiness, nausea, URI
INTERACTIONS Fluconazole, indomethacin, ketoconazole, phenobarbital, rifamycin
NC/PT If surgery needed, alert surgeon to drug use; volume replacement may be needed. Not for use in pregnancy (barrier contraceptives advised), breast-feeding. Pt should use caution in situations that could lead to fluid loss, maintain hydration, take safety precautions w/ CNS effects.

lovastatin (Altoprev, Mevacor)

CLASS Antihyperlipidemic, statin
PREG/CONT X/NA

IND & DOSE Tx of familial hypercholesterolemia, type II hyperlipidemia (ER only); to slow progression of atherosclerosis in pts w/ CAD; tx of primary hypercholesterolemia. *Adult:* 20 mg/day PO in evening w/ meals. Maint, 10–80 mg/day PO; max, 80 mg/day. For ER tablets, 10–60 mg/day PO single dose in evening. **As adjunct to diet to reduce total cholesterol, LDLs,**

apolipoprotein B in heterozygous familial hypercholesterolemia. *Adolescent boy, postmenarchal girl, 10–17 yr:* 10–40 mg/day PO; may increase to max 40 mg/day.

ADJUST DOSE Renal impairment
ADV EFF Abd pain, cataracts, cramps, constipation, flatulence, headache, nausea, **rhabdomyolysis**
INTERACTIONS Amiodarone, azole antifungals, cyclosporine, gemfibrozil, grapefruit juice, itraconazole, ketoconazole, other statins, verapamil
NC/PT Monitor LFTs. Not for use in pregnancy (barrier contraceptives advised). Pt should not cut, crush, or chew ER tablets; take in evening for best effects; follow diet, exercise program; get periodic eye exams; report muscle pain w/ fever, unusual bleeding.

loxapine hydrochloride, loxapine succinate
(Adasuve, Loxitane)

CLASS Antipsychotic, dopaminergic blocker
PREG/CONT C/NA

BBW Increased risk of mortality when antipsychotics used in elderly pts w/ dementia-related psychosis. Avoid this use; not approved for this use. Increased risk of potentially fatal bronchospasm w/ inhaled form; available only through limited release program; monitor pt closely.

IND & DOSE Tx of schizophrenia. *Adult:* 10 mg PO bid; max, 50 mg/day. Increase fairly rapidly over first 7–10 days until symptoms controlled; range, 60–100 mg/day PO. Dosage over 250 mg/day PO not recommended. For maint: range, 20–60 mg/day PO. **Acute tx of agitation associated w/ schizophrenia, bipolar disorder.** *Adult:* 10 mg/24 hr by oral inhalation using inhaler.

ADJUST DOSE Elderly pts
ADV EFF Bone marrow suppression, **bronchospasm**, drowsiness, dry mouth, extrapyramidal symptoms,

gynecomastia, **laryngospasm,** photosensitivity, rash, **refractory arrhythmias**
INTERACTIONS CNS drugs, drugs that affect airway disease (inhaled form)
NC/PT Ensure hydration of elderly pts. Monitor CBC; stop if seizure. Screen pulmonary hx and examine pt before using inhaled form; inhaled form available only through restricted access program. Pt should take safety precautions w/ CNS effects, avoid sun exposure, report unusual bleeding, infections, palpitations. Name confusion w/ *Loxitane* (loxapine), *Lexapro* (escitalopram), *Soriatane* (acitretin); use caution.

---

lucinactant (Surfaxin)
CLASS Lung surfactant
PREG/CONT Unkn/NA

IND & DOSE Px of RDS in premature infants at high risk for RDS.
Infant: 5.8 mL/kg birth weight intratracheally. Up to four doses within first 48 hr of life; space no less than 16 hr.
ADV EFF Acute change in lung compliance, ET tube obstruction, ET tube reflux, oxygen desaturation
NC/PT Ensure proper placement of ET tube. Warm vial, shake vigorously before use; discard after 2 hr. Do not suction for 1 hr after dosing. Monitor color, breath sounds, oximetry, blood gases continually. Incorporate teaching into parents' comprehensive teaching plan for premature infant.

---

lurasidone hydrochloride (Latuda)
CLASS Atypical antipsychotic
PREG/CONT B/NA

BBW Increased risk of mortality when antipsychotics used in elderly pts w/ dementia-related psychosis. Avoid this use; not approved for this use. Increased risk of suicidality in child, adolescent, young adult; monitor accordingly.

IND & DOSE Tx of schizophrenia.
Adult: 40 mg/day PO w/ food; may titrate to max 80 mg/day PO.
ADJUST DOSE Hepatic, renal impairment
ADV EFF Akathisia, dystonia, hyperglycemia, **NMS,** n/v/d, parkinsonism, **suicidality,** weight gain
INTERACTIONS Alcohol, grapefruit juice, strong CYP3A4 inducers/inhibitors
NC/PT Dispense least amount possible to suicidal pts. Not for use in breast-feeding. Pt should take safety measures w/ CNS effects, monitor serum glucose/weight gain, avoid alcohol, report increased thirst/appetite, thoughts of suicide.

---

macitentan (Opsumit)
CLASS Endothelin receptor blocker, pulmonary hypertension drug
PREG/CONT X/NA

BBW Known teratogen; life-threatening birth defects possible. Available by limited access program for women. Monthly pregnancy tests required.
IND & DOSE Tx of pulmonary artery hypertension. *Adult:* 10 mg/day PO.
ADV EFF Anemia, bronchitis, decreased Hgb, headache, **hepatotoxicity,** nasopharyngitis, **pulmonary edema,** reduced sperm count, UTI
INTERACTIONS Ketoconazole, rifampin, ritonavir; avoid these combinations
NC/PT Ensure proper dx, negative monthly pregnancy test for women. Monitor LFTs, Hgb, respiratory status. Female pt should avoid pregnancy (contraceptives required), breast-feeding; males should be aware of reduced sperm count. Pt should monitor activity tolerance; report difficulty breathing, color changes in urine/stool, extreme fatigue.

magnesium salts, magnesia, magnesium citrate (Citroma), magnesium hydroxide (Milk of Magnesia), magnesium oxide (Mag-Ox)

CLASS Antacid, laxative
PREG/CONT C; A (antacids); B (laxative)/NA

IND & DOSE *Laxative. Adult:* 300 mL (citrate) PO w/ full glass of water, or 15–60 mL (hydroxide) PO w/ liquid. *Child 12 and older:* 30–60 mL (400 mg/5 mL) (hydroxide) PO w/ water or 15–30 mL/day (800 mg/5 mL) PO once daily at bedtime, or eight 311-mg tablets PO once daily at bedtime or in divided doses. *Child 6–11 yr:* 15–30 mL (400 mg/5 mL) (hydroxide) PO once daily at bedtime, or 7.5–15 mL (800 mg/5 mL) PO once daily at bedtime, or four 311-mg tablets/day PO at bedtime. *Child 2–5 yr:* 5–15 mL (400 mg/5 mL) PO once daily at bedtime, or two 311-mg tablets/day PO at bedtime. *Antacid. Adult:* 5–15 mL (hydroxide) qid or 622–1,244-mg tablets PO qid (adult, pt over 12 yr). *Supplemental magnesium replacement. Adult:* Magnesium oxide capsules, 140 mg PO tid–qid. Tablets, 400–800 mg/day PO.
ADV EFF Dizziness, hypermagnesemia, n/v/d, perianal irritation
INTERACTIONS Fluoroquinolones, ketoconazole, nitrofurantoin, penicillamine, tetracyclines
NC/PT Pt should avoid other oral drugs within 1–2 hr of antacids, take between meals and at bedtime, chew antacid tablet thoroughly, avoid long-term laxative use, avoid laxatives if abd pain, n/v occur, maintain hydration, report rectal bleeding, weakness.

DANGEROUS DRUG

magnesium sulfate (generic)

CLASS Antiepileptic, electrolyte, laxative
PREG/CONT A; B (laxative)/NA

IND & DOSE *Control of hypertension w/ acute nephritis. Child:* 100 mg/kg (0.8 mEq/kg or 0.2 mL/kg of 50% sol) IM q 4–6 hr as needed. Or, 20–40 mg/kg (0.16–0.32 mEq/kg or 0.1–0.2 mL/kg of 20% sol) IM. Or, for severe symptoms, 100–200 mg/kg of 1%–3% sol IV over 1 hr w/ half of dose given in first 15–20 min (seizure control). *Laxative. Adult:* 10–30 g/day PO. *Child 6–11 yr:* 5–10 g/day PO; 15–30 mL/day PO. *Child 2–5 yr:* 2.5–5 g/day PO; 5–15 mL/day PO. *Tx of arrhythmias. Adult:* 3–4 g IV over several min; then 3–20 mg/min continuous infusion for 5–48 hr. *Tx of eclampsia, severe preeclampsia. Adult:* 10–14 g IV. May infuse 4–5 g in 250 mL 5% dextrose injection or normal saline while giving IM doses up to 10 g (5 g or 10 mL of undiluted 50% sol in each buttock). Or, may give initial 4 g IV by diluting 50% sol to 10% or 20%; may inject diluted fluid (40 mL of 10% or 20 mL of 20% sol) IV over 3–4 min. Then inject 4–5 g (8–10 mL of 50% sol) IM into alternate buttocks q 4 hr as needed depending on patellar reflex, respiratory function. Or, after initial IV dose, may give 1–2 g/hr by constant IV infusion. Continue until paroxysms stop. To control seizures, optimal serum magnesium level is 6 mg/100 mL; max, 30–40 g/24 hr. *Correction of hypomagnesemia. Adult:* 1 g IM or IV q 6 hr for four doses (32.5 mEq/24 hr); up to 246 mg/kg IM within 4 hr or 5 g (40 mEq)/1,000 mL D₅W or normal saline IV infused over 3 hr for severe cases. *Parenteral nutrition. Adult:* 8–24 mEq/day IV.
ADJUST DOSE Renal impairment

ADV EFF Dizziness, excessive bowel activity, fainting, magnesium intoxication, perianal irritation, weakness
INTERACTIONS Adult, aminoglycosides, amphotericin B, cisplatin, cyclosporine, digoxin, diuretics, NMJ blockers
NC/PT Monitor serum magnesium level during parenteral tx; normal limits, 1.5–3 mEq/L. Save IV use in eclampsia for life-threatening situations. Monitor knee-jerk reflex before repeated parenteral administration. If knee-jerk reflex suppressed, do not give. Use as temporary relief of constipation; stop if diarrhea occurs.

mannitol (Osmitrol)
CLASS Diagnostic agent, osmotic diuretic, urinary irrigant
PREG/CONT B/NA

IND & DOSE Px of oliguria in renal failure. *Adult:* 50–100 g IV as 5%–25% sol. Tx of oliguria in renal failure. *Adult:* 50–100 g IV as 15%–25% sol. To reduce intracranial pressure, cerebral edema. *Adult:* 1.5–2 g/kg IV as 15%–25% sol over 30–60 min. Reduced pressure should be evident in 15 min. Reduction of IOP. *Adult:* 1.5–2 g/kg IV infusion as 25%, 20%, or 15% sol over 30 min. If used preop, give 60–90 min before surgery for max effect. Adjunct tx to promote diuresis in intoxication. *Adult:* Max 200 g IV mannitol w/ other fluids, electrolytes. To measure GFR. *Adult:* Dilute 100 mL of 20% sol w/ 180 mL sodium chloride injection. Infuse this 280 mL of 7.2% sol IV at 20 mL/min. Collect urine w/ catheter for specified time to measure mannitol excreted in mg/min. Draw blood at start and end of time for mannitol measurement in mg/mL plasma. Test dose of mannitol in pts w/ inadequate renal function. *Adult:* 0.2 g/kg IV (about 50 mL of 25% sol, 75 mL of 20% sol) in 3–5 min to produce urine flow of 30–50 mL/hr. If urine flow not increased,

repeat dose. If no response to second dose, reevaluate situation.
ADV EFF Anorexia, diuresis, dizziness, dry mouth, n/v, **seizures**, thirst
NC/PT Do not give electrolyte-free mannitol w/ blood. If blood must be given, add at least 20 mEq sodium chloride to each liter mannitol sol; use filter. Monitor serum electrolytes periodically. Pt should use sugarless lozenges for dry mouth, take safety precautions w/ CNS effects.

maprotiline hydrochloride (generic)
CLASS TCA
PREG/CONT B/NA

BBW Increased risk of suicidal thinking, behavior in children, adolescents, young adults; monitor accordingly.
IND & DOSE Tx of mild to moderate depression. *Adult:* 75 mg/day PO in outpts; after 2 wk may increase gradually in 25-mg increments. Usual dose, 150 mg/day. Tx of severe depression. *Adult:* 100–150 mg/day PO in inpts; may gradually increase to 225 mg/day. Maint tx of depression. *Adult:* Use lowest effective dose, usually 75–150 mg/day PO.
ADJUST DOSE Elderly pts
ADV EFF Confusion, constipation, disturbed conc, dry mouth, gynecomastia, **MI**, orthostatic hypotension, peripheral neuropathy, photosensitivity, rash, restlessness, sedation, **stroke**, urine retention
INTERACTIONS Alcohol, anticholinergics, phenothiazines, sympathomimetics, thyroid medication
NC/PT Limit access to depressed/potentially suicidal pts. Expect clinical response in 3 wk. Give at bedtime if orthostatic hypotension occurs. Not for use in pregnancy (barrier contraceptives advised). Pt should avoid alcohol, sun exposure; report numbness/tingling, chest pain, thoughts of suicide.

198   maraviroc (Selzentry)

maraviroc (Selzentry)

CLASS Antiviral, CCR5 coreceptor antagonist
PREG/CONT B/NA

BBW Risk of severe hepatotoxicity, possibly preceded by systemic allergic reaction (rash, eosinophilia, elevated IgE level). Immediately evaluate, support pt w/ s&sx of hepatitis, allergic reaction.

IND & DOSE Combination antiretroviral tx of pts infected only w/ detectable CCR5-tropic HIV-1. *Adult, child over 16 yr:* W/ strong CYP3A inhibitors, protease inhibitors (except tipranavir/ritonavir), delavirdine, 150 mg PO bid. W/ tipranavir/ritonavir, nevirapine, enfuvirtide, nucleoside reverse transcriptase inhibitors, other drugs that are not strong CYP3A inhibitors, 300 mg PO bid. W/ efavirenz, rifampin, carbamazepine, phenobarbital, phenytoin, 600 mg PO bid.

ADJUST DOSE Renal impairment
ADV EFF Abd pain, cough, dizziness, fever, headache, **hepatotoxicity**, musculoskeletal symptoms, rash
INTERACTIONS CYP3A inducers/inhibitors, St. John's wort
NC/PT Give w/ other antiretrovirals. Monitor LFTs, CD4. Use caution in pregnancy; not for use in breast-feeding. Pt should swallow tablet whole and not cut, crush, or chew it; take precautions to prevent spread (drug not a cure); avoid St. John's wort; take safety precautions w/ CNS effects.

mecasermin (Increlex)

CLASS Insulin-like growth factor-1
PREG/CONT C/NA

IND & DOSE Long-term tx of growth failure in child w/ severe primary insulin growth factor-1 deficiency or w/ growth hormone gene deletion who has developed neutralizing antibodies to growth hormone. *Child 2 yr and over:* Initially, 0.04–0.08 mg/kg (40–80 mcg/kg) bid by subcut injection shortly before meal or snack; may be increased by 0.04 mg/kg/dose to max of 0.12 mg/kg bid.

ADV EFF Hypersensitivity reactions, hypoglycemia, **intracranial hypertension**, progression of scoliosis, slipped capital femoral epiphysis, tonsillar hypertrophy
NC/PT Monitor blood glucose, tonsils. Ensure given just before meal or snack. Pt should avoid pregnancy, breast-feeding; learn proper administration/disposal of needles, syringes; report difficulty breathing/swallowing, sudden limb or hip/knee pain, injection site pain, rash.

DANGEROUS DRUG

mechlorethamine hydrochloride (Mustargen, Valchlor)

CLASS Alkylating agent, antineoplastic, nitrogen mustard
PREG/CONT D/NA

BBW Handle drug with caution; use chemo-safe nonpermeable gloves. Drug highly toxic and a vesicant. Avoid inhaling dust, vapors; avoid contact w/ skin, mucous membranes (especially eyes). If eye contact, immediately irrigate w/ copious amount of ophthalmic irrigating sol, get ophthalmologic consultation. If skin contact, irrigate w/ copious amount of water for 15 min, then apply 2% sodium thiosulfate. Monitor injection site for extravasation. Painful inflammation/induration, skin sloughing possible. If leakage, promptly infiltrate w/ sterile isotonic sodium thiosulfate (1/6M), apply ice compress for 6–12 hr. Notify physician.

IND & DOSE Palliative tx of bronchogenic carcinoma, Hodgkin disease, lymphosarcoma, CML, chronic lymphocytic leukemia, mycosis fungoides, polycythemia vera.

Adult: Total 0.4 mg/kg IV for each course as single dose or in two to four divided doses of 0.1–0.2 mg/kg/day. Give at night if sedation needed for side effects. Interval between courses usually 3–4 wk. **Palliative tx of effusion secondary to metastatic carcinoma.** *Adult:* Dose, preparation for intracavity use vary greatly; usual dose, 0.2–0.4 mg/kg. **Tx of stage 1A, 1B mycosis fungoides–type T-cell lymphoma after direct skin tx.** *Adult:* Apply thin film to affected areas of skin; avoid eyes and mucous membranes.

ADV EFF Anorexia, **bone marrow suppression,** dizziness, drowsiness, impaired fertility, n/v/d, thrombophlebitis, weakness

INTERACTIONS Adalimumab, denosumab, infliximab, leflunomide, natalizumab, pimecrolimus, roflumilast

NC/PT Avoid skin contact w/ powder for injection. Premedicate w/ antiemetics, sedatives. Monitor CBC closely, injection site for extravasation. Maintain hydration. Not for use in pregnancy (contraceptives advised). Pt should have safety precautions w/ CNS changes; avoid smoking, open flames when using topical gel until gel dries (very flammable); report burning at IV site, fever.

---

meclizine hydrochloride
(Antivert, Bonine, Dramamine)

CLASS Anticholinergic, antiemetic, antihistamine, anti-motion sickness

PREG/CONT B/NA

IND & DOSE Px, tx of motion sickness. *Adult, child over 12 yr:* 25–50 mg/day PO 1 hr before travel. **Tx of vertigo.** *Adult, child over 12 yr:* 25–100 mg/day PO.

ADJUST DOSE Elderly pts

ADV EFF Anorexia, confusion, drowsiness, dry mouth, nausea, **respiratory depression to death,** urinary difficulty/frequency

INTERACTIONS Alcohol, CNS depressants

NC/PT For anti–motion sickness, works best if used before motion. Pt should avoid alcohol, take safety precautions w/ CNS experience, use sugarless lozenges for dry mouth, report difficulty breathing.

---

medroxyPROGESTERone acetate (Depo-Provera, depo-subQ provera 104, Provera)

CLASS Antineoplastic, contraceptive, hormone, progestin

PREG/CONT X/NA

BBW Before tx, rule out pregnancy; caution pt to avoid pregnancy and have frequent medical follow-up. Alert pt using contraceptive injections that drug does not protect from HIV, other STDs, and to take precautions. *Depo-Provera* use may result in significant bone density loss; drug should not be used for longer than 2 yr unless other contraception form is adequate.

IND & DOSE Contraception. *Adult:* 150 mg IM q 3 mo. For *depo-subQ provera:* 104 mg subcut into thigh or abdomen q 12–14 wk. **Tx of secondary amenorrhea.** *Adult:* 5–10 mg/day PO for 5–10 days. **Tx of abnormal uterine bleeding.** *Adult:* 5–10 mg/day PO for 5–10 days, starting on 16th or 21st day of menstrual cycle. **Tx of endometrial, renal carcinoma.** *Adult:* 400–1,000 mg/ wk IM. **To reduce endometrial hyperplasia.** *Adult:* 5–10 mg/day PO for 12–14 consecutive days/mo. Start on 1st or 16th day of cycle. **Mgt of endometriosis-associated pain.** *Adult:* 104 mg subcut *(depo-subQ Provera)* into anterior thigh or abdomen q 12–14 wk for no longer than 2 yr.

ADV EFF Amenorrhea, breakthrough bleeding, edema, fluid retention, menstrual flow changes, rash,

thromboembolic events, vision changes, weight changes
NC/PT Arrange for pretreatment, periodic (at least annual) complete hx, physical. Not for use in pregnancy. Pt should know drug does not protect against STDs, HIV; protection is still required. Pt should mark calendar for tx days, report sudden vision loss, swelling, severe headache.

mefenamic acid (Ponstel)
CLASS NSAID
PREG/CONT C/NA

BBW Increased risk of CV events, GI bleeding; monitor accordingly. Do not use for periop pain in CABG surgery.
IND & DOSE Tx of acute pain. *Adult, child over 14 yr:* 500 mg PO, then 250 mg q hr as needed for up to 1 wk. **Tx of primary dysmenorrhea.** *Adult, child over 14 yr:* 500 mg PO, then 250 mg q 6 hr starting w/ bleeding onset. Can initiate at start of menses, then for 2–3 days.
ADJUST DOSE Elderly pts, renal impairment (not recommended)
ADV EFF Anaphylactoid reactions to anaphylactic shock, bone marrow suppression, constipation, diarrhea, dizziness, dyspepsia, edema, GI pain, headache, nausea, rash, renal impairment
INTERACTIONS ASA, anticoagulants, methotrexate, NSAIDs
NC/PT Pt should take w/ food, use safety precautions w/ CNS effects, stop drug and report rash, diarrhea, black tarry stools.

DANGEROUS DRUG
(AS ANTINEOPLASTIC)

megestrol acetate (Megace)
CLASS Antineoplastic, hormone, progestin
PREG/CONT X (suspension); D (tablets)/NA

BBW Caution pt not to use if pregnant; fetal risks. Advise barrier con-

traceptives. Risk of thromboembolic events, stop drug at sx of thrombosis.
IND & DOSE Palliative tx of breast cancer. *Adult:* 160 mg/day PO (40 mg qid). **Palliative tx of endometrial cancer.** *Adult:* 40–320 mg/day PO. **Tx of cachexia w/ HIV.** *Adult:* 800 mg/day PO; range, 400–800 mg/day (suspension only) or 625 mg/day PO (ES suspension)
ADV EFF Amenorrhea, breakthrough bleeding, dizziness, edema, fluid retention, menstrual flow changes, photosensitivity, rash, somnolence, **thromboembolic events,** vision changes, weight changes
NC/PT Stop if thromboembolic events. Store suspension in cool place; shake well before use. Not for use in pregnancy (barrier contraceptives advised). Pt should avoid sun exposure; take safety precautions w/ CNS effects; report chest/leg pain, swelling, numbness/tingling, severe headache.

meloxicam (Mobic)
CLASS NSAID
PREG/CONT C (1st, 2nd trimesters); D (3rd trimester)/NA

BBW Increased risk of CV events, GI bleeding; monitor accordingly. Do not use for periop pain in CABG surgery.
IND & DOSE Relief of s&sx of osteoarthritis, rheumatoid arthritis. *Adult:* 7.5 mg/day PO. Max, 15 mg/day. **Relief of s&sx of pauciarticular/polyarticular course juvenile rheumatoid arthritis.** *Child 2 yr and older:* 0.125 mg/kg/day PO; max, 7.5 mg (oral suspension)
ADV EFF Anaphylactic shock, bone marrow suppression, diarrhea, dizziness, dyspepsia, edema, GI pain, headache, insomnia, nausea, rash
INTERACTIONS ACE inhibitors, aspirin, anticoagulants, diuretics, lithium, methotrexate, oral corticosteroids
NC/PT Pt should take w/ food, use safety precautions w/ CNS effects,

report difficulty breathing, swelling, black tarry stools.

DANGEROUS DRUG
melphalan (Alkeran)
CLASS Alkylating agent, antineoplastic, nitrogen mustard
PREG/CONT D/NA

BBW Arrange for blood tests to evaluate hematopoietic function before and wkly during tx; severe bone marrow suppression possible. Caution pt to avoid pregnancy during tx; drug considered mutagenic.

IND & DOSE Tx of multiple myeloma. *Adult:* 6 mg/day PO. After 2–3 wk, stop for up to 4 wk; monitor blood counts. When counts rising, start maint of 2 mg/day PO. Or, 16 mg/m² as single IV infusion over 15–20 min at 2-wk intervals for four doses, then at 4-wk intervals. Tx of epithelial ovarian carcinoma. *Adult:* 0.2 mg/kg/ day PO for 5 days as single course. Repeat courses q 4–5 wk.

ADJUST DOSE Renal impairment
ADV EFF Alopecia, amenorrhea, anaphylaxis, bone marrow suppression, cancer, n/v, pulmonary fibrosis, rash
NC/PT Refrigerate tablets in glass bottle. Monitor CBC regularly; dose adjustment may be needed. Maintain hydration. Give antiemetics for severe nausea. Not for use in pregnancy (barrier contraceptives advised). Pt should cover head at temp extremes (hair loss possible), avoid exposure to infection, report bleeding, signs of infection.

memantine hydrochloride (Namenda)
CLASS Alzheimer drug; *N*-methyl-*D*-aspartate receptor antagonist
PREG/CONT B/NA

IND & DOSE Tx of moderate to severe Alzheimer-type dementia.

Adult: 5 mg/day PO. Increase at wkly intervals to 5 mg PO bid (10 mg/day), 15 mg/day PO (5-mg and 10-mg doses) w/ at least 1 wk between increases. Target, 20 mg/day (10 mg bid). ER form: 7 mg/day PO; may increase by 7 mg/day after at least 1 wk. Maint, 28 mg/day

ADJUST DOSE Renal impairment
ADV EFF Confusion, constipation, cough, dizziness, fatigue, headache
INTERACTIONS Amantadine, carbonic anhydrase inhibitors, dextromethorphan, ketamine, sodium bicarbonate, urine alkalinizers
NC/PT Obtain baseline functional profile. Not a cure; medical follow-up needed. Pt should swallow ER tablet whole and not cut, crush, or chew it; take safety precaution w/ CNS effects; report lack of improvement, swelling, respiratory problems.

menotropins (Menopur, Repronex)
CLASS Fertility drug, hormone
PREG/CONT X/NA

IND & DOSE To induce ovulation in anovulatory women, w/ HCG. *Adult:* 225 units IM; then 75–150 units/day subcut to max 450 units/day for no longer than 12 days (*Repronex*) or 20 days (*Menopur*). Or, pts who have received GnRH agonists or pituitary suppression: 150 international units/day subcut or IM (*Repronex*) for first 5 days; max, 450 international units/day. Use no longer than 12 days.

ADV EFF Dizziness, febrile reactions, multiple births, ovarian enlargement, ovarian overstimulation, thromboembolic events
NC/PT Must follow w/ HCG when clinical evidence shows sufficient follicular maturation based on urine excretion of estrogens. Dissolve contents of 1–6 vials in 1–2 mL sterile saline; give immediately. Monitor for ovarian overstimulation; admit pt to hosp for tx. Risk of multiple births. Teach proper administration, disposal

of needles, syringes. Pt should mark calendar of tx days, report severe abd pain, fever.

meperidine hydrochloride (Demerol, Meperitab)

CLASS Opioid agonist analgesic
PREG/CONT B; D (long-term use)/NA

IND & DOSE Relief of moderate to severe acute pain. *Adult:* 50–150 mg IM, subcut, or PO q 3–4 hr as needed. May give diluted subcut by slow IV injection. IM route preferred for repeated injections. *Child:* 1.1–1.75 mg/kg IM, subcut, or PO up to adult dose q 3–4 hr as needed. **Preop medication.** *Adult:* 50–100 mg IM or subcut 30–90 min before anesthesia. *Child:* 1.1–2.2 mg/kg IM or subcut, up to adult dose, 30–90 min before anesthesia. **Anesthesia support.** *Adult:* Dilute to 10 mg/mL; give repeated doses by slow IV injection. Or, dilute to 1 mg/mL; infuse continuously. **Obstetric analgesia.** *Adult:* When contractions regular, 50–100 mg IM or subcut; repeat q 1–3 hr.
ADJUST DOSE Elderly, debilitated pts; hepatic, renal impairment
ADV EFF Apnea, cardiac arrest, circulatory depression, constipation, dizziness, light-headedness, n/v, respiratory arrest/depression, shock, sweating
INTERACTIONS Alcohol, barbiturate anesthetics, CNS depressants, MAOIs, phenothiazines. Incompatible w/ sols of barbiturates, aminophylline, heparin, iodide, morphine sulfate, methicillin, phenytoin, sodium bicarbonate, sulfadiazine, sulfisoxazole
NC/PT Contraindicated in preterm infants. May give diluted sol by slow IV injection. IM route preferred for repeated injections. Have opioid antagonist, facilities for assisted or controlled respiration on hand during parenteral administration. Pt should take safety precautions w/ CNS effects; use laxative if constipated; take drug 4–6 hr before next feeding if breast-feeding; report difficulty breathing.

meprobamate (generic)

CLASS Anxiolytic
PREG/CONT D/C-IV

IND & DOSE Mgt of anxiety disorders. *Adult:* 1,200–1,600 mg/day PO in three or four divided doses. Max, 2,400 mg/day. *Child 6–12 yr:* 100–200 mg PO bid–tid.
ADJUST DOSE Elderly pts
ADV EFF Ataxia, bone marrow suppression, dependence w/ withdrawal reactions, dizziness, drowsiness, headache, impaired vision, hypotensive crisis, n/v/d, rash, suicidality, vertigo
INTERACTIONS Alcohol, CNS depressants, barbiturates, opioids
NC/PT Dispense least amount possible to depressed/addiction-prone pts. Withdraw gradually over 2 wk after long-term use. Not for use in pregnancy (barrier contraceptives advised). Pt should avoid alcohol, take safety precautions w/ CNS effects, report thoughts of suicide.

mercaptopurine (Purinethol)

CLASS Antimetabolite, antineoplastic
PREG/CONT D/NA

BBW Reserve for pts w/ established dx of acute lymphatic leukemia; serious adverse effects possible.
IND & DOSE Maint tx of acute leukemia (lymphocytic, lymphoblastic). *Adult, child:* Induction, 2.5 mg/kg/day PO (about 100–200 mg in adult, 50 mg in average 5-yr-old); may increase to 5 mg/kg/day. Maint tx after complete hematologic

remission, 1.5–2.5 mg/kg/ day PO as single daily dose.

ADJUST DOSE Renal impairment
ADV EFF Bone marrow depression, hepatosplenic T-cell lymphoma, hepatotoxicity, hyperuricemia, immunosuppression, n/v, stomatitis
INTERACTIONS Allopurinol, TNF blockers

NC/PT Monitor CBC regularly; dose adjustment may be needed. Not for use in pregnancy (barrier contraceptives advised), breast-feeding. Maintain hydration. Pt should get regular checkups, report night sweats, fever, abd pain, weight loss. Name confusion between *Purinethol* (mercaptopurine) and propylthiouracil; use caution.

---

meropenem (Merrem IV)
CLASS Carbapenem antibiotic
PREG/CONT B/NA

IND & DOSE Tx of meningitis, intra-abdominal infections caused by susceptible strains. *Adult:* 1 g IV q 8 hr. *Child 3 mo and older:* For meningitis: Over 50 kg, 2 g IV q 8 hr; under 50 kg, 40 mg/kg IV q 8 hr. For intra-abdominal infections: Over 50 kg, 1 g IV q 8 hr; under 50 kg, 20 mg/kg IV q 8 hr. Tx of skin/skin-structure infections caused by susceptible strains. *Adult:* 500 mg IV q 8 hr. *Child 3 mo and older:* Over 50 kg, 500 mg IV q 8 hr; under 50 kg, 10 mg/kg IV q 8 hr.

ADJUST DOSE Renal impairment
ADV EFF Abd pain, anorexia, flatulence, headache, n/v/d, phlebitis, **pseudomembranous colitis**, rash, superinfections
INTERACTIONS Probenecid, valproic acid

NC/PT Culture before tx. Do not mix in sol w/ other drugs. Stop if s&sx of colitis. Pt should report severe diarrhea, pain at injection site.

---

mesalamine (Apriso, Asacol, Lialda, Pentasa, Rowasa)
CLASS Anti-inflammatory
PREG/CONT B/NA

IND & DOSE Tx of active mild to moderate ulcerative colitis. *Adult:* 2–4 1.2-g tablets PO once daily w/ food for total 2.4–4.8 g (*Lialda*). Or, 1.5 g/day PO (4 capsules) in a.m. for up to 6 mo (*Apriso*). Or, 1 g PO qid for total daily dose of 4 g for up to 8 wk (*Pentasa*). Or, 1.6 g/day PO in divided doses (*Asacol*). Or, 800 mg PO tid for 6 wk (*Asacol HD*). Tx of active, distal, mild to moderate ulcerative colitis/ proctitis, proctosigmoiditis. *Adult:* 60-mL units in 1 rectal instillation (4 g) once/day, preferably at bedtime, retained for approximately 8 hr for 3–6 wk. Effects may occur within 3–21 days. Or, 1 g (1 suppository) bid retained for 1–3 hr or longer. Usual course, 3–6 wk.

ADV EFF Abd pain, cramps, fatigue, fever, flatulence, flulike sx, gas, headache, malaise
NC/PT Products vary; use caution to differentiate doses. Teach proper rectal suppository, retention enema administration. Pt should swallow tablet whole and not cut, crush, or chew it; report severe abd pain, difficulty breathing. Name confusion w/ mesalamine, methenamine, memantine; use caution.

---

mesna (Mesnex)
CLASS Cytoprotective
PREG/CONT B/NA

IND & DOSE Px to reduce incidence of ifosfamide-induced hemorrhagic cystitis. *Adult:* 20% ifosfamide dose IV at time of ifosfamide infusion and at 4 and 8 hr after; timing must be exact.

ADV EFF Abd pain, alopecia, anemia, anorexia, constipation, fatigue, fever, n/v, thrombocytopenia

NC/PT Helps prevent chemotherapy complications. Timing critical to balance chemotherapy effects. May give antiemetics. Pt should report severe abd pain.

metaproterenol sulfate (generic)

CLASS Antiasthmatic, beta₂-selective agonist, bronchodilator
PREG/CONT C/NA

IND & DOSE Px, tx of bronchial asthma, reversible bronchospasm. *Adult, child 12 yr and older:* 20 mg PO tid to qid. *Child over 9–under 12 yr, over 27 kg:* 20 mg PO tid to qid. *Child 6–9 yr, under 27 kg:* 10 mg PO tid to qid.
ADJUST DOSE Elderly pts
ADV EFF Anxiety, apprehension, CNS stimulation, fear, flushing, heartburn, n/v, pallor, sweating, tachycardia
NC/PT Switch to syrup if swallowing difficult. Do not exceed recommended dose. Protect tablets from moisture. Pt should take safety precautions w/ CNS effects, report chest pain, difficulty breathing.

metaxalone (Skelaxin)

CLASS Skeletal muscle relaxant (centrally acting)
PREG/CONT C/NA

IND & DOSE Adjunct for relief of discomfort associated w/ acute, painful musculoskeletal disorders. *Adult, child 12 yr and older:* 800 mg PO tid to qid.
ADV EFF Dizziness, drowsiness, hemolytic anemia, leukopenia, lightheadedness, nausea
INTERACTIONS Alcohol, CNS depressants
NC/PT Arrange for other tx for muscle spasm relief. Pt should take safety precautions w/ CNS effects, avoid alcohol, report rash, yellowing of skin/eyes.

DANGEROUS DRUG

metformin hydrochloride (Fortamet, Glucophage, Glumetza, Riomet)

CLASS Antidiabetic
PREG/CONT B/NA

BBW Risk of severe lactic acidosis. Monitor pt; treat if suspicion of lactic acidosis.
IND & DOSE Adjunct to diet to lower blood glucose in type 2 diabetes, alone or w/ sulfonylurea. *Adult:* 500 mg PO bid or 850 mg PO once daily; max, 2,550 mg/day in divided doses. ER tablet: 1,000 mg/day PO w/ evening meal; max, 2,000 mg/day (2,500 *Fortamet*). *Child 10–16 yr:* 500 mg bid w/ meals. Max, 2,000 mg/day in divided doses. ER form not recommended for child.
ADJUST DOSE Elderly pts, renal impairment
ADV EFF Allergic skin reactions, anorexia, gastric discomfort, heartburn, hypoglycemia, **lactic acidosis**, n/v/d
INTERACTIONS Alcohol, amiloride, celery, cimetidine, coriander, dandelion root, digoxin, fenugreek, furosemide, garlic, ginseng, iodinated contrast media, juniper berries, sulfonylureas, vancomycin
NC/PT Monitor serum glucose frequently to determine drug effectiveness, dose. Arrange for transfer to insulin during high-stress periods. Not for use in pregnancy. Pt should swallow ER tablet whole and not cut, crush, or chew it; take at night if GI problems; avoid alcohol; continue diet, exercise program; report all herbs used (so dose adjustment can be made), hypoglycemic episodes, urine/stool color changes.

DANGEROUS DRUG

methadone hydrochloride (Dolophine, Methadose)

CLASS Opioid agonist analgesic
PREG/CONT C/C-II

BBW Use for opioid addiction should be part of approved program; deaths have occurred during start of tx for opioid dependence. Carefully determine all drugs pt taking. Have emergency services on standby. Monitor for prolonged QT interval, especially at higher doses.
IND & DOSE Relief of severe pain unresponsive to nonopioid analgesics. *Adult:* 2.5–10 mg IM, subcut, or PO q 8–12 hr as needed. **Detoxification, temporary maint tx of opioid addiction.** *Adult:* 20–30 mg PO or parenteral; PO preferred. Increase to suppress withdrawal s&sx; 40 mg/day in single or divided doses is usual stabilizing dose. Continue stabilizing doses for 2–3 days, then gradually decrease q 1 or 2 days. Provide sufficient amount to keep withdrawal sx tolerable. Max, 21 days' tx; do not repeat earlier than 4 wk after completion of previous course. For maint tx: For heavy heroin users up until hospital admission, initially 20 mg PO 4–8 hr after heroin stopped or 40 mg PO in single dose; may give additional 10-mg doses if needed to suppress withdrawal syndrome. Adjust dose to max 120 mg/day PO.
ADJUST DOSE Elderly pts, impaired adults
ADV EFF Apnea, cardiac arrest, circulatory depression, constipation, dizziness, light-headedness, n/v, **prolonged QT interval, respiratory arrest, respiratory depression, shock,** sweating
INTERACTIONS Barbiturate anesthetics, HIV antiretrovirals, hydantoins, protease inhibitors, QT-prolonging drugs, rifampin, urine acidifiers
NC/PT Have opioid antagonist, equipment for assisted or controlled

respiration on hand during parenteral administration. Not for use in pregnancy (barrier contraceptives advised). Pt should take drug 4–6 hr before next feeding if breast-feeding, avoid alcohol, take safety precautions w/ CNS effects, report difficulty breathing, severe n/v.

methazolamide (generic)

CLASS Carbonic anhydrase inhibitor, glaucoma drug
PREG/CONT C/NA

IND & DOSE Tx of ocular conditions where lowering IOP is beneficial. *Adult:* 50–100 mg PO bid-tid.
ADJUST DOSE Hepatic, renal impairment
ADV EFF Anorexia, **bone marrow suppression,** dizziness, drowsiness, fatigue, GI disturbances, kidney stones, photosensitivity, **Stevens-Johnson syndrome,** taste alteration, tingling, tinnitus
INTERACTIONS Aspirin, corticosteroids
NC/PT Monitor IOP regularly. Pt should take safety precautions w/ CNS effects; avoid exposure sun, infection; report fever, rash.

methenamine (generic), methenamine hippurate (Hiprex, Urex)

CLASS Antibacterial, urinary tract anti-infective
PREG/CONT C/NA

IND & DOSE To suppress, eliminate bacteriuria associated w/ UTIs. *Adult:* 1 g methenamine PO qid after meals and at bedtime, or 1 g hippurate PO bid. *Child 6–12 yr:* 500 mg methenamine PO qid, or 0.5–1 g hippurate PO bid. *Child under 6 yr:* 50 mg/kg/day PO methenamine divided into three doses.
ADV EFF Bladder irritation, dysuria, **hepatotoxicity** (hippurate), nausea, rash

NC/PT Culture before tx. Maintain hydration. Monitor LFTs w/ hippurate form. Use additional measures for UTIs. It should take w/ food, report rash, stool/urine color changes. Name confusion between methimazole and mesalamine; use caution.

methimazole (Tapazole)
CLASS Antithyroid drug
PREG/CONT D/NA

IND & DOSE Tx of hyperthyroidism; palliation in certain thyroid cancers. *Adult:* 15–60 mg/day PO in three equal doses q 8 hr. Maint, 5–15 mg/day PO. *Child:* 0.4 mg/kg/day PO, then maint of approximately ½ initial dose. Or, initially, 0.5–0.7 mg/kg/day or 15–20 mg/m²/day in three divided doses, then maint of ⅓–⅔ initial dose, starting when pt becomes euthyroid. Max, 30 mg/24 hr.

ADV EFF Bone marrow suppression, dizziness, neuritis, paresthesia, rash, vertigo, weakness
INTERACTIONS Cardiac glycosides, metoprolol, oral anticoagulants, propranolol, theophylline
NC/PT Monitor CBC, thyroid function. Tx will be long-term. Not for use in pregnancy (barrier contraceptives advised), breast-feeding. Pt should take safety precautions w/ CNS effects, report unusual bleeding/bruising, signs of infection.

methocarbamol (Robaxin)
CLASS Skeletal muscle relaxant
PREG/CONT C/NA

IND & DOSE Relief of discomfort associated w/ acute, painful musculoskeletal conditions. *Adult:* 1.5 g PO qid. For first 48–72 hr, 6 g/day or up to 8 g/day recommended. Maint, 1 g PO qid, or 750 mg q 4 hr, or 1.5 g tid for total 4–4.5 g/day. Or, 1 g IM or IV; may need 2–3 g in severe cases. Do not use 3 g/day for more than 3 days. **Control of neuromuscular manifestations of tetanus.** *Adult:* Up to 24 g/day PO or 1 g IM or IV; may need 2–3 g IV for no longer than 3 days. *Child:* 15 mg/kg IV repeated q 6 hr as needed.

ADV EFF Bradycardia, discolored urine, dizziness, drowsiness, headache, nausea, urticaria
NC/PT Have pt remain recumbent during and for at least 15 min after IV injection. For IM, do not inject more than 5 mL into each gluteal region; repeat at 8-hr intervals. Switch from parenteral to oral route as soon as possible. Not for use in pregnancy. Urine may darken to green, brown, black on standing. Pt should take safety precautions w/ CNS effects, avoid alcohol. Name confusion between methocarbamol and mephobarbital; use caution.

methotrexate (Rheumatrex, Trexall)
CLASS Antimetabolite, antineoplastic, antipsoriatic, antirheumatic
PREG/CONT X/NA

BBW Arrange for CBC, urinalysis, LFTs/renal function tests, chest X-ray before, during, and for several wk after tx; severe toxicity possible. Rule out pregnancy before starting tx; counsel pt on severe risks of fetal abnormalities. Reserve use for life-threatening neoplastic diseases, severe psoriasis/rheumatoid arthritis unresponsive to other tx. Monitor LFTs carefully w/ long-term use; serious hepatotoxicity possible. High risk of serious opportunistic infections; monitor closely during tx. Use cautiously w/ malignant lymphomas, rapidly growing tumors; worsening of malignancy possible.

IND & DOSE Tx of choriocarcinoma, other trophoblastic diseases. *Adult:* 15–30 mg PO or IM daily for 5-day course. Repeat course three to

five times w/ rest periods of 1 wk or longer between courses until toxic symptoms subside. **Tx of leukemia.** *Adult:* Induction: 3.3 mg/m² methotrexate PO or IM w/ 60 mg/m² prednisone daily for 4–6 wks. Maint, 30 mg/m² methotrexate PO or IM twice wkly or 2.5 mg/kg IV q 14 days. **Tx of meningeal leukemia.** *Adult:* Give methotrexate intrathecally as px in lymphocytic leukemia. 12 mg/m² (max, 15 mg) intrathecally at intervals of 2–5 days; repeat until CSF cell count normal, then give one additional dose. *Child:* 3 yr or older, 12 mg intrathecally q 2–5 days. 2–3 yr, 10 mg intrathecally q 2–5 days. 1–2 yr, 8 mg intrathecally q 2–5 days. Under 1 yr, 6 mg intrathecally q 2–5 days. **Tx of lymphomas.** *Adult:* Burkitt tumor (stages I, II), 10–25 mg/day PO for 4–8 days. Stage III, use w/ other neoplastic drugs. All usually require several courses of tx w/ 7- to 10-day rest periods between doses. **Tx of mycosis fungoides.** *Adult:* 2.5–10 mg/day PO for wks or mos, or 10 mg IM once wkly, or 25 mg IM twice wkly. Can also give IV w/ combination chemotherapy regimens in advanced disease. **Tx of osteosarcoma.** *Adult:* 12 g/m² or up to 15 g/m² IV to give peak serum conc of 1,000 micromol. Must use as part of cytotoxic regimen w/ leucovorin rescue. **Tx of severe psoriasis.** *Adult:* 10–25 mg/wk PO, IM, or IV as single wkly dose; max, 30 mg/wk. Or, 2.5 mg PO at 12-hr intervals for three doses each wk. **Tx of severe rheumatoid arthritis.** *Adult:* Single doses of 7.5 mg/wk PO or divided dose of 2.5 mg PO at 12-hr intervals for three doses as a course once wkly. Max, 20 mg/wk. **Tx of polyarticular course juvenile rheumatoid arthritis.** *Child 2–16 yr:* 10 mg/m² PO wkly; max, 20 mg/m²/wk.
ADV EFF Alopecia, **anaphylaxis,** blurred vision, chills, dizziness, fatigue, fertility alterations, fever, **interstitial pneumonitis,** n/v/d, rash, **renal failure, severe bone marrow**

depression, sudden death, ulcerative stomatitis
INTERACTIONS Alcohol, digoxin, NSAIDs (serious to fatal reactions), phenytoin, probenecid, salicylates, sulfonamides, theophylline
NC/PT Monitor CBC, LFTs, renal/pulmonary function regularly. Have leucovorin or levoleucovorin on hand as antidote for methotrexate overdose or when large doses used. Not for use in pregnancy (men, women should use contraceptives during, for 3 mo after tx). Give antiemetic for n/v. Pt should avoid alcohol, NSAIDs; cover head at temp extremes (hair loss possible); perform frequent mouth care; take safety precautions w/ CNS effects; report urine changes, abd pain, black tarry stools, unusual bleeding.

---

methoxsalen (8-MOP, Oxsoralen, Uvadex)
CLASS Psoralen
PREG/CONT C/NA

BBW Reserve use for severe/disabling disorders unresponsive to traditional tx; risk of eye/skin damage, melanoma. Brand names not interchangeable; use extreme caution.
IND & DOSE Tx of disabling psoriasis; repigmentation of vitiliginous skin; cutaneous T-cell lymphoma. *Adult:* Dose varies by weight. Must time tx w/ UV exposure; see manufacturer's details.
ADV EFF Depression, dizziness, headache, itching, leg cramps, **melanoma, ocular/skin damage,** swelling
INTERACTIONS Anthralin, coal tar/coal tar derivatives, fluoroquinolones, griseofulvin, methylene blue, nalidixic acid, phenothiazines, sulfonamides, tetracyclines, thiazides/certain organic staining dyes
NC/PT Do not use w/ actinic degeneration; basal cell carcinomas; radiation, arsenic tx; hepatic, cardiac disease. Alert pt to adverse effects, including ocular damage, melanoma. Must time tx w/ UV light exposure. Pt

should mark calendar for tx days, take safety precautions if dizzy, report vision changes.

methscopolamine bromide (Pamine)
CLASS Anticholinergic, antispasmodic
PREG/CONT C/NA

IND & DOSE Adjunct tx of peptic ulcer. *Adult:* 2.5 mg PO 30 min before meals, 2.5–5 mg PO at bedtime.
ADV EFF Altered taste perception, blurred vision, decreased sweating, dry mouth, dysphagia, n/v, urinary hesitancy, urine retention
INTERACTIONS Anticholinergics, antipsychotics, haloperidol, TCAs
NC/PT Pt should maintain adequate hydration, empty bladder before each dose, avoid hot environments, use sugarless lozenges for dry mouth, take safety precautions w/ vision changes, report difficulty swallowing, palpitations.

methsuximide (Celontin)
CLASS Antiepileptic, succinimide
PREG/CONT C/NA

IND & DOSE Control of absence seizures. *Adult:* 300 mg/day PO for first wk; titrate to max 1.2 g/day.
ADV EFF Aggression, ataxia, **blood dyscrasias**, blurred vision, dizziness, drowsiness, headache, nervousness **hepatotoxicity**, n/v/d, **SLE, Stevens-Johnson syndrome, suicidality**
INTERACTIONS Other antiepileptics
NC/PT Monitor CBC, LFTs w/ long-term tx. Not for use in pregnancy (barrier contraceptives advised). Pt should take safety precaution w/ CNS changes, thoughts of suicide.

methyldopa, methyldopate hydrochloride (generic)
CLASS Antihypertensive, sympatholytic
PREG/CONT B (oral); C (IV)/NA

IND & DOSE Tx of hypertension. *Adult:* 250 mg PO bid–tid in first 48 hr; maint, 500 mg–2 g/day PO in two to four doses. If given w/ other antihypertensives, limit initial dose to 500 mg/day in divided doses. *Child:* 10 mg/kg/day PO in two to four doses. Max, 65 mg/kg/day PO or 3 g/day PO, whichever less. Tx of hypertensive crisis. *Adult:* 250–500 mg IV q 6 hr as needed; max, 1 g q 6 hr. Switch to oral tx as soon as control attained. *Child:* 20–40 mg/kg/day IV in divided doses q 6 hr. Max, 65 mg/kg or 3 g/day, whichever less.
ADJUST DOSE Elderly pts, renal impairment
ADV EFF Asthenia, bradycardia, constipation, decreased mental acuity, distention, headache, **hemolytic anemia, hepatotoxicity, HF, myocarditis,** n/v, rash, sedation, weakness
INTERACTIONS General anesthetics, levodopa, lithium, sympathomimetics
NC/PT Give IV slowly over 30–60 min; monitor injection site. Monitor CBC, LFTs periodically. Monitor BP carefully when stopping; hypertension usually returns within 48 hr. Pt should take safety precautions w/ CNS effects, report urine/stool color changes, rash, unusual tiredness.

methylene blue (Methblue 65)
CLASS Antidote, diagnostic agent, urinary tract anti-infective
PREG/CONT C/NA

IND & DOSE Tx of cyanide poisoning, drug-induced methemoglobinemia; GU antiseptic for cystitis, urethritis *Adult, child:* 65–130 mg PO tid

w/ full glass of water. Or, 1–2 mg/kg IV or 25–50 mg/m² IV injected over several min. May repeat after 1 hr.
ADV EFF Blue-green stool, confusion, discolored urine, dizziness, headache
INTERACTIONS SSRIs
NC/PT Give IV slowly over several min; do not give subcut or intrathecally. Contact w/ skin will dye skin blue; may remove stain w/ hypochlorite sol. Use other measures to decrease UTI incidence. Urine, stool may turn blue-green. Pt should take safety measures w/ CNS effects, report severe n/v.

---

methylergonovine maleate (generic)
CLASS Ergot derivative, oxytocic
PREG/CONT C/NA

IND & DOSE Routine mgt after delivery of placenta; tx of postpartum atony, hemorrhage; subinvolution of uterus; uterine stimulation during second stage of labor after delivery of anterior shoulder. *Adult:* 0.2 mg IM or IV slowly over at least 60 sec, after delivery of placenta/anterior shoulder, or during puerperium. May repeat q 2–4 hr, then 0.2 mg PO three or four times/day in puerperium for up to 1 wk.
ADV EFF Dizziness, headache, hypertension, nausea
INTERACTIONS CYP3A4 inhibitors, ergot alkaloids, vasoconstrictors
NC/PT Reserve IV use for emergency; monitor BP/bleeding postpartum; use for no longer than 1 wk. Pt should report increased vaginal bleeding, numb/cold extremities.

---

methylnaltrexone bromide (Relistor)
CLASS Opioid receptor antagonist, laxative
PREG/CONT B/NA

IND & DOSE Tx of opioid-induced constipation in pts in palliative care

in whom other laxatives do not work. *Adult:* 62–114 kg, 12 mg subcut q other day; 38–under 62 kg, 8 mg subcut q other day. If weight not in above range, 0.15 mg/kg subcut q other day.
ADJUST DOSE Renal impairment
ADV EFF Abd pain, diarrhea, dizziness, flatulence, **GI perforation**, hyperhidrosis, nausea
NC/PT Teach proper administration, disposal of needles, syringes. Use caution in pregnancy, breast-feeding. Pt should take safety precautions w/ dizziness, report acute abd pain, severe diarrhea.

---

methylphenidate hydrochloride (Concerta, Daytrana, Metadate, Methylin, Ritalin)
CLASS CNS stimulant
PREG/CONT C/C-II

BBW Potential for abuse; use caution w/ emotionally unstable pts.
IND & DOSE Tx of narcolepsy (*Ritalin, Ritalin SR, Metadate ER, Methylin*); tx of attention-deficit disorders, hyperkinetic syndrome, minimal brain dysfunction in child, adult w/ behavioral syndrome. *Adult:* Range, 10–60 mg/day PO. ER: 18 mg/day PO in a.m. May increase by 18 mg/day at 1-wk intervals; max, 54 mg/day (*Concerta*). Or, 10- to 20-mg/day increments to max 60 mg/day (*Metadate CD, Ritalin LA*). *Child 13–17 yr:* 18 mg/day PO in a.m. Titrate to max 72 mg/day PO; do not exceed 2 mg/kg/day. Or, 10–30 mg/day transdermal patch; apply 2 hr before effect needed, remove after 9 hr. *Child 6–12 yr:* 5 mg PO before breakfast, lunch w/ gradual increments of 5–10 mg wkly; max, 60 mg/day. ER: Use adult dose up to max 54 mg/day PO. Or, 10–30 mg/day transdermal patch; apply 2 hr before effect needed, remove after 9 hr.
ADV EFF Abd pain, angina, anorexia, cardiac arrhythmias, changes in P/BP,

growth changes, insomnia, nausea, nervousness, rash

INTERACTIONS Alcohol, MAOIs, oral anticoagulants, phenytoin, SSRIs, TCAs

NC/PT Ensure proper dx; rule out underlying cardiac problems. Baseline ECG recommended. Stop tx periodically to evaluate sx. Monitor growth in children. Monitor BP frequently when starting tx. Pt should swallow ER tablet whole and not cut, crush, or chew it; take before 6 p.m. to avoid sleep disturbances; apply patch to clean, dry area of hip (remove old patch before applying new one); avoid heating pads on patch; keep in secure place; report chest pain, nervousness, insomnia.

---

methyLPREDNISolone (Medrol), methyLPREDNISolone acetate (Depo-Medrol), methyLPREDNISolone sodium succinate (Solu-Medrol)
CLASS Corticosteroid, hormone
PREG/CONT C/NA

IND & DOSE Short-term mgt of inflammatory/allergic disorders, thrombocytopenic purpura, erythroblastoma, ulcerative colitis, acute exacerbations of MS, trichinosis w/ neurologic/cardiac involvement; px of n/v w/ chemotherapy. *Adult:* 4–48 mg/day PO. Alternate-day tx: twice usual dose q other a.m. Or, 10–40 mg IV over several min. Or, high-dose tx: 30 mg/kg IV infused over 10–30 min; repeat q 4–6 hr but not longer than 72 hr. *Child:* Minimum dose, 0.5 mg/kg/day PO; base dose on actual response. **Maint tx of rheumatoid arthritis.** *Adult:* 40–120 mg/wk IM. **Adrenogenital syndrome.** *Adult:* 40 mg IM q 2 wk. **Dermatologic lesions.** *Adult:* 40–120 mg/wk IM for 1–4 wk. **Asthma, allergic rhinitis.** *Adult:* 80–120 mg IM. **Intralesional.** *Adult:* 20–60 mg. **Intra-articular.**

Adult: dose depends on site of injection: 4–10 mg (small joints); 10–40 mg (medium); 20–80 mg (large).

ADV EFF Aggravation of infections, amenorrhea, **anaphylactic reactions**, edema, fluid retention, headache, hyperglycemia, hypotension, immunosuppression, impaired healing, increased appetite, **shock**, vertigo

INTERACTIONS Azole antifungals, edrophonium, erythromycin, live vaccines, neostigmine, phenytoin, pyridostigmine, rifampin, salicylates, troleandomycin

NC/PT Individualize dose based on severity, response. Give daily dose before 9 a.m. to minimize adrenal suppression. For maint, reduce initial dose in small increments at intervals until lowest satisfactory clinical dose reached. If long-term tx needed, consider alternate-day therapy w/ short-acting corticosteroid. After long-term tx, withdraw slowly to prevent adrenal insufficiency. Monitor serum glucose. Pt should avoid exposure to infections, report signs of infection, black tarry stools.

---

metoclopramide (Reglan)
CLASS Antiemetic, dopaminergic, GI stimulant
PREG/CONT B/NA

BBW Long-term tx associated w/ permanent tardive dyskinesia; risk increases w/ pts over 60 yr, especially women. Use smallest dose possible. Max, 3 mo of tx.

IND & DOSE Relief of sx of gastroparesis. *Adult:* 10 mg PO 30 min before each meal and at bedtime for 2–8 wk; severe, 10 mg IM or IV for up to 10 days until sx subside. **Tx of symptomatic gastroesophageal reflux.** *Adult:* 10–15 mg PO up to four times/day 30 min before meals and at bedtime for max 12 wk. **Px of postop n/v.** *Adult:* 10–20 mg IM at end of surgery. **Px of chemotherapy-induced vomiting.** *Adult:* IV infusion over at least 15 min. First dose 30 min before

chemotherapy; repeat q 2 hr for two doses, then q 3 hr for three doses. For highly emetogenic drugs (cisplatin, dacarbazine), initial two doses, 1–2 mg/kg. If extrapyramidal symptoms, give 50 mg diphenhydramine IM. **Facilitation of small-bowel intubation, gastric emptying.** *Adult:* 10 mg (2 mL) by direct IV injection over 1–2 min. *Child 6–14 yr:* 2.5–5 mg by direct IV injection over 1–2 min. *Child under 6 yr:* 0.1 mg/kg by direct IV injection over 1–2 min.
ADV EFF Diarrhea, drowsiness, extrapyramidal reactions, fatigue, lassitude, nausea, restlessness
INTERACTIONS Alcohol, CNS depressants, cyclosporine, digoxin, succinylcholine
NC/PT Monitor BP w/ IV use. Give diphenhydramine for extrapyramidal reactions. Pt should take safety precautions w/ CNS effects; report involuntary movements, severe diarrhea.

metolazone (Zaroxolyn)
CLASS Thiazide diuretic
PREG/CONT B/NA

BBW Do not interchange *Zaroxolyn* w/ other formulations; not therapeutically equivalent.
IND & DOSE Tx of hypertension. *Adult:* 2.5–5 mg/day PO. **Tx of edema from systemic disease.** *Adult:* 5–20 mg/day PO.
ADV EFF Anorexia, **bone marrow depression,** dizziness, dry mouth, nocturia, n/v/d, orthostatic hypotension, photophobia, polyuria, vertigo
INTERACTIONS Antidiabetics, cholestyramine, colestipol, diazoxide, dofetilide, lithium
NC/PT Withdraw drug 2–3 days before elective surgery; for emergency surgery, reduce preanesthetic/anesthetic dose. Pt should take early in day to avoid sleep interruption; avoid sun exposure; weigh self daily, report changes of 3 lb or more/day; report unusual bleeding.

DANGEROUS DRUG

metoprolol, metoprolol succinate, metoprolol tartrate (Lopressor)
CLASS Antihypertensive, selective beta blocker
PREG/CONT C/NA

BBW Do not stop abruptly after long-term tx (hypersensitivity to catecholamines possible, causing angina exacerbation, MI, ventricular arrhythmias). Taper gradually over 2 wk w/ monitoring. Pts w/ bronchospastic diseases should not, in general, receive beta blockers. Use w/ caution only in pts unresponsive to or intolerant of other antihypertensives.
IND & DOSE Tx of hypertension. *Adult:* 100 mg/day PO; maint, 100–450 mg/day PO. Or, 25–100 mg/day ER tablet PO; max, 400 mg/day. **Tx of angina pectoris.** *Adult:* 100 mg/day PO in two divided doses; range, 100–400 mg/day. Or, 100 mg/day ER tablet PO. **Early tx of MI.** *Adult:* 3 IV boluses of 5 mg each at 2-min intervals; then 50 mg PO 15 min after last IV dose and q 6 hr for 48 hr. Then maint of 100 mg PO bid. **Late tx of MI.** *Adult:* 100 mg PO bid as soon as possible after infarct, continuing for at least 3 mo–3 yr. **Tx of HF.** *Adult:* 12.5–25 mg ER tablet PO for 2 wk; max, 200 mg/day.
ADV EFF ANA development, **bronchospasm,** cardiac arrhythmias, constipation, decreased exercise tolerance/libido, dizziness, ED, flatulence, gastric pain, HF, **laryngospasm,** n/v/d, paresthesia
INTERACTIONS Barbiturates, cimetidine, clonidine, epinephrine, hydralazine, lidocaine, methimazole, NSAIDs, prazosin, propylthiouracil, rifampin, verapamil
NC/PT Monitor cardiac function w/ IV use. Pt should swallow ER tablet whole and not cut, crush, or chew it; take safety precautions w/ CNS effects; report difficulty breathing, swelling.

metreleptin (Myalept)

CLASS Leptin analogue
PREG/CONT C/NA

BBW Risk of development of anti-metreleptin antibodies, w/ loss of drug efficacy and worsening metabolic issues, severe infections; test for antibodies in pts with severe infection or loss of efficacy. Risk of T-cell lymphoma; assess risk in pts with hematologic abnormalities and/or acquired generalized lipodystrophy.

IND & DOSE Adjunct to diet as replacement tx in leptin deficiency in pts w/ congenital or acquired lipodystrophy. *Adult, child 40 kg or less:* 0.06 mg/kg/day subcut; max, 0.13 mg/kg. *Males over 40 kg:* 2.5 mg/kg/day subcut; max 10 mg/day. *Females over 40 kg:* 5 mg/kg/day subcut; max 10 mg/day.

ADV EFF Abd pain, autoimmune disorder progression, **benzyl alcohol toxicity**, headache, hypersensitivity reactions, hypoglycemia, **T-cell lymphoma**, weight loss

NC/PT Ensure proper use of drug; only use for approved indication. Monitor for infections; test for antibody development. Dilute with Bacteriostatic Water for Injection or Sterile Water for Injection; avoid benzyl alcohol when using drug in neonates, infants. Pt should learn proper reconstitution, subcut administration, proper disposal of syringes; avoid pregnancy, breastfeeding; report difficulty breathing, dizziness, fever, sx of infection.

metronidazole (Flagyl, MetroCream, MetroGel)

CLASS Amebicide, antibiotic, antiprotozoal
PREG/CONT B/NA

BBW Avoid use unless needed; possibly carcinogenic.

IND & DOSE Tx of amebiasis. *Adult:* 750 mg PO tid for 5–10 days. *Child:* 35–50 mg/kg/day PO in three divided doses for 10 days. **Tx of antibiotic-associated pseudomembranous colitis.** *Adult:* 1–2 g/day PO in three to four divided doses for 7–10 days. **Tx of gardnerella vaginalis.** *Adult:* 500 mg PO bid for 7 days. **Tx of giardiasis.** *Adult:* 250 mg PO tid for 7 days. **Tx of trichomoniasis.** *Adult:* 2 g PO in 1 day (1-day tx) or 250 mg PO tid for 7 days. **Bacterial vaginosis.** Nonpregnant women, 750 mg PO daily for 7 days, or 1 applicator intravaginally one to two times/day for 5 days. Pregnant women, 750 mg/day PO for 7 days; avoid in first trimester. **Tx of anaerobic bacterial infection.** *Adult:* 15 mg/kg IV infused over 1 hr, then 7.5 mg/kg infused over 1 hr q 6 hr for 7–10 days; max, 4 g/day. **Preop, intraop, postop px for pts undergoing colorectal surgery.** *Adult:* 15 mg/kg infused IV over 30–60 min, completed about 1 hr before surgery; then 7.5 mg/kg infused over 30–60 min at 6- to 12-hr intervals after initial dose during day of surgery only. **Tx of inflammatory papules, pustules, erythema of rosacea.** Apply, rub in thin film bid (a.m. and p.m.) to entire affected areas after washing; for 9 wk.

ADV EFF Anorexia, ataxia, darkened urine, dizziness, dry mouth, headache, injection-site reactions, n/v/d, superinfections, unpleasant metallic taste

INTERACTIONS Alcohol, barbiturates, disulfiram, oral anticoagulants

NC/PT Urine may darken. Pt should take full course; take orally w/ food; avoid alcohol or alcohol-containing preparations during and for 24–72 after tx (severe reactions possible); use sugarless lozenges for dry mouth/metallic taste; report severe GI problems, fever.

metyrosine (Demser)

CLASS Enzyme inhibitor
PREG/CONT C/NA

IND & DOSE Mgt of pheochromocytoma. *Adult, child over 12 yr:* 250–500 mg PO qid. **Preop preparation**

for pheochromocytoma surgery.
Adult, child over 12 yr: 2–3 g/day PO for 5–7 days; max, 4 g/day.
ADV EFF Anxiety, diarrhea, dysuria, extrapyramidal effects, gynecomastia, hypotension, insomnia, sedation
INTERACTIONS Alcohol, CNS depressants, haloperidol, phenothiazines
NC/PT Maintain hydration. Antidiarrheals may be needed. Give supportive care throughout surgery. Monitor for hypotension. Pt should avoid alcohol.

DANGEROUS DRUG

mexiletine hydrochloride (Mexitil)
CLASS Antiarrhythmic
PREG/CONT C/NA

BBW Reserve for life-threatening arrhythmias; possible serious proarrhythmic effects.
IND & DOSE Tx of documented life-threatening ventricular arrhythmias. *Adult:* 200 mg PO q 8 hr. Increase in 50- to 100-mg increments q 2–3 days until desired antiarrhythmic effect. Max, 1,200 mg/day PO. Rapid control, 400 mg loading dose, then 200 mg PO q 8 hr. Transferring from other antiarrhythmics: Lidocaine, stop lidocaine w/ first mexiletine dose; leave IV line open until adequate arrhythmia suppression ensured. Quinidine sulfate, initially 200 mg PO 6–12 hr after last quinidine dose. Procainamide, initially 200 mg PO 3–6 hr after last procainamide dose. Disopyramide, 200 mg PO 6–12 hr after last disopyramide dose.
ADV EFF Cardiac arrhythmias, chest pain, coordination difficulties, dizziness, dyspnea, headache, heartburn, light-headedness, n/v, rash, tremors, visual disturbances
INTERACTIONS Hydantoins, propafenone, rifampin, theophylline
NC/PT Monitor for safe, effective serum level (0.5–2 mcg/mL); monitor cardiac rhythm frequently. Pt should

not stop without consulting prescriber, take safety precautions w/ CNS effects, report chest pain, excessive tremors, lack of coordination.

DANGEROUS DRUG

micafungin sodium (Mycamine)
CLASS Antifungal, echinocandin
PREG/CONT C/NA

IND & DOSE Tx of esophageal candidiasis. *Adult:* 150 mg/day by IV infusion over 1 hr for 10–30 days. Px of candidal infections in pts undergoing hematopoietic stem-cell transplantation. *Adult:* 50 mg/day by IV infusion over 1 hr for about 19 days. Tx of systemic candidal infections. *Adult:* 100 mg/day by IV infusion over 1 hr for 10–47 days based on infection.
ADV EFF Headache, hemolytic anemia, hepatotoxicity, nausea, phlebitis, renal toxicity, serious hypersensitivity reaction
INTERACTIONS Nifedipine, sirolimus
NC/PT Obtain baseline, periodic CBC, LFTs, renal function tests. Monitor injection site for phlebitis. Not for use in pregnancy (contraceptives advised), breast-feeding. Pt should get periodic blood tests, report difficulty breathing, urine/stool color changes, pain at IV site.

DANGEROUS DRUG

miconazole nitrate (Breeze Mist, Fungoid Tincture, Lotrimin AF, Monistat)
CLASS Antifungal
PREG/CONT B/NA

IND & DOSE Local tx of vulvovaginal candidiasis (moniliasis). *Adult:* 1 suppository intravaginally once daily at bedtime for 3 days (Monistat). Or, 1 applicator cream or 1 suppository intravaginally daily at bedtime for

7 days *(Monistat 7)*. Repeat course if needed. Alternatively, one 1,200-mg vaginal suppository at bedtime for 1 dose. **Topical tx of susceptible fungal infections.** *Adult, child over 2 yr:* Cream/lotion, cover affected areas a.m. and p.m. Powder, spray or sprinkle powder liberally over affected area a.m. and p.m.

ADV EFF Local irritation/burning, nausea, rash

NC/PT Culture before tx. Monitor response. PT should take full tx course; insert vaginal suppositories high into vagina; practice good hygiene to prevent spread, reinfection; report rash, pelvic pain.

DANGEROUS DRUG

midazolam hydrochloride (generic)

CLASS Benzodiazepine, CNS depressant
PREG/CONT D/C-IV

BBW Only personnel trained in general anesthesia should give. Have equipment for maintaining airway, resuscitation on hand; respiratory depression/arrest possible. Give IV w/ continuous monitoring of respiratory, CV function. Individualize dose; use lower dose in elderly/debilitated pts. Adjust according to other premedication use.

IND & DOSE **Preop sedation, anxiety, amnesia.** *Adult:* Over 60 yr or debilitated, 20–50 mcg/kg IM 1 hr before surgery; usual dose, 1–3 mg. Under 60 yr, 70–80 mcg/kg IM 1 hr before surgery; usual dose, 5 mg. *Child 6 mo–16 yr:* 0.1–0.15 mg/kg IM; max, 10 mg/dose. **Conscious sedation for short procedures.** *Adult:* Over 60 yr, 1–1.5 mg IV initially. Maint, 25% initial dose; total dose, 3.5 mg. Under 60 yr, 1–2.5 mg IV initially. Maint, 25% of initial dose; total dose, 5 mg. *Child over 12 yr:* 1–2.5 mg IV; maint, 25% of initial dose. **Conscious sedation for short procedures before anesthesia.** *Child 6–12 yr:* Initially, 25–50 mcg/kg

IV. May give up to 400 mcg/kg; max, 10 mg/dose. *6 mo–5 yr:* 50–100 mcg/kg IV; max, 6 mg total dose. **Induction of anesthesia.** *Adult:* Over 55 yr, 150–300 mcg/kg IV as initial dose. Under 55 yr, 300–350 mcg/kg IV (to total 600 mcg/kg). Debilitated adult, 200–250 mcg/kg IV as initial dose. **Sedation in critical care areas.** *Adult:* 10–50 mcg/kg (0.5–4 mg usual dose) as loading dose. May repeat q 10–15 min; continuous infusion of 20–100 mcg/kg/hr to sustain effect. **Sedation in critical care areas for intubated child.** *Neonates over 32 wks' gestation:* 60 mcg/kg/hr IV. *Neonates under 32 wks' gestation:* 30 mcg/kg/hr IV.

ADV EFF Amnesia, bradycardia, confusion, disorientation, drowsiness, sedation, incontinence, injection-site reactions, n/v/d, rash, **respiratory depression,** slurred speech

INTERACTIONS Alcohol, antihistamines, carbamazepine, CNS depressants, grapefruit juice, opioids, phenobarbital, phenytoin, protease inhibitors, rifabutin, rifampin

NC/PT Do not give intra-arterially; may cause arteriospasm, gangrene. Keep resuscitative facilities on hand; have flumazenil available as antidote if overdose. Monitor P, BP, R during administration. Monitor level of consciousness for 2–6 hr after use. Do not let pt drive after use. Provide written information (amnesia likely). Pt should take safety precautions w/ CNS effects, avoid alcohol, grapefruit juice before receiving drug; report visual/hearing disturbances, persistent drowsiness.

---

midodrine (generic)

CLASS Antihypotensive, alpha agonist
PREG/CONT C/NA

BBW Use only w/ firm dx of orthostatic hypotension that interferes w/ daily activities; systolic pressure increase can cause serious problems.

IND & DOSE Tx of severe ortho-static hypotension. *Adult:* 10 mg PO tid while upright.

ADJUST DOSE Renal impairment

ADV EFF Bradycardia, dizziness, increased IOP, paresthesia, pruritus, supine hypertension, syncope, urine retention

INTERACTIONS Corticosteroids, digoxin, sympathomimetics, vaso-constrictors

NC/PT Monitor BP, orthostatic BP carefully. Monitor IOP w/ long term use. Pt should take safety precautions w/ CNS effects, empty bladder before taking, avoid OTC cold/allergy remedies, report headache, fainting, numbness/tingling.

---

mifepristone (Korlym, Mifeprex)
CLASS Abortifacient
PREG/CONT X/NA

BBW Serious, fatal infection possible after abortion; monitor for sustained fever, prolonged heavy bleeding, severe abd pain. Urge pt to seek emergency medical help if these occur. Rule out pregnancy before tx and if tx stopped for 14 days or longer (with *Korlym*).

IND & DOSE Pregnancy termination through 49 days gestational age. *Adult:* Day 1, 600 mg (3 tablets) PO as single dose. Day 3, if termination not confirmed, 400 mcg PO (2 tablets) misoprostol (*Cytotec*). Day 14, evaluate for termination; if unsuccessful, surgical intervention suggested. **To control hyperglycemia secondary to hypercortisolism in adults w/ Cushing's syndrome and type 2 diabetes or glucose intolerance who have failed other tx and are not candidates for surgery.** *Adult:* 300 mg/day PO with meal; max, 1,200 mg/day (*Korlym*).

ADV EFF Abd pain, dizziness, headache, n/v/d, **potentially serious to fatal infection,** heavy uterine bleeding

NC/PT Alert pt that menses usually begins within 5 days of tx and lasts for 1–2 wk; arrange to follow drug within 48 hr w/ prostaglandin (*Cytotec*) as appropriate. Ensure abortion complete or that other measures are used to complete abortion if drug effects insufficient. Give analgesic, antiemetic as needed for comfort. Ensure pt follow-up; serious to fatal infections possible. Pt treated for hyperglycemia should take w/ meals; continue other tx for Cushing's syndrome. Not for use in pregnancy with this indication (contraceptives advised). Pt should swallow tablet whole, and not cut, crush, or chew it; immediately report sustained fever, severe abd pain, prolonged heavy bleeding, dizziness on arising, persistent malaise. Name confusion between mifepristone and misoprostol, *Mifeprex* and *Mirapex* (pramipexole); use caution.

DANGEROUS DRUG

miglitol (Glyset)
CLASS Alpha-glucosidase inhibitor, antidiabetic
PREG/CONT B/NA

IND & DOSE Adjunct to diet, exercise to lower blood glucose in type 2 diabetes as monotherapy or w/ sulfonylurea. *Adult:* 25 mg PO tid at first bite of each meal. After 4–8 wk, start maint: 50 mg PO tid at first bite of each meal. Max, 100 mg PO tid. If combined w/ sulfonylurea, monitor blood glucose; adjust doses accordingly.

ADV EFF Abd pain, anorexia, flatulence, hypoglycemia, n/v/d

INTERACTIONS Celery, charcoal, coriander, dandelion root, digestive enzymes, fenugreek, garlic, ginseng, juniper berries, propranolol, ranitidine

NC/PT Ensure thorough diabetic teaching, diet/exercise program. Pt should take w/ first bite of each meal, monitor blood glucose, report severe abd pain.

miglustat (Zavesca)
CLASS Enzyme inhibitor
PREG/CONT X/NA

IND & DOSE Tx of mild to moderate type 1 Gaucher disease. *Adult:* 100 mg PO tid.
ADJUST DOSE Elderly pts, renal impairment
ADV EFF Diarrhea, GI complaints, male infertility, peripheral neuropathy, reduced platelet count, tremor, weight loss
NC/PT Not for use in pregnancy, breast-feeding; men should use barrier contraceptives during tx. Pt should use antidiarrheals for severe diarrhea, report unusual bleeding, increasing tremors.

DANGEROUS DRUG

milrinone lactate (generic)
CLASS Inotropic
PREG/CONT C/NA

IND & DOSE Short-term mgt of pts w/ acute decompensated HF. *Adult:* 50 mcg/kg IV bolus over 10 min. Maint infusion, 0.375–0.75 mcg/kg/min IV. Max, 1.13 mcg/kg/day.
ADJUST DOSE Renal impairment
ADV EFF Headache, hypotension, **death**, ventricular arrhythmias
INTERACTIONS Furosemide in sol
NC/PT Do not mix in sol w/ other drugs. Monitor rhythm, BP, P, I & O, electrolytes carefully. Pt should report pain at injection site, chest pain.

---

milnacipran (Savella)
CLASS Selective serotonin and norepinephrine reuptake inhibitor
PREG/CONT C/NA

BBW Increased risk of suicidality; monitor accordingly.
IND & DOSE Mgt of fibromyalgia. *Adult:* 12.5 mg/day PO; increase over 1 wk to target 50 mg PO bid.
ADJUST DOSE Elderly pts, renal impairment
ADV EFF Bleeding, constipation, dizziness, dry mouth, headache, hypertension, insomnia, nausea, **NMS**, palpitations, **seizures, serotonin syndrome**
INTERACTIONS Alcohol, clonidine, digoxin, epinephrine, MAOIs, norepinephrine, tramadol, triptans
NC/PT Do not use w/ uncontrolled narrow-angle glaucoma. Not for use in breast-feeding. Taper when stopping to avoid withdrawal reactions. Pt should avoid alcohol, take safety precautions w/ CNS effects, report bleeding, rapid heart rate, thoughts of suicide.

---

minocycline hydrochloride (Arestin, Dynacin, Minocin)
CLASS Tetracycline
PREG/CONT D/NA

IND & DOSE Infections caused by susceptible bacteria. *Adult:* Initially, 200 mg PO or IV, then 100 mg q 12 hr PO or IV. Or, 100–200 mg PO initially, then 50 mg PO qid. *Adult (ER):* 91–136 kg, 135 mg/day PO; 60–90 kg, 90 mg/day PO; 45–59 kg, 45 mg/day PO. *Child over 8 yr:* 4 mg/kg PO, then 2 mg/kg PO q 12 hr. **Tx of syphilis.** *Adult:* 100 mg PO q 12 hr for 10–15 days. **Tx of urethral, endocervical, rectal infections.** *Adult:* 100 mg PO q 12 hr for 7 days. **Tx of gonococcal urethritis in men.** *Adult:* 100 mg PO bid for 5 days. **Tx of gonorrhea.** *Adult:* 200 mg PO, then 100 mg q 12 hr for 4 days. Obtain post-tx cultures within 2–3 days. **Tx of meningococcal carrier state.** *Adult:* 100 mg PO q 12 hr for 5 days. **Tx of periodontitis.** *Adult:* Unit dose cartridge discharged in subgingival area. **Tx of moderate to severe acne vulgaris.** *Adult, child 12 yr and older:* 1 mg/kg/day PO for up to 12 wk (ER form).

ADJUST DOSE Elderly pts, renal impairment
ADV EFF Anorexia; **bone marrow depression;** discoloring/inadequate calcification of primary teeth of fetus if used by pregnant women, of permanent teeth if used during dental development; glossitis; **liver failure;** n/v/d; phototoxic reactions; rash; superinfections
INTERACTIONS Alkali, antacids, dairy products, food, digoxin, hormonal contraceptives, iron, penicillin
NC/PT Culture before tx. Give w/ food for GI upset. Use IV only if oral not possible; switch to oral as soon as feasible. Additional form of contraception advised; hormonal contraceptives may be ineffective. Pt should avoid sun exposure, report rash, urine/stool color changes, watery diarrhea.

---

minoxidil (Rogaine)
CLASS Antihypertensive, vasodilator
PREG/CONT C/NA

BBW Arrange for echocardiographic evaluation of possible pericardial effusion if using oral drug; more vigorous diuretic therapy, dialysis, other tx (including minoxidil withdrawal) may be needed. Increased risk of exacerbation of angina, malignant hypertension. When first administering, hospitalize pt, monitor closely; use w/ beta blocker and/or diuretic to decrease risk.
IND & DOSE Tx of severe hypertension. *Adult, child 12 yr and older:* 5 mg/day PO as single dose. Range, usually 10–40 mg/day PO; max, 100 mg/day. Concomitant therapy w/ diuretics: Add hydrochlorothiazide 50 mg PO bid, or chlorthalidone 50–100 mg/day PO, or furosemide 40 mg PO bid. Concomitant therapy w/ beta-adrenergic blockers, other sympatholytics: Add propranolol 80–160 mg/day PO; other beta blockers (dose equivalent to above); methyldopa 250–750 mg PO bid (start methyldopa at least 24 hr before minoxidil); clonidine 0.1–0.2 mg PO bid. *Child under 12 yr:* General guidelines: 0.2 mg/kg/day PO as single dose. Range, 0.25–1 mg/kg/day; max, 50 mg/day. Topical tx of alopecia areata, male-pattern alopecia. *Adult:* 1 mL to total affected scalp areas bid. Total daily max, 2 mL. May need 4 mo of tx to see results; balding returns if untreated 3–4 mo.
ADJUST DOSE Elderly pts, renal impairment
ADV EFF Bronchitis, dry scalp, eczema, edema, fatigue, headache, hypertrichosis, local irritation, pruritus, **Stevens-Johnson syndrome,** tachycardia, URI
NC/PT Monitor pt closely. Withdraw slowly. Do not apply other topical drugs to topically treated area. Enhanced/darkening of body, facial hair possible. Twice daily use will be needed to maintain hair growth; baldness will return if drug stopped. Pt should take P, report increase over 20 beats above normal; report weight gain of more than 3 lb in one day; wash hands thoroughly after applying topical form; avoid applying more than prescribed, not apply to inflamed or broken skin.

---

mipomersen sodium (Kynamro)
CLASS Lipid-lowering drug, oligonucleotide inhibitor
PREG/CONT B/NA

BBW May cause transaminase increases, hepatotoxicity, hepatic steatosis; available only through restricted access program.
IND & DOSE Adjunct to other lipid-lowering drugs, diet to reduce LDL, total cholesterol, non-HDL cholesterol in pts with familial hypercholesterolemia. *Adult:* 200 mg/wk subcut.
ADJUST DOSE Hepatic impairment

ADV EFF Arthralgia, chills, fatigue, flulike illness, injection-site reactions, **hepatotoxicity**, malaise, myalgia
NC/PT Available only through limited access program. Monitor LFTs before and frequently during therapy. Rotate injection sites; review continued diet, exercise, other drugs to lower lipids. Not for use in pregnancy (contraceptives advised), breastfeeding. Pt should learn proper injection technique, disposal of syringes; rotate injection sites; refrigerate drug, protect from light; report urine/stool color changes, extreme fatigue.

---

mirabegron (Myrbetriq)
CLASS Beta-adrenergic agonist
PREG/CONT C/NA

IND & DOSE Tx of overactive bladder. *Adult:* 25 mg/day PO; max, 50 mg/day.
ADJUST DOSE Hepatic, renal impairment
ADV EFF Dizziness, headache, hypertension, nasopharyngitis, UTI
INTERACTIONS Anticholinergics, desipramine, digoxin, flecainamide, metoprolol, propafenone
NC/PT Ensure dx; rule out obstruction, infection. Monitor BP; check for urine retention. Not for use in breast-feeding. Pt should swallow tablet whole and not cut, crush, or chew it; take w/ full glass of water; use safety precautions w/ dizziness; report urinary tract sx, fever, persistent headache.

---

mirtazapine (Remeron)
CLASS Antidepressant
PREG/CONT C/NA

BBW Ensure depressed/potentially suicidal pts have access only to limited quantity. Increased risk of suicidality in children, adolescents, young adults. Observe for clinical worsening of depressive disorders, suicidality, unusual changes in behavior, espe-

cially when starting tx or changing dose.
IND & DOSE Tx of major depressive disorder. *Adult:* 15 mg/day PO as single dose in evening. May increase up to 45 mg/day as needed. Change dose only at intervals of more than 1–2 wk. Continue tx for up to 6 mo for acute episodes.
ADJUST DOSE Elderly pts; hepatic, renal impairment
ADV EFF Agranulocytosis, confusion, constipation, dry mouth, disturbed concentration, dizziness, dysphagia, gynecomastia, **heart block**, increased appetite, **MI**, neutropenia, photosensitivity, **stroke**, urine retention, weight gain
INTERACTIONS Alcohol, CNS depressants, MAOIs
NC/PT Do not give within 14 days of MAOIs; serious reactions possible. CBC needed if fever, signs of infection. Pt should take safety precautions w/ CNS effects; avoid alcohol, sun exposure; use sugarless lozenges for dry mouth; report signs of infection, chest pain, thoughts of suicide.

---

misoprostol (Cytotec)
CLASS Prostaglandin
PREG/CONT X/NA

BBW Arrange for serum pregnancy test for women of childbearing age. Women must have negative test within 2 wk of starting tx; drug possible abortifacient.
IND & DOSE Px of NSAID (including aspirin)-induced gastric ulcers in pts at high risk for gastric ulcer complications. *Adult:* 100–200 mcg PO four times/day w/ food.
ADJUST DOSE Elderly pts, renal impairment
ADV EFF Abd pain, dysmenorrhea, flatulence, miscarriage, n/v/d
NC/PT Explain high risk of miscarriage if used in pregnancy (contraceptives advised). Pt should take drug w/ NSAID, not share drug w/ others, report severe diarrhea, pregnancy.

Name confusion between misoprostol and mifepristone; use caution.

DANGEROUS DRUG

mitomycin (generic)
CLASS Antineoplastic antibiotic
PREG/CONT D/NA

BBW Monitor CBC, renal/pulmonary function tests frequently at start of tx; risk of bone marrow suppression, hemolytic uremic syndrome w/ renal failure. Adverse effects may require decreased dose or drug stoppage; consult physician.

IND & DOSE Palliative tx of disseminated adenocarcinoma of stomach, pancreas. *Adult:* 20 mg/m² IV as single dose q 6 to 8 wk; adjust according to hematologic profile.

ADV EFF Acute respiratory distress syndrome, alopecia, anorexia, bone marrow toxicity, confusion, drowsiness, fatigue, hemolytic uremic syndrome, injection-site reactions, n/v/d, pulmonary toxicity

NC/PT Do not give IM, subcut. Monitor injection site for extravasation. Not for use in pregnancy (barrier contraceptives advised). Pt should mark calendar for tx days, cover head at temp extremes (hair loss possible), take safety precautions w/ CNS effects, report difficulty breathing, unusual bleeding.

---

mitotane (Lysodren)
CLASS Antineoplastic
PREG/CONT C/NA

BBW Stop temporarily during stress; adrenal hormone replacement may be needed.

IND & DOSE Tx of inoperable adrenocortical carcinoma. *Adult:* 2–6 g/day PO in divided doses; gradually increase to target 9–10 g/day.

ADV EFF Anorexia, dizziness, lethargy, n/v, orthostatic hypotension, rash, somnolence, visual disturbances

INTERACTIONS Warfarin
NC/PT Give antiemetics if needed. Pt should take safety precautions w/ CNS effects.

DANGEROUS DRUG

mitoxantrone hydrochloride (generic)
CLASS Antineoplastic, MS drug
PREG/CONT D/NA

BBW Monitor CBC and LFTs carefully before and frequently during tx; dose adjustment possible if myelosuppression severe. Monitor IV site for extravasation; if extravasation occurs, stop and immediately restart at another site. Evaluate left ventricular ejection fraction (LVEF) before each dose when treating MS. Evaluate yearly after tx ends to detect late cardiac toxic effects; decreased LVEF, frank HF possible. Monitor BP, P, cardiac output regularly during tx; start supportive care for HF at first sign of failure.

IND & DOSE Tx of acute nonlymphocytic leukemia as part of comb tx. *Adult:* 12 mg/m²/day IV on days 1–3, w/ 100 mg/m² cytarabine for 7 days as continuous infusion on days 1–7. Consolidation tx: Mitoxantrone 12 mg/m² IV on days 1, 2, w/ cytarabine 100 mg/m² as continuous 24-hr infusion on days 1–5. First course given 6 wk after induction tx if needed. Second course generally given 4 wk after first course. Tx of pain in advanced prostate cancer. *Adult:* 12–14 mg/m² as short IV infusion q 21 days. Tx of MS. *Adult:* 12 mg/m² IV over 5–15 min q 3 mo; max cumulative lifetime dose, 140 mg/m².

ADV EFF Alopecia, bone marrow depression, cough, fever, headache, HF, hyperuricemia, n/v/d

NC/PT Handle drug w/ great care; gloves, gowns, goggles recommended. If drug contacts skin, wash immediately w/ warm water. Clean spills w/ calcium hypochlorite sol. Monitor CBC, uric acid level, LFTs. Not for use in pregnancy (barrier contraceptives advised). Urine, whites of eyes may appear blue; should pass w/ time. Pt should avoid exposure to infection, mark calendar for tx days, cover head at temp extremes (hair loss possible), report swelling, signs of infection, unusual bleeding.

modafinil (Provigil)
CLASS CNS stimulant, narcolepsy drug
PREG/CONT C/C-IV

IND & DOSE Tx of narcolepsy; improvement in wakefulness in pts w/ obstructive sleep apnea/hypopnea syndrome. *Adult:* 200 mg/day PO. Max, 400 mg/day. **Tx of shift-work sleep disorder.** *Adult:* 200 mg/day PO 1 hr before start of shift.
ADJUST DOSE Elderly pts, hepatic impairment
ADV EFF Anorexia, anxiety, dry mouth, headache, insomnia, nervousness, **Stevens-Johnson syndrome**
INTERACTIONS Hormonal contraceptives, phenytoin, TCAs, triazolam, warfarin
NC/PT Ensure accurate dx. Distribute least feasible amount of drug at any time to decrease risk of overdose. Monitor LFTs. Not for use in pregnancy (barrier contraceptives advised); pt using hormonal contraceptives should use second method (drug affects hormonal contraceptives). Pt should take safety precautions w/ CNS effects, report rash.

moexipril (Univasc)
CLASS ACE inhibitor, antihypertensive
PREG/CONT D/NA

BBW Do not give during pregnancy; serious fetal injury or death possible.
IND & DOSE Tx of hypertension. *Adult:* 7.5 mg/day PO 1 hr before meal; maint. 7.5–30 mg/day PO 1 hr before meals. If pt receiving diuretic,

stop diuretic for 2 or 3 days before starting moexepril. If diuretic cannot be stopped, start w/ 3.75 mg; monitor for symptomatic hypotension.
ADJUST DOSE Elderly pts, renal impairment
ADV EFF Aphthous ulcers, cough, diarrhea, dizziness, dysgeusia, flulike syndrome, flushing, gastric irritation, **MI, pancytopenia**, peptic ulcers, proteinuria, pruritus, rash
INTERACTIONS Diuretics, lithium, potassium supplements
NC/PT Alert surgeon if surgery required; volume support may be needed. Monitor for BP fall w/ drop in fluid volume. Not for use in pregnancy (barrier contraceptives advised). Pt should perform mouth care for mouth ulcers, take safety precautions w/ CNS effects, report chest pain, signs of infection.

montelukast sodium (Singulair)
CLASS Antiasthmatic, leukotriene receptor antagonist
PREG/CONT B/NA

IND & DOSE Px, long-term tx of asthma in pts 12 mo and older; relief of seasonal allergic rhinitis sx in pts 2 yr and older; relief of perennial allergic rhinitis sx in pts 6 mo and older; px of exercise-induced bronchoconstriction in pts 6 yr and older. *Adult, child 15 yr and older:* 10 mg/day PO in p.m. For exercise-induced bronchoconstriction, dose taken 2 hr before exercise; not repeated for at least 24 hr. *Child 6–14 yr:* 5 mg/day chewable tablet PO in p.m. *Child 2–5 yr:* 4 mg/day chewable tablet PO in p.m. *Child 6–23 mo:* 1 packet (4 mg)/day PO. For asthma only, 4 mg granules/day PO in p.m.
ADV EFF Abd pain, behavior/mood changes, dizziness, fatigue, headache, nausea, URI
INTERACTIONS Phenobarbital
NC/PT Give in p.m. continually for best results. Not for acute asthma

attacks. Pt should have rescue medication for acute asthma, take safety precautions w/ CNS effects, report increased incidence of acute attacks, changes in behavior/mood.

DANGEROUS DRUG

morphine sulfate (Avinza, DepoDur, Duramorph, Infumorph, Kadian, MS Contin, Roxanol)

CLASS Opioid agonist analgesic
PREG/CONT C/C-II

BBW Caution pt not to chew, crush CR, ER, SR forms; ensure appropriate use of forms. Do not substitute *Infumorph* for *Duramorph*; conc differs significantly, serious overdose possible. Ensure pt observed for at least 24 hr in fully equipped, staffed environment if given by epidural, intrathecal route; risk of serious adverse effects. Liposome preparation for lumbar epidural injection only; do not give liposome intrathecally, IV, IM.

IND & DOSE Relief of moderate to severe pain; analgesic adjunct during anesthesia; preop medication. *Adult:* 5–30 mg PO q 4 hr. CR, ER, SR: 30 mg q 8–12 hr PO or as directed by physician. *Kadian,* 20–100 mg/day PO. *MS Contin,* 200 mg PO q 12 hr. *Avinza,* 30 mg/day PO; if opioid-naive, increase by 30-mg (or lower) increments q 4 days. Or, 10 mg (range, 5–20 mg) IM or subcut q 4 hr. Or, 10 mg IV q 4 hr (range, 5–15 mg); usual daily dose, 12–120 mg. Or, 10–20 mg rectally q 4 hr. *Child:* 0.1–0.2 mg/kg (max, 15 mg/dose) IM or subcut q 4 hr. Or, 0.05 to 0.1 mg/kg (max, 10 mg/dose) slowly IV. **Relief of intractable pain.** *Adult:* 5 mg injected in lumbar region provides relief for up to 24 hr; max, 10 mg/24 hr. For continuous infusion, initial dose of 2–4 mg/24 hr recommended. Or, intrathecally, w/ dosage 1/10 epidural dosage; single injection of 0.2–1 mg

may provide satisfactory relief for up to 24 hr. Do not inject more than 2 mL of 5 mg/10-mL ampule or more than 1 mL of 10 mg/10-mL ampule. Use only in lumbar area. Repeated intrathecal injections not recommended.
Tx of pain after major surgery. *Adult:* 10–15 mg liposome injection by lumbar epidural injection using catheter or needle before major surgery or after clamping umbilical cord during cesarean birth.
ADJUST DOSE Elderly pts, impaired adults
ADV EFF Apnea, bronchospasm, cardiac arrest, circulatory depression, dizziness, drowsiness, impaired mental capacity, injection-site irritation, laryngospasm, light-headedness, n/v, respiratory arrest/depression, sedation, shock, sweating
INTERACTIONS Alcohol, barbiturate anesthetics
NC/PT Have opioid antagonist, facilities for assisted or controlled respiration on hand during IV administration. Pt should lie down during IV use. Use caution when injecting IM, subcut into chilled areas and in pts w/ hypotension, shock; impaired perfusion may delay absorption. Excessive amount may be absorbed w/ repeated doses when circulation restored. Pt should swallow CR, ER, SR forms whole and not cut, crush, or chew them; store in secure place; take safety precautions w/ CNS effects, report difficulty breathing.

---

moxifloxacin hydrochloride (Avelox, Moxeza, Vigamox)
CLASS Fluoroquinolone
PREG/CONT C/NA

BBW Increased risk of tendonitis, tendon rupture, especially in pts over 60 yr, pts taking corticosteroids, pts w/ kidney, heart, lung transplant. Risk of exacerbated weakness in pts w/ myasthenia gravis; avoid use w/ hx of myasthenia gravis.

IND & DOSE Tx of bacterial infections in adults caused by susceptible strains. *Pneumonia:* 400 mg/day PO, IV for 7–14 days. *Sinusitis:* 400 mg/day PO, IV for 10 days. *Acute exacerbation of chronic bronchitis:* 400 mg/day PO, IV for 5 days. *Uncomplicated skin, skin-structure infections:* 400 mg/day PO IV for 7 days. *Complicated skin, skin-structure infections:* 400 mg/day PO, IV for 7–21 days. *Complicated intra-abdominal infections:* 400 mg PO, IV for 5–14 days.

ADV EFF Bone marrow suppression, cough, dizziness, drowsiness, headache, insomnia, n/v/d, photosensitivity, **prolonged QT interval,** rash, vision changes

INTERACTIONS Risk of prolonged QT w/ amiodarone, phenothiazines, procainamide, quinidine, sotalol; do not combine. Antacids, didanosine, NSAIDs, sucralfate

NC/PT Culture before tx. Pt should take oral drug 4 hr before or 8 hr after antacids; stop if severe diarrhea, rash; take safety precautions w/ CNS effects; avoid sun exposure; report rash, unusual bleeding, severe GI problems.

---

mycophenolate mofetil
(CellCept), mycophenolate sodium (Myfortic)
CLASS Immunosuppressant
PREG/CONT D/NA

BBW Risk of serious to life-threatening infection. Protect from exposure to infections; maintain sterile technique for invasive procedures. Monitor for possible lymphoma development related to drug action.

IND & DOSE Px of organ rejection in allogeneic transplants. Renal. *Adult:* 1 g bid PO, IV (over at least 2 hr) as soon as possible after transplant. Or, 720 mg PO bid on empty stomach (*Myfortic*). *Child:* 600 mg/m² oral suspension PO bid; max daily dose, 2 g/10 mL. Or, 400 mg/m² PO bid; max, 720 mg bid (*Myfortic*). Car-

diac. *Adult:* 1.5 g PO bid, or IV (over at least 2 hr). Hepatic. *Adult:* I g IV bid over at least 2 hr, or 1.5 g PO bid.

ADJUST DOSE Elderly pts; hepatic, renal impairment; cardiac dysfx
ADV EFF Anorexia, **bone marrow suppression,** constipation, headache, **hepatotoxicity,** hypertension, infection, insomnia, n/v/d, photosensitivity, **renal impairment**
INTERACTIONS Antacids, cholestyramine, phenytoin, theophylline
NC/PT Intended for use w/ corticosteroids, cyclosporine. Do not mix w/ other drugs in infusion. Monitor LFTs, renal function regularly. Do not confuse two brand names; not interchangeable. Not for use in pregnancy (barrier contraceptives advised). Pt should swallow DR form whole and not cut, crush, or chew it; avoid exposure to sun, infection; get cancer screening; report signs of infection, unusual bleeding.

---

nabilone (Cesamet)
CLASS Antiemetic, cannabinoid
PREG/CONT C/C-II

IND & DOSE Tx of n/v associated w/ chemotherapy in pts unresponsive to conventional antiemetics. *Adult:* 1–2 mg PO bid. Give initial dose 1–3 hr before chemotherapy. Max, 6 mg/day PO divided tid. May give daily during each chemotherapy cycle and for 48 hr after last dose in cycle, if needed. Risk of altered mental state; supervise pt closely.

ADV EFF Ataxia, concentration difficulties, drowsiness, dry mouth, euphoria, orthostatic hypotension, vertigo

INTERACTIONS Alcohol, amitriptyline, amoxapine, amphetamines, anticholinergics, antihistamines, atropine, barbiturates, benzodiazepines, buspirone, CNS depressants, cocaine, desipramine, lithium, muscle relaxants, opioids, scopolamine, sympathomimetics, TCAs

NC/PT Risk of altered mental state; supervise pt closely; stop w/ sx of psychotic reaction. Use caution in pregnancy, breast-feeding. Warn pt possible altered mental state may persist for 2–3 days after use. Pt should take safety measures w/ CNS effects, avoid alcohol, report all drugs used (interactions possible), chest pain, psychotic episodes.

nabumetone (generic)
CLASS NSAID
PREG/CONT C (1st, 2nd trimesters); D (3rd trimester)/NA

BBW Increased risk of CV events, GI bleeding; monitor accordingly. Not for use for perio pain after CABG surgery.
IND & DOSE Tx of s&sx of rheumatoid arthritis, osteoarthritis. *Adult:* 1,000 mg PO as single dose w/ or without food; 1,500–2,000 mg/day has been used.
ADJUST DOSE Renal impairment
ADV EFF Anaphylactic shock, bone marrow suppression, bronchospasm, dizziness, dyspepsia, GI pain, headache, insomnia, n/v/d, rash, renal impairment
INTERACTIONS Aspirin, warfarin
NC/PT Pt should take w/ food, take safety precautions w/ CNS effects, report swelling, signs of infection, difficulty breathing.

nadolol (Corgard)
CLASS Antianginal, antihypertensive, beta blocker
PREG/CONT C/NA

IND & DOSE Tx of hypertension; mgt of angina. *Adult:* 40 mg/day PO; gradually increase in 40- to 80-mg increments. Maint, 40–80 mg/day.
ADJUST DOSE Elderly pts, renal failure
ADV EFF Cardiac arrhythmias, constipation, decreased exercise tolerance/libido, diarrhea, dizziness, ED, flatulence, gastric pain, HF, laryngo-spasm, n/v/d, **pulmonary edema, stroke**
INTERACTIONS Alpha-adrenergic blockers, clonidine, dihydroergotamine, epinephrine, ergotamine, lidocaine, NSAIDs, theophylline, verapamil
NC/PT To discontinue, reduce gradually over 1–2 wk. Alert surgeon if surgery required; volume replacement may be needed. Pt should take safety precautions w/ CNS effects, report difficulty breathing, numbness, confusion.

nafarelin acetate (Synarel)
CLASS GnRH
PREG/CONT X/NA

IND & DOSE Tx of endometriosis. *Adult:* 400 mcg/day: One spray (200 mcg) into one nostril in a.m., 1 spray into other nostril in p.m. Start tx between days 2, 4 of menstrual cycle. May give 800-mcg dose as 1 spray into each nostril in a.m. (total of 2 sprays) and again in p.m. for pts w/ persistent regular menstruation after 2 mo of tx. Retreatment not recommended. **Tx of central precocious puberty.** *Child:* 1,600 mcg/day: Two sprays (400 mcg) in each nostril in a.m., 2 sprays in each nostril in p.m.; may increase to 1,800 mcg/day. If 1,800 mcg needed, give 3 sprays into alternating nostrils three times/day. Continue until resumption of puberty desired.
ADV EFF Androgenic effects, dizziness, headache, hypoestrogenic effects, nasal irritation, rash
NC/PT Rule out pregnancy before tx. Store upright, protected from light. Begin endometriosis tx during menstrual period, between days 2, 4. Advise barrier contraceptives. Low estrogen effects, masculinizing effects possible (some may not be reversible). If nasal decongestant used, use at least 2 hr before dose. Pt should not interrupt tx; report nasal irritation, unusual bleeding.

DANGEROUS DRUG

nalbuphine hydrochloride (Nubain)

CLASS Opioid agonist-antagonist analgesic
PREG/CONT B; D (long-term use, high doses)/NA

IND & DOSE Relief of moderate to severe pain. *Adult, 70 kg:* 10 mg IM, IV, subcut q 3–6 hr as needed. **Supplement to balanced anesthesia.** *Adult:* Induction, 0.3–3 mg/kg IV over 10–15 min; maint, 0.25–0.5 mg/kg IV.
ADJUST DOSE Hepatic, renal impairment
ADV EFF Bradycardia, dizziness, drowsiness, dry mouth, headache, hypotension, n/v, **respiratory depression,** sweating, vertigo
INTERACTIONS Barbiturate anesthetics
NC/PT Taper when stopping after prolonged use to avoid withdrawal symptoms. Have opioid antagonist, facilities for assisted or controlled respiration on hand for respiratory depression. Pt should take safety precautions w/ CNS effects, report difficulty breathing.

naloxone hydrochloride (generic)

CLASS Diagnostic agent, opioid antagonist
PREG/CONT C/NA

IND & DOSE Complete, partial reversal of opioid depression from opioid overdose. *Adult:* 0.4–2 mg IV; may repeat at 2- to 3-min intervals. If no response after 10 mg, question dx. May use IM, subcut if IV route unavailable. *Child:* 0.01 mg/kg IV, IM, subcut. May give subsequent 0.1 mg/kg if needed. **Reversal of postop opioid depression.** *Adult:* 0.1–0.2 mg IV at 2- to 3-min intervals until desired degree of reversal. *Child:* Inject in increments of 0.005–0.01 mg IV at 2- to

3-min intervals to desired degree of reversal.
ADV EFF Hypertension, hypotension, n/v, **pulmonary edema,** sweating, tachycardia, tremors, **ventricular fibrillation**
NC/PT Monitor continually after use. Maintain open airway, provide life support as needed. Pt should report sweating, tremors.

naltrexone hydrochloride (ReVia, Vivitrol)

CLASS Opioid antagonist
PREG/CONT C/NA

BBW Obtain periodic LFTs during tx; stop tx if increasing hepatic impairment (risk of hepatocellular injury).
IND & DOSE Naloxone challenge. *Adult:* Draw 2 mL (0.8 mg) into syringe; inject 0.5 mL (0.2 mg) IV. Leave needle in vein; observe for 30 sec. If no withdrawal s&sx, inject remaining 1.5 mL (0.6 mg); observe for 20 min for withdrawal s&sx. Or, 2 mL (0.8 mg) naloxone subcut; observe for withdrawal s&sx for 20 min. If withdrawal s&sx occur or if any doubt pt opioid free, do not administer naltrexone. **Adjunct to tx of alcohol/opioid dependence.** *Adult:* 50 mg/day PO. Or, 380 mg IM q 4 wk into upper outer quadrant of gluteal muscle *(Vivitrol);* alternate buttock w/ each dose. **Px of relapse to opioid dependence after opioid detoxification.** *Adult:* 25 mg PO. Observe for 1 hr. If no s&sx, complete dose w/ 25 mg; maint, 50 mg/24 hr PO. Can use flexible dosing schedule w/ 100 mg q other day or 150 mg q third day.
ADV EFF Abd pain, anxiety, chills, delayed ejaculation, joint/muscle pain, headache, **hepatocellular injury,** increased thirst, insomnia, n/v, nervousness
INTERACTIONS Opioid-containing products
NC/PT Do not use until pt opioid free for 7–10 days; check urine opioid

levels. Do not give until pt has passed naloxone challenge. Ensure active participation in comprehensive tx program. Large opioid doses may overcome blocking effect but could cause serious injury, death. Pt should wear medical ID, take safety precautions w/ CNS effects, report unusual bleeding, urine/stool color changes.

naproxen (Naprelan, Naprosyn), naproxen sodium (Aleve, Anaprox)
CLASS Analgesic, NSAID
PREG/CONT C/NA

BBW Increased risk of CV events, GI bleeding; monitor accordingly. Contraindicated for periop pain after CABG surgery; serious complications possible.
IND & DOSE Tx of rheumatoid arthritis, osteoarthritis, ankylosing spondylitis. *Adult:* 375–500 mg DR tablet PO bid; or 750–1,000 mg/day CR tablet PO; or 275–550 mg naproxen sodium PO bid (may increase to 1.65 g/day for limited time); or 250–500 mg naproxen PO bid; or 250 mg (10 mL), 375 mg (15 mL), 500 mg (20 mL) naproxen suspension PO bid. Tx of acute gout. *Adult:* 1,000–1,500 mg/day CR tablet PO; or 825 mg naproxen sodium PO then 275 mg q 8 hr until attack subsides; or 750 mg naproxen PO then 250 mg q 8 hr until attack subsides. Tx of mild to moderate pain. *Adult:* 1,000 mg/day CR tablet PO; or 550 mg naproxen sodium PO then 275 mg q 6–8 hr; or 500 mg naproxen PO then 500 mg q 12 hr; or 250 mg naproxen PO q 6–8 hr; or OTC products 200 mg PO q 8–12 hr w/ full glass of liquid while sx persist (max, 600 mg/24 hr). Tx of juvenile arthritis. *Child:* 10 mg/kg/day naproxen PO in two divided doses.
ADJUST DOSE Elderly pts
ADV EFF Anaphylactoid reactions to anaphylactic shock, bone marrow suppression, bronchospasm, dizzi-

ness, dyspepsia, GI pain, headache, insomnia, nausea, somnolence
INTERACTIONS Lithium
NC/PT Pt should not cut, crush, or chew DR, CR forms; take w/ food for GI upset; take safety precautions w/ CNS effects; report difficulty breathing, swelling, black tarry stools.

naratriptan (Amerge)
CLASS Antimigraine, triptan
PREG/CONT C/NA

IND & DOSE Tx of acute migraine attacks. *Adult:* 1 or 2.5 mg PO; may repeat in 4 hr if needed. Max, 5 mg/24 hr.
ADJUST DOSE Hepatic, renal impairment
ADV EFF Chest pain, **CV events**, dizziness, drowsiness, headache, neck/throat/jaw discomfort
INTERACTIONS Ergots, hormonal contraceptives, SSRIs
NC/PT For acute attack only; not for px. Monitor BP w/ known CAD. Not for use in pregnancy (barrier contraceptives advised). Pt should take safety measures w/ CNS effects, continue usual migraine measures, report chest pain, visual changes, severe pain.

natalizumab (Tysabri)
CLASS Monoclonal antibody, MS drug
PREG/CONT C/NA

BBW Increased risk of possibly fatal progressive multifocal leukoencephalopathy (PML). Monitor closely for PML; stop drug immediately if signs occur. Drug available only to prescribers and pts in TOUCH prescribing program; pts must understand risks, need for close monitoring. Risk increases w/ number of infusions. Risk of immune reconstitution inflammatory syndrome in pts who developed PML and stopped drug.
IND & DOSE Tx of relapsing MS; tx of Crohn's disease in pts

unresponsive to other tx. *Adult:*
300 mg by IV infusion over 1 hr q 4 wk.
ADV EFF Abd pain, **anaphylactic reactions,** arthralgia, depression, diarrhea, dizziness, fatigue, gastroenteritis, **hepatotoxicity,** increased WBCs, lower respiratory tract infections, **PML**
INTERACTIONS Corticosteroids, TNF blockers
NC/PT Withhold drug at s&sx of PML. Ensure pt not immune-suppressed or taking immunosuppressants. Refrigerate vials, protect from light. Monitor continually during infusion. Not for use in pregnancy (barrier contraceptives advised), breast-feeding. Pt should mark calendar of tx days, avoid exposure to infection, report signs of infection, changes in eyesight/thinking.

DANGEROUS DRUG

nateglinide (Starlix)
CLASS Antidiabetic, meglitinide
PREG/CONT C/NA

IND & DOSE Adjunct to diet, exercise to lower blood glucose in type 2 diabetes, alone or w/ metformin, thiazolidinedione. *Adult:* 120 mg PO tid 1–30 min before meals; may try 60 mg PO tid if pt near HbA$_{1c}$ goal.
ADV EFF Dizziness, headache, hypoglycemia, nausea, URI
INTERACTIONS Beta blockers, MAOIs, NSAIDs, salicylates
NC/PT Monitor serum glucose, HbA$_{1c}$ frequently to determine effectiveness of drug, dose being used. Arrange for thorough diabetic teaching program; ensure diet, exercise protocols. Pt should report unusual bleeding, severe abd pain.

nebivolol (Bystolic)
CLASS Antihypertensive, beta blocker
PREG/CONT C/NA

IND & DOSE Tx of hypertension. *Adult:* 5 mg/day PO; may increase at 2-wk intervals to max 40 mg/day PO

ADJUST DOSE Hepatic, renal impairment
ADV EFF Bradycardia, chest pain, dizziness, dyspnea, headache, hypotension
INTERACTIONS Antiarrhythmics, beta blockers, catecholamine-depleting drugs, clonidine, CYP2D6 inducers/inhibitors, digoxin, diltiazem, verapamil
NC/PT Do not stop abruptly after long-term tx; taper gradually over 2 wk while monitoring pt. Use caution in pregnancy; not for use in breast-feeding. Pt should take safety precautions w/ CNS effects, report difficulty breathing, fainting.

nefazodone (generic)
CLASS Antidepressant
PREG/CONT C/NA

BBW Increased risk of suicidality in children, adolescents, young adults; monitor accordingly. Risk of severe to fatal liver failure; do not use if s&sx of hepatic impairment. Monitor closely; stop at first sign of liver failure.
IND & DOSE Tx of depression. *Adult:* 200 mg/day PO in divided doses; range, 300–600 mg/day.
ADJUST DOSE Elderly pts, hepatic impairment
ADV EFF Abnormal vision, agitation, asthenia, confusion, constipation, dizziness, dry mouth, **hepatic failure,** insomnia, light-headedness, mania, nausea, orthostatic hypotension, priapism, seizures, **suicidality**
INTERACTIONS MAOIs, triazolam. Contraindicated w/ astemizole, carbamazepine, cisapride, pimozide, terfenadine.
NC/PT Monitor LFTs before, regularly during tx. Ensure no MAOI use within 14 days. Use caution in pregnancy, breast-feeding. Pt should avoid antihistamines, take safety precautions w/ CNS effects, report all drugs being used, urine/stool color changes, thoughts of suicide.

DANGEROUS DRUG

nelarabine (Arranon)

CLASS Antimitotic, antineoplastic
PREG/CONT D/NA

BBW Monitor for neurologic toxicity including neuropathies, demyelinating disorders. Stop if neurotoxicity; effects may not be reversible.
IND & DOSE Tx of T-cell acute lymphoblastic anemia, T-cell lymphoblastic lymphoma. *Adult:* 1,500 mg/m² IV over 2 hr on days 1, 3, 5; repeat q 21 days. *Child:* 650 mg/m²/day IV over 1 hr for 5 consecutive days; repeat q 21 days.
ADJUST DOSE Hepatic, renal impairment
ADV EFF Bone marrow suppression, constipation, cough, dizziness, fatigue, fever, **neurotoxicity,** n/v/d, somnolence
INTERACTIONS Live vaccines
NC/PT Monitor neuro function before, regularly during tx; stop if sign of neurotoxicity. Not for use in pregnancy (barrier contraceptives advised). Pt should avoid exposure to infection, take safety precautions w/ CNS effects, report numbness/tingling, unusual bleeding, signs of infection.

nelfinavir mesylate (Viracept)

CLASS Antiviral, protease inhibitor
PREG/CONT B/NA

IND & DOSE Tx of HIV infection w/ other drugs. *Adult, child over 13 yr:* 750 mg PO tid, or 1,250 mg PO bid. Max, 2,500 mg/day. *Child 2–13 yr:* 45–55 mg/kg PO bid, or 25–35 mg/kg PO tid.
ADV EFF Anorexia, anemia, diarrhea, dizziness, GI pain, nausea, **seizures,** sexual dysfx
INTERACTIONS Carbamazepine, dexamethasone, grapefruit juice, hormonal contraceptives, pheno-barbital, phenytoin, rifabutin, St. John's wort. Avoid use w/ amiodarone, ergot derivatives, lovastatin, midazolam, pimozide, rifampin, quinidine, simvastatin, triazolam.
NC/PT Given w/ other antivirals. Interferes w/ hormonal contraceptives (barrier contraceptives advised). Pt should take w/ light meal, snack; avoid grapefruit juice, St. John's wort; take safety precautions w/ CNS effects; use precautions to avoid infections, prevent transmission (drug not a cure). Name confusion between *Viracept* (nelfinavir) and *Viramune* (nevirapine); use caution.

neomycin sulfate (Mycifradin, Neo-fradin, Neo-Tabs)

CLASS Aminoglycoside
PREG/CONT D/NA

IND & DOSE Preop suppression of GI bacteria for colorectal surgery. *Adult:* See manufacturer's recommendations for complex 3-day regimen that includes oral erythromycin, bisacodyl, magnesium sulfate, enemas, dietary restrictions. **Adjunct tx in hepatic coma to reduce ammonia-forming bacteria in GI tract.** *Adult:* 12 g/day PO in divided doses for 5–6 days as adjunct to protein-free diet, supportive tx. *Child:* 50–100 mg/kg/day PO in divided doses for 5–6 days as adjunct to protein-free diet, supportive tx.
ADJUST DOSE Elderly pts, renal failure
ADV EFF Anorexia, leukemoid reaction, n/v, ototoxicity, pain, rash, superinfection
INTERACTIONS Beta-lactam antibiotics, citrate-anticoagulated blood, carbenicillin, cephalosporins, digoxin, diuretics, NMJ blockers, other aminoglycosides, penicillins, succinylcholine, ticarcillin
NC/PT Ensure hydration. Pt should report hearing changes, dizziness.

neostigmine bromide
(generic), neostigmine
methylsulfate
(Prostigmin)

CLASS Antidote,
parasympathomimetic, urinary
tract drug
PREG/CONT C/NA

IND & DOSE Px of postop distention,
urine retention. *Adult:* 0.25 mg methylsulfate subcut, IM as soon as possible postop. Repeat q 4–6 hr for
2–3 days. **Tx of postop distention.**
Adult: 1 mL 1:2,000 sol (0.5 mg) methylsulfate subcut, IM. **Tx of urine retention.** *Adult:* 1 mL 1:2,000 sol (0.5 mg)
methylsulfate subcut, IM. After bladder
emptied, continue 0.5-mg injections
q 3 hr for at least five injections. **Symptomatic control of myasthenia gravis.**
Adult: 1 mL 1:2,000 sol (0.5 mg) subcut, IM. Use w/ atropine to counteract
adverse muscarinic effects. Or, 15–
375 mg/day tablets PO; average dose,
150 mg/day. *Child:* 0.01–0.04 mg/kg
per dose IM, IV, subcut q 2–3 hr as
needed. Or, 2 mg/kg/day tablets PO q
3–4 hr as needed. **Antidote for NMJ
blockers.** *Adult:* 0.6–1.2 mg atropine IV
several min before slow neostigmine IV
injection of 0.5–2 mg. Repeat as needed.
Max, 5 mg. *Child:* 0.008–0.025 mg/kg
atropine IV several min before slow
neostigmine IV injection of 0.025–
0.08 mg/kg.
ADV EFF Abd cramps, **bronchospasm, cardiac arrest,** cardiac arrhythmias, dizziness, drowsiness, dysphagia, increased
peristalsis, increased pharyngeal/tracheobronchial secretions,
increased salivation/lacrimation, **laryngospasm,** miosis, nausea, urinary
frequency/incontinence, vomiting
INTERACTIONS Aminoglycosides,
corticosteroids, succinylcholine
NC/PT Have atropine sulfate on
hand as antidote and antagonist in
case of cholinergic crisis, hypersensitivity reaction. Stop drug, consult
physician for excessive salivation,
emesis, frequent urination, diarrhea.
Give IV slowly. Pt should take safety
precautions w/ CNS effects, report
excessive sweating/salivation,
difficulty breathing, muscle
weakness.

nesiritide (Natrecor)
CLASS Human B-type
natriuretic peptide, vasodilator
PREG/CONT C/NA

IND & DOSE Tx of acutely decompensated HF. *Adult:* 2 mcg/kg IV bolus, then 0.01 mcg/kg/min IV infusion
for no longer than 48 hr.
ADV EFF Azotemia, headache, hypotension, tachycardia
INTERACTIONS ACE inhibitors
NC/PT Replace reconstituted drug q
24 hr. Monitor continuously during
administration. Monitor renal function
regularly. Maintain hydration.

nevirapine (Viramune)
CLASS Antiviral, nonnucleoside
reverse transcriptase inhibitor
PREG/CONT B/NA

BBW Monitor LFTs, renal function
before, during tx. Stop if s&sx of hepatic impairment; severe to lifethreatening hepatotoxicity possible
(greatest risk at 6–18 wk of tx). Monitor closely. Do not give if severe rash
occurs, especially w/ fever, blisters,
lesions, swelling, general malaise;
stop if rash recurs on rechallenge. Severe to life-threatening reactions possible; risk greatest at 6–18 wk of tx.
IND & DOSE Tx of HIV-1 infection
w/ other drugs. *Adult:* 200 mg/day
PO for 14 days; if no rash, then
200 mg PO bid. Or, 400 mg/day PO
ER tablet. Max, 400 mg/day. *Child
15 days and over:* 150 mg/m² PO once
daily for 14 days, then 150 mg/m² PO
bid.
ADV EFF Fat redistribution, headache, **hepatic impairment including
hepatitis, hepatic necrosis,** n/v/d,

rash, **Stevens-Johnson syndrome, toxic epidermal necrolysis**
INTERACTIONS Clarithromycin, hormonal contraceptives, itraconazole, ketoconazole, protease inhibitors, rifampin, St. John's wort
NC/PT Give w/ nucleoside analogues. Do not switch to ER form until pt stabilized on immediate-release form (14 days). Shake suspension gently before use; rinse oral dosing cup and have pt drink rinse. Not for use in pregnancy (barrier contraceptives advised). Pt should swallow ER tablet whole and not cut, crush, or chew it; be aware drug not a cure, continue preventive measures, other drugs for HIV; report rash, urine/stool color changes. Name confusion between *Viramune* (nevirapine) and *Viracept* (nelfinavir); use caution.

niacin (Niacor, Niaspan, Slo-Niacin)

CLASS Antihyperlipidemic, vitamin
PREG/CONT C/NA

IND & DOSE Tx of dyslipidemias. *Adult, child over 16 yr:* 100 mg PO tid, increased to 1,000 mg PO tid (immediate-release form); 500 mg/day PO at bedtime for 4 wk, then 1,000 mg/day PO at bedtime for another 4 wk (ER form); titrate to pt response, tolerance. Max, 2,000 mg/day; 1,000–2,000 mg/day PO (SR form). *Child under 16 yr:* 100–250 mg/day PO in three divided doses w/ meals; may increase at 2- to 3-wk intervals to max 10 mg/kg/day (immediate-release form). **Tx of CAD, post MI.** *Adult:* 500 mg/day PO at bedtime, titrated at 4-wk intervals to max 1,000–2,000 mg/day. **Tx of pellagra.** *Adult, child:* 50–100 mg PO tid to max 500 mg/day.
ADV EFF Flushing, GI upset, glucose intolerance, hyperuricemia, n/v/d, rash
INTERACTIONS Anticoagulants, antihypertensives, bile acid sequestrants, statins, vasoactive drugs

NC/PT Do not substitute ER form for immediate-release form at equivalent doses; severe hepatotoxicity possible. ASA 325 mg 30 min before dose may help flushing. Pt should take at bedtime, avoid hot foods/beverages, alcohol around dose time to decrease flushing; maintain diet, exercise program; report rash, unusual bleeding/bruising.

niCARdipine hydrochloride (Cardene)

CLASS Antianginal, antihypertensive, calcium channel blocker
PREG/CONT C/NA

IND & DOSE Tx of chronic, stable angina. *Adult:* Immediate-release only, 20 mg PO tid; range, 20–40 mg PO tid. **Tx of hypertension.** *Adult:* Immediate-release, 20 mg PO tid; range, 20–40 mg tid. SR, 30 mg PO bid; range, 30–60 mg bid. Or, 5 mg/hr IV. Increase by 2.5 mg/hr IV q 15 min to max 15 mg/hr. For rapid reduction, begin infusion at 5 mg/hr; switch to oral form as soon as possible.
ADJUST DOSE Hepatic, renal impairment
ADV EFF Asthenia, bradycardia, dizziness, flushing, headache, heart block, light-headedness, nausea
INTERACTIONS Cyclosporine, nitrates
NC/PT Monitor closely when titrating to therapeutic dose. Pt should have small, frequent meals for GI complaints; take safety precautions w/ CNS effects; report irregular heartbeat, shortness of breath.

nicotine (Nicoderm, Nicotrol)

CLASS Smoking deterrent
PREG/CONT D/NA

IND & DOSE Temporary aid to give up cigarette smoking. *Adult:* Apply transdermal system, 5–21 mg, q 24 hr. *Nicoderm:* 21 mg/day for first

6 wk; 14 mg/day for next 2 wk; 7 mg/day for next 2 wk. *Nicotrol:* 15 mg/day for first 6 wk; 10 mg/day for next 2 wk; 5 mg/day for last 2 wk. Or nasal spray, 1 spray in each nostril as needed, one to two doses/hr; max, five doses/hr, 40 doses/day. Or nasal inhaler, 1 spray in each nostril, one to two doses/hr. Max, 5 doses/hr, 40 doses/day; use for no longer than 6 mo. Treat for 12 wk, then wean over next 6–12 wk.

ADV EFF Cough, dizziness, GI upset, headache, insomnia, light-headedness, local reaction to patch

INTERACTIONS Adrenergic agonists, adrenergic blockers, caffeine, furosemide, imipramine, pentazocine, theophylline

NC/PT Ensure pt has stopped smoking, is using behavioral modification program. Protect dermal system from heat. Apply to nonhairy, clean, dry skin. Remove old system before applying new one; rotate sites. Wrap old system in foil pouch, fold over, dispose of immediately. If nasal spray contacts skin, flush immediately. Dispose of bottle w/ cap on. Pt should take safety precautions w/ CNS effects, report burning/swelling at dermal system site, chest pain.

nicotine polacrilex
(Nicorette, Nicotine Gum)
CLASS Smoking deterrent
PREG/CONT C/NA

IND & DOSE Temporary aid to give up cigarette smoking. *Adult:* Chewing gum—under 25 cigarettes/day, 2 mg; over 25 cigarettes/day, 4 mg. Have pt chew one piece when urge to smoke occurs; 10 pieces daily often needed during first month. Max, 24 pieces/day no longer than 4 mo. Lozenge—2 mg if first cigarette over 30 min after waking; 4 mg if first cigarette within 30 min of waking. Wk 1–6, 1 lozenge q 1–2 hr; wk 7–9, 1 lozenge q 2–4 hr; wk 10–12, 1 lozenge

q 4–8 hr. Max, 5 lozenges in 6 hr or 20/day.

ADV EFF Dizziness, GI upset, headache, hiccups, light-headedness, mouth/throat soreness, n/v

INTERACTIONS Adrenergic agonists, adrenergic blockers, caffeine, furosemide, imipramine, pentazocine, theophylline

NC/PT For gum, have pt chew each piece slowly until it tingles, then place between cheek and gum. When tingle gone, have pt chew again, repeat process. Gum usually lasts for about 30 min to promote even, slow, buccal absorption of nicotine. For lozenge, have pt place in mouth, let dissolve over 20–30 min. Pt should avoid eating, drinking anything but water for 15 min before use. Taper use at 3 mo. Pt should not smoke (behavioral tx program advised), take safety precautions w/ CNS effects, report hearing/vision changes, chest pain.

NIFEdipine (Adalat, Nifediac, Procardia)
CLASS Antianginal, antihypertensive, calcium channel blocker
PREG/CONT C/NA

IND & DOSE Tx of angina. *Adult:* 10 mg PO tid; range, 10–20 mg tid. Max, 180 mg/day. Tx of hypertension. *Adult:* 30–60 mg/day ER tablet PO; max, 90–120 mg/day.

ADV EFF Angina, asthenia, AV block, constipation, cough, dizziness, fatigue, flushing, headache, light-headedness, mood changes, nasal congestion, nervousness, n/v, peripheral edema, tremor, weakness

INTERACTIONS Cimetidine, grapefruit juice

NC/PT Monitor closely while adjusting dose. Pt should swallow ER tablet whole and not cut, crush, or chew it; avoid grapefruit juice; take safety precautions w/ CNS effects; report irregular heartbeat, swelling of hands/feet.

nilotinib (Tasigna)

CLASS Antineoplastic, kinase inhibitor
PREG/CONT D/NA

BBW Risk of prolonged QT interval, sudden death. Increased risk w/ hypokalemia, hypomagnesemia, known prolonged QT interval, use of strong CYP3A4 inhibitors.

IND & DOSE Tx of Philadelphia chromosome–positive CML. *Adult*: 300–400 mg PO bid 12 hr apart on empty stomach.

ADJUST DOSE Hepatic impairment
ADV EFF Abd pain, anorexia, **bone marrow suppression,** constipation, fatigue, headache, **hepatic dysfx,** nasopharyngitis, n/v/d, pain, **prolonged QT,** rash, **sudden death, tumor lysis syndrome**

INTERACTIONS Proton pump inhibitors, QT-prolonging drugs, strong CYP3A4 inducers/inhibitors, St. John's wort

NC/PT Obtain baseline, periodic ECG, QT measurement. Not for use in pregnancy (barrier contraceptives advised), breast-feeding, long-term tx. Pt should avoid exposure to infection; report all drugs/herbs being used, urine/stool color changes, signs of infection, unusual bleeding.

nimodipine (Nymalize)

CLASS Calcium channel blocker
PREG/CONT C/NA

BBW Do not give parenterally; serious to fatal reactions have occurred.
IND & DOSE To improve neurologic outcomes after subarachnoid hemorrhage from ruptured aneurysm. *Adult*: 60 mg PO q 4 hr for 21 days.
ADJUST DOSE Hepatic impairment
ADV EFF Bradycardia, hypotension, diarrhea
INTERACTIONS Antihypertensives, CYP3A4 inducers/inhibitors
NC/PT If pt unable to swallow capsule, may extract drug from capsule

using syringe, give through NG or PEG tube, then flush w/ normal saline. Do not give parenterally. Monitor carefully; provide life support as needed.

nisoldipine (Sular)

CLASS Antihypertensive, calcium channel blocker
PREG/CONT C/NA

IND & DOSE Tx of hypertension. *Adult*: 17 mg/day PO; increase in wkly increments of 8.5 mg/wk until BP controlled; range, 17–34 mg/day PO Max, 34 mg/day.
ADJUST DOSE Elderly pts, hepatic impairment
ADV EFF **Angina,** asthenia, dizziness, edema, fatigue, headache, high-fat meals, light-headedness, **MI,** nausea
INTERACTIONS Cimetidine, cyclosporine, grapefruit juice, quinidine
NC/PT Monitor closely when titrating to therapeutic dose. Pt should swallow tablet whole and not cut, crush, or chew it; take w/ meals; avoid grapefruit juice, high-fat meals; report chest pain, shortness of breath.

nitazoxanide (Alinia)

CLASS Antiprotozoal
PREG/CONT B/NA

IND & DOSE Tx of diarrhea caused by *Giardia lamblia.* *Adult, child 12 yr and older*: 500 mg PO q 12 hr w/ food, or 25 mL (500 mg) suspension PO q 12 hr w/ food. *Child 4–11 yr*: 10 mL (200 mg) suspension PO q 12 hr w/ food. *Child 1–3 yr*: 5 mL (100 mg) suspension PO q 12 hr w/ food. Tx of diarrhea caused by *Cryptosporidium parvum.* *Child 4–11 yr*: 10 mL (200 mg) PO q 12 hr w/ food. *Child 1–3 yr*: 5 mL (100 mg) suspension PO q 12 hr w/ food.
ADV EFF Abd pain, diarrhea, headache, vomiting
NC/PT Culture before tx. Ensure hydration. Pt should take w/ food, report continued diarrhea, vomiting.

nitrofurantoin (Macrobid, Macrodantin)

CLASS Antibacterial, urinary tract anti-infective
PREG/CONT B/NA

IND & DOSE Tx of UTIs. *Adult:* 50–100 mg PO qid for 10–14 days, or 100 mg PO bid for 7 days *(Macrobid)*. Max, 400 mg/day. *Child over 1 mo:* 5–7 mg/kg/day in four divided doses PO. **Long-term suppression of UTIs.** *Adult:* 50–100 mg PO at bedtime. *Child:* 1 mg/kg/day PO in one or two doses.
ADV EFF Abd pain, **bone marrow suppression,** dizziness, drowsiness, **hepatotoxicity,** n/v/d, **pulmonary hypersensitivity,** rash, **Stevens-Johnson syndrome,** superinfections
NC/PT Culture before tx. Monitor CBC, LFTs regularly. Monitor pulmonary function. Urine may be brown or yellow-green. Pt should take w/ food or milk, complete full course, take safety precautions w/ CNS effects, report difficulty breathing.

nitroglycerin (Minitran, Nitrek, Nitro-Bid, Nitro-Dur, Nitrolingual Pumpspray, Nitrostat, Nitro-Time, Rectiv)

CLASS Antianginal, nitrate
PREG/CONT C/NA

IND & DOSE Tx of acute anginal attack. *Adult:* 1 sublingual tablet under tongue or in buccal pouch at first sign of anginal attack, let dissolve; repeat q 5 min until relief obtained. No more than 3 tablets/15 min. Or, for translingual spray: Spray preparation delivers 0.4 mg/metered dose. At onset of attack, one to two metered doses sprayed into oral mucosa; no more than three doses/15 min. **Px of angina attacks.** *Adult:* Sublingual, 1 tablet 5–10 min before activities that might precipitate attack. Buccal, 1 tablet between lip, gum; allow to dissolve over 3–5 min. Tablet should not be chewed/

swallowed. Initial dose, 1 mg q 5 hr while awake; maint, 2 mg tid. SR tablet, 2.5–9 mg q 12 hr; max, 26 mg qid. Topical, ½ inch q 8 hr. Increase by ½ inch to achieve desired results. Usual dose, 1–2 inches q 8 hr; max 4–5 inches q 4 hr has been used. 1 inch ½ 15 mg nitroglycerin. Transdermal, one patch applied each day. Translingual spray, one to two metered doses sprayed into oral mucosa 5–10 min before activity that might precipitate attack. **Tx of moderate to severe pain associated w/ anal fissure.** *Adult:* 1 inch ointment intra-anally q 12 hr for 3 wk *(Rectiv)*. **Tx of periop hypertension, HF associated w/ MI, angina unresponsive to nitrates, beta blockers.** *Adult:* 5 mcg/min IV through infusion pump. Increase by 5-mcg/min increments q 3–5 min as needed. If no response at 20 mcg/min, increase increments to 10–20 mcg/min.
ADV EFF Abd pain, angina, apprehension, faintness, headache, **hypotension,** local reaction to topical use, n/v, rash
INTERACTIONS Ergots, heparin, sildenafil, tadalafil, vardenafil
NC/PT Review proper administration of each form. Sublingual should "fizzle" under tongue; replace q 6 mo. Withdraw gradually after long-term use. Pt may relieve headache by lying down. Pt should not cut, crush, or chew SR tablet; apply topical to clean, dry, hair-free area (remove old patch before applying new one); take safety precautions w/ CNS effects; report unrelieved chest pain, severe headache. Name confusion between *NitroBid* (nitroglycerin) and *Nicotrol* (nicotine), nitroglycerin and nitroprusside; use caution.

nitroprusside sodium (Nitropress)

CLASS Antihypertensive, vasodilator
PREG/CONT C/NA

BBW Monitor BP closely. Do not let BP drop too rapidly; do not lower systolic BP below 60 mm Hg. Monitor blood acid-base balance (metabolic acidosis early sign of cyanide toxicity), serum thiocyanate level daily during prolonged tx, especially w/ renal impairment.

IND & DOSE Tx of hypertensive crises; controlled hypotension during anesthesia; tx of acute HF. *Adult, child:* Not on antihypertensive: Average dose, 3 mcg/kg/min IV; range, 0.3–10 mcg/kg/min. At this rate, diastolic BP usually lowered by 30%–40% below pretreatment diastolic level. Use smaller doses in pts on antihypertensive. Max infusion rate, 10 mcg/kg/min. If this rate does not reduce BP within 10 min, stop drug.

ADJUST DOSE Elderly pts, renal impairment

ADV EFF Abd pain, apprehension, cyanide toxicity, diaphoresis, faintness, headache, hypotension, muscle twitching, n/v, restlessness

NC/PT Do not mix in sol w/ other drugs. Monitor BP, IV frequently. Have amyl nitrate inhalation, materials to make 3% sodium nitrite sol, sodium thiosulfate on hand for nitroprusside overdose and depletion of body stores of sulfur, leading to cyanide toxicity. Pt should report chest pain, pain at injection site.

---

nizatidine (Axid)

CLASS Histamine-2 antagonist
PREG/CONT B/NA

IND & DOSE Short-term tx of active duodenal ulcer, benign gastric ulcer. *Adult:* 300 mg PO daily at bedtime. **Maint tx of healed duodenal ulcer; tx of GERD.** *Adult:* 150 mg PO daily at bedtime. **Px of heartburn, acid indigestion.** *Adult:* 75 mg PO w/ water 30–60 min before problematic food, beverages.

ADJUST DOSE Elderly pts; hepatic, renal impairment

ADV EFF Bone marrow suppression, cardiac arrest, confusion, diarrhea, dizziness, ED, gynecomastia, hallucinations, headache, hepatic dysfx, somnolence

INTERACTIONS Aspirin
NC/PT Monitor LFTs, renal function, CBC w/ long-term use. Switch to oral sol if swallowing difficult. Pt should take drug at bedtime; avoid OTC drugs that may contain same ingredients; have regular medical follow-up; report unusual bleeding, dark tarry stools.

---

norepinephrine bitartrate (Levophed)

CLASS Cardiac stimulant, sympathomimetic, vasopressor
PREG/CONT C/NA

BBW Have phentolamine on standby for extravasation (5–10 mg phentolamine in 10–15 mL saline to infiltrate affected area).

IND & DOSE To restore BP in controlling certain acute hypotensive states; adjunct in cardiac arrest. *Adult:* Add 4 mL sol (1 mg/mL) to 1,000 mL 5% dextrose sol for conc of 4 mcg base/mL. Give 8–12 mcg base/min IV. Adjust gradually to maintain desired BP (usually 80–100 mm Hg systolic). Average maint, 2–4 mcg base/min.

ADV EFF Bradycardia, headache, hypertension

INTERACTIONS Methyldopa, phenothiazines, reserpine, TCAs
NC/PT Give whole blood, plasma separately, if indicated. Give IV infusions into large vein, preferably antecubital fossa, to prevent extravasation. Monitor BP q 2 min from start of infusion until desired BP achieved, then monitor q 5 min if infusion continued. Do not give pink, brown sols. Monitor for extravasation.

---

norethindrone acetate (Aygestin)

CLASS Progestin
PREG/CONT X/NA

IND & DOSE Tx of amenorrhea; abnormal uterine bleeding. *Adult:* 2.5–10 mg PO for 5–10 days during second half of theoretical menstrual cycle. *Tx of endometriosis. Adult:* 5 mg/day PO for 2 wk; increase in increments of 2.5 mg/day q 2 wk to max 15 mg/day.

ADV EFF Acne, amenorrhea, breakthrough bleeding/spotting, dizziness, edema, insomnia, menstrual changes, **PE,** photosensitivity, rash, **thromboembolic disorders,** vision changes/blindness, weight increase

NC/PT Stop if sudden vision loss, s&sx of thromboembolic event. Pt should mark calendar of tx days, avoid sun exposure, take safety precautions w/ CNS effects, report calf swelling/pain, chest pain, vision changes, difficulty breathing.

---

norfloxacin (Noroxin)
CLASS Fluoroquinolone, urinary tract anti-infective
PREG/CONT C/NA

BBW Increased risk of tendonitis, tendon rupture, especially in pts over 60 yr, those taking corticosteroids, kidney/heart/lung transplant pts. Risk of severe muscle weakness if used w/ myasthenia gravis; do not use w/ hx of myasthenia gravis.

IND & DOSE *Tx of infections in adults caused by susceptible bacteria. Uncomplicated UTI:* 400 mg PO q 12 hr for 7–10 days; max, 800 mg/day. *Uncomplicated cystitis:* 400 mg PO q 12 hr for 3 days. *Complicated UTI:* 400 mg PO q 12 hr for 10–21 days. *Uncomplicated gonorrhea:* 800 mg PO as single dose. *Prostatitis:* 400 mg PO q 12 hr for 28 days.

ADJUST DOSE Elderly pts, renal impairment

ADV EFF Bone marrow suppression, dizziness, drowsiness, dry mouth, fatigue, fever, headache, **hepatic impairment,** nausea, photosensitivity, **prolonged QT interval,** rash

INTERACTIONS Antacids, cyclosporine, iron salts, QT-prolonging drugs, St. John's wort, sucralfate, theophyllines

NC/PT Culture before tx. Ensure hydration. Pt should take on empty stomach 1 hr before or 2 hr after meals, milk, dairy; avoid antacids within 2 hr of dose; avoid St. John's wort; take safety precautions w/ CNS effects, report tendon pain, signs of infection. Name confusion between *Noroxin* and *Neurontin* (gabapentin); use caution.

---

norgestrel (generic)
CLASS Hormonal contraceptive, progestin
PREG/CONT X/NA

IND & DOSE *To prevent pregnancy.* 1 tablet PO daily, starting on first day of menstruation, at same time each day, q day of year. For one missed dose, 1 tablet as soon as pt remembers, then next tablet at usual time. For two consecutive missed doses, pt takes one of missed tablets, discards other, takes daily tablet at usual time. For three consecutive missed doses, pt should discontinue immediately, use additional form of birth control until menses, or pregnancy ruled out.

ADV EFF Breakthrough bleeding/spotting, breast tenderness, **cerebral hemorrhage,** corneal curvature changes, edema, menstrual changes, migraine, **MI, PE,** thrombophlebitis

INTERACTIONS Barbiturates, carbamazepine, griseofulvin, hydantoins, penicillins, rifampin, St. John's wort, tetracyclines

NC/PT Arrange for pretreatment, periodic complete physical, Pap test. Start no earlier than 4 wk postpartum. Stop if s&sx of thrombotic event, sudden vision loss. Not for use in pregnancy. Review all drugs pt taking; additional contraceptive measure may be needed. Pt should avoid sun exposure, St John's wort; take safety precautions w/ CNS effects; report calf swelling/pain, vision loss, difficulty breathing.

nortriptyline hydrochloride (Aventyl, Pamelor)
CLASS TCA
PREG/CONT D/NA

BBW Limit access in depressed, potentially suicidal pts. Risk of suicidality in children, adolescents, young adults; monitor accordingly.
IND & DOSE Tx of depression.
Adult: 25 PO mg tid–qid. Max, 150 mg/day. *Child 12 yr and over:* 30–50 mg/day PO in divided doses.
ADJUST DOSE Elderly pts
ADV EFF Atropine-like effects, **bone marrow depression**, constipation, disturbed concentration, dry mouth, glossitis, gynecomastia, hyperglycemia, orthostatic hypotension, photosensitivity, **seizures, stroke**, urine retention
INTERACTIONS Alcohol, cimetidine, clonidine, fluoxetine, MAOIs, sympathomimetics
NC/PT Monitor CBC. Pt should take at bedtime if drowsiness an issue; avoid sun exposure, alcohol; take safety precautions w/ CNS effects; use sugarless lozenges for dry mouth; report thoughts of suicide.

nystatin (Mycostatin, Nilstat, NySert)
CLASS Antifungal
PREG/CONT C/NA

IND & DOSE Local tx of vaginal candidiasis (moniliasis). *Adult:* 1 tablet (100,000 units) or 1 applicator cream (100,000 units) vaginally daily–bid for 2 wk. Tx of cutaneous/mucocutaneous mycotic infections caused by *Candida albicans*, other *Candida* sp. *Adult:* Apply to affected area two to three times daily until healing complete. For fungal foot infection, dust powder on feet, in shoes/socks. Tx of oropharyngeal candidiasis. *Adult, child over 1 yr:* 500,000–1,000,000 units PO tid for at least 48 hr after clinical cure, or 400,000–600,000 units suspension four times/day for 14 days and for at least 48 hr after sx subside.
ADV EFF GI distress, local reactions at application site, n/v/d
NC/PT Culture before tx. Pt should complete full course of tx; hold suspension in mouth as long as possible (can be made into popsicle for longer retention); clean affected area before topical application; use appropriate hygiene to prevent reinfection; report worsening of condition.

obinutuzumab (Gazyva)
CLASS Antineoplastic, monoclonal antibody
PREG/CONT C/NA

BBW Risk of reactivation of hepatitis B, fulminant hepatitis, progressive multifocal leukoencephalopathy (PML), death. Monitor closely.
IND & DOSE Tx of previously untreated chronic lymphocytic leukemia, w/ chlorambucil. *Adult:* 6-day cycle: 100 mg IV on day 1, cycle 1; 900 mg IV on day 2, cycle 1; 1,000 mg IV on day 8 and 15, cycle 1; 1,000 mg IV on day 1 of cycles 2–6.
ADV EFF Cough, bone marrow suppression, fever, **hepatotoxicity**, infusion reactions, n/v/d, PML, tumor lysis syndrome
NC/PT Premedicate with glucocorticoids, acetaminophen, antihistamine. For pt with large tumor load, premedicate w/ antihyperuricemics; ensure adequate hydration. Dilute and administer as IV infusion, not IV push or bolus. Do not give live vaccines before or during tx. Monitor LFTs; stop drug w/ sx of hepatotoxicity. Monitor CBC; watch for PML. Pt should avoid pregnancy during and for 12 mo after tx; avoid breast-feeding; take safety measures w/ drug reaction; report color changes in urine/stool, severe n/v/d, fever, dizziness, CNS changes.

octreotide acetate
(Sandostatin)
CLASS Antidiarrheal, hormone
PREG/CONT B/NA

IND & DOSE Symptomatic tx of carcinoid tumors. *Adult:* First 2 wk: 100–600 mcg/day subcut in two to four divided doses; mean daily dose, 300 mcg. **Tx of watery diarrhea of VI-Pomas.** *Adult:* 200–300 mcg subcut in two to four divided doses during first 2 wk to control symptoms. Depot injection, 20 mg IM q 4 wk. *Child:* 1–10 mcg/kg/day subcut. Range, 150–750 mcg subcut. **Tx of acromegaly.** *Adult:* 50 mcg tid subcut, adjusted up to 100–500 mcg tid. Withdraw for 4 wk once yrly. Depot injection: 20 mg IM intragluteally q 4 wk.
ADV EFF Abd pain, asthenia, anxiety, bradycardia, cholelithiasis, dizziness, fatigue, flushing, injection-site pain, hyperglycemia, hypoglycemia, light-headedness, n/v/d
NC/PT Give subcut; rotate sites. Give depot injections deep IM; avoid deltoid region. Arrange to withdraw for 4 wk (8 wk for depot injection) once yrly for acromegaly. Monitor blood glucose, gallbladder ultrasound. Pt should take safety precautions w/ CNS effects, report severe abd pain, severe pain at injection site. Name confusion between *Sandostatin* (octreotide) and *Sandimmune* (cyclosporine); use caution.

ofatumumab (Arzerra)
CLASS Antineoplastic, cytotoxic
PREG/CONT C/NA

IND & DOSE Tx of chronic lymphocytic leukemia refractory to standard tx. *Adult:* 12 doses total, 300 mg IV then, in 1 wk, 2,000 mg/wk IV for 7 doses; then, in 4 wk, 2,000 mg IV q 4 wk for 4 doses.
ADV EFF Anemia, ataxia, bone marrow suppression, bronchitis, cough, diarrhea, dizziness, dyspnea, fatigue,

fever, **hepatitis B reactivation**, infusion reactions, intestinal obstruction, nausea, **progressive multifocal leukoencephalopathy**, URI, vision problems
INTERACTIONS Live vaccines
NC/PT Premedicate w/ acetaminophen, IV antihistamine, IV corticosteroids. Monitor CBC regularly. Not for use in pregnancy (contraceptives advised). Pt should avoid exposure to infection, take safety precautions w/ CNS effects, report difficulty breathing, unusual bleeding, signs of infection.

ofloxacin (Floxin, Ocuflox)
CLASS Fluoroquinolone
PREG/CONT C/NA

BBW Increased risk of tendinitis, tendon rupture. Risk higher in pts over 60 yr, women, pts w/ kidney/heart/lung transplant. Risk of exacerbated muscle weakness, sometimes severe, w/ myasthenia gravis; do not give w/ hx of myasthenia gravis.
IND & DOSE Tx of infections caused by susceptible bacteria strains. Uncomplicated UTIs: *Adult:* 200 mg q 12 hr PO for 3–7 days. Complicated UTIs: *Adult:* 200 mg PO bid for 10 days. **Bacterial exacerbations of COPD, community-acquired pneumonia, mild to moderate skin infections.** *Adult:* 400 mg PO q 12 hr for 10 days. **Prostatitis.** *Adult:* 300 mg PO q 12 hr for 6 wk. **Acute, uncomplicated gonorrhea.** *Adult:* 400 mg PO as single dose. **Cervicitis, urethritis.** *Adult:* 300 mg PO q 12 hr for 7 days. **Ocular infections.** *Adult:* 1–2 drops/eye as indicated. **Otic infections.** *Adult, child over 12 yr:* 10 drops in affected ear tid for 10–14 days. *Child 1–12 yr w/ tympanostomy tubes:* 5 drops in affected ear bid for 10 days. **Swimmer's ear.** *Adult:* 10 drops/day (1.5 mg) in affected ear for 7 days. *Child 12 yr and older:* 10 drops in affected ear bid for 10 days. *Child 6 mo–under 12 yr:* 5 drops in affected

ear bid for 10 day. **Chronic suppurative otitis media.** *Adult, child:* 10 drops in affected ear bid for 14 days.
ADJUST DOSE Elderly pts, renal impairment
ADV EFF Bone marrow suppression, dizziness, drowsiness, headache, **hepatic impairment**, insomnia, n/v/d, photosensitivity, prolonged QT, tendinitis, tendon rupture
INTERACTIONS Antacids, iron salts, QT-prolonging drugs, St. John's wort, sucralfate, zinc
NC/PT Culture before tx. Teach proper administration of eye/eardrops. Pt should take oral drug 1 hr before or 2 hr after meals on empty stomach; avoid antacids within 2 hr of ofloxacin; drink plenty of fluids; avoid sun exposure; take safety precautions w/ CNS effects; report tendon pain, severe GI upset.

olanzapine (Zyprexa)
CLASS Antipsychotic, dopaminergic blocker
PREG/CONT C/NA

BBW Increased risk of death when used in elderly pts w/ dementia-related psychosis; drug not approved for this use. Risk of severe sedation, including coma/delirium, after each injection of *Zyprexa Relprevv.* Monitor pt for at least 3 hr after each injection, w/ ready access to emergency services. Because of risk, drug available only through *Zyprexa Relprevv* Patient Care Program.
IND & DOSE Tx of schizophrenia.
Adult: 5–10 mg/day PO. Increase to 10 mg/day PO within several days; max, 20 mg/day. Or long-acting injection *(Zyprexa Relprevv):* 150, 210, or 300 mg IM q 2 wk, or 300 or 405 mg IM q 4 wk. *Child 13–17 yr:* 2.5–5 mg/day PO; target, 10 mg/day. **Tx of bipolar mania.** *Adult:* 10–15 mg/day PO. Max, 20 mg/day; maint, 5–20 mg/day PO. *Child 13–17 yr:* 2.5–5 mg/day PO; target, 10 mg/day. **Tx of agitation associated w/ schizophrenia, mania.**

Adult: 10 mg IM; range, 5–10 mg. May repeat in 2 hr if needed; max, 30 mg/24 hr. **Tx-resistant depression.** *Adult:* 5 mg/day PO w/ fluoxetine 20 mg/day PO; range, 5–12.5 mg/day olanzapine w/ 20–50 mg/day PO fluoxetine.
ADJUST DOSE Elderly/debilitated pts
ADV EFF Constipation, dizziness, fever, headache, hyperglycemia, **NMS**, orthostatic hypotension, somnolence, weight gain
INTERACTIONS Alcohol, anticholinergics, antihypertensives, benzodiazepines, carbamazepine, CNS drugs, dopamine agonists, fluvoxamine, levodopa, omeprazole, rifampin, smoking
NC/PT Dispense 1 wk at a time. Use care to distinguish short-term from long-term IM form. Monitor serum glucose, lipids. Not for use in pregnancy. Pt should peel back (not push through) foil on blister pack of disintegrating tablet, remove w/ dry hands; avoid alcohol; report all drugs being used (many interactions possible); take safety precautions w/ CNS effects, orthostatic hypotension; report fever, flulike symptoms. Name confusion between *Zyprexa* (olanzapine) and *Zyrtec* (cetirizine); use caution.

olmesartan medoxomil (Benicar)
CLASS Antihypertensive, ARB
PREG/CONT D/NA

BBW Rule out pregnancy before tx; suggest barrier contraceptives. Fetal injury, death have occurred.
IND & DOSE Tx of hypertension. *Adult, child 6–16 yr, 35 kg or more:* 20 mg/day PO; may titrate to 40 mg/day after 2 wk. *Child 6–16 yr, 20–under 35 kg:* 10 mg/day PO; max, 20 mg/day PO.
ADV EFF Abd/back pain, angioedema, bronchitis, cough, dizziness, drowsiness, flulike symptoms, headache, n/v/d, URI

NC/PT Alert surgeon if surgery scheduled; fluid volume expansion may be needed. Not for use in pregnancy (barrier contraceptives advised), breast-feeding. Pt should use caution in situations that may lead to BP drop (excessive hypotension possible); take safety precautions w/ CNS effects; report swelling.

olsalazine sodium
(Dipentum)
CLASS Anti-inflammatory
PREG/CONT C/NA

IND & DOSE Maint of remission of ulcerative colitis in pts resistant to sulfasalazine. *Adult:* 1 g/day PO in divided doses w/ meals.
ADJUST DOSE Renal impairment
ADV EFF Abd pain, diarrhea, headache, itching, rash
INTERACTIONS Heparin, 6-mercaptopurine, thioguanine, varicella vaccine, warfarin
NC/PT Not for use in breast-feeding. Pt should always take w/ food, report diarrhea.

omacetaxine mepesuccinate (Synribo)
CLASS Antineoplastic, protein synthesis inhibitor
PREG/CONT D/NA

IND & DOSE Tx of adult w/ accelerated CML w/ resistance or intolerance to two or more kinase inhibitors. *Adult:* 1.25 mg/m² subcut bid for 14 consecutive days of 28-day cycle, then 1.25 mg/m² subcut bid for 7 consecutive days of 28-day cycle.
ADV EFF Bleeding, fatigue, fever, hair loss, hyperglycemia, injection-site reactions, n/v/d, **severe myelosuppression**
NC/PT Monitor bone marrow function frequently; dosage adjustment may be needed. Monitor blood glucose. Not for use in pregnancy, breast-feeding.; Pt should avoid expo-

sure to infections; be aware fatigue, bleeding, hair loss possible; report unusual bleeding, fever, s&sx of infection, rash.

omalizumab (Xolair)
CLASS Antiasthmatic, monoclonal antibody
PREG/CONT B/NA

BBW Anaphylaxis w/ bronchospasm, hypotension, syncope, urticaria, edema possible. Monitor closely after each dose; have emergency equipment on hand.
IND & DOSE To decrease asthma exacerbation in pts w/ moderate to severe asthma, positive skin test to perennial airborne allergens. *Adult, child over 12 yr:* 150–375 mg subcut q 2–4 wk.
ADV EFF Anaphylaxis, cancer, injection-site reactions, pain
NC/PT Base dose on weight, pretreatment immunoglobulin E level. Monitor after each injection for anaphylaxis. Not for use in breast-feeding. Pt should have appropriate cancer screening, report difficulty breathing, tongue swelling, rash, chest tightness.

omega-3-acid ethyl esters (Lovaza)
CLASS Lipid-lowering drug, omega-3 fatty acid
PREG/CONT C/NA

IND & DOSE Adjunct to diet to reduce very high (over 500 mg/dL) triglycerides. *Adult:* 4 g/day PO as single dose (4 capsules) or divided into two doses (2 capsules PO bid).
ADV EFF Back pain, eructation, dyspepsia, flulike symptoms, infection, taste changes
INTERACTIONS Anticoagulants
NC/PT Monitor serum triglycerides. Ensure use of diet, exercise program. Not for use in pregnancy, breast-feeding. Name confusion between *Omacor*

(former brand name of omega-3-acid ethyl esters) and *Amicar* (aminocaproic acid). Although *Omacor* has been changed to *Lovaza*, confusion possible; use caution.

omeprazole (Prilosec, Zegerid)

CLASS Proton pump inhibitor
PREG/CONT C/NA

IND & DOSE **Tx of active duodenal ulcer.** *Adult:* 20 mg/day PO for 2–8 wk. **Tx of active gastric ulcer.** *Adult:* 40 mg/day PO for 4–8 wk. **Tx of severe erosive esophagitis, poorly responsive GERD.** *Adult:* 20 mg/day PO for 4–8 wk. **Tx of pathologic hypersecretory conditions.** *Adult:* 60 mg/day PO. Up to 120 mg/day has been used. **Tx of frequent heartburn.** 20 mg/day (*Prilosec OTC* tablet) PO in a.m. before eating for 14 days. May repeat 14-day course q 4 mo. **Upper GI bleeding in critically ill pts.** *Adult:* 40 mg/day PO then 40 mg PO in 6–8 hr on day 1, then 40 mg/day for up to 14 days (*Zegerid*). **GERD, other acid-related disorders.** *Adult, child 2 yr and over:* 20 kg or more, 20 mg daily PO; 11–under 20 kg, 10 mg daily PO; 5–10 kg, 5 mg daily PO.
ADV EFF Abd pain, bone fractures, *Clostridium difficile* diarrhea, dizziness, headache, n/v/d, pneumonia, rash, URI
INTERACTIONS Benzodiazepines, clopidogrel, phenytoin, sucralfate, warfarin
NC/PT If sx persist after 8 wk, re-evaluate. Pt should take w/ meals; swallow capsule whole and not cut, crush, or chew it; if cannot swallow, open capsules, sprinkle contents on applesauce, swallow immediately; take safety precautions w/ CNS effects; report severe diarrhea, fever.

ondansetron hydrochloride (Zofran, Zuplenz)

CLASS Antiemetic
PREG/CONT B/NA

IND & DOSE **Px of chemotherapy-induced n/v.** *Adult:* Three 0.15-mg/kg doses IV: First dose over 15 min starting 30 min before chemotherapy; subsequent doses over 4 and 8 hr. Or, single 32-mg dose infused over 15 min starting 30 min before chemotherapy. Or, 8 mg PO 30 min before chemotherapy, then 8 mg PO 8 hr later; give 8 mg PO q 12 hr for 1–2 days after chemotherapy. For highly emetogenic chemotherapy, 24 mg PO 30 min before chemotherapy. *Child 6 mo–18 yr:* Three 0.15-mg/kg doses IV over 15 min starting 30 min before chemotherapy, then 4 and 8 hr later. *Child 4–11 yr:* 4 mg PO 30 min before chemotherapy, 4 mg PO at 4 and 8 hr, then 4 mg PO tid for 1–2 days after chemotherapy. **Px of n/v associated w/ radiotherapy.** *Adult:* 8 mg PO tid. For total-body radiotherapy, give 1–2 hr before radiation each day. For single high-dose radiotherapy to abdomen, give 1–2 hr before radiotherapy, then q 8 hr for 1–2 days after therapy. For daily fractionated radiotherapy to abdomen, give 1–2 hr before tx, then q 8 hr for each day tx given. **Px of postop n/v.** *Adult:* 4 mg undiluted IV, preferably over 2–5 min, or as single IM dose immediately before anesthesia induction. Or, 16 mg PO 1 hr before anesthesia. *Child 1 mo–12 yr:* Single dose of 4 mg IV if over 40 kg, 0.1 mg/kg IV if under 40 kg, preferably 2–5 min before or after anesthesia induction. Infuse over at least 30 sec.
ADJUST DOSE Hepatic impairment
ADV EFF Abd pain, diarrhea, dizziness, drowsiness, headache, myalgia, pain at injection site, **prolong QT interval**, weakness
INTERACTIONS QT-prolonging drugs

NC/PT Obtain baseline ECG for QT interval. Ensure timing to correspond w/ surgery, chemotherapy. For *Zofran* orally disintegrating tablet, pt should peel foil back over (do not push through) one blister, immediately place on tongue, swallow w/ saliva. For *Zuplenz*, pt should use dry hands, fold pouch along dotted line, carefully tear pouch along edge, remove film, place on tongue, swallow after it dissolves, then wash hands. Pt should take safety precautions w/ CNS effects; report pain at injection site, palpitations.

DANGEROUS DRUG

opium preparations
**(Opium Tincture,
Deodorized; Paregoric)**
CLASS Antidiarrheal, opioid
agonist
PREG/CONT C/C-III (Paregoric);
C/C-II (Opium Tincture,
Deodorized)

IND & DOSE Tx of diarrhea. *Adult:*
5–10 mL *Paregoric* PO daily–qid (5 mL equivalent to 2 mg morphine), or 0.6 mL *Opium Tincture* qid. Max, 6 mL/day. *Child:* 0.25–0.5 mL/kg *Paregoric* PO daily–qid.
ADJUST DOSE Elderly pts, impaired adults
ADV EFF Bronchospasm, **cardiac arrest**, constipation, dizziness, drowsiness, flushing, **laryngospasm**, light-headedness, n/v, **respiratory arrest**, sedation, **shock**, sweating, ureteral spasm, vision changes
INTERACTIONS Barbiturate general anesthetics
NC/PT *Opium Tincture, Deodorized,* contains 25 times more morphine than *Paregoric*; do not confuse dosage (severe toxicity possible). Do not use in preterm infants. Pt should take 4–6 hr before next feeding if breast-feeding; not take left-over medication; take safety precautions w/ CNS effects; use laxative if constipated; report difficulty breathing. Name confusion between *Paregoric* (camphorated

tincture of opium) and *Opium Tincture, Deodorized*; use caution.

oprelvekin (Neumega)
CLASS Interleukin
PREG/CONT C/NA

BBW Severe allergic reactions, including anaphylaxis, possible; monitor w/ each dose.
IND & DOSE Px of severe thrombocytopenia; to reduce need for platelet transfusions after myelosuppressive chemotherapy in pts w/ nonmyeloid malignancies. *Adult:* 50 mcg/kg/day subcut starting day 1 after chemotherapy for 14–21 days.
ADJUST DOSE Renal impairment
ADV EFF Anemia, **anaphylaxis**, **capillary leak syndrome**, cardiac arrhythmias, dyspnea, edema, fluid retention, papilledema
NC/PT Obtain baseline, periodical CBC. Monitor for anaphylaxis; stop immediately if it occurs. Not for use in pregnancy, breast-feeding. Teach proper administration, disposal of needles, syringes. Pt should mark calendar of injection days, report difficulty breathing, weight gain, fluid retention, vision changes.

orlistat (Alli, Xenical)
CLASS Lipase inhibitor, weight
loss drug
PREG/CONT B/NA

BBW Severe allergic reactions, including anaphylaxis, possible; monitor w/ each dose.
IND & DOSE Tx of obesity as part of weight loss program. *Adult:* 120 mg PO tid w/ each fat-containing meal. OTC, 60 mg PO w/ each fat-containing meal; max, 3 capsules/day. *Child 12 yr and over:* 120 mg PO tid w/ fat-containing meals. OTC not for use in children.
ADV EFF Dry mouth, flatulence, incontinence, loose stools, **severe hepatic injury**, vitamin deficiency

INTERACTIONS Fat-soluble vitamins, oral anticoagulants, pravastatin
NC/PT Increased risk of severe hepatic injury; monitor LFTs before, periodically during tx. Ensure diet, exercise program. Not for use in pregnancy (contraceptives advised). Pt should use sugarless lozenges for dry mouth, use fat-soluble vitamins (take separately from orlistat doses), report right upper quadrant pain, urine/stool color changes.

orphenadrine citrate
(Banflex, Flexon, Norflex)
CLASS Skeletal muscle relaxant
PREG/CONT C/NA

IND & DOSE Relief of discomfort associated w/ acute, painful musculoskeletal conditions. *Adult:* 60 mg IV, IM. May repeat q 12 hr. Inject IV over 5 min. Or, 100 mg PO a.m. and p.m.
ADJUST DOSE Elderly pts
ADV EFF Confusion, constipation, decreased sweating, dizziness, dry mouth, flushing, gastric irritation, headache, n/v, tachycardia, urinary hesitancy, urine retention
INTERACTIONS Alcohol, anticholinergics, haloperidol, phenothiazines
NC/PT Ensure pt supine during IV injection and for at least 15 min after; assist from supine position after tx. Pt should swallow SR tablet whole and not cut, crush, or chew it; empty bladder before each dose; use caution in hot weather (sweating reduced); avoid alcohol; take safety precautions w/ CNS effects; use sugarless lozenges for dry mouth; report difficulty swallowing, severe GI upset.

oseltamivir phosphate
(Tamiflu)
CLASS Antiviral, neuraminidase inhibitor
PREG/CONT C/NA

IND & DOSE Tx of uncomplicated illness due to influenza virus (A or

B). *Adult, child 13 yr and older:* 75 mg PO bid for 5 days, starting within 2 days of sx onset. *Child 1–12 yr:* 30–75 mg suspension PO bid for 5 days based on weight. *Child 2 wk–under 1 yr:* 3 mg/kg PO bid for 5 days. **Px of influenza A and B infection.** *Adult, child 13 yr and older:* 75 mg/day PO for at least 10 days; begin within 2 days of exposure. *Child 1–12 yr:* Over 40 kg, 75 mg/day PO; 23–40 kg, 60 mg/day PO; 15–23 kg, 45 mg/day PO; 15 kg or less, 30 mg/day PO. Continue for 10 days. *Child 6–11 mo:* 25 mg/day PO for 10 days. *Child 3–5 mo:* 20 mg/day PO for 10 days.
ADJUST DOSE Renal impairment
ADV EFF Anorexia, dizziness, headache, n/v, rhinitis
NC/PT Give within 2 days of exposure or sx onset. Pt should complete full course; refrigerate sol, shake well before each use; take safety precautions w/ dizziness; report severe GI problems.

ospemifene (Osphena)
CLASS Estrogen modulator
PREG/CONT X/NA

BBW Increased risk of endometrial cancer in women w/ uterus and unopposed estrogens; addition of progestin strongly advised. Increased risk of stroke, DVT; monitor accordingly.
IND & DOSE Tx of moderate to severe dyspareunia (painful intercourse) related to vulvar/vaginal atrophy due to menopause. *Adult:* 60 mg once/day with food.
ADV EFF DVT, hot flashes, hyperhidrosis, muscle spasms, PE, vaginal discharge
INTERACTIONS Estrogen, fluconazole, other estrogen modulators, rifampin
NC/PT Rule out pregnancy (contraceptives advised). Not for use in breast-feeding. Combine w/ progestin in women w/ intact uterus; ensure annual pelvic/breast exam, mammogram. Monitor for DVT, PE, other

thrombotic events. Reevaluate need for drug q 3–6 mo. Pt should take once/day, schedule annual complete exam and mammogram, report vision/speech changes, difficulty breathing, vaginal bleeding, chest pain, severe leg pain.

oxacillin sodium
(generic)

CLASS Penicillinase-resistant penicillin
PREG/CONT B/NA

BBW Increased risk of infection by multiple drug-resistant strains; weigh benefit/risk before use.
IND & DOSE Infections due to penicillinase-producing staphylococci; to initiate tx when staphylococcal infection suspected. *Adult, child 40 kg or more:* 250–500 mg IV q 4–6 hr; up to 1 g q 4–6 hr in severe infections. Max, 6 g/day. *Child under 40 kg:* 50–100 mg/kg/day IV in equally divided doses q 4–6 hr. *Neonates 2 kg or more:* 25–50 mg/kg IV q 8 hr. *Neonates under 2 kg:* 25–50 mg/kg IV q 12 hr.
ADV EFF Anaphylaxis, bone marrow suppression, fever, gastritis, nephritis, n/v/d, pain, phlebitis, rash, seizures, sore mouth, superinfections, wheezing
INTERACTIONS Aminoglycosides, tetracyclines
NC/PT Culture before tx. Do not mix in same IV sol as other antibiotics. Be prepared for serious hypersensitivity reactions. Treat superinfections. Pt should avoid exposure to infection, use mouth care for sore mouth, report rash, difficulty breathing, signs of infection.

oxaliplatin (Eloxatin)

CLASS Antineoplastic
PREG/CONT D/NA

BBW Risk of serious to fatal anaphylactic reactions.

IND & DOSE Tx of metastatic colon/rectum cancer as first-line tx or after progression after other tx. *Adult:* 85 mg/m² IV infusion in 250–500 mL D₅W w/ leucovorin 200 mg/m² in D₅W both over 2 hr followed by 5-FU 400 mg/m² IV bolus over 2–4 min, followed by 5-FU 600 mg/m² IV infusion in 500 mL D₅W as 22-hr continuous infusion on day 1. Then leucovorin 200 mg/m² IV infusion over 2 hr followed by 5-FU 400 mg/m² bolus over 2–4 min, followed by 5-FU 600 mg/m² IV infusion in 500 mL D₅W as 22-hr continuous infusion on day 2. Repeat cycle q 2 wk.
ADV EFF Abd pain, anaphylaxis, anorexia, constipation, cough, dyspnea, fatigue, hyperglycemia, hypokalemia, injection-site reactions, neuropathy, n/v/d, paresthesia, pulmonary fibrosis, RPLS
INTERACTIONS Nephrotoxic drugs
NC/PT Premedicate w/ antiemetics, dexamethasone. Monitor for potentially dangerous anaphylactic reactions. Monitor respiratory/neurologic function. Not for use in pregnancy, breast-feeding. Pt should take safety precautions w/ CNS effects, report severe headache, vision changes, difficulty breathing, numbness/tingling.

oxandrolone (Oxandrin)

CLASS Anabolic steroid
PREG/CONT X/C-III

BBW Monitor LFTs, serum electrolytes periodically. Consult physician for corrective measures; risk of peliosis hepatitis, liver cell tumors. Measure cholesterol periodically in pts at high risk for CAD; lipids may increase.
IND & DOSE Relief of bone pain w/ osteoporosis; adjunct tx to promote weight gain after weight loss due to extensive trauma; to offset protein catabolism associated w/ prolonged corticosteroid use; HIV wasting syndrome; HIV-associated muscle weakness. *Adult:* 2.5 mg PO

bid–qid; max, 20 mg. May need 2–4 wk to evaluate response. *Child:* Total daily dose, 0.1 mg/kg or less, or 0.045 mg/lb or less PO; may repeat intermittently.

ADV EFF Abd fullness, acne, anorexia, blood lipid changes, burning of tongue, excitation, gynecomastia, **hepatitis** in females, **intra-abdominal hemorrhage, liver cell tumors, liver failure,** virilization of prepubertal males

NC/PT May need 2–4 wk to evaluate response. Monitor effect on child w/ long-bone X-rays q 3–6 mo; stop drug well before bone age reaches norm for pt's chronologic age. Monitor LFTs, serum electrolytes, blood lipids. Not for use in pregnancy (barrier contraceptives advised). Pt should take w/ food, report urine/stool color changes, abd pain, severe n/v.

---

oxaprozin (Daypro), oxaprozin potassium (Daypro Alta)
CLASS NSAID
PREG/CONT C/NA

BBW Increased risk of CV events, GI bleeding; monitor accordingly. Contraindicated for periop pain associated w/ CABG surgery.
IND & DOSE Tx of osteoarthritis. *Adult:* 1,200 mg/day PO. Use initial 600 mg w/ low body weight or milder disease. **Tx of rheumatoid arthritis.** *Adult:* 1,200 mg/day PO. **Tx of juvenile rheumatoid arthritis.** *Child 6–16 yr:* 600–1,200 mg/day PO based on body weight.
ADJUST DOSE Renal impairment
ADV EFF Anaphylactoid reactions to anaphylactic shock, constipation, dizziness, dyspepsia, n/v/d, platelet inhibition, rash
NC/PT Pt should take w/ food, take safety precautions w/ dizziness, report unusual bleeding, black tarry stools.

---

oxazepam (generic)
CLASS Anxiolytic, benzodiazepine
PREG/CONT D/C-IV

IND & DOSE Mgt of anxiety disorders, alcohol withdrawal. *Adult, child over 12 yr:* 10–15 mg PO or up to 30 mg PO tid–qid, depending on severity of anxiety sx. Higher range recommended in alcoholics.
ADJUST DOSE Elderly, debilitated pts
ADV EFF Apathy, bradycardia, constipation, **CV collapse,** depression, diarrhea, disorientation, dizziness, drowsiness, dry mouth, fatigue, fever, hiccups, lethargy, light-headedness
INTERACTIONS Alcohol, CNS depressants, theophylline
NC/PT Taper gradually after long-term tx, especially in pts w/ epilepsy. Pt should take safety precautions w/ CNS effects, report vision changes, fainting, rash.

---

oxcarbazepine (Oxtellar XR, Trileptal)
CLASS Antiepileptic
PREG/CONT C/NA

BBW Monitor serum sodium before and periodically during tx; serious hyponatremia can occur. Teach pt to report sx (nausea, headache, malaise, lethargy, confusion).
IND & DOSE Tx of partial seizures. *Adult:* 300 mg PO bid; may increase to total 1,200 mg PO bid if clinically needed as adjunct tx. Converting to monotherapy: 300 mg PO bid started while reducing dose of other antiepileptics; reduce other drugs over 3–6 wk while increasing oxcarbazepine over 2–4 wk to max 2,400 mg/day. Starting as monotherapy: 300 mg PO bid; increase by 300 mg/day q third day until desired dose of 1,200 mg/day reached. Or 600 mg/day PO ER form; increase at weekly intervals of 600 mg/day to target 2,400 mg/day.

Adjunct tx of partial seizures. *Child 4–16 yr:* 8–10 mg/kg/day PO in two equally divided doses; max, 600 mg/day. *Child 2–4 yr over 20 kg:* 8–10 mg/kg/day PO; max, 600 mg/day. *Child 2–4 yr under 20 kg:* 16–20 mg/kg/day PO; max, 600 mg/day.
Monotherapy for partial seizures in epileptic child. *Child 4–16 yr:* 8–10 mg/kg/day PO in two divided doses. If pt taking another antiepileptic, slowly withdraw that drug over 3–6 wk. Then, increase oxcarbazepine in 10-mg/kg/day increments at wkly intervals to desired level. If pt not taking another antiepileptic, increase dose by 5 mg/kg/day q third day.
ADJUST DOSE Elderly pts, renal impairment
ADV EFF Bradycardia, **bronchospasm**, confusion, disturbed coordination, dizziness, drowsiness, hypertension, hyponatremia, hypotension, impaired fertility, n/v, **pulmonary edema, suicidality**, unsteadiness
INTERACTIONS Alcohol, carbamazepine, felodipine, hormonal contraceptives, phenobarbital, phenytoin, valproic acid, verapamil
NC/PT Monitor for hyponatremia. Taper slowly if stopping or switching to other antiepileptic. Not for use in pregnancy (barrier contraceptives advised). Pt should swallow ER tablets whole, not cut, crush, or chew them; take safety precautions w/ CNS effects; avoid alcohol; wear medical ID; report unusual bleeding, difficulty breathing, thoughts of suicide, headache, confusion, lethargy.

---

oxybutynin chloride
(Ditropan, Gelnique, Oxytrol)
CLASS Anticholinergic, urinary antispasmodic
PREG/CONT B/NA

IND & DOSE Relief of bladder instability sx; tx of overactive bladder (ER form). *Adult:* 5 mg PO bid or tid; max, 5 mg qid. ER tablets, 5 mg daily; max, 30 mg/day. Transdermal patch, 1 patch applied to dry, intact skin on abdomen, hip, or buttock q 3–4 days (twice wkly). (OTC form available for women 18 yr and older.) Topical gel, 1 mL applied to thigh, abdomen, or upper arm q 24 hr. *Child over 6 yr:* 5 mg ER tablets PO daily; max, 20 mg/day. *Child over 5 yr:* 5 mg PO bid; max, 5 mg tid.
ADJUST DOSE Elderly pts
ADV EFF Blurred vision, decreased sweating, dizziness, drowsiness, dry mouth, tachycardia, urinary hesitancy
INTERACTIONS Amantadine, haloperidol, nitrofurantoin, phenothiazines
NC/PT Arrange for cystometry, other diagnostic tests before, during tx. Monitor vision periodically. Periodic bladder exams needed. Pt should swallow ER tablet whole and not cut, crush, or chew it; apply gel to thigh, abdomen, or upper arm (rotate sites); apply patch to dry, intact skin on abdomen, hip, or buttock (remove old patch before applying new one); take safety precautions w/ CNS effects; report vision changes vision, vomiting.

DANGEROUS DRUG

oxycodone hydrochloride (M-oxy, Oxecta, OxyContin, OxyFAST, OxyIR, Roxicodone)
CLASS Opioid agonist analgesic
PREG/CONT B/C-II

BBW OxyFAST, Roxicodone Intensol highly concentrated preparations; use extreme care. Drug has abuse potential; monitor accordingly. Concurrent use of CYP3A4 inhibitors may result in increased drug effects, potentially fatal respiratory depression.
IND & DOSE Relief of moderate to moderately severe pain. *Adult:* Tablets, 5–15 mg PO q 4–6 hr; opioid-naïve, 10–30 mg PO q 4 hr. Capsules, 5 mg PO q 6 hr. Tablets in aversion technology, 5–15 mg PO q 4 hr as needed. Oral sol, 10–30 mg PO q 4 hr

as needed. **Tx of breakthrough pain.** *Adult:* Immediate-release (*OxyIR*), 5 mg PO q 4 hr. **Mgt of moderate to severe pain when continuous, around-the-clock analgesic needed for extended period.** *Adult:* CR tablets, 10 mg PO q 12 hr for pts taking nonopioid analgesics and requiring around-the-clock tx for extended period. Adjust q 1–2 days as needed by increasing by 25% to 50%.

ADJUST DOSE Elderly pts, impaired adults

ADV EFF Bronchospasm, **cardiac arrest,** constipation, dizziness, drowsiness, flushing, **laryngospasm,** light-headedness, n/v, **respiratory arrest,** sedation, **shock,** sweating, ureteral spasm, vision changes

INTERACTIONS Barbiturate general anesthetics, opioids, protease inhibitors; avoid these combinations

NC/PT CR form not for child. Use pediatric formulas to determine child dose for immediate-release form. Have opioid antagonist, facilities for assisted, controlled respiration on hand. Pt should swallow CR form whole and not cut, crush, or chew it; take 4–6 hr before next feeding if breast-feeding; take safety precautions w/ CNS effects; use laxative for constipation; report difficulty breathing, fainting.

oxymetazoline (Afrin, Dristan, Neo-Synephrine 12 Hour Extra Moisturizing, Vicks Sinex 12-Hour)

CLASS Nasal decongestant
PREG/CONT C/NA

BBW Monitor BP carefully; pts w/ hypertension may experience increased hypertension related to vasoconstriction. If nasal decongestant needed, pseudoephedrine is drug of choice.

IND & DOSE Symptomatic relief of nasal, nasopharyngeal mucosal congestion. *Adult, child over 6 yr:* 2–3 sprays of 0.05% sol in each nos-

tril bid a.m. and p.m. or q 10–12 hr for up to 3 days.

ADV EFF Anxiety, arrhythmias, **CV collapse,** dizziness, drowsiness, dysuria, fear, headache, hypertension, light-headedness, nausea, painful urination, rebound congestion, restlessness, tenseness

INTERACTIONS MAOIs, methyldopa, TCAs, urine acidifiers/alkalinizers

NC/PT Systemic adverse effects less common because drug not generally absorbed systemically. Review proper administration. Rebound congestion possible. Pt should avoid prolonged use (over 3 days), smoky rooms; drink plenty of fluids; use humidifier; take safety precautions w/ CNS effects; report excessive nervousness.

oxymetholone (Anadrol-50)

CLASS Anabolic steroid
PREG/CONT X/C-III

BBW Monitor LFTs, serum electrolytes during tx. Consult physician for corrective measures; risk of peliosis hepatis, liver cell tumors. Measure cholesterol in pts at high risk for CAD; lipids may increase.

IND & DOSE Tx of anemias, including congenital aplastic, hypoplastic. *Adult, child:* 1–5 mg/kg/day PO. Give for minimum trial of 3–6 mo.

ADV EFF Abd fullness, acne, anorexia, blood lipid changes, burning of tongue, confusion, excitation, gynecomastia, **intra-abdominal hemorrhage, hepatitis,** hirsutism in females, hyperglycemia, insomnia, **liver cell tumors, liver failure,** virilization of prepubertal males

INTERACTIONS Oral anticoagulants, oral antidiabetics

NC/PT Use w/ extreme caution; risk of serious disruption of growth/development; weigh benefits, risks. Monitor LFTs, lipids, bone age in children. Not for use in pregnancy (barrier contraceptives advised). Pt should take w/ food; monitor glucose closely if diabetic; take safety precautions w/ CNS effects; report severe nausea, urine/stool color changes.

DANGEROUS DRUG

oxymorphone hydrochloride (Opana)

CLASS Opioid agonist analgesic
PREG/CONT C/C-II

BBW Ensure pt swallows ER form whole; cutting, crushing, chewing could cause rapid release and fatal overdose. ER form has abuse potential; monitor accordingly. ER form indicated only for around-the-clock use over extended period. Do not give PRN. Pt must not consume alcohol in any form while taking oxycodone; risk of serious serum drug level increase, potentially fatal overdose.

IND & DOSE Relief of moderate to moderately severe acute pain. *Adult:* 10–20 mg PO q 4–6 hr. **Relief of moderate to moderately severe pain in pts needing around-the-clock tx.** *Adult:* 5 mg ER tablet PO q 12 hr; may increase in 5- to 10-mg increments q 3–7 days. **Preop medication; anesthesia support; obstetric analgesia; relief of anxiety in pts w/ pulmonary edema associated w/ left ventricular dysfx.** *Adult:* 0.5 mg IV or 1–1.5 mg IM, subcut q 4–6 hr as needed. For analgesia during labor, 0.5–1 mg IM.

ADJUST DOSE Elderly pts, impaired adults, renal impairment

ADV EFF Cardiac arrest, bronchospasm, constipation, dizziness, dry mouth, euphoria, flushing, hypertension, hypotension, **laryngospasm,** n/v, **respiratory arrest,** sedation, **shock,** sweating, urine retention

INTERACTIONS Alcohol, barbiturate anesthetics, CNS depressants

NC/PT Have opioid antagonist, facilities for assisted, controlled respiration on hand during parenteral administration. Pt should swallow ER tablet whole and not cut, crush, or chew it; take 4–6 hr before next feeding if breast-feeding; avoid alcohol; use laxative for constipation; take safety precautions w/ CNS effects; report difficulty breathing.

DANGEROUS DRUG

oxytocin (Pitocin)

CLASS Hormone, oxytocic
PREG/CONT X/NA

BBW Reserve for medical use, not elective induction.

IND & DOSE Induction, stimulation of labor. *Adult:* 0.5–2 milliunits/min (0.0005–0.002 units/min) by IV infusion through infusion pump. Increase in increments of no more than 1–2 milliunits/min at 30- to 60-min intervals until contraction pattern similar to normal labor established. Rates exceeding 9–10 milliunits/min rarely needed. **Control of postpartum uterine bleeding.** *Adult:* Add 10–40 units to 1,000 mL nondydrating diluent, infuse IV at rate to control uterine atony. Or, 10 units IM after delivery of placenta. **Tx of incomplete, inevitable abortion.** *Adult:* 10 units oxytocin w/ 500 mL physiologic saline sol or 5% dextrose in physiologic saline IV infused at 10–20 milliunits (20–40 drops)/min. Max, 30 units in 12 hr.

ADV EFF Afibrinogenemia, anaphylactic reaction, cardiac arrhythmias, fetal bradycardia, **maternal death,** neonatal jaundice, n/v, **severe water intoxication**

NC/PT Ensure fetal position/size, absence of complications. Continuously observe pt receiving IV oxytocin for induction, stimulation of labor; fetal monitoring preferred. Regulate rate to establish uterine contractions. Stop at first sign of hypersensitivity reactions.

DANGEROUS DRUG

paclitaxel (Abraxane)

CLASS Antimitotic, antineoplastic

PREG/CONT D/NA

BBW Do not give unless blood counts within acceptable range. Premedicate w/ one of following to prevent severe hypersensitivity reactions: Oral dexamethasone 20 mg 12 hr and 6 hr before paclitaxel, 10 mg if AIDS-related Kaposi sarcoma; diphenhydramine 50 mg IV 30–60 min before paclitaxel; cimetidine 300 mg IV or ranitidine 50 mg IV 30–60 min before paclitaxel. Do not substitute *Abraxane* for other paclitaxel formulations.

IND & DOSE Tx of ovarian cancer after failure of other tx. *Adult:* Previously untreated, 135 mg/m² IV over 24 hr or 175 mg/m² IV over 3 hr q 3 wk, then 75 mg/m² IV cisplatin Previously treated, 135 mg/m² or 175 mg/m² IV over 3 hr q 3 wk. Tx of breast cancer after failure of combination tx. *Adult:* 175 mg/m² IV over 3 hr q 3 wk for four courses after failure of chemotherapy; 175 mg/m² IV over 3 hr q 3 wk after initial chemotherapy failure or relapse within 6 mo; or 260 mg/m² IV over 30 min q 3 wk. Tx of AIDS-related Kaposi sarcoma. *Adult:* 135 mg/m² IV over 3 hr q 3 wk or 100 mg/m² IV over 3 hr q 2 wk. Tx of non-small-cell-lung cancer. *Adult:* 135 mg/m² IV over 24 hr, then 75 mg/m² cisplatin IV q 3 wk. Adjunct tx sequential to doxorubicin-containing regimen for node-positive breast cancer. *Adult:* 175 mg/m² IV over 3 hr q 3 wk for four courses, with doxorubicin regimen.

ADV EFF Alopecia, arthralgia, **bone marrow depression, hypersensitivity reactions, infection,** myalgia, n/v, peripheral neuropathies

INTERACTIONS Cisplatin, cyclosporine, dexamethasone, diazepam, etoposide, ketoconazole, quinidine,

teniposide, testosterone, verapamil, vincristine

NC/PT Monitor CBC carefully; dose based on response. Premedicate to decrease risk of hypersensitivity reactions. Not for use in pregnancy (barrier contraceptives advised). Pt should avoid exposure to infections; mark calendar of tx days; take safety precautions w/ CNS effects; cover head at temp extremes (hair loss possible); report signs of infection, difficulty breathing.

palifermin (Kepivance)

CLASS Keratinocyte growth factor

PREG/CONT C/NA

IND & DOSE To decrease incidence, duration of severe oral mucositis in pts w/ hematologic malignancies receiving myelotoxic chemotherapy requiring hematopoietic stem-cell support. *Adult:* 60 mcg/kg/day by IV bolus for 3 consecutive days before and 3 consecutive days after chemotherapy regimen.

ADV EFF Edema, erythema, pruritus, rash, taste alterations, tongue swelling

INTERACTIONS Heparin, myelotoxic chemotherapy

NC/PT Risk of tumor growth stimulation; monitor accordingly. Not for use in breast-feeding. Provide nutrition support w/ taste changes, skin care for rash. Pt should report pain at infusion site, severe rash.

paliperidone (Invega)

CLASS Atypical antipsychotic, benzisoxazole

PREG/CONT C/NA

BBW Avoid use in elderly pts w/ dementia-related psychosis; increased risk of CV death. Drug not approved for this use.

IND & DOSE Tx of schizophrenia, schizoaffective disorder. *Adult:* 6 mg/day PO in a.m.; max, 12 mg/day PO. Tx of schizophrenia. *Adult:* 234 mg IM, then 156 mg IM in 1 wk, both in deltoid; 117 mg IM 1 wk later in gluteal or deltoid. Maint, 39–234 mg/mo IM. *Child 12–17 yr:* 51 kg or more, 3 mg/day PO; range, 3–12 mg/day PO. Under 56 kg, 3 mg/day PO; range, 3–6 mg/day.
ADJUST DOSE Renal impairment
ADV EFF Akathisia, dizziness, dry mouth, dystonia, extrapyramidal disorders, hyperglycemia, impaired thinking, **increased mortality in geriatric pts w/ dementia-related psychosis**, NMS, orthostatic hypotension, **prolonged QT interval, suicidality,** tachycardia, weight gain
INTERACTIONS Alcohol, antihypertensives, CNS depressants, dopamine agonist, levodopa, QT-prolonging drugs
NC/PT Monitor for hyperglycemia, weight gain. Tablet matrix may appear in stool. Not for use in pregnancy, breast-feeding. Pt should swallow tablet whole and not cut, crush, or chew it; avoid alcohol; take safety precautions w/ CNS effects; report fever, thoughts of suicide.

palivizumab (Synagis)
CLASS Antiviral, monoclonal antibody
PREG/CONT C/NA

IND & DOSE Px of serious lower respiratory tract disease caused by RSV in children at high risk for RSV disease. *Child:* 15 mg/kg IM as single injection monthly during RSV season; give first dose before start of RSV season.
ADV EFF Chills, fever, malaise, pharyngitis, **severe anaphylactoid reaction**
INTERACTIONS Immunosuppressants
NC/PT Give preferably in anterolateral aspect of thigh; do not use gluteal muscle. For cardiopulmonary bypass pts, give as soon as possible following procedure, even if under 1 mo since previous dose. Monitor for anaphylaxis, infection. Caregivers should protect from infection, report fever, difficulty breathing.

palonosetron hydrochloride (Aloxi)
CLASS Antiemetic, selective serotonin receptor antagonist
PREG/CONT B/NA

IND & DOSE Px of acute/delayed n/v associated w/ chemotherapy. *Adult:* 0.25 mg IV as single dose over 30 sec 30 min before start of chemotherapy, or 0.5 mg PO 1 hr before start of chemotherapy. Px of postop n/v. *Adult:* 0.075 mg IV as single dose over 10 sec immediately before anesthesia induction.
ADV EFF Arrhythmias, constipation, drowsiness, flulike sx, headache, somnolence
NC/PT Coordinate dose timing. Pt should take safety precautions, analgesic for headache; report severe constipation, fever.

pamidronate disodium (Aredia)
CLASS Bisphosphonate, calcium regulator
PREG/CONT D/NA

IND & DOSE Tx of hypercalcemia. *Adult:* 60–90 mg IV over 2–24 hr as single dose; max, 90 mg/dose. Tx of Paget disease. *Adult:* 30 mg/day IV as 4-hr infusion on 3 consecutive days for total dose of 90 mg; max, 90 mg/dose. Tx of osteolytic bone lesions. *Adult:* 90 mg IV as 2-hr infusion q 3–4 wk. For bone lesions caused by multiple myeloma, monthly 4-hr infusion; max, 90 mg/dose.
ADJUST DOSE Renal impairment

ADV EFF Bone pain, diarrhea, headache, hypocalcemia, nausea, **osteonecrosis of jaw**

NC/PT Have calcium on hand for hypocalcemic tetany. Monitor serum calcium regularly. Dental exam needed before tx for cancer pts at risk for osteonecrosis of jaw. Maintain hydration, nutrition. Pt should not take foods high in calcium, calcium supplements within 2 hr of dose; report muscle twitching, severe diarrhea.

---

pancrelipase (Creon, Pancreaze, Pertyze, Ultresa, Viokace)

CLASS Digestive enzyme
PREG/CONT C/NA

IND & DOSE Replacement tx in pts w/ deficient exocrine pancreatic secretions. *Adult:* 4,000–20,000 units (usually 1–3 capsules/tablets) PO w/ each meal, snacks; may increase to 8 capsules/tablets in severe cases. *Viokace:* 500 units/kg/meal PO to max 2,500 units/kg/meal. Pts w/ pancreatectomy or obstruction, 72,000 units lipase meal PO while consuming 100 g/day fat (*Creon*). *Child 4 yr and older:* 500 units lipase/kg/meal PO to max 2,500 units/kg/meal. *Child 1–under 4 yr:* 1,000 units/kg/meal PO to max 2,500 units/kg/meal or 10,000 units/kg/day. *Child up to 1 yr:* 3,000 units lipase PO/120 mL formula or breast-feeding session; 2,000–4,000 units/feeding PO (*Ultresa*).
ADV EFF Abd cramps, diarrhea, hyperuricemia, nausea
NC/PT Do not mix capsules directly into infant formula, breast milk; follow dose w/ formula, breast milk. *Creon* and *Viokace* are not interchangeable. Pt should not crush or chew enteric-coated capsules; may open *Ultresa* capsules and sprinkle contents on food. Pt should report difficulty breathing, joint pain.

---

panitumumab (Vectibix)

CLASS Monoclonal antibody, antineoplastic
PREG/CONT C/NA

BBW Monitor for possibly severe infusion reactions, dermatologic toxicity, pulmonary fibrosis.
IND & DOSE Tx of epidermal growth factor receptor–expressing metastatic colorectal carcinoma w/ disease progressing w/ or after chemotherapy regimens. *Adult:* 6 mg/kg IV over 60 min q 14 days; give doses larger than 1,000 mg over 90 min.
ADV EFF Abd pain, constipation, dermatologic toxicity, diarrhea, electrolyte depletion, fatigue, hypomagnesemia, **infusion reactions, pulmonary fibrosis**
NC/PT Monitor electrolytes, respiratory function. Monitor constantly during infusion; stop if infusion reaction. Men, women should use barrier contraceptives during and for 6 mo after tx; not for use in breast-feeding. Pt should report difficulty breathing, pain at injection site, fever, rash.

---

pantoprazole (Protonix)

CLASS Proton pump inhibitor
PREG/CONT B/NA

IND & DOSE Tx of GERD; maint tx of erosive esophagitis; tx of pathological hypersecretory disorders. *Adult:* 40 mg/day PO for 8 wk or less for maint healing of erosive esophagitis. May repeat 8-wk course if no healing. Give continually for hypersecretory conditions: 40 mg/day IV bid up to 240 mg/day (2-yr duration) or 40 mg/day IV for 7–10 days. For severe hypersecretory syndromes, 80 mg q 12 hr (up to 240 mg/day) PO, IV (6-day duration).
ADJUST DOSE Hepatic impairment
ADV EFF Abd pain, bone loss, *Clostridium difficile* diarrhea, dizziness,

headache, insomnia, n/v/d, pneumonia, URI

NC/PT Further evaluation needed after 4 wk of tx for GERD. Switch from IV to oral as soon as possible. Pt should swallow tablet whole and not cut, crush, or chew it; take safety measures for dizziness; report severe diarrhea/headache, fever.

---

paricalcitol (Zemplar)
CLASS Vitamin
PREG/CONT C/NA

IND & DOSE Px, tx of secondary hyperparathyroidism associated w/ chronic renal failure. *Adult:* 0.04–0.1 mcg/kg injected during dialysis, no more often than q three wk. Pts not on dialysis: 1–2 mcg/day PO, or 2–4 mcg PO three times/wk based on parathyroid level.

ADV EFF Arthralgia, chills, dry mouth, fever, flulike sx, **GI hemorrhage,** n/v

INTERACTIONS Aluminum-containing antacids, ketoconazole

NC/PT Arrange for calcium supplements; restrict phosphorus intake. Not for use in breast-feeding. Pt should avoid vitamin D; report changes in thinking, appetite/weight loss, increased thirst.

---

paroxetine hydrochloride (Paxil), paroxetine mesylate (Brisdelle, Pexeva)
CLASS Antidepressant, SSRI
PREG/CONT C/NA

BBW Risk of increased suicidality in children, adolescents, young adults; monitor accordingly.

IND & DOSE Tx of depression. *Adult:* 20 mg/day PO; range, 20–50 mg/day. Or, 25–62.5 mg/day CR form. Tx of OCD. *Adult:* 20 mg/day PO. May increase in 10-mg/day increments; max, 60 mg/day. Tx of panic disorder. *Adult:* 10 mg/day PO; range,

10–60 mg/day. Or 12.5–75 mg/day CR tablet; max, 75 mg/day. Tx of social anxiety disorder. *Adult:* 20 mg/day PO in a.m. Or, 12.5 mg/day PO CR form; max, 60 mg/day or 37.5 mg/day CR form. Tx of generalized anxiety disorder. *Adult:* 20 mg/day PO; range, 20–50 mg/day. Tx of PMDD. *Adult:* 12.5 mg/day PO in a.m.; range, 12.5–25 mg/day. May give daily or just during luteal phase of cycle. Tx of PTSD. *Adult:* 20 mg/day PO as single dose; range, 20–50 mg/day. Tx of vasomotor sx of menopause (hot flashes). *Adult:* 7.5 mg/day PO at bedtime (*Brisdelle*).

ADJUST DOSE Elderly pts; hepatic, renal impairment

ADV EFF Anxiety, asthenia, constipation, diarrhea, MAOIs, phenobarbital, dry mouth, ejaculatory disorders, headache, insomnia, nervousness, somnolence, **suicidality**

INTERACTIONS Digoxin, fosamprenavir, MAOIs, phenobarbital, phenytoin, procyclidine, ritonavir, serotonergics, St. John's wort, tryptophan, warfarin

NC/PT Do not give within 14 days of MAOIs. Not for use in pregnancy, breast-feeding. Pt should take in evening; swallow CR tablet whole and not cut, crush, or chew it; shake suspension before use; take safety precautions w/ CNS effects; avoid St. John's wort; report blurred vision, thoughts of suicide.

---

pazopanib (Votrient)
CLASS Antineoplastic, kinase inhibitor
PREG/CONT D/NA

BBW Risk of severe to fatal hepatotoxicity. Monitor LFTs regularly; adjust dose accordingly.

IND & DOSE Tx of advanced renal cell carcinoma; tx of soft-tissue sarcoma progressed after prior tx. *Adult:* 800 mg/day PO without food.

ADJUST DOSE Hepatic impairment

ADV EFF Anorexia, **arterial throm-botic events**, GI perforation, hair color changes, **hemorrhagic events**, hepatotoxicity, hypertension, impaired wound healing, hypothyroidism, n/v, prolonged QT interval, proteinuria
INTERACTIONS CYP3A4 inducers/inhibitors, simvastatin
NC/PT Not for use in pregnancy. Hair may lose pigmentation. Provide nutrition support for n/v. Pt should take on empty stomach at least 1 hr before, 2 hr after meal; report all drugs, OTC, herbs used (many drug interactions possible), report urine/stool color changes, yellowing of skin, eyes.

pegaptanib (Macugen)
CLASS Monoclonal antibody
PREG/CONT B/NA

IND & DOSE Tx of neovascular (wet) age-related macular degeneration. *Adult:* 0.3 mg q 6 wk by intravitreous injection into affected eye.
ADV EFF Anaphylaxis; **endophthalmitis;** eye discharge, pain; infection; increased IOP; retinal detachment; traumatic cataract; vision changes; vitreous floaters
NC/PT Monitor IOP. Pt should mark calendar of tx days, report eye redness, sensitivity to light, sudden vision change.

DANGEROUS DRUG
pegaspargase (Oncaspar)
CLASS Antineoplastic
PREG/CONT C/NA

IND & DOSE Tx of ALL. *Adult:* 2,500 international units/m² IM, IV q 14 days.
ADV EFF Anaphylaxis, bone marrow depression, coagulopathy, glucose intolerance, hepatic impairment, **pancreatitis,** renal toxicity
NC/PT IM route preferred; reserve IV for extreme situations. Monitor

LFTs, renal function. Not for use in breast-feeding. Pt should report excessive thirst, severe headache, acute shortness of breath, difficulty breathing.

pegfilgrastim (Neulasta)
CLASS Colony stimulating factor
PREG/CONT C/NA

IND & DOSE To decrease incidence of infection in pts w/ nonmyeloid malignancies receiving myelosuppressive anticancer drugs. *Adult, child over 45 kg:* 6 mg subcut as single dose once per chemotherapy cycle. Do not give within 14 days before and 24 hr after cytotoxic therapy.
ADV EFF Acute respiratory distress syndrome, alopecia, anorexia, arthralgia, **bone marrow suppression,** bone pain, dizziness, dyspepsia, edema, fatigue, fever, generalized weakness, mucositis, n/v/d, **splenic rupture,** stomatitis
INTERACTIONS Lithium
NC/PT Monitor CBC. Protect from light. Do not shake syringe. Sol should be free of particulate matter, not discolored. Pt should cover head at temp extremes (hair loss possible), avoid exposure to infection, report signs of infection, difficulty breathing, pain at injection site. Name confusion between *Neulasta* (pegfilgrastim) and *Neumega* (oprelvekin); use caution.

peginterferon alfa-2a (Pegasys)
CLASS Interferon
PREG/CONT X/NA

BBW May cause, aggravate life-threatening to fatal neuropsychiatric, autoimmune, ischemic, infectious disorders. Monitor closely; stop w/ persistent s&sx. Risk of serious fetal defects when used w/ ribavirin; men, women should avoid pregnancy.

IND & DOSE Tx of hepatitis C in pts w/ compensated liver disease and not treated w/ interferon alfa. *Adult:* 180 mcg subcut wkly for 48 wk w/ ribavirin.

ADJUST DOSE Hepatic, renal impairment

ADV EFF Asthenia, **bone marrow suppression, colitis,** fatigue, fever, headache, **hemolytic anemia, hepatic impairment, infections,** myalgia, **neuropsychiatric events, pancreatitis, pulmonary events, suicidality**

INTERACTIONS Azathioprine, didanosine, methadone, nucleoside analogues, theophylline, zidovudine

NC/PT Monitor closely; adverse effects may require stopping. Safety in pts w/ hepatitis B, concomitant hepatitis C/HIV not established. Not for use in pregnancy; men, women should use two forms of contraception during, for 6 mo after tx. Store in refrigerator. Teach proper administration, disposal of needles, syringes. Pt should avoid exposure to infection, report severe abd pain, bloody diarrhea, signs of infection, thoughts of suicide, difficulty breathing.

---

peginterferon alfa-2b
(Peg-Intron, Sylatron)
CLASS Interferon
PREG/CONT C/NA

BBW May cause, aggravate life-threatening to fatal neuropsychiatric, autoimmune, ischemic, infectious disorders. Monitor closely; stop w/ persistent s&sx. Risk of serious fetal defects when used w/ ribavirin; men, women should avoid pregnancy.

IND & DOSE Tx of chronic hepatitis C in pts w/ compensated livers; tx of genotype-1 chronic hepatitis C in combination w/ other drugs. *Adult:* 1.5 mcg/kg/wk subcut; may give w/ ribavirin 800–1,400 mg/day PO. *Child 3 yr and older:* 60 mcg/kg/wk subcut; may give w/ ribavirin 15 mg/kg/day PO.

ADJUST DOSE Hepatic, renal impairment

ADV EFF Asthenia, **bone marrow suppression, colitis,** fatigue, fever, headache, **hemolytic anemia, hepatic impairment, infections,** ischemic cerebral events, myalgia, **neuropsychiatric events, pancreatitis, pulmonary events, suicidality**

INTERACTIONS Azathioprine, didanosine, methadone, nucleoside analogues, theophylline, zidovudine

NC/PT Monitor closely; adverse effects may require stopping. Safety in pts w/ hepatitis B, concomitant hepatitis C/HIV not established. Not for use in pregnancy; men, women should use two forms of contraception during, for 6 mo after tx. Store in refrigerator. Teach proper administration, disposal of needles, syringes. Pt should avoid exposure to infection, report severe abd pain, bloody diarrhea, signs of infection, thoughts of suicide, difficulty breathing.

---

pegloticase (Krystexxa)
CLASS PEGylated uric-acid specific enzyme
PREG/CONT C/NA

BBW Severe anaphylaxis, infusion reactions have occurred; premedicate, closely monitor. Monitor serum uric acid level.

IND & DOSE Tx of chronic gout in pts refractory to conventional tx. *Adult:* 8 mg by IV infusion over no less than 120 min q 2 wk.

ADJUST DOSE Renal impairment

ADV EFF **Anaphylaxis,** chest pain, constipation, ecchymosis, gout flares, HF, infusion reactions, nasopharyngitis, vomiting

NC/PT Monitor serum uric acid level. Premedicate w/ antihistamines, corticosteroids. Contraindicated w/ G6PD deficiencies. Alert pt gout flares may occur up to 3 mo after starting tx. Not for use in breast-feeding. Pt should report difficulty breathing, edema.

pegvisomant (Somavert)

CLASS Human growth hormone analogue
PREG/CONT C/NA

IND & DOSE Tx of acromegaly in pts w/ inadequate response to surgery, radiation. *Adult:* 40 mg subcut as loading dose, then 10 mg/day subcut.
ADV EFF Diarrhea, dizziness, edema, **hepatic impairment**, infection, injection-site reactions, nausea, pain, peripheral edema, sinusitis
INTERACTIONS Opioids
NC/PT Local reactions to injection common; rotate sites regularly. Monitor for infection. Monitor liver function. Teach proper administration, disposal of needles, syringes. Not for use in breast-feeding.

DANGEROUS DRUG

pemetrexed (Alimta)

CLASS Antifolate antineoplastic
PREG/CONT D/NA

IND & DOSE Tx of unresectable malignant mesothelioma; tx of locally advanced, metastatic nonsmall-cell lung cancer. *Adult:* 500 mg/m² IV infused over 10 min on day 1, then 75 mg/m² cisplatin (tx of mesothelioma only) IV over 2 hr; repeat cycle q 21 days.
ADJUST DOSE Renal, hepatic impairment
ADV EFF Anorexia, **bone marrow suppression**, constipation, fatigue, n/v/d, **renal impairment**, stomatitis
INTERACTIONS Nephrotoxic drugs, NSAIDs
NC/PT Pretreat w/ corticosteroid, folic acid, vitamin B₁₂. Monitor CBC; dosage adjustment based on response. Not for use in pregnancy (barrier contraceptives advised), breast-feeding. Pt should avoid NSAIDs, exposure to infection; report unusual bleeding, severe GI sx.

penbutolol sulfate (Levatol)

CLASS Antihypertensive, beta blocker
PREG/CONT C/NA

IND & DOSE Tx of mild to moderate hypertension. *Adult:* 20 mg/day PO.
ADV EFF Bradycardia, **bronchospasm**, cardiac arrhythmias, constipation, decreased exercise tolerance/libido, dizziness, dyspnea, ED, fatigue, gastric pain, HF, **laryngospasm**, n/v/d, **pulmonary edema**, rash, **stroke**
INTERACTIONS Beta blockers, calcium channel blockers, epinephrine, ergots, insulin, NSAIDs, prazosin, sympathomimetics, verapamil
NC/PT Taper gradually after long-term tx. Pt should take safety precautions w/ CNS effects, report difficulty breathing, numbness/tingling, swelling.

penicillamine (Cuprimine, Depen)

CLASS Antirheumatic, chelate
PREG/CONT D/NA

BBW Because of severe toxicity, including bone marrow suppression, renal damage, reserve use for serious cases; monitor closely.
IND & DOSE Tx of severe, active rheumatoid arthritis, Wilson disease, cystinuria when other measures fail. *Adult:* 125–250 mg/day PO; max, 1 g/day
ADV EFF Agitation, anxiety, **bone marrow suppression**, fever, **myasthenia gravis**, paresthesia, rash, **renal toxicity**, tinnitus
INTERACTIONS Gold salts, nephrotoxic drugs
NC/PT Monitor CBC, renal function twice/wk. Assess neurologic functioning; stop if increasing weakness. Not for use in pregnancy (barrier contraceptives advised), breast-feeding. Pt should avoid exposure to infection,

report signs of infection, muscle weakness, edema.

penicillin G benzathine
(Bicillin L-A, Permapen)
CLASS Penicillin antibiotic
PREG/CONT B/NA

BBW Not for IV use. Do not inject or mix w/ other IV sols. Inadvertent IV administration has caused cardiorespiratory arrest, death.
IND & DOSE Tx of streptococcal infections. *Adult:* 1.2 million units IM. *Older child:* 900,000 units IM. *Child under 27 kg:* 300,000–600,000 units IM. **Tx of early syphilis.** *Adult:* 2.4 million units IM. **Tx of syphilis lasting longer than 1 yr.** *Adult:* 7.2 million units as 2.4 million units IM wkly for 3 wk. **Tx of yaws, bejel, pinta, erysipeloid.** *Adult:* 1.2 million units IM as single dose. **Tx of congenital syphilis.** *Child 2–12 yr:* Adjust dose based on adult schedule. *Child under 2 yr:* 50,000 units/kg body weight IM. **Px of rheumatic fever, chorea.** *Adult:* 1.2 million units IM q mo; or 600,000 units q 2 wk.
ADV EFF Anaphylaxis, bone marrow suppression, gastritis, glossitis, n/v/d, pain, phlebitis, rash, superinfections
INTERACTIONS Amikacin, gentamicin, neomycin, tetracyclines, tobramycin
NC/PT Culture before tx. Use IM only: Upper outer quadrant of buttock (adults), midlateral aspect of thigh (infants, small children). Pt should report difficulty breathing, rash, pain at injection site.

penicillin G potassium, penicillin G sodium
(Pfizerpen)
CLASS Penicillin antibiotic
PREG/CONT B/NA

IND & DOSE Tx of meningococcal meningitis. *Adult:* 1–2 million units q 2 hr IM, or 20–30 million units/day by continuous IV infusion. *Child:* 200,000–300,000 units/kg/day IV q

6 hr. *Infants under 7 days:* 50,000 units/kg/day IV in divided doses q 12 hr. **Tx of actinomycosis.** *Adult:* 1–6 million units/day IM in divided doses q 4–6 hr for 6 wk, or IV for cervicofacial cases. Or, 10–20 million units/day IV for thoracic, abd diseases. **Tx of clostridial infections.** *Adult:* 20 million units/day in divided doses q 4–6 hr IM or IV w/ antitoxin. **Tx of fusospirochetal infections (Vincent disease).** *Adult:* 5–10 million units/day IM or IV in divided doses q 4–6 hr. **Tx of rat-bite fever.** *Adult:* 12–20 million units/day IM or IV in divided doses q 4–6 hr for 3–4 wk. **Tx of Listeria infections.** *Adult:* 15–20 million units/day IM or IV in divided doses q 4–6 hr for 2 or 4 wk (meningitis, endocarditis, respectively). **Tx of Pasteurella infections.** *Adult:* 4–6 million units/day IM or IV in divided doses q 4–6 hr for 2 wk. **Tx of erysipeloid endocarditis.** *Adult:* 12–20 million units/day IM or IV in divided doses q 4–6 hr for 4–6 wk. **Tx of diphtheria (adjunct tx w/ antitoxin to prevent carrier state).** *Adult:* 2–3 million units/day IM or IV in divided doses q 4–6 hr for 10–12 days. **Tx of anthrax.** *Adult:* Minimum 5 million units/day IM or IV in divided doses. **Tx of streptococcal infections.** *Adult:* 5–24 million units/day IM or IV in divided doses q 4–6 hr. *Child:* 150,000 units/kg/day IM or IV q 4–6 hr. *Child under 7 days:* 75,000 units/kg/day IV in divided doses q 8 hr. **Tx of syphilis.** *Adult:* 18–24 million units/day IV q 4–6 hr for 10–14 days, then benzathine penicillin G 2.4 million units IM wkly for 3 wk. **Tx of gonorrhea.** 10 million units/day IV q 4–6 hr until improvement. **Tx of group B streptococci.** *Child:* 100,000 units/kg/ day IV.
ADV EFF Anaphylaxis, bone marrow suppression, gastritis, glossitis, n/v/d, pain, phlebitis, rash, superinfections
INTERACTIONS Amikacin, gentamicin, neomycin, tetracyclines, tobramycin

NC/PT Culture before tx. Smallest volume possible for IM use. Have emergency equipment on hand w/ IV infusion. Monitor serum electrolytes w/ penicillin potassium. Pt should report difficulty breathing, rash, unusual bleeding, signs of infection.

penicillin G procaine (Wycillin)
CLASS Penicillin antibiotic
PREG/CONT B/NA

IND & DOSE Tx of moderately severe infections caused by sensitive strains of streptococci, pneumococci, staphylococci. *Adult:* 600,000–1 million units/day IM for minimum 10 days. Tx of bacterial endocarditis (group A streptococci). *Adult:* 600,000–1 million units/day IM. Tx of fusospirochetal infections, rat-bite fever, erysipeloid, anthrax. *Adult:* 600,000–1 million units/day IM. Tx of diphtheria. *Adult:* 300,000–600,000 units/day IM w/ antitoxin. Tx of diphtheria carrier state. *Adult:* 300,000 units/day IM for 10 days. Tx of syphilis. *Adult, child over 12 yr:* 600,000 units/day IM for 8 days, 10–15 days for late-stage syphilis. Tx of neurosyphilis. *Adult:* 2.4 million units/day IM w/ 500 mg probenecid PO qid for 10–14 days, then 2.4 million units benzathine penicillin G IM after completion of tx regimen. Tx of congenital syphilis. *Child under 32 kg:* 50,000 units/kg/day IM for 10 days. Tx of group A streptococcal, staphylococcal pneumonia. *Child under 27 kg:* 300,000 units/day IM.
ADV EFF Anaphylaxis, bone marrow suppression, gastritis, glossitis, n/v/d, pain, phlebitis, rash, superinfections
INTERACTIONS Amikacin, gentamicin, neomycin, tetracyclines, tobramycin
NC/PT Culture before tx. IM route only in upper outer quadrant of buttock; midlateral aspect of thigh may be preferred for infants, small children. Pt should report difficulty breathing, rash, unusual bleeding, signs of infection.

penicillin V (generic)
CLASS Penicillin antibiotic
PREG/CONT B/NA

IND & DOSE Tx of fusospirochetal infections, staphylococcal infections of skin, soft tissues. *Adult, child over 12 yr:* 250–500 mg PO q 6–8 hr. Tx of streptococcal infections. *Adult, child over 12 yr:* 125–250 mg PO q 6–8 hr for 10 days. Tx of pneumococcal infections. *Adult, child over 12 yr:* 250–500 mg PO q 6 hr until afebrile for 48 hr. Px of rheumatic fever/chorea recurrence. *Adult, child over 12 yr:* 25–250 mg PO bid. Tx of Lyme disease. *Adult, child over 12 yr:* 500 mg PO qid for 10–20 days. Tx of mild, uncomplicated cutaneous anthrax. *Adult, child over 12 yr:* 200–500 mg PO qid. *Child 2–12 yr:* 25–50 mg/kg/day PO in two or four divided doses. Px of anthrax px. *Adult, child over 9 yr:* 7.5 mg/kg PO qid. *Child under 9 yr:* 50 mg/kg/day PO in four divided doses. Px of *Streptococcus pneumoniae* septicemia in sickle cell anemia. *Child 6–9 yr:* 250 mg PO bid. *Child 3 mo–5 yr:* 125 mg PO bid.
ADV EFF Anaphylaxis, bone marrow suppression, gastritis, glossitis, n/v/d, pain, phlebitis, rash, superinfections
INTERACTIONS Tetracyclines
NC/PT Culture before tx. Stable for max 14 days. Pt should take w/ water, not w/ milk, fruit juices, soft drinks; refrigerate suspension; report difficulty breathing, rash, unusual bleeding, signs of infection.

pentamidine isethionate (NebuPent, Pentam 300)

CLASS Antiprotozoal
PREG/CONT C/NA

IND & DOSE Tx of *Pneumocystis jiroveci* pneumonia. *Adult, child:* 4 mg/kg/day for 14–21 days by deep IM injection or IV infusion over 60–120 min. Px of *P. jiroveci* pneumonia. *Adult, child:* 300 mg once q 4 wk through *Respirgard II* nebulizer.
ADV EFF Acute renal failure, anorexia, cough, dizziness, fatigue, fever, hypotension, **laryngospasm**, metallic taste (inhalation), **severe hypotension**, pain at injection site, rash, Stevens-Johnson syndrome
NC/PT Culture before tx. Drug a biohazard; use safe handling procedures. Monitor CBC, LFTs, renal function. Have pt in supine position for parenteral administration. Pt should take safety precautions w/ hypotension, CNS effects; learn proper use, care of *Respirgard II*; report difficulty breathing, rash.

---

pentazocine (Talwin)

CLASS Opioid agonist-antagonist
PREG/CONT C/C-IV

BBW Pentazocine/naloxone for oral use only; can be lethal if injected.
IND & DOSE Relief of moderate to severe pain; preanesthetic (parenteral). *Adult, child over 12 yr:* 50 mg PO q 3–4 hr; max, 600 mg/24 hr. Or, 30 mg IM, subcut or IV. May repeat q 3–4 hr; max, 360 mg/24 hr. *Women in labor:* 30 mg IM as single dose. Or, 20 mg IV two to three times at 2- to 3-hr intervals.
ADJUST DOSE Elderly pts, impaired adults
ADV EFF Bronchospasm, cardiac arrest, constipation, dizziness, euphoria, hypotension, light-headedness, **laryngospasm**, n/v, pain at injection site, sedation, **shock**, sweating, urine retention
INTERACTIONS Alcohol, barbiturate anesthetics, CNS depressants, methadone, opioids
NC/PT Doses over 30 mg IV or 60 mg IM, subcut not recommended. Oral form especially abused in combination w/ tripelennamine ("Ts and Blues"); serious, fatal consequences. Have opioid antagonist, equipment for assisted, controlled respiration on hand during parenteral administration. Withdraw gradually after 4–5 days. Pt should avoid alcohol, OTC products; use laxative for constipation, take safety precautions w/ CNS effects; report difficulty breathing.

---

pentobarbital (Nembutal)

CLASS Antiepileptic, barbiturate, sedative-hypnotic
PREG/CONT D/C-II

BBW Do not administer intra-arterially; may produce arteriospasm, thrombosis, gangrene.
IND & DOSE Sedative-hypnotic, preanesthetic, emergency antiseizure. *Adult:* Give by slow IV injection (max, 50 mg/min); 100 mg in 70-kg adult. Wait at least 1 min for full effect. Base dose on response. May give additional small increments to max 200–500 mg. Minimize dose in seizure states to avoid compounding possible depression after seizures. Or, 150–200 mg IM. *Child:* Reduce initial adult dose based on age, weight, condition. Or, 25–80 mg or 2–6 mg/kg IM; max, 100 mg.
ADJUST DOSE Elderly pts, debilitated adults
ADV EFF Agitation, apnea, ataxia, bradycardia, **bronchospasm**, CNS depression, **circulatory collapse**, confusion, dizziness, hallucinations, hyperkinesia, hypotension, hypoventilation, insomnia, **laryngospasm**, pain/necrosis at injection

site, somnolence, **Stevens-Johnson syndrome**, syncope, **withdrawal syndrome**
INTERACTIONS Alcohol, beta-adrenergic blockers, CNS depressants, corticosteroids, doxycycline, estrogens, hormonal contraceptives, metronidazole, oral anticoagulants, phenylbutazones, quinidine, theophylline
NC/PT Use caution in children; may produce irritability, aggression, inappropriate tearfulness. Give slowly IV or by deep IM injection. Monitor continuously during IV use; monitor injection site for irritation. Taper gradually w/ long-term use. Pt should take safety precautions for CNS effects; report difficulty breathing, rash.

---

pentosan polysulfate sodium (Elmiron)
CLASS Bladder protectant
PREG/CONT B/NA

IND & DOSE Relief of bladder pain associated w/ interstitial cystitis.
Adult: 100 mg PO tid on empty stomach.

ADV EFF Abd pain, alopecia, bleeding, diarrhea, dizziness, dyspepsia, liver function changes, nausea
INTERACTIONS Anticoagulants, aspirin, NSAIDs
NC/PT Use caution w/ hepatic insufficiency. Drug a heparin; use caution if surgery needed. Pt should cover head at temp extremes (hair loss possible), report unusual bleeding, urine/stool color changes.

---

pentostatin (Nipent)
CLASS Antineoplastic antibiotic
PREG/CONT D/NA

BBW Associated w/ fatal pulmonary toxicity, bone marrow depression.
IND & DOSE Tx of alpha interferon–refractory hairy cell leukemia, chronic lymphocytic leukemia, cuta-

neous/peripheral T-cell lymphoma.
Adult: 4 mg/m² IV q other wk.
ADJUST DOSE Renal impairment
ADV EFF Abd pain, anorexia, **bone marrow suppression**, chills, cough, dizziness, dyspepsia, n/v, **pulmonary toxicity**, rash
INTERACTIONS Allopurinol, cyclophosphamide, fludarabine, vidarabine
NC/PT Toxic drug; use special precautions in handling. Monitor CBC regularly; monitor pulmonary function. Not for use in pregnancy, breastfeeding. Pt should mark calendar of tx days, avoid exposure to infection, report difficulty breathing, signs of infection.

---

pentoxifylline (Trental)
CLASS Hemorrheologic, xanthine
PREG/CONT C/NA

IND & DOSE Tx of intermittent claudication. *Adult:* 400 mg PO tid w/ meals for at least 8 wk.
ADJUST DOSE Renal impairment
ADV EFF Angina, anxiety, dizziness, dyspepsia, headache, nausea, rash
INTERACTIONS Anticoagulants, theophylline
NC/PT Pt should take w/ meals; swallow tablet whole and not cut, crush, or chew it; take safety precautions w/ CNS effects; report chest pain.

---

perampanel (Fycompa)
CLASS Antiepileptic, glutamate receptor antagonist
PREG/CONT C/NA

BBW Risk of serious to life-threatening psychiatric, behavioral reactions; monitor pt closely especially when starting drug or changing dose.
IND & DOSE Adjunct tx of partial-onset seizures. *Adult, child 12 yr and older:* 2 mg/day PO at bedtime, 4 mg/day PO at bedtime if also on enzyme-inducing antiepileptics; max, 12 mg/day PO.

ADJUST DOSE Mild to moderate hepatic impairment: severe hepatic, renal impairment; dialysis (not recommended)

ADV EFF Ataxia, balance disorders, falls, fatigue, gait disturbances, irritability, nausea, **serious psychiatric/ behavioral reactions**, somnolence, **suicidality**, weight gain

INTERACTIONS Alcohol, carbamazepine, CNS depressants, hormonal contraceptives, oxcarbazepine, phenytoin, rifampin, St. John's wort

NC/PT Monitor closely when starting tx or changing dose; taper gradually after long-term use. Not for use in pregnancy, breast-feeding. Protect from falls; advise pt to avoid driving, operating dangerous machinery. Pt should take once a day at bedtime; not stop drug suddenly; avoid alcohol, St John's wort; use caution to avoid falls, injury; be aware behavior changes, suicidal thoughts possible; report severe dizziness, trouble walking, suicidal thoughts, behavior changes.

---

perindopril erbumine (Aceon)

CLASS ACE inhibitor, antihypertensive
PREG/CONT D/NA

BBW Serious fetal injury possible; advise barrier contraceptives.

IND & DOSE Tx of hypertension. *Adult:* 4 mg/day PO; max, 16 mg/day. Tx of pts w/ stable CAD to reduce risk of CV mortality, nonfatal MI. *Adult:* 4 mg/day PO for 2 wk; maint, 8 mg/day PO.

ADJUST DOSE Elderly pts, renal impairment

ADV EFF Airway obstruction, angioedema, bone marrow suppression, diarrhea, dizziness, fatigue, gastric irritation, headache, insomnia, nausea, orthostatic hypotension, somnolence

INTERACTIONS Indomethacin, lithium, potassium-sparing diuretics, potassium supplements

NC/PT Have epinephrine on hand for angioedema of face, neck. Alert surgeons; volume replacement may be needed if surgery required. Use caution in conditions w/ possible BP drop (diarrhea, sweating, vomiting, dehydration). Not for use in pregnancy (barrier contraceptives advised). Pt should avoid potassium supplements, OTC drugs that might increase BP; take safety precautions w/ CNS effects; report difficulty breathing, signs of infection, swelling of face, neck.

---

pertuzumab (Perjeta)

CLASS Antiepileptic, HER2/NEU receptor antagonist
PREG/CONT D/NA

BBW Risk of embryo-fetal and/or birth defects; not for use in pregnancy.

IND & DOSE Adjunct tx of pts w/ HER2-positive metastatic breast cancer who have not received prior HER2 therapy or tx for metastatic disease, w/ trastuzumab and docetaxel. *Adult:* 840 mg IV over 60 min, then 420 mg IV over 30–60 min q 3 wk, w/ trastuzumab and docetaxel.

ADV EFF Alopecia, fatigue, infusion reaction, left ventricular (LV) dysfunction, neutropenia, n/v, peripheral neuropathy, rash

NC/PT Perform HER2 testing before use; ensure concurrent use of trastuzumab, docetaxel. Infuse first dose over 60 min, subsequent doses over 30–60 min; do not give as bolus. Not for use in pregnancy (contraceptives advised during and for 6 mo after tx), breast-feeding. Monitor for infusion reactions, LV dysfunction. Pt should mark calendar for injection days; be aware hair loss possible; report difficulty breathing, numbness/tingling, fever, s&sx of infection.

phenazopyridine hydrochloride (Azo-Standard, Baridium, Pyridium, Urinary Pain Relief)

CLASS Urinary analgesic
PREG/CONT B/NA

IND & DOSE Symptomatic relief of s&sx of lower urinary tract irritation. *Adult, child over 12 yr:* 100–200 mg PO tid after meals for max 2 days. *Child 6–12 yr:* 12 mg/kg/day divided into three doses PO for max 2 days.
ADJUST DOSE Elderly pts, renal impairment
ADV EFF GI disturbances, headache, rash, yellowish orange urine
NC/PT May permanently stain contact lenses. Stop if skin, sclera become yellow; may indicate drug accumulation. Urine may be yellowish orange; will stain fabric. Pt should take after meals and not take longer than 2 days, report unusual bleeding, fever.

phenelzine sulfate (Nardil)

CLASS Antidepressant, MAOI
PREG/CONT C/NA

BBW Increased risk of suicidality in children, adolescents, young adults; monitor accordingly.
IND & DOSE Tx of depression in pts unresponsive to other tx. *Adult:* 15 mg PO tid. Rapidly increase to at least 60 mg/day. After max benefit achieved, reduce dose slowly over several wk. Maint, 15 mg/day or q other day PO.
ADJUST DOSE Elderly pts
ADV EFF Abd pain, anorexia, blurred vision, confusion, constipation, dizziness, drowsiness, dry mouth, headache, hyperreflexia, **hypertensive crisis**, hypomania, hypotension, insomnia, jitteriness, **liver toxicity**, n/v/d, orthostatic hypoten-

sion, suicidal thoughts, twitching, vertigo
INTERACTIONS Alcohol, amphetamines, antidiabetics, beta blockers, dextromethorphan, meperidine, SSRIs, sympathomimetics, TCAs, thiazides, tyramine-containing foods
NC/PT Have phentolamine/other alpha-adrenergic blocker on hand for hypertensive crisis. Monitor LFTs, BP regularly. Pt should avoid diet high in tyramine-containing foods during; for 2 wk after tx; avoid alcohol, OTC appetite suppressants; take safety precautions w/ CNS effects; change position slowly if orthostatic hypotension; report rash, urine/stool color changes, thoughts of suicide.

DANGEROUS DRUG
phenobarbital (Bellatal, Solfoton), phenobarbital sodium (Luminal Sodium)

CLASS Antiepileptic, barbiturate, sedative-hypnotic
PREG/CONT D/C-IV

BBW Increased risk of suicidality in children, adolescents, young adults; monitor accordingly.
IND & DOSE Sedation. *Adult:* 30–120 mg/day PO in two to three divided doses; max, 400 mg/24 hr. Or, 30–120 mg/day IM or IV in two to three divided doses. *Child:* 6 mg/kg/day PO in divided doses. Preop sedation. *Adult:* 100–200 mg IM 60–90 min before surgery. *Child:* 1–3 mg/kg IM or IV 60–90 min before surgery. Hypnotic. *Adult:* 100–320 mg PO at bedtime, or 100–320 mg IM or IV. Antiepileptic. *Adult:* 60–300 mg/day PO. *Child:* 3–6 mg/kg/day PO. Or, 4–6 mg/kg/day IM or IV for 7–10 days to blood level of 10–15 mcg/mL. Or, 10–15 mg/kg/day IV or IM. Tx of acute seizures. *Adult:* 200–320 mg IM or IV repeated in 6 hr if needed. Tx of status epilepticus. *Child:* 15–20 mg/kg IV over 10–15 min.

ADJUST DOSE Elderly pts, debilitated adults; hepatic, renal impairment

ADV EFF Agitation, apnea, ataxia, bradycardia, **bronchospasm**, CNS depression, **circulatory collapse**, confusion, dizziness, hallucinations, hypotension, hypoventilation, hyperkinesia, insomnia, **laryngospasm**, pain/necrosis at injection site, somnolence, **Stevens-Johnson syndrome**, syncope, **withdrawal syndrome**

INTERACTIONS Alcohol, beta-adrenergic blockers, CNS depressants, corticosteroids, doxycycline, felodipine, fenoprofen, estrogens, hormonal contraceptives, metronidazole, oral anticoagulants, phenylbutazones, quinidine, theophylline, valproic acid

NC/PT Use caution in children; may produce irritability, aggression, inappropriate tearfulness. Do not give intra-arterially; arteriospasm, thrombosis, gangrene possible. Give slowly IV or by slow IM injection. Monitor continuously during IV use; monitor injection site for irritation. Taper gradually w/ long-term use. Not for use in pregnancy (contraceptives advised). Pt should take safety precautions w/ CNS effects; not take longer than 2 wk for insomnia; wear medical ID for seizure disorder; report difficulty breathing, rash, thoughts of suicide.

DANGEROUS DRUG

phentolamine mesylate (OraVerse)
CLASS Alpha blocker, diagnostic agent
PREG/CONT C/NA

IND & DOSE Px, control of hypertensive episodes in pheochromocytoma. *Adult:* For preop reduction of elevated BP, 5 mg IV or IM 1–2 hr before surgery; repeat if necessary. Give 5 mg IV during surgery as indicated to control paroxysms of hypertension, other epinephrine toxicity effects. *Child:* 1 mg IV or IM 1–2 hr before surgery; repeat if necessary. Give 1 mg IV during surgery as indicated for epinephrine toxicity. **Px of tissue necrosis, sloughing after IV dopamine extravasation.** *Adult:* Infiltrate 10–15 mL normal saline injection containing 5–10 mg phentolamine. *Child:* Infiltrate 0.1–0.2 mg/kg to max 10 mg. **Px of tissue necrosis, sloughing after IV norepinephrine extravasation.** *Adult:* 10 mg phentolamine added to each liter IV fluids containing norepinephrine. **Dx of pheochromocytoma.** *Adult:* Use only to confirm evidence after risks carefully considered. Usual dose, 5 mg IM or IV. **Reversal of soft-tissue anesthesia.** *Adult:* 0.2–0.8 mg based on amount of local anesthetic given, injected into anesthetized area. *Child 6 yr and older, over 30 kg:* Adult dose w/ max 0.4 mg. *Child 6 yr and older, 15–30 kg:* Max, 0.2 mg.

ADV EFF Acute, prolonged hypotension; arrhythmias; dizziness; **MI**; nausea; weakness

INTERACTIONS Ephedrine, epinephrine

NC/PT Give *OraVerse* after dental procedure, using same location as local anesthetic. Monitor P, BP closely. Pt should take safety precautions w/ CNS effects, hypotension; report palpitations, chest pain.

DANGEROUS DRUG

phenylephrine hydrochloride (Neo-Synephrine, PediaCare Children's Decongestant, Sudafed PE, Vicks Sinex Ultra Fine Mist)
CLASS Alpha agonist, nasal decongestant, ophthalmic mydriatic, sympathomimetic
PREG/CONT C/NA

BBW Protect parenteral sol from light. Do not give unless sol is clear; discard unused sol.
IND & DOSE Tx of mild to moderate hypotension. *Adult:* 1–10 mg subcut,

---

IM; max initial dose, 5 mg. Or, 0.1 or 0.5 mg IV; max initial dose, 0.5 mg. Do not repeat more often than q 10–15 min; 0.5 mg IV should raise BP for 15 min. **Tx of severe hypotension, shock.** *Adult:* For continuous infusion, add 10 mg to 500 mL dextrose or normal saline injection. Start at 100–180 mcg/min (based on drop factor of 20 drops/mL [100–180 drops/min]). When BP stabilized, maint, 40–60 mcg/min. **Spinal anesthesia.** *Adult:* 2–3 mg subcut or IM 3–4 min before spinal anesthetic injection. **Hypotensive emergencies during anesthesia.** *Adult:* 0.2 mg IV; max, 0.5 mg/dose. *Child:* 0.5–1 mg/11.3 kg subcut, IM. **Prolongation of spinal anesthesia.** *Adult:* Adding 2–5 mg to anesthetic sol increases motor block duration by as much as 50%. **Vasoconstrictor for regional anesthesia.** *Adult:* 1:20,000 concentration (add 1 mg phenylephrine to q 20 mL local anesthetic sol). **Tx of paroxysmal supraventricular tachycardia.** *Adult:* Rapid IV injection (within 20–30 sec) recommended. Max initial dose, 0.5 mg. Subsequent doses should not exceed preceding dose by more than 0.1–0.2 mg; should never exceed 1 mg. Use only after other tx failed. **Tx of nasal congestion.** *Adult:* 2–3 sprays, drops of 0.25% or 0.5% sol in each nostril q 3–4 hr. In severe cases, may need 0.5% or 1% sol. Or, 10 mg PO bid–qid. Or, 1–2 tablets PO q 4 hr. Or, 1 strip q 4 hr; max, 6 strips/24 hr. Place 1 strip on tongue; let dissolve. Or, 10 mL liquid q 6 hr. *Child 6 yr and older:* 2–3 sprays 0.25% sol in each nostril no more than q 4 hr. Or, 1 tablet PO q 4 hr. *Child 2–5 yr:* 2–3 drops 0.125% sol in each nostril q 4 hr PRN. Or, 1 dropperful (5 mL [2.5 mg]) 0.25% oral drops q 4 hr; max, 6 mL (15 mg)/day. **Vasoconstriction, pupil dilation.** *Adult:* 1 drop 2.5% or 10% sol on upper limbus. May repeat in 1 hr. **Tx of uveitis to prevent posterior synechiae.** *Adult:* 1 drop 2.5% or 10% sol on surface of cornea w/ atropine.

Max, three times. **Tx of wide-angle glaucoma.** *Adult:* 1 drop 2.5% or 10% sol on upper surface of cornea repeated as necessary, w/ miotics. **Intraocular surgery.** *Adult:* 2.5% or 10% sol in eye 30–60 min before procedure. **Refraction.** *Adult:* 1 drop of cycloplegic then, in 5 min, 1 drop phenylephrine 2.5% sol and, in 10 min, another drop of cycloplegic. **Ophthalmoscopic exam.** *Adult:* 1 drop 2.5% sol in each eye. Mydriasis produced in 15–30 min, lasting 4–6 hr. **Tx of minor eye irritation.** *Adult:* 1–2 drops 0.12% sol in eye bid–qid as needed.

ADJUST DOSE Elderly pts

ADV EFF Anorexia, anxiety, blurred vision, cardiac arrhythmias, decreased urine output, dizziness, drowsiness, dysuria, fear, headache, light-headedness, local stinging w/ ophthalmic sol, nausea, pallor, rebound congestion w/ nasal sol, urine incontinence

INTERACTIONS Halogenated anesthetics, MAOIs, methyldopa, oxytocics, sympathomimetics, TCAs

NC/PT Have alpha-adrenergic blocker on hand. If extravasation, infiltrate area w/ phentolamine (5–10 mg in 10–15 mL saline) using fine hypodermic needle; usually effective if area infiltrated within 12 hr of extravasation. Five mg IM should raise BP for 1–2 hr; 0.5 mg IV, for 15 min. Do not give within 14 days of MAOIs. Monitor closely during administration. Teach proper administration of nasal sol, eyedrops. Pt should not use longer than prescribed; take safety precautions w/ CNS effects; report chest pain, palpitations, vision changes.

---

phenytoin (Dilantin, Phenytek)

CLASS Antiarrhythmic, antiepileptic, hydantoin
PREG/CONT D/NA

BBW Give IV slowly to prevent severe hypotension, venous irritation;

small margin of safety between full therapeutic, toxic doses. Continually monitor cardiac rhythm; check BP frequently, regularly during infusion. Suggest use of fosphenytoin sodium if IV route needed.

IND & DOSE Tx of status epilepticus. *Adult:* 10–15 mg/kg by slow IV. Maint, 100 mg PO IV q 6–8 hr; max infusion rate, 50 mg/min. *Child:* Dose based on children's formulas; may also calculate infants', children's doses based on 10–15 mg/kg IV in divided doses of 5–10 mg/kg. For neonates, 15–20 mg/kg IV in divided doses of 5–10 mg/kg recommended.

Px of seizures during neurosurgery. *Adult:* 100–200 mg IM q 4 hr during surgery, postop; not preferred route.

Tx of tonic-clonic, psychomotor seizures. *Adult:* Loading dose in hospitalized pts: 1 g phenytoin capsules (phenytoin sodium, prompt) divided into three doses (400 mg, 300 mg, 300 mg) and given PO q 2 hr. When control established, may consider once-a-day dosing w/ 300 mg PO. W/ no previous tx: Initially, 100 mg PO tid; maint, 300–400 mg/day. *Child not previously treated:* 5 mg/kg/day PO in two to three equally divided doses. Max, 300 mg/day; maint, 4–8 mg/kg. Child older than 6 yr may need minimum adult dose (300 mg/day).

IM tx in pt previously stabilized on oral dose. *Adult:* Increase dose by 50% over oral dose. When returning to oral dose, decrease dose by 50% of original oral dose for 1 wk to prevent excessive plasma level.

ADJUST DOSE Elderly pts, hepatic impairment

ADV EFF Aplastic anemia, ataxia, dizziness, drowsiness, dysarthria, **frank malignant lymphoma, bullous/exfoliative/purpuric dermatitis, CV collapse,** gum hyperplasia, **hematopoietic complications,** insomnia, irritation, **liver damage, lupus erythematosus,** mental confusion, nausea, nystagmus, **Stevens-Johnson syndrome**

INTERACTIONS Acetaminophen, alcohol, allopurinol, amiodarone, anti-neoplastics, atracurium, benzodiazepines, carbamazepine, cardiac glycosides, chloramphenicol, cimetidine, corticosteroids, cyclosporine, diazoxide, disopyramide, disulfiram, doxycycline, estrogens, fluconazole, folic acid, furosemide, haloperidol, hormonal contraceptives, isoniazid, levodopa, loxapine, methadone, metronidazole, metyrapone, mexiletine, miconazole, nitrofurantoin, omeprazole, pancuronium, phenacemide, phenothiazide, phenylbutazone, primidone, pyridoxine, quinidine, rifampin, sucralfate, sulfonamides, sulfonylureas, theophylline, trimethoprim, valproic acid, vecuronium

NC/PT Monitor for therapeutic serum level (10–20 mcg/mL). Enteral tube feedings may delay absorption. Provide 2-hr window between *Dilantin* doses, tube feedings. Reduce dose, stop phenytoin, or substitute other antiepileptic gradually; stopping abruptly may precipitate status epilepticus. Stop if rash, depressed blood count, enlarged lymph nodes, hypersensitivity reaction, signs of liver damage, Peyronie disease (induration of corpora cavernosa of penis); start another antiepileptic promptly. Have lymph node enlargement during tx evaluated carefully. Lymphadenopathy that simulates Hodgkin lymphoma has occurred; lymph node hyperplasia may progress to lymphoma. Not for use in pregnancy (contraceptives advised). Pt should have regular dental care; take safety precautions for CNS effects; wear medical ID; report rash, unusual bleeding, urine/stool color changes, thoughts of suicide.

---

pilocarpine hydrochloride (Salagen)

CLASS Parasympathomimetic

PREG/CONT C/NA

IND & DOSE Tx of sx of xerostomia from salivary gland dysfx caused by radiation for head/neck cancer.

Adult: 5–10 mg PO tid. **Tx of dry mouth in Sjögren syndrome.** Adult: 5 mg PO qid.
ADJUST DOSE Severe hepatic impairment
ADV EFF Bronchospasm, headache, hypertension, hypotension, n/v/d, renal colic, sweating, tearing, visual changes
INTERACTIONS Anticholinergics, beta blockers
NC/PT Maintain hydration. Not for use in breast-feeding. Pt should take safety precautions w/ vision changes, report dehydration, difficulty breathing.

pimozide (Orap)
CLASS Antipsychotic, diphenylbutylpiperidine
PREG/CONT C/NA

IND & DOSE **To suppress severely compromising motor, phonic tics in Tourette syndrome.** Adult: 1–2 mg/day PO; max, 10 mg/day.
ADJUST DOSE Severe hepatic impairment
ADV EFF Akathisia, asthenia, dry mouth, extrapyramidal effects, fever, headache, increased salivation, motor restlessness, **NMS, prolonged QT interval,** sedation, somnolence, tardive dyskinesia
INTERACTIONS Amphetamines, antifungals, citalopram, escitalopram, grapefruit juice, methylphenidate, nefazodone, pemoline, protease inhibitors, sertraline, QT-prolonging drugs, strong CYP2D6 inhibitors
NC/PT Ensure correct dx. Obtain baseline, periodic ECG. Not for use in breast-feeding. Check pt's drugs closely; numerous drug interactions w/ contraindications. Pt should take safety precautions w/ CNS effects, avoid grapefruit juice.

pindolol (Visken)
CLASS Antihypertensive, beta blocker
PREG/CONT B/NA

IND & DOSE **Tx of hypertension.** Adult: 5 mg PO bid; max, 60 mg/day. Usual maint, 5 mg PO tid.
ADV EFF Arrhythmias, **bronchospasm,** constipation, decreased exercise tolerance/libido, fatigue, flatulence, gastric pain, serum glucose changes, **HF, laryngospasm,** n/v/d
INTERACTIONS Clonidine, epinephrine, ergots, ibuprofen, indomethacin, insulin, lidocaine, naproxen, piroxicam, prazosin, sulindac, theophyllines, thioridazine, verapamil
NC/PT When stopping, taper gradually over 2 wk w/ monitoring. Pt should take safety precautions w/ CNS effects, report difficulty breathing, swelling. Name confusion between pindolol and Plendil (felodipine); use caution.

pioglitazone (Actos)
CLASS Antidiabetic, thiazolidinedione
PREG/CONT C/NA

BBW Thiazolidinediones cause or worsen HF in some pts; pioglitazone not recommended for pts w/ symptomatic HF (contraindicated in NYHA Class III, IV HF). After starting or increasing, watch carefully for HF s&sx. If they occur, manage HF according to current standards of care. Pioglitazone may be reduced or stopped. Increased risk of bladder cancer when used for longer than 1 yr; monitor accordingly.
IND & DOSE **Adjunct to diet, exercise to improve glucose control in type 2 diabetes as monotherapy or w/ insulin, sulfonylurea, metformin.** Adult: 15–30 mg/day PO; max, 45 mg daily PO.
ADJUST DOSE Hepatic impairment

ADV EFF Aggravated diabetes, fatigue, headache, **hepatic injury, hyperglycemia, hypoglycemia,** infections, myalgia, pain
INTERACTIONS Celery, coriander, dandelion root, fenugreek, garlic, ginseng, hormonal contraceptives, juniper berries
NC/PT Interferes w/ hormonal contraceptives; suggest alternative birth control method or consider higher contraceptive dose. Increased risk of bladder cancer when used for longer than 1 yr; monitor accordingly. Monitor blood glucose regularly; ensure complete diabetic teaching, support. Pt should take without regard to meals, report infections, difficulty breathing. Name confusion between *Actos* (pioglitazone) and *Actonel* (risedronate); use caution.

piroxicam (Feldene)
CLASS NSAID
PREG/CONT C/NA

BBW Increased risk of CV events, GI bleeding; monitor accordingly. Contraindicated for periop pain after CABG surgery.
IND & DOSE Relief of s&sx of acute/chronic rheumatoid arthritis, osteoarthritis. *Adult:* 20 mg/day PO.
ADV EFF Anaphylactoid reactions to anaphylactic shock, bone marrow suppression, bronchospasm, constipation, dizziness, dyspepsia, edema, fatigue, GI pain, headache, insomnia, nausea, rash, somnolence
INTERACTIONS Beta blockers, cholestyramine, lithium, oral anticoagulants
NC/PT Take w/ food or milk; use safety precautions w/ CNS effects; report swelling, difficulty breathing, rash.

pitavastatin (Livalo)
CLASS Antihyperlipidemic, statin
PREG/CONT X/NA

IND & DOSE To reduce elevated total cholesterol, LDLs, apolipoprotein B, triglycerides, increase HDL in primary hyperlipidemia, mixed dyslipidemia. *Adult:* 2 mg/day PO; max, 4 mg/day.
ADJUST DOSE Renal impairment (pts on dialysis)
ADV EFF Back pain, constipation, diarrhea, flulike sx, headache, **liver toxicity,** myalgias, **rhabdomyolysis**
INTERACTIONS Alcohol, cyclosporine, erythromycin, fibrates, lopinavir/ritonavir, niacin, rifampin
NC/PT Monitor LFTs regularly. Ensure diet, exercise program. Not for use in pregnancy (barrier contraceptives advised), breast-feeding. Pt should get regular blood tests, avoid alcohol, report severe muscle pain w/ fever, weakness, urine/stool color changes.

plasma protein fraction (Plasmanate, Plasma-Plex, Protenate)
CLASS Blood product, plasma protein
PREG/CONT C/NA

IND & DOSE Tx of hypovolemic shock. *Adult:* Initially, 250–500 mL IV. Max, 10 mL/min; do not exceed 5–8 mL/min as plasma volume nears normal. Tx of hypoproteinemia. *Adult:* 1,000–1,500 mL IV daily; max, 5–8 mL/min. Adjust rate based on pt response.
ADV EFF Chills, fever, **HF,** hypotension, n/v, **pulmonary edema after rapid infusion,** rash
INTERACTIONS Alcohol, cyclosporine, erythromycin, fibrates, lopinavir/ritonavir, niacin, rifampin
NC/PT Infusion only provides symptomatic relief of hypoproteinemia; consider need for whole blood based on pt's clinical condition. Give IV without regard to blood type. Monitor closely during infusion. Pt should report headache, difficulty breathing.

plerixafor (Mozobil)

CLASS Hematopoietic stem-cell mobilizer
PREG/CONT D/NA

IND & DOSE To mobilize hematopoietic stem cells to peripheral blood for collection, subsequent autologous transplantation in pts w/ non-Hodgkin lymphoma/multiple myeloma, w/ granulocyte-colony stimulating factor (G-CSF). *Adult:* 0.24 mg/kg subcut for up to 4 consecutive days; start after pt has received G-CSF once daily for 4 days. Give approximately 11 hours before apheresis.

ADJUST DOSE Renal impairment
ADV EFF Dizziness, headache, injection-site reactions, n/v/d, orthostatic hypotension, rash, splenic rupture
NC/PT Do not use in leukemia; may mobilize leukemic cells. Not for use in pregnancy (barrier contraceptives advised), breast-feeding. Pt should report rash, injection-site reactions, difficulty breathing, edema.

polidocanol (Asclera)

CLASS Sclerosing agent
PREG/CONT C/NA

IND & DOSE Tx of uncomplicated spider, reticular veins in lower extremities. *Adult:* 0.1–0.3 mL as IV injection at varicose vein site; max volume/session, 10 mL.
ADV EFF Anaphylaxis, injection-site reactions
NC/PT Do not inject intra-arterially. Have emergency equipment on hand. Advise compression stockings, support hose on treated legs continuously for 2 to 3 days, then for 2 to 3 wk during the day; walk for 15–20 min immediately after procedure and daily for next few days.

poly-L-lactic acid (Sculptra)

CLASS Polymer
PREG/CONT Unkn/NA

IND & DOSE To restore, correct sx of lipoatrophy in pts w/ HIV syndrome. *Adult:* 0.1–0.2 mL injected intradermally at each injection site. May need up to 20 injections/cheek; retreat periodically.
ADV EFF Injection-site reactions
NC/PT Do not use if signs of skin infection. Apply ice packs to area immediately after injection and for first 24 hr. Massage injection sites daily. Monitor pt on anticoagulants for increased bleeding.

DANGEROUS DRUG

polymyxin B sulfate (generic)

CLASS Antibiotic
PREG/CONT C/NA

BBW Monitor renal function carefully; nephrotoxicity possible. Avoid concurrent use of other nephrotoxics. Neurotoxicity can cause respiratory paralysis; monitor accordingly. IV, intrathecal administration for hospitalized pts only.
IND & DOSE Tx of acute infections caused by susceptible bacteria strains when less toxic drugs contraindicated. *Adult, child over 2 yr:* 15,000–25,000 units/kg/day IV q 12 hr; max, 25,000 units/kg/day. *Infants:* 40,000 units/kg/day IV, IM. Tx of meningeal infections caused by *Pseudomonas aeruginosa. Adult, child over 2 yr:* 50,000 units/day intrathecally for 3–4 days; then 50,000 units q other day for at least 2 wk after CSF cultures negative, glucose content normal. *Infants:* 20,000 units/day intrathecally for 3–4 days or 25,000 units q other day. Continue w/ 25,000 units once q other day for at least 2 wk after CSF cultures negative, glucose content normal.

ADJUST DOSE Renal impairment
ADV EFF Apnea, **nephrotoxicity, neurotoxicity,** pain at injection site, rash, superinfections, thrombophlebitis
INTERACTIONS Aminoglycosides, nephrotoxic drugs, NMJ blockers
NC/PT Culture before tx. Monitor renal function regularly. IM route may cause severe pain. Treat superinfections. Pt should take safety precautions w/ CNS effects, report swelling, difficulty breathing, vision changes.

pomalidomide (Pomalyst)
CLASS Antineoplastic, thalidomide analogue
PREG/CONT X/NA

BBW Known human teratogen. Can cause severe, life-threatening birth defects; not for use in pregnancy. Risk of DVT, PE in pts treated w/ multiple myeloma.
IND & DOSE Tx of multiple myeloma in pts who have had disease progression after at least two other therapies. *Adult:* 4 mg/day PO on days 1–21 of repeated 28-day cycle until progression occurs.
ADJUST DOSE Severe hepatic, renal impairment
ADV EFF Anemia, asthenia, back pain, confusion, constipation, diarrhea, dizziness, **DVT,** dyspnea, fatigue, nausea, neuropathy, **neutropenia, PE,** URI
NC/PT Available only through restricted access program. Rule out pregnancy before starting drug. Ensure monthly negative pregnancy test; recommend highly effective contraceptive measures for men, women. Not for use in breast-feeding. Monitor for DVT, PE. Obtain baseline, periodic CBC. Pt should take drug once/day at about same time each day; swallow capsule whole w/ water and not cut, crush, or chew it; obtain monthly pregnancy test; avoid donating blood during and for 1 mo after tx; take safety precautions w/ CNS effects; report extreme fatigue, difficulty breathing, calf pain.

DANGEROUS DRUG
ponatinib (Iclusig)
CLASS Antineoplastic, kinase inhibitor
PREG/CONT D/NA

BBW Risk of vascular occlusion, HF, hepatotoxicity, any of which can lead to death.
IND & DOSE Tx of T3151-positive CML or T3151-positive ALL. *Adult:* 45 mg/day with food; adjust based on toxicity.
ADJUST DOSE Severe hepatic impairment
ADV EFF Abd pain, arrhythmias, arthralgia, compromised wound healing, constipation, fever, fluid retention, **HF, hepatotoxicity,** hypertension, myelosuppression, neuropathies, n/v, pancreatitis, **vascular occlusions,** vision changes
INTERACTIONS CYP3A inhibitors
NC/PT Ensure proper dx. Monitor LFTs, lipase, cardiac function, CBC, BP, vision. Ensure adequate hydration; correct uric acid levels. Pt should avoid pregnancy (serious fetal harm possible), breast-feeding; report fever, extreme fatigue, color changes in urine/stool, headache, vision changes.

poractant alfa (Curosurf)
CLASS Lung surfactant
PREG/CONT Unkn/NA

IND & DOSE Rescue tx of infants w/ RDS. *Infants:* Entire contents of vial (2.5 mL/kg birth weight) intratracheally, ½ of dose into each bronchi. Give first dose as soon as possible after RDS dx and when pt on ventilator. May need up to two subsequent doses of 1.25 mL/kg birth weight at 12-hr intervals. Max total dose, 5 mL/kg (sum of initial, two repeat doses).

ADV EFF Bradycardia, flushing, hyperbilirubinemia, hypotension, infections, **intraventricular hemorrhage, patent ductus arteriosus, pneumothorax,** sepsis
NC/PT Ensure ET tube in correct position, w/ bilateral chest movement, lung sounds. Store in refrigerator; protect from light. Enter vial only once. Instill slowly; inject ¼ of dose over 2–3 sec. Do not suction infant for 1 hr after completion of full dose; do not flush catheter. Maintain appropriate interventions for critically ill infant.

DANGEROUS DRUG

porfimer sodium
(Photofrin)
CLASS Antineoplastic
PREG/CONT C/NA

IND & DOSE Photodynamic tx for palliation of pts w/ completely/partially obstructing esophageal/transitional cancer who cannot be treated w/ laser alone; transitional cell carcinoma in situ of urinary bladder; endobronchial non-small-cell lung cancer; high-grade dysplasia of Barrett esophagus. *Adult:* 2 mg/kg as slow IV injection over 3–5 min; laser tx must follow in 40–50 hr and again in 96–120 hr.
ADV EFF Abd pain, anemia, **bleeding,** chest pain, constipation, dyspnea, GI perforation, n/v, photosensitivity, **pleural effusion, respiratory toxicity**
NC/PT Monitor for pleural effusion, respiratory complications. Avoid contact w/ drug. Protect pt from light exposure for 30 days after tx; photosensitivity may last up to 90 days. Pt should report difficulty breathing/swallowing, unusual bleeding.

DANGEROUS DRUG

posaconazole (Noxafil)
CLASS Antifungal
PREG/CONT C/NA

IND & DOSE Px of invasive *Aspergillus, Candida* infections in immu-

nosuppressed pts. *Adult, child 13 yr and older:* 200 mg (5 mL) PO tid. Tx of oropharyngeal candidiasis. *Adult, child 13 yr and older:* 100 mg (2.5 mL) PO bid on day 1; then 100 mg/day PO for 13 days. For refractory infection, 400 mg (10 mL) PO bid; duration based on pt response.
ADJUST DOSE Hepatic impairment
ADV EFF Abd pain, anemia, constipation, cough, dizziness, dyspnea, epistaxis, fatigue, fever, headache, **hepatotoxicity,** insomnia, n/v/d, **prolonged QT interval,** rash
INTERACTIONS Calcium channel blockers, cimetidine, cyclosporine, ergots, midazolam, phenytoin, quinidine, rifabutin, sirolimus, statins, tacrolimus, vincristine, vinblastine
NC/PT Culture before tx. Obtain baseline ECG; monitor LFTs. Shake bottle well before use. Give w/ full meal or nutritional supplement. Maintain hydration, nutrition. Not for use in pregnancy, breast-feeding. Pt should report fever, urine/stool color changes.

DANGEROUS DRUG

potassium acetate,
potassium chloride,
potassium gluconate
(Kaon-Cl, Kaylixir, K-Dur, K-G Elixir, Klorvess, Klotrix, Tri-K)
CLASS Electrolyte
PREG/CONT C/NA

IND & DOSE Px of potassium deficiency. *Adult:* 16–24 mEq/day PO. Tx of potassium deficiency. 40–100 mEq/day PO or IV. *Child:* 2–3 mEq/kg/day or 40 mEq/m²/day PO or IV; 2–6 mEq/kg/hr PO or IV for newborns.
ADJUST DOSE Elderly pts, renal impairment
ADV EFF Abd pain, hyperkalemia, n/v/d, tissue sloughing, venospasm
INTERACTIONS Potassium-sparing diuretics, salt substitutes using potassium

NC/PT Obtain baseline, periodic serial serum potassium level. Dilute in dextrose sol to 40–80 mEq/L; do not give undiluted. Monitor for cardiac arrhythmias during IV infusion. Monitor injection site carefully. Wax tablet matrix may appear in stool. Pt should swallow tablet whole and not cut, crush, or chew it; take w/ food or after meals; avoid salt substitutes, report tingling in hands/feet, black tarry stools, pain at IV injection site.

pralatrexate (Folotyn)
CLASS Folate analogue metabolic inhibitor, antineoplastic
PREG/CONT X/NA

IND & DOSE Tx of relapsed, refractory peripheral T-cell lymphoma.
Adult: 30 mg/m²/wk as IV push over 3–5 min for 6 wk in 7-wk cycle.
ADJUST DOSE Elderly pts, renal impairment
ADV EFF Bone marrow suppression, dehydration, dyspnea, fatigue, mucositis, n/v/d, night sweats, pain, rash, serious to fatal dermatologic reactions, tumor lysis syndrome
NC/PT Monitor CBC, skin. Pt should also receive vitamin B₁₂ (1 mg IM q 8–10 wk) and folic acid (1–1.25 mg/day PO). Maintain hydration. Not for use in pregnancy (contraceptives advised), breast-feeding. Provide skin care. Pt should avoid exposure to infection, report signs of infection, unusual bleeding, rash.

pralidoxime chloride (Protopam Chloride)
CLASS Antidote
PREG/CONT C/NA

IND & DOSE Antidote in poisoning due to organophosphate pesticides, chemicals w/ anticholinesterase activity. **Adult:** Atropine 2–4 mg IV. If cyanotic, 2–4 mg atropine IM while improving ventilation; repeat q 5–10 min until signs of atropine toxicity appear. Maintain atropinization for at least 48 hr. Give pralidoxime concomitantly: Initially, 1–2 g pralidoxime IV, preferably as 15–30 min infusion in 100 mL saline. After 1 hr, give second dose of 1–2 g IV if muscle weakness not relieved. Give additional doses cautiously q 10–12 hr. If IV route not feasible or pulmonary edema present, give IM or subcut. **Child 16 yr and under:** Loading dose, 20–50 mg/kg (max, 2,000 mg/dose) IV over 15–30 min, then continuous IV infusion of 10–20 mg/kg/hr. Or, 20–50 mg/kg (max, 2,000 mg/dose) IV over 15–30 min. Give second dose of 20–50 mg/kg in 1 hr if muscle weakness not relieved. May repeat dosing q 10–12 hr as needed. Or, for pt 40 kg and over, 1,800 mg IM/course of tx; under 40 kg, 15 mg/kg IM q 15 min if needed, to total of three doses (45 mg/kg). **Adjunct to atropine in poisoning by nerve agents w/ anticholinesterase activity. Adult:** Give atropine, pralidoxime as soon as possible after exposure. Use autoinjectors, giving atropine first. Repeat both atropine, pralidoxime after 15 min. If sx after additional 15 min, repeat injections. If sx persist after third set of injections, seek medical help. **Tx of anticholinesterase overdose of myasthenia gravis drugs. Adult:** 1–2 g IV, then increments of 250 mg q 5 min.
ADV EFF Blurred vision, diplopia, dizziness, drowsiness, headache, pain at injection site, transient LFT increases
NC/PT For acute organophosphate poisoning, remove secretions, maintain patent airway, provide artificial ventilation as needed; then begin tx. After skin exposure to organophosphate poisoning, remove clothing, thoroughly wash hair/skin w/ sodium bicarbonate or alcohol as soon as possible. Give by slow IV infusion. Have IV sodium thiopental or diazepam on hand if seizures occur. Pt should report pain at injection site, vision changes.

pramipexole dihydrochloride
(Mirapex)

CLASS Antiparkinsonian, dopamine receptor agonist
PREG/CONT C/NA

BBW Use extreme caution in pts w/ hx of hypotension, hallucinations, confusion, dyskinesias.

IND & DOSE Tx of sx of Parkinson disease. *Adult:* 0.125 mg PO tid for 1 wk; wk 2, 0.25 mg PO tid; wk 3, 0.5 mg PO tid; wk 4, 0.75 mg PO tid; wk 5, 1 mg PO tid; wk 6, 1.25 mg PO tid; wk 7, 1.5 mg PO tid. Once levels established, may use ER tablets for once-a-day dosing. Tx of restless legs syndrome (*Mirapex*). *Adult:* 0.125 mg/day PO 2–3 hr before bedtime. May increase q 4–7 days, if needed, to 0.25 mg/day; max, 0.5 mg/day.
ADJUST DOSE Renal impairment
ADV EFF Asthenia, constipation, dizziness, extrapyramidal sx, headache, insomnia, orthostatic hypotension, somnolence
INTERACTIONS Cimetidine, diltiazem, dopamine antagonists, levodopa, quinidine, quinine, ranitidine, triamterene, verapamil
NC/PT Give w/ extreme caution to pts w/ hx of hypotension, hallucinations, confusion, dyskinesia. Taper gradually over at least 1 wk when stopping. Not for use in pregnancy (barrier contraceptives advised). Pt should swallow ER tablet whole and not cut, crush, or chew it; take safety precautions w/ CNS effects; report hallucinations, swelling.

DANGEROUS DRUG

pramlintide acetate
(Symlin)

CLASS Amylinomimetic, antidiabetic
PREG/CONT C/NA

BBW Severe hypoglycemia associated w/ combined use of insulin, pramlintide; usually seen within 3 hr of pramlintide injection. Monitor accordingly.

IND & DOSE Adjunct tx in pts w/ type 1, 2 diabetes who use mealtime insulin and have failed to achieve desired glucose control. *Adult w/ type 1 diabetes:* 15 mcg subcut before major meals; titrate at 15-mcg increments to maint of 30 or 60 mcg as tolerated. *Adult w/ type 2 diabetes:* 60–120 mcg subcut immediately before major meals.
ADV EFF Cough, dizziness, hypoglycemia, injection-site reactions, n/v
INTERACTIONS Anticholinergics, oral drugs
NC/PT Doses of oral drugs, insulins will need reduction, usually by 50% based on pt response. Drug affects gastric emptying; if rapid effect needed, give oral medication 1 hr before or 2 hr after pramlintide. Inject subcut more than 2 inches away from insulin injection site. Rotate sites. Do not mix in syringe w/ insulin. Use caution in pregnancy, breast-feeding. Store unopened vial in refrigerator; may store opened vial at room temp. Teach proper administration, disposal of needles, syringes. Pt should not take if not going to eat; avoid alcohol; continue diet, exercise, other diabetes tx; monitor blood glucose level; report hypoglycemic reactions, injection-site pain/swelling.

DANGEROUS DRUG

prasugrel (Effient)

CLASS Platelet inhibitor
PREG/CONT B/NA

BBW Risk of serious to fatal bleeding; do not use w/ active bleeding or hx of TIA, stroke. Risk increased w/ age older than 75 yr, weight under 60 kg, bleeding tendency, warfarin/NSAID use. Do not use in likely candidates for CABG surgery; if pts taking drug need CABG, stop prasugrel at least 7 days before surgery. Suspect bleeding in pt who becomes hypotensive and has undergone invasive procedure. If possible, control bleeding without stopping prasugrel; stopping prematurely increases risk of thrombotic episodes.

IND & DOSE To reduce risk of thrombotic CV events (including stent thrombosis) in pts w/ acute coronary syndrome who are to be managed w/ percutaneous coronary intervention. *Adult:* 60 mg PO as single dose, then 10 mg/day PO without regard to food. Use 5 mg/day in pt weighing under 60 kg. Pt should also receive aspirin (75–325 mg/day).

ADV EFF Bleeding, fatigue, fever, headache, hyperlipidemia, hypertension, pain, rash, **risk of thrombotic episodes if stopped prematurely, thrombotic thrombocytopenic purpura**

INTERACTIONS NSAIDs

NC/PT Ensure pt also receives aspirin. Limit invasive procedures; monitor for bleeding. Stop drug 7 days before planned surgery. Protect from injury. Not for use in pregnancy (barrier contraceptives advised), breast-feeding. Do not stop prematurely; risk of rebound thrombotic events. Pt should wear medical ID; inform all health care providers about pramlintide use, increased risk of bleeding; report excessive bleeding, fever, purple skin patches; pink, brown urine, black or bloody stools.

---

pravastatin sodium
(Pravachol)
CLASS Antihyperlipidemic, statin
PREG/CONT X/NA

IND & DOSE Adjunct to diet in tx of elevated total cholesterol, LDL cholesterol; px of MI in pts at risk for first MI; to slow progression of CAD in pts w/ clinically evident CAD; to reduce risk of stroke, MI. *Adult:* 40 mg/day PO at bedtime. Max, 80 mg/day. *Adult on immunosuppressants:* 10 mg/day PO; max, 20 mg/day. **Tx of heterozygous familial hypercholesterolemia**

as adjunct to diet, exercise: *Child 14–18 yr:* 40 mg/day PO. *Child 8–13 yr:* 20 mg/day PO.

ADJUST DOSE Elderly pts; hepatic, renal impairment

ADV EFF Abd pain, blurred vision, cataracts, constipation, cramps, dizziness, flatulence, LFT elevations, n/v, **rhabdomyolysis**

INTERACTIONS Bile acid sequestrants, cyclosporine, digoxin, erythromycin, gemfibrozil, itraconazole, niacin, warfarin

NC/PT Ensure diet, exercise program for CAD. Not for use in pregnancy (barrier contraceptives advised), breast-feeding. Pt should take at bedtime, have periodic eye exams, report severe GI upset, urine/stool color changes, muscle pain.

---

praziquantel (Biltricide)
CLASS Anthelmintic
PREG/CONT B/NA

IND & DOSE Tx of *Schistosoma* infections, liver flukes. *Adult, child over 4 yr:* Three doses of 20–25 mg/kg PO as one-day tx, w/ 4–6 hr between doses.

ADV EFF Abd pain, dizziness, fever, malaise, nausea, urticaria

INTERACTIONS Chloroquine, CP450 inducers, grapefruit juice

NC/PT Give w/ food; GI upset common. Pt should swallow tablet whole and not cut, crush, or chew it; avoid grapefruit juice.

---

prazosin hydrochloride
(Minipress)
CLASS Alpha blocker, antihypertensive
PREG/CONT C/NA

IND & DOSE Tx of hypertension. *Adult:* 1 mg PO bid–tid. Increase to total 20 mg/day in divided doses; range, 6–15 mg/day. If using w/ other antihypertensives, reduce dose to 1–2 mg PO tid, titrate to control BP.

ADV EFF Abd pain, dizziness, drowsiness, dry mouth, headache, hypotension, lack of energy, nausea, paresthesia, weakness
INTERACTIONS Beta blockers, sildenafil, tadalafil, vardenafil, verapamil
NC/PT First dose may cause syncope w/ sudden loss of consciousness; limit first dose to 1 mg PO, give at bedtime. Pt should take safety precautions w/ CNS effects, use sugarless lozenges for dry mouth, report fainting.

---

prednisoLONE, prednisoLONE acetate, prednisoLONE sodium phosphate (Hydrocortone, Orapred, Pred Forte, Pred Mild, Prelone)
CLASS Corticosteroid, antiinflammatory
PREG/CONT C/NA

IND & DOSE Mgt of inflammatory disorders; tx of hypercalcemia of cancer. *Adult:* 5–60 mg/day PO based on condition. *Child:* 0.14–2 mg/kg/day PO in three to four divided doses. **Mgt of acute MS exacerbations.** *Adult:* 200 mg/day PO for 1 wk, then 80 mg q other day for 1 mo (sodium phosphate). **Mgt of nephrotic syndrome.** *Child:* 60 mg/m²/day PO in three divided doses for 4 wk (sodium phosphate). Then single doses for 4 wk. Or, 40 mg/m²/day PO. **Mgt of inflammation of eyelid, conjunctiva, cornea, globe.** *Adult, child:* 2 drops qid. For Pred Mild/Forte, sodium phosphate, 1–2 drops q hr during day, q 2 hr at night. W/ favorable results, 1 drop q 4 hr, then 1 drop three to four times/day to control sx.

ADV EFF Aggravation of infections, amenorrhea, **anaphylactic reactions**, edema, fluid retention, headache, hyperglycemia, hypotension, immunosuppression, impaired healing, increased appetite, **shock**, vertigo

INTERACTIONS Ambenonium, barbiturates, cyclosporine, edrophonium, estrogens, hormonal contraceptives, ketoconazole, neostigmine, phenytoin, pyridostigmine, rifampin, salicylates
NC/PT Individualize dose, depending on severity, response. Give daily dose before 9 a.m. to minimize adrenal suppression. For maint, reduce initial dose in small increments at intervals until lowest satisfactory dose reached. If long-term tx needed, consider alternate-day tx w/ short-acting corticosteroid. After long-term tx, withdraw slowly to prevent adrenal insufficiency. Monitor serum glucose level. Pt should avoid exposure to infection, bright light (eyes may be sensitive); learn proper eyedrop technique; report signs of infection, black tarry stools.

---

predniSONE (Prednisone Intensol Concentrate, Rayos)
CLASS Corticosteroid
PREG/CONT C/NA

IND & DOSE Mgt of inflammatory disorders; tx of hypercalcemia of cancer; replacement tx w/ adrenal insufficiency. *Adult:* 5–60 mg/day PO titrated based on response. *Child:* 0.05–2 mg/kg/day PO or 4–5 mg/m²/day PO in equal divided doses q 12 hr. **Mgt of acute MS exacerbations.** *Adult:* 200 mg/day PO for 1 wk, then 80 mg PO q other day for 1 mo.

ADV EFF Aggravation of infections, amenorrhea, **anaphylactic reactions**, edema, fluid retention, headache, hyperglycemia, hypotension, immunosuppression, impaired healing, increased appetite, **shock**, vertigo
INTERACTIONS Barbiturates, cyclosporine, edrophonium, estrogens, hormonal contraceptives, ketoconazole, neostigmine, phenytoin, pyridostigmine, rifampin, salicylates, troleandomycin

NC/PT Individualize dose, depending on severity, response. Give daily dose before 9 a.m. to minimize adrenal suppression. For maint, reduce initial dose in small increments at intervals until lowest satisfactory dose reached. If long-term tx needed, consider alternate-day tx w/ short-acting corticosteroid. After long-term tx, withdraw slowly to prevent adrenal insufficiency. Monitor blood glucose level. Pt should avoid exposure to infections, report signs of infection, worsening of condition.

pregabalin (Lyrica)

CLASS Analgesic, antiepileptic, calcium channel modulator
PREG/CONT C/C-V

BBW Increased risk of suicidal ideation; monitor accordingly.
IND & DOSE Mgt of neuropathic pain. *Adult:* 100 mg PO tid. Max, 300 mg/day. Mgt of postherpetic neuralgia. *Adult:* 75–150 mg PO bid or 50–100 mg PO tid; max, 600 mg/day. Adjunct tx for partial-onset seizures. 150–600 mg/day PO divided into two to three doses. Mgt of fibromyalgia. *Adult:* 75–150 mg PO bid. Max, 450 mg/day. Mgt of neuropathic pain associated w/ spinal cord injuries. *Adult:* 75 mg PO bid. Increase to 150 mg PO bid within 1 wk; may increase to 300 mg PO bid if insufficient relief.
ADJUST DOSE Renal impairment
ADV EFF Angioedema, confusion, constipation, dizziness, dry mouth, infection, neuropathy, peripheral edema, somnolence, thrombocytopenia, weight gain
INTERACTIONS Alcohol, CNS depressants, pioglitazone, rosiglitazone
NC/PT Taper when stopping. Not for use in pregnancy (barrier contraceptives advised), breast-feeding. Men should not father child during tx. Pt should take safety measures w/ CNS effects, avoid alcohol, report vision changes, weight gain, increased bleeding, thoughts of suicide.

primidone (Mysoline)

CLASS Antiepileptic
PREG/CONT D/NA

BBW Increased risk of suicidal ideation; monitor accordingly.
IND & DOSE Control of tonic-clonic, psychomotor, focal epileptic seizures. *Adult w/ no previous tx:* Days 1–3, 100–125 mg PO at bedtime; days 4–6, 100–125 mg PO bid; days 7–9, 100–125 mg PO tid; day 10, maint, 250 mg tid. Max, 500 mg qid (2 g/day). *Adult on other epileptics:* 100–125 mg PO at bedtime. When primidone alone desired, do not complete transition in under 2 wk. *Child under 8 yr:* Days 1–3, 50 mg PO at bedtime; days 4–6, 50 mg PO bid; days 7–9, 100 mg PO bid; day 10, maint, 125–250 mg tid or 10–25 mg/kg/day in divided doses.
ADV EFF Anorexia, ataxia, fatigue, hyperirritability, megaloblastic anemia, nausea, rash
INTERACTIONS Acetazolamide, alcohol, carbamazepine, isoniazid, nicotinamide, phenytoin, succinimides
NC/PT Taper when stopping; evaluate for therapeutic serum level (5–12 mcg/mL). Monitor CBC, folic acid for megaloblastic anemia. Not for use in pregnancy (barrier contraceptives advised). Pt should take safety measures w/ CNS effects, wear medical ID, avoid alcohol, report rash, fever, thoughts of suicide.

probenecid (Probalan)

CLASS Antigout, uricosuric
PREG/CONT B/NA

IND & DOSE Tx of hyperuricemia associated w/ gout, gouty arthritis. *Adult:* 0.25 g PO bid for 1 wk, then 0.5 g PO bid. Max, 2–3 g/day. Adjuvant to tx w/ penicillins, cephalosporins. *Adult:* 2 g/day PO in divided doses. *Child 2–14 yr:* Initially, 25 mg/kg PO, then 40 mg/kg/day in four divided doses. Tx of gonorrhea.

Adult: Single 1-g dose PO 30 min before penicillin. *Child under 45 kg:* 23 mg/kg PO in one single dose 30 min before penicillin.

ADJUST DOSE Elderly pts, renal impairment

ADV EFF Anaphylaxis, anemia, anorexia, dizziness, n/v, rash, urinary frequency

INTERACTIONS Acyclovir, allopurinol, benzodiazepines, clofibrate, dapsone, dyphylline, methotrexate, NSAIDs, rifampin, sulfonamides, thiopental, zidovudine

NC/PT Check urine alkalinity; urates crystallize in acidic urine. Sodium bicarbonate, potassium citrate may be ordered to alkalinize urine. Pt should take w/ meals, antacids; drink 2.5–3 L fluid/day; take safety precautions w/ dizziness; report dark urine, painful urination.

DANGEROUS DRUG

procarbazine hydrochloride (Matulane)
CLASS Antineoplastic
PREG/CONT D/NA

IND & DOSE Part of MOPP regimen for tx of stage III, IV Hodgkin lymphoma. *Adult:* 2–4 mg/kg/day PO for first wk, then 4–6 mg/kg/day PO. Maint, 1–2 mg/kg/day PO.

ADJUST DOSE Elderly pts, renal impairment

ADV EFF Bone marrow suppression, confusion, diarrhea, fever, hallucinations, **hepatotoxicity, hypertensive crisis,** pneumonitis

INTERACTIONS Alcohol, anticholinergics, antihistamines, MAOIs, oral anticoagulants, TCAs

NC/PT Monitor CBC, LFTs; do not give within 14 days of MAOIs. Not for use in pregnancy (barrier contraceptives advised), breast-feeding. Pt should follow prescription carefully; avoid exposure to infection, injury; report severe headache, unusual bleeding, signs of infection.

---

prochlorperazine (Compro), prochlorperazine edisylate, prochlorperazine maleate (Procomp)
CLASS Antiemetic, antipsychotic, dopaminergic blocker, phenothiazine
PREG/CONT C/NA

BBW Increased risk of death if used to treat dementia-related psychosis in elderly pts; not approved for this use.

IND & DOSE Mgt of manifestations of psychotic disorders. *Adult:* 5–10 mg PO tid or qid. Range, 50–75 mg/day for mild/moderate disturbances, 100–150 mg/day PO for more severe disturbances. For immediate control of severely disturbed adults, 10–20 mg IM repeated q 2–4 hr (q hour for resistant cases). *Child 2–12 yr:* 2.5 mg PO or rectally bid–tid; max, 25 mg/day (6–12 yr), 20 mg/day (2–5 yr). *Child under 12 yr:* 0.132 mg/kg by deep IM injection. Switch to oral as soon as possible (usually after one dose). **Tx of emesis.** *Adult:* 5–10 mg PO tid–qid; or 15 mg SR on arising; or 25 mg rectally bid; or 5–10 mg IM initially, then q 3–4 hr (max, 40 mg/day). *Child over 2 yr:* 18.2–38.6 kg, 2.5 mg PO or rectally tid or 5 mg bid; max, 15 mg/day. 13.6–17.7 kg, 2.5 mg PO or rectally bid–tid; max, 10 mg/day. 9.1–13.2 kg, 2.5 mg PO or rectally daily–bid; max, 7.5 mg/day. *Child 2 yr and older, at least 9.1 kg:* 0.132 mg/kg IM (usually at least one dose). **Mgt of n/v related to surgery.** *Adult:* 5–10 mg IM 1–2 hr before anesthesia or periop and postop (may repeat once in 30 min); or 5–10 mg IV 15 min before anesthesia or periop and postop (may repeat once); or 20 mg/L isotonic sol added to IV infusion 15 min before anesthesia. **Tx of nonpsychotic anxiety.** *Adult:* 5 mg PO tid or qid; max, 20 mg/day for no more than 12 wk.

ADV EFF Akathisia, **aplastic anemia, bone marrow suppression, bronchospasm,** dizziness, drowsiness, dystonia, **HF, laryngospasm, NMS,** photosensitivity, pink to red-brown urine, pseudoparkinsonism, rash, **refractory arrhythmias,** tardive dyskinesia
INTERACTIONS Alcohol, anticholinergics, barbiturate anesthetics
NC/PT Monitor CBC, renal function; elderly pts may be more susceptible to adverse reactions. Maintain hydration. Avoid skin contact w/ oral sol. Give IM injection deep into upper outer quadrant of buttock. Urine may be pink to red-brown. Pt should avoid sun exposure, take safety precautions w/ CNS effects, report unusual bleeding, swelling, fever.

---

progesterone (Crinone, Endometrin, Prometrium)
CLASS Hormone, progestin
PREG/CONT B (oral), X (injection)/NA

BBW Do not use for px of CV disease. Not effective for this use; may actually increase risk of CV disease. Increased risk of dementia; weigh risks. Increased risk of invasive breast cancer; monitor pt closely.
IND & DOSE Tx of primary amenorrhea. *Adult:* 5–10 mg/day IM for 6–8 consecutive days. Or, 400 mg PO in p.m. for 10 days. **Tx of secondary amenorrhea.** *Adult:* 4%–8% gel, 45–90 mg q other day; max, six doses. **Mgt of uterine bleeding.** *Adult:* 5–10 mg/day IM for six doses. If estrogen given, begin treatment after 2 wk of estrogen tx. **Tx of endometrial hyperplasia.** *Adult:* 200 mg/day PO in p.m. for 12 days/28 day cycle w/ daily conjugated estrogen. **Tx of infertility.** *Adult:* 90 mg vaginally daily in women needing progesterone supplementation; 90 mg vaginally bid for replacement. Continue for 10–12 wk into pregnancy if it occurs. **Support for embryo implantation.**

Adult: 100 mg vaginally two to three times daily starting at oocyte retrieval, continuing for up to 10 wk.
ADV EFF Abd cramps, amenorrhea; breakthrough bleeding, spotting; breast tenderness; cervical erosion; change in menstrual flow, weight; constipation; dizziness; headache; **PE;** photosensitivity; rash; somnolence; **thromboembolic/thrombotic disease**
INTERACTIONS Grapefruit juice
NC/PT Obtain baseline, periodic (at least annual) hx, physical exam. Insert intrauterine system during or immediately after menstrual period. Give IM by deep injection. Stop at first sign of thromboembolic problems. Not for use in pregnancy (contact prescriber if pregnancy occurs). Pt should perform monthly breast self-exams; avoid grapefruit juice, sun exposure; stop if sudden vision loss, difficulty breathing, leg pain/swelling.

DANGEROUS DRUG

promethazine hydrochloride (Phenadoz, Phenergan, Promethegan)
CLASS Antiemetic, antihistamine, anti–motion sickness drug, dopaminergic blocker, phenothiazine, sedative-hypnotic
PREG/CONT C/NA

BBW Do not give to child under 2 yr; risk of fatal respiratory depression. Use lowest effective dose, caution in child 2 yr and older. Give IM injection deep into muscle. Do not give subcut; tissue necrosis possible. Do not give intra-arterially; arteriospasm, limb gangrene possible. If IV route used, limit drug conc, rate of administration; ensure open IV line.
IND & DOSE Relief of allergy s&sx. *Adult:* 25 mg PO, rectally, preferably at bedtime. If needed, 12.5 mg PO before meals and at bedtime. Or, 25 mg IM or IV for serious reactions. May repeat within 2 hr if needed. *Child over*

2 yr: 25 mg PO at bedtime or 6.25–12.5 mg tid. **Tx, px of motion sickness.** *Adult:* 25 mg PO bid 30–60 min before travel; repeat in 8–12 hr if needed. Then, 25 mg on rising and before evening meal. *Child over 2 yr:* 12.5–25 mg PO, rectally bid. **Tx, px of n/v.** *Adult:* 25 mg PO; repeat doses of 12.5–25 mg as needed q 4–6 hr. Give rectally or parenterally if PO not tolerated. Or, 12.5–25 mg IM or IV; max, q 4–6 hr. *Child over 2 yr:* 0.5 mg/lb body weight IM q 4–6 hr as needed. **Sedation, postop sedation, adjunctive use w/ analgesics.** *Adult:* 25–50 mg PO, IM or IV. *Child over 2 yr:* 12.5–25 mg PO rectally at bedtime. For postop sedation, 12.5–25 mg PO, IV or IM, rectally. **Preop use.** *Adult:* 50 mg PO night before surgery. *Child over 2 yr:* 0.5 mg/lb body weight PO. **Obstetric sedation.** *Adult:* 50 mg IM or IV in early stages. When labor established, 25–75 mg w/ reduced opioid dose. May repeat once or twice at 4-hr intervals. Max within 24 hr, 100 mg.

ADV EFF Agranulocytosis, confusion, dizziness, drowsiness, dysuria, epigastric distress, excitation, hypotension, **pancytopenia,** photosensitivity, poor coordination, thickened bronchial secretions, urinary frequency

INTERACTIONS Alcohol, anticholinergics, methohexital, phenobarbital anesthetic, thiopental

NC/PT Do not give subcut, deep IM. Maintain hydration. Pt should take safety precautions w/ CNS effects, avoid sun exposure, report unusual bleeding, rash, dark urine.

DANGEROUS DRUG

propafenone hydrochloride (Rythmol)

CLASS Antiarrhythmic
PREG/CONT C/NA

BBW Arrange for periodic ECG to monitor effects on cardiac conduction; risk of serious proarrhythmias.

Monitor pt response carefully, especially at start of tx; increase dosage at minimum of 3- to 4-day intervals.
IND & DOSE Tx of documented life-threatening ventricular arrhythmias; tx of paroxysmal supraventricular tachycardia w/ disabling s&sx in pts w/out structural heart disease. *Adult:* 150 mg PO q 8 hr (450 mg/day). May increase at minimum of 3- to 4-day intervals to 225 mg PO q 8 hr (675 mg/day) to max 300 mg PO q 8 hr (900 mg/day). **To prolong time to recurrence of symptomatic atrial fibrillation in pts w/ structural heart disease.** *Adult:* 225 mg ER tablet PO q 12 hr; titrate at 5-day intervals to max 425 mg q 12 hr.

ADJUST DOSE Elderly pts; hepatic, renal impairment

ADV EFF Agranulocytosis, arrhythmias, blurred vision, constipation, dizziness, headache, **cardiac arrest, coma,** fatigue, headache, **HF,** n/v, unusual taste

INTERACTIONS Beta blockers, cimetidine, cyclosporine, digoxin, quinidine, ritonavir, SSRIs, theophylline, warfarin

NC/PT .Monitor ECG periodically. Not for use in pregnancy. Pt should swallow ER tablet whole and not cut, crush, or chew it; take around the clock; use safety precautions w/ CNS effects; report difficulty breathing, fainting, palpitations.

---

propantheline bromide (generic)

CLASS Anticholinergic, antispasmodic, parasympatholytic
PREG/CONT C/NA

IND & DOSE Adjunct tx in peptic ulcer. *Adult:* 7.5–15 mg PO 30 min before meals and at bedtime. *Child:* 1.5 mg/kg/day PO in divided doses tid q qid.

ADJUST DOSE Elderly pts; hepatic, renal impairment

ADV EFF Blurred vision, decreased sweating, drowsiness, dry mouth, headache, n/v, urine retention
INTERACTIONS Antacids, anticholinergics, digoxin, phenothiazines
NC/PT Risk of heat prostration; maintain hydration. Pt should swallow ER tablet whole and not cut, crush, or chew it; take 30 min before meals and at bedtime; empty bladder before each dose; use sugarless lozenges for dry mouth; take safety precautions for CNS effects; report rash, eye pain.

DANGEROUS DRUG

propofol disodium
(Diprivan)
CLASS Sedative/hypnotic
PREG/CONT B/NA

IND & DOSE Induction of general anesthesia. *Adult:* 2–2.5 mg/kg IV at 40 mg/10 sec. *Children 3–16 yr:* 2.5–3.5 mg/kg IV over 20–30 sec. Induction of general anesthesia in neurosurgery. *Adult:* 1–2 mg/kg IV at 20 mg/10 sec. Induction of general anesthesia in cardiac surgery. *Adult:* 0.5–1.5 mg/kg IV at 20 mg/10 sec. Maintenance of general anesthesia. *Adult:* 100–200 mcg/kg/min IV or 25–50 mg intermittant IV bolus, based on pt response. *Children 3–16 yr:* 125–150 mcg/kg/min IV, based on pt response. Monitored anesthesia care. *Adult:* 25–75 mcg/kg/min IV, based on pt response. ICU sedation of intubated pts. *Adult:* 5–50 mcg/kg/min IV as continuous infusion.
ADJUST DOSE Elderly, debilitated pts
ADV EFF Anxiety, **apnea,** chills, confusion, dry mouth, **hypoxemia,** injection-site reactions, **loss of responsiveness, MI, respiratory depression**
INTERACTIONS Benzodiazepines, opioid analgesics
NC/PT Monitor continuously. Perform frequent BP checks, oximetry; give oxygen; have emergency equipment on standby; ensure pt safety

w/ CNS effects; taper after prolonged ICU use. Pt should be aware of sedation effects (do not drive; avoid important decisions, tasks requiring alertness); report difficulty breathing, chest pain, pain at injection site.

DANGEROUS DRUG

propranolol hydrochloride (Inderal, InnoPran XL)
CLASS Antianginal, antiarrhythmic, antihypertensive, beta blocker
PREG/CONT C/NA

BBW Do not stop abruptly after long-term tx (hypersensitivity to catecholamines possible, causing angina exacerbation, MI, ventricular arrhythmias). Taper gradually over 2 wk w/ monitoring.
IND & DOSE Tx of hypertension. *Adult:* 40 mg PO regular propranolol bid, or 80 mg (SR, ER) PO daily initially; range, 120–240 mg/day bid or tid or 120–160 mg (SR, ER) daily (max, 640 mg/day). Tx of angina. *Adult:* 80–320 mg/day PO divided bid, tid, or qid, or 80 mg (SR, ER) daily initially; usual dose, 160 mg/day (max, 320 mg/day). Mgt of IHSS. *Adult:* 20–40 mg PO tid or qid, or 80–160 mg PO (SR, ER) daily. Post-MI. *Adult:* 120 mg/day PO divided tid. After 1 mo, may titrate to 180–240 mg/day PO tid or qid (max, 240 mg/day). Mgt of pheochromocytoma s&sx. *Adult:* Preop, 60 mg/day PO for 3 days in divided doses; inoperable tumor, 30 mg/day in divided doses. Px of migraine. *Adult:* 80 mg/day PO (SR, ER) once or in divided doses; range, 160–240 mg/day. Mgt of essential tremor. *Adult:* 40 mg PO bid; maint, 120 mg/day (max, 320 mg/day). Tx of arrhythmias. *Adult:* 10–30 mg PO tid or qid, or 1–3 mg IV w/ careful monitoring; max, 1 mg/min. May give second dose in 2 min, then do not repeat for 4 hr.

ADV EFF Arrhythmias, **broncho-spasm,** constipation, decreased exercise tolerance/libido, fever, flatulence, gastric pain, serum glucose changes, **HF, laryngospasm,** n/v/d, **stroke**

INTERACTIONS Barbiturates, clonidine, epinephrine, ergots, ibuprofen, indomethacin, insulin, lidocaine, methimazole, naproxen, phenothiazines, piroxicam, prazosin, propylthiouracil, sulindac, theophyllines, thioridazine, verapamil

NC/PT Provide continuous cardiac, regular BP monitoring w/ IV form. Change to oral form as soon as possible. Taper when stopping. Pt should take w/ food, take safety precautions w/ CNS effects, report difficulty breathing, swelling, numbness/tingling.

propylthiouracil (PTU) (generic)

CLASS Antithyroid drug
PREG/CONT D/NA

BBW Associated w/ severe, possibly fatal, liver injury. Monitor carefully for liver adverse effects, especially during first 6 mo of tx. Do not use in child unless allergic to or intolerant of other tx; risk of liver toxicity higher in children. Drug of choice when antithyroid tx needed during or just before first trimester (fetal abnormalities are associated w/ methimazole).

IND & DOSE Tx of hyperthyroidism. *Adult:* 300 mg/day PO in divided doses q 8 hr, up to 400–900 mg/day in severe cases. Range, 100–150 mg/day in divided doses q 8 hr. *Child 6 and older intolerant to other tx:* 50 mg/ day PO in divided doses q 8 hr.

ADV EFF Agranulocytosis, drowsiness, epigastric distress, fever, neuritis, n/v, paresthesia, rash, **severe liver injury,** vertigo

INTERACTIONS Cardiac glycosides, metoprolol, oral anticoagulants, propranolol, theophylline

NC/PT Monitor TSH, T_3/T_4. Prolonged tx will be needed. Alert sur-geon that drug may increase risk of bleeding. Pt should take around the clock, use safety precautions w/ CNS effects, report signs of infection, urine/stool color changes. Name confusion between propylthiouracil and *Purinethol* (mercaptopurine); use extreme caution.

protamine sulfate (generic)

CLASS Heparin antagonist
PREG/CONT C/NA

BBW Keep emergency equipment on hand in case of anaphylactic reaction. Pt should take around the clock.

IND & DOSE Tx of heparin over-dose. *Adult, child:* 1 mg IV neutralizes not less than 100 heparin units.

ADV EFF Anaphylaxis, hypotension, n/v, rash

NC/PT Monitor coagulation studies to adjust dose; screen for heparin rebound and response. Pt should report difficulty breathing, dizziness.

DANGEROUS DRUG
protein C concentrate (Ceprotin)

CLASS Anticoagulant, blood product
PREG/CONT C/NA

IND & DOSE Replacement tx for pts w/ severe congenital protein C deficiency. *Adult, child:* 100–120 international units/kg by IV injection. Then 60–80 international units/kg IV q 6 hr for three more doses. Maint, 45–60 international units/kg IV q 6–12 hr.

ADV EFF Anaphylactoid reaction, bleeding, hemothorax, hypotension, light-headedness, pruritus, rash

NC/PT Risk of disease transmission w/ blood products. Protect from light. Monitor for bleeding. Pt should report difficulty breathing, hives, rash, unusual bleeding.

prothrombin complex concentrate (Kcentra, Octaplex)

CLASS Vitamin K anticoagulant reversal agent
PREG/CONT C/NA

BBW Risk of thromboembolic complications. Monitor closely; consider need to resume anticoagulant therapy when risks outweigh benefits.
IND & DOSE Urgent reversal of acquired coagulation factor deficiency from warfarin overactivity w/ major bleeding. *Adult:* INR of 2 to less than 4, 25 units/kg IV; max, 2,500 units. INR of 4–6, 35 units/kg IV; max, 3,500 units. INR greater than 6, 50 units/kg IV; max, 5,000 units.
ADV EFF Arthralgia, **blood-related infections**, DVT, headache, hypotension, n/v, **serious hypersensitivity reactions, stroke**
NC/PT Monitor INR during and after tx. Monitor for hypersensitivity reactions, sx of thrombotic events. Pt should know risks of receiving blood products. Risks in pregnancy, breast-feeding unknown. Pt should report difficulty breathing, chest pain, acute leg pain, numbness or tingling, vision or speech changes, abnormal swelling.

protriptyline hydrochloride (Vivactil)

CLASS TCA
PREG/CONT C/NA

BBW Limit drug access in depressed, potentially suicidal pts. Increased risk of suicidality in children, adolescents, young adults; monitor accordingly.
IND & DOSE Relief of sx of depression. *Adult:* 15–40 mg/day PO in three to four divided doses; max, 60 mg/day.
ADJUST DOSE Elderly pts

ADV EFF Anticholinergic effects, **bone marrow suppression**, constipation, dry mouth, extrapyramidal effects, **MI**, orthostatic hypotension, photosensitivity, rash, **stroke**
INTERACTIONS Alcohol, cimetidine, clonidine, fluoxetine, MAOIs, ranitidine, sympathomimetics, tramadol
NC/PT Do not stop suddenly. Monitor CBC periodically. Not for use in pregnancy (contraceptives advised). Pt should avoid sun exposure, take safety precautions w/ CNS effects, use sugarless lozenges for dry mouth, report thoughts of suicide, excessive sedation.

pseudoephedrine hydrochloride, pseudoephedrine sulfate (Efidac/24, Genaphed, Sudafed, Unifed)

CLASS Nasal decongestant, sympathomimetic
PREG/CONT C/NA

BBW Administer cautiously to pts with CV disease, diabetes, hyperthyroidism, glaucoma, hypertension, over 65 yr; increased sensitivity to sympathetic amines possible in these pts.
IND & DOSE Relief of nasal congestion. *Adult, child over 12 yr:* 60 mg PO q 4–6 hr (ER, 120 mg PO q 12 hr; CR, 240 mg/day PO); max, 240 mg/24 hr. *Child 6–12 yr:* 30 mg PO q 4–6 hr; max, 120 mg/24 hr. *Child 2–5 yr:* 15 mg PO (syrup) q 4–6 hr; max, 60 mg/24 hr.
ADJUST DOSE Elderly pts
ADV EFF Arrhythmias, anxiety, dizziness, drowsiness, fear, headache, hypertension, n/v, pallor, restlessness, **seizures,** tenseness, tremors
INTERACTIONS MAOIs, methyldopa, urine acidifiers/alkalinizers
NC/PT Avoid prolonged use. Underlying medical problems may be

causing congestion. Pt should swallow ER tablet whole and not cut, crush, or chew it; take safety precautions w/ CNS effects; report sweating, sleeplessness.

pyrantel pamoate
(Pin-Rid, Pin-X, Reese's Pinworm)
CLASS Anthelmintic
PREG/CONT C/NA

IND & DOSE Tx of enterobiasis, ascariasis. *Adult, child over 2 yr:* 11 mg/kg (5 mg/lb) PO as single oral dose. Max total dose, 1 g.
ADJUST DOSE Hepatic impairment
ADV EFF Abd cramps, anorexia, dizziness, drowsiness, headache, n/v/d
INTERACTIONS Piperazine, theophylline
NC/PT Culture before tx. Pt should shake suspension well; take w/ fruit juice, milk; use strict hand washing, hygiene measures; launder undergarments, bed linens, nightclothes daily; disinfect toilet facilities daily, bathroom floors periodically; take safety precautions w/ CNS effects; report severe headache.

pyrazinamide (generic)
CLASS Antituberculotic
PREG/CONT C/NA

IND & DOSE Tx of active, drug-resistant TB. *Adult, child:* 15–30 mg/kg/day PO; max, 2 g/day. Always use w/ up to four other antituberculotics; give for first 2 mo of 6-mo tx program.
ADV EFF Bone marrow suppression, gouty arthritis, hepatotoxicity, n/v, photosensitivity, rash
INTERACTIONS Piperazine, theophylline
NC/PT Give only w/ other antituberculotics. Monitor LFTs during tx. Pt should have regular medical follow-up,

report unusual bleeding, urine/stool color changes, severe joint pain.

pyridostigmine bromide
(Mestinon, Regonol)
CLASS Antimyasthenic, cholinesterase inhibitor
PREG/CONT C/NA

IND & DOSE Control of myasthenia gravis sx. *Adult:* 600 mg PO over 24 hr; range, 60–1,500 mg. Or, 180–540 mg (ER) PO daily, bid. As supplement to oral dose preop, postop, during labor/myasthenic crisis, etc: Give 1/30 oral dose IM or very slow IV. May give 1 hr before second stage of labor completed. *Child:* 7 mg/kg/day PO divided into five or six doses (over 30 days); 5 mg/kg/day PO divided into five or six doses (29 days or younger). *Neonates w/ myasthenic mothers who have difficulty swallowing, sucking, breathing.* 0.05–0.15 mg/kg IM. Change to syrup as soon as possible. *Military w/ threat of sarin nerve gas exposure. Adult:* 30 mg PO q 8 hr starting several hr before exposure; stop if exposure occurs. *Antidote for NMJ blocker.* Atropine sulfate 0.6–1.2 mg IV immediately before slow IV injection of pyridostigmine 0.1–0.25 mg/kg; 10–20 mg pyridostigmine usually suffices. Full recovery usually within 15 min; may take 30 min.
ADV EFF Abd cramps, anaphylaxis, bradycardia, bronchospasm, cardiac arrhythmias, dysphagia, increased respiratory secretions/lacrimation/salivation, laryngospasm, urinary frequency/incontinence
INTERACTIONS Corticosteroids, succinylcholine
NC/PT Have atropine on hand as antidote. Give IV slowly. Pt should swallow ER tablet whole and not cut, crush, or chew it; report difficulty breathing, excessive sweating.

quazepam (Doral)

CLASS Benzodiazepine, sedative-hypnotic
PREG/CONT X/C-IV

IND & DOSE Tx of insomnia. *Adult:* 7.5–15 mg PO at bedtime.
ADJUST DOSE Elderly, debilitated pts
ADV EFF Anaphylaxis, angioedema, apathy, bradycardia, **CV collapse,** constipation, depression, diarrhea, disorientation, dizziness, drowsiness, dry mouth, fatigue, fever, hiccups, lethargy, light-headedness
INTERACTIONS Alcohol, aminophylline, anticonvulsants, antihistamines, cimetidine, disulfiram, hormonal contraceptives, psychotropics, smoking, theophylline
NC/PT Monitor LFTs, CBC, renal function w/ long-term tx. Taper gradually after long-term use. Not for use in pregnancy (barrier contraceptives advised). Pt should take safety precautions w/ CNS effects, report rash, swelling, vision changes, difficulty breathing.

quetiapine fumarate (Seroquel)

CLASS Antipsychotic
PREG/CONT C/NA

BBW Do not use in elderly pts w/ dementia-related psychosis; increased risk of CV mortality, including stroke, MI. Increased risk of suicidality in children, adolescents, young adults; monitor accordingly. Not approved for use in children.
IND & DOSE Tx of schizophrenia. *Adult:* 25 mg PO bid. Increase in increments of 25–50 mg bid–tid on days 2, 3. Range by day 4, 300–400 mg/day in two to three divided doses; max, 800 mg/day. Once stabilized, switch to ER, 300 mg/day PO in p.m.; range, 400–800 mg/day. *Child 13–17 yr:* Divided dose bid. Total dose: day 1, 50 mg PO; day 2, 100 mg; day 3, 200 mg; day 4, 300 mg; day 5, 400 mg.

Range, 400–800 mg/day. **Tx of manic episodes of bipolar 1 disorder.** *Adult:* 100 mg/day PO divided bid on day 1; increase to 400 mg/day PO in bid divided doses by day 4, using 100-mg/day increments. Range, 400–800 mg/day in divided doses. ER: 300 mg/day PO on day 1; 600 mg on day 2; may adjust to 800 mg on day 3 if needed. *Child 10–17 yr:* 50 mg PO on day 1, 100 mg on day 2, 200 mg on day 3, 300 mg on day 4, 400 mg on day 5. Max, 600 mg/day. **Tx of depressive episodes of bipolar 1 disorder.** *Adult:* 50 mg (ER) PO on day 1, then 100 mg at bedtime on day 2; increase to desired dose of 300 mg/day by day 4. **Tx of major depressive disorder.** *Adult:* 50 mg (ER) PO at bedtime; on day 3, increase to 150 mg in evening. Range, 150–300 mg/day.
ADJUST DOSE Elderly, debilitated pts; hepatic impairment
ADV EFF Dizziness, drowsiness, dry mouth, headache, hyperglycemia, **NMS,** orthostatic hypotension, **prolonged QT interval,** sweating
INTERACTIONS Alcohol, anticholinergics, antihypertensives, carbamazepine, CNS depressants, dopamine antagonists, glucocorticoids, levodopa, lorazepam, phenobarbital, phenytoin, QT-prolonging drugs, rifampin, thioridazine
NC/PT Monitor for hyperglycemia. Ensure hydration in elderly pts. Not for use in pregnancy (barrier contraceptives advised). Pt should swallow ER tablet whole and not cut, crush, or chew it; avoid alcohol; take safety precautions w/ CNS effects; report fever, unusual bleeding, rash, suicidal thoughts.

quinapril hydrochloride (Accupril)

CLASS ACE inhibitor, antihypertensive
PREG/CONT D/NA

BBW Should not be used during pregnancy; advise barrier contraceptives.

IND & DOSE Tx of hypertension.
Adult: 10 or 20 mg/day PO; maint, 20–80 mg/day PO. **Adjunct tx of HF.**
Adult: 5 mg PO bid; range, 10–20 mg PO bid.

ADJUST DOSE Elderly pts, renal impairment

ADV EFF Angioedema, cough, dizziness, headache, orthostatic hypotension, LFT changes, rash

INTERACTIONS Lithium, potassium-sparing diuretics, tetracycline

NC/PT Alert surgeon to drug use; volume replacement may be needed after surgery. Maintain hydration. Pt should use care in situations that may lead to BP drop; take safety precautions w/ dizziness, hypotension; report fever, difficulty breathing, swelling of lips/tongue.

DANGEROUS DRUG

quinidine gluconate, quinidine sulfate
(generic)
CLASS Antiarrhythmic
PREG/CONT C/NA

IND & DOSE Tx of atrial arrhythmias; paroxysmal, chronic ventricular tachycardia. *Adult:* 400–600 mg (sulfate) PO q 2–3 hr until paroxysm terminated. *Child:* 30 mg/kg/24 h PO in five equally divided doses. **Conversion of atrial fibrillation (AF).** *Adult:* 648 mg (gluconate) PO q 8 hr; may increase after three to four doses if needed. Or, 324 mg (gluconate) PO q 8 hr for 2 days, then 648 mg PO q 8 hr for 2 days. Or, 5–10 mg/kg (gluconate) IV. For ER, 300 mg (sulfate) PO q 8–12 hr; may increase cautiously if serum level is in therapeutic range. For immediate-release, 400 mg (sulfate) PO q 6 hr; may increase after four to five doses if no conversion. **To convert relapse into AF.** *Adult:* 324 mg (gluconate) PO q 8–12 hr. For ER, 300 mg (sulfate) PO q 8–12 hr. For immediate-release, 200 mg (sulfate) PO q 6 hr. **Tx of *Plasmodium falciparum* malaria.** *Adult:* 24 mg/kg gluconate IV in 250 mL normal saline infused over 4 hr;

then 12 mg/kg IV infused over 4 hr q 8 hr for 7 days. Or, 10 mg/kg gluconate in 5 mL/kg IV as loading dose; then maint IV infusion of 20 mcg/kg/min. May switch to same oral dose of sulfate q 8 hr for 72 hr or until parasitemia decreased to 1% or less.

ADJUST DOSE Hepatic, renal impairment

ADV EFF Bone marrow suppression, cardiac arrhythmias, cinchonism, diarrhea, headache, hepatic impairment, light-headedness, nausea, rash, vision changes

INTERACTIONS Amiodarone, cimetidine, digoxin, grapefruit juice, hydantoins, NMJ blockers, oral anticoagulants, phenobarbital, rifampin, sodium bicarbonate, succinylcholine, sucralfate, TCAs, verapamil

NC/PT Give test dose of 200 mg PO or 200 mg IV for idiosyncratic reaction. Ensure pts w/ atrial flutter, fibrillation digitalized before starting quinidine. Monitor for safe, effective serum level (2–6 mcg/mL). Pt should swallow ER tablet whole and not cut, crush, or chew it; wear medical ID; take safety precautions w/ CNS effects; report vision disturbances, unusual bleeding, signs of infection.

---

quinine sulfate
(Qualaquin)
CLASS Antimalarial, cinchonan
PREG/CONT C/NA

BBW Not for tx, px of nocturnal leg cramps; serious to life-threatening hematologic reactions possible. No evidence for therapeutic effectiveness for nocturnal leg cramps.
IND & DOSE Tx of uncomplicated *Plasmodium falciparum* malaria.
Adult: 648 mg (two capsules) PO q 8 hr for 7 days.

ADJUST DOSE Renal impairment
ADV EFF Abd pain, anaphylaxis, blindness, blurred vision, cardiac arrhythmias, deafness, dizziness, headache, hearing impairment, hypoglycemia, n/v/d, prolonged QT

interval, sweating, tinnitus, **thrombocytopenia including idiopathic thrombocytopenic purpura**, vertigo
INTERACTIONS CYP3A4 inducers/inhibitors, digoxin, NMJ blockers, QT-prolonging drugs, rifampin
NC/PT Monitor LFTs, renal function, blood glucose, CBC. Use caution in pregnancy, breast-feeding. Pt should report unusual bleeding, difficulty breathing, palpitations, fainting.

---

rabeprazole sodium
(AcipHex)
CLASS Proton pump inhibitor
PREG/CONT B/NA

IND & DOSE Tx of GERD. *Adult, child 12 yr and older:* 20 mg/day PO for 4–8 wk; maint, 20 mg/day PO. *Child 1–11 yr:* 15 kg or more, 10 mg/day PO; less than 15 kg, 5 mg/day PO up to 12 wk. **Healing of duodenal ulcer.** *Adult:* 20 mg PO daily for up to 4 wk. **Tx of pathological hypersecretory conditions.** *Adult:* 60 mg PO daily–bid. *Helicobacter pylori* **eradication.** *Adult:* 20 mg PO bid w/ amoxicillin 1,000 mg PO bid and clarithromycin 500 mg PO bid w/ meals for 7 days.
ADJUST DOSE Hepatic impairment
ADV EFF Asthenia, bone loss, *Clostridium difficile* diarrhea, diarrhea, dizziness, dry mouth, headache, hypomagnesemia, n/v, pneumonia, URI sx
INTERACTIONS Azole antifungals, digoxin, warfarin
NC/PT Pt should swallow tablet whole and not cut, crush, or chew it; maintain other tx for condition; take safety precautions w/ CNS effects; maintain nutrition; report worsening of condition, severe diarrhea.

---

radium Ra 223 dichloride (Xofigo)
CLASS Antineoplastic, radioactive particle–emitting agent
PREG/CONT X/NA

IND & DOSE Tx of castration-resistant prostate cancer w/ symptomatic bone metastases and no known visceral metastatic disease. *Adult:* 50 kBq (1.35 microcurie)/kg by slow IV injection (over 1 min) at 4-wk intervals for six injections.
ADV EFF Bone marrow suppression, n/v/d, peripheral edema
NC/PT Ensure proper dx, proper handling of drug. Monitor CBC; provide supportive measures. Use universal precautions with body fluids. Pt should use gloves when handling body fluids; flush toilet several times; avoid pregnancy (men should use barrier contraceptives during and for 6 mo after use); report extreme fatigue, bleeding, severe vomiting, diarrhea.

---

raloxifene hydrochloride (Evista)
CLASS Selective estrogen receptor modulator
PREG/CONT X/NA

BBW Increased risk of DVT, PE; monitor accordingly. Increased risk of stroke, CV events in women w/ documented CAD; weigh benefits/risks before use in these women.
IND & DOSE Px, tx of osteoporosis in postmenopausal women; to reduce risk of invasive breast cancer in postmenopausal women w/ osteoporosis and high risk of invasive breast cancer. *Adult:* 60 mg/day PO.
ADV EFF Depression, dizziness, edema, flulike sx, hot flashes, lightheadedness, rash, vaginal bleeding, **venous thromboembolism**
INTERACTIONS Cholestyramine, oral anticoagulants
NC/PT Obtain periodic CBC. Provide comfort measures for effects. Not for use in pregnancy (contraceptives advised). Pt should take safety precautions w/ CNS effects; report difficulty breathing, numbness/tingling, pain/swelling in legs.

raltegravir (Isentress)
CLASS Antiretroviral, integrase inhibitor
PREG/CONT C/NA

IND & DOSE Tx of HIV-1 infection. *Adult, child 12 yr and older:* 400 mg PO bid w/ other antivirals, without regard to food. If given w/ rifampin, 800 mg PO bid without regard to food. *Child 6–under 12 yr:* 25 kg or more, 400 mg PO bid or up to 300 mg PO bid chewable tablet; under 25 kg, chewable tablets weight-based to max 300 mg PO bid. *Child 2–under 6 yr:* 40 kg or more, 300 mg PO bid; 28–under 40 kg, 200 mg PO bid; 20–under 28 kg, 150 mg PO bid; 14–under 20 kg, 100 mg PO bid; 10–under 14 kg, 75 mg PO bid; under 10 kg, not recommended. *Child 4 wk–under 2 yr:* 14–under 20 kg, 5 mL (100 mg) PO bid; 11–under 14 kg, 4 mL (80 mg) PO bid; 8–under 11 kg, 3 mL (60 mg) PO bid; 6–under 8 kg, 2 mL (40 mg) PO bid; 4–under 6 kg, 1.5 mL (30 mg) PO bid; 3–less than 4 kg, 1 mL (20 mg) PO bid.
ADV EFF Diarrhea, dizziness, headache, fever, n/v, rhabdomyolysis
INTERACTIONS Rifampin, St. John's wort
NC/PT Ensure pt taking other antivirals. Not for use in pregnancy, breast-feeding. Calculate weight-based use of chewable tablets for child. Pt should not let prescription run out or stop temporarily (virus could become resistant to antivirals); take precautions to avoid spread (drug not a cure); avoid St. John's wort; report signs of infection, unexplained muscle pain/weakness.

ramelteon (Rozerem)
CLASS Melatonin receptor agonist, sedative-hypnotic
PREG/CONT C/NA

IND & DOSE Tx of insomnia. *Adult:* 8 mg PO within 30 min of bedtime.
ADJUST DOSE Hepatic impairment

ADV EFF Amenorrhea, **anaphylaxis**, **angioedema**, decreased testosterone, depression, diarrhea, galactorrhea, headache, insomnia, **suicidality**
INTERACTIONS Clarithromycin, fluconazole, fluvoxamine, itraconazole, ketoconazole, nefazodone, nelfinavir, ritonavir
NC/PT Not for use in pregnancy, breast-feeding. Pt should take 30 min before bed, avoid activities after taking, plan on 8 or more hr sleep, report difficulty breathing, swelling, thoughts of suicide.

ramipril (Altace)
CLASS ACE inhibitor, antihypertensive
PREG/CONT D/NA

BBW Not for use in pregnancy; risk of fetal harm. Advise contraceptives.
IND & DOSE Tx of hypertension. *Adult:* 2.5 mg PO daily; range, 2.5–20 mg/day. **Tx of HF first few days post MI.** *Adult:* 2.5 mg PO bid; if hypotensive, may use 1.25 mg PO bid; target dose, 5 mg PO bid. **To decrease risk of MI, stroke, death from CV disease.** *Adult 55 yr and older:* 2.5 mg/day PO for 1 wk, then 5 mg/day PO for 3 wk; maint, 10 mg PO daily.
ADJUST DOSE Elderly pts, renal impairment
ADV EFF **Agranulocytosis, angioedema,** aphthous ulcers, **bone marrow suppression,** cough, dizziness, dysgeusia, gastric irritation, **HF,** light-headedness, proteinuria, rash, **Stevens-Johnson syndrome,** tachycardia
INTERACTIONS Capsaicin, lithium
NC/PT Stop diuretics 2-3 days before tx. Not for use in pregnancy (barrier contraceptives advised). Alert surgeon of ramipril use; volume replacement may be needed postop. Stable for 24 hr at room temp, 48 hr if refrigerated. Pt should open capsules, sprinkle contents over small amount of applesauce or mix in applesauce/water; take safety precautions

w/ CNS effects; use caution in situations that could lead to fluid loss, decreased BP; maintain hydration; report unusual bleeding, swelling, rash.

ranibizumab (Lucentis)
CLASS Monoclonal antibody, ophthalmic agent
PREG/CONT C/NA

IND & DOSE Tx of neovascular (wet) age-related macular degeneration; macular edema after retinal vein occlusion. 0.5 mg (0.05 mL) by intravitreal injection q 1–3 mo.
ADV EFF Conjunctival hemorrhage, eye pain, hypersensitivity reactions, increased IOP, intraocular inflammation, ocular infection, vision changes, vitreous floaters
NC/PT Monitor carefully for detached retina, increased IOP. Pt should be anesthetized before injection, receive antibiotic. Pt should report increased light sensitivity, vision changes, painful eye.

ranitidine hydrochloride (Zantac)
CLASS Gastric acid secretion inhibitor, histamine-2 antagonist
PREG/CONT B/NA

IND & DOSE Tx of active duodenal ulcer. *Adult:* 150 mg PO bid for 4–8 wk, or 300 mg PO once daily at bedtime, or 50 mg IM or IV q 6–8 hr *or* by intermittent IV infusion, diluted to 100 mL and infused over 15–20 min. Max, 400 mg/day; maint, 150 mg PO at bedtime. *Child 1 mo–16 yr:* 2–4 mg/kg PO bid for tx; once daily for maint. Max, 3,000 mg/day (tx), 1,500 mg/day (maint). Or, 2–4 mg/kg/day IV or IM q 6–8 hr; max, 50 mg q 6–8 hr. Tx of active gastric ulcer. *Adult:* 150 mg PO bid, or 50 mg IM or IV q 6-8 hr. Tx of pathologic hypersecretory syndrome, GERD maint, esophagitis, benign gastric ulcer. *Adult:* 150 mg PO bid;

max, 6 g/day. Tx of heartburn, acid indigestion. *Adult:* 75 mg PO as needed.
ADJUST DOSE Elderly pts, renal impairment
ADV EFF Abd pain, bradycardia, bone marrow suppression, constipation, headache, n/v/d, pain at injection site, rash
INTERACTIONS Warfarin
NC/PT Give IM undiluted into large muscle; give oral drug w/ meals and at bedtime. May continue antacids for pain relief. Pt should report unusual bleeding, signs of infection. Name confusion w/ *Zantac* (ranitidine), *Zyrtec* (cetirizine), *Xanax* (alprazolam); use caution.

ranolazine (Ranexa)
CLASS Antianginal, piperazineacetamide
PREG/CONT C/NA

IND & DOSE Tx of chronic angina. *Adult:* 500 mg PO bid; max, 1,000 mg bid.
ADJUST DOSE Hepatic impairment (not recommended)
ADV EFF Constipation, dizziness, headache, nausea, prolonged QT interval
INTERACTIONS Antipsychotics, digoxin, diltiazem, grapefruit juice, HIV protease inhibitors, ketoconazole, macrolide antibiotics, QT-prolonging drugs, rifampin, TCAs, verapamil
NC/PT Obtain baseline ECG, LFTs, renal function. Continue other antianginals. Not for use in pregnancy (contraception advised), breast-feeding. Pt should swallow tablet whole and not cut, crush, or chew it; take safety measures w/ dizziness; avoid grapefruit juice; use laxative for severe constipation; report fainting, palpitations.

rasagiline (Azilect)
CLASS Antiparkinsonian, MAO type B inhibitor
PREG/CONT C/NA

IND & DOSE Tx of s&sx of idiopathic Parkinson disease. *Adult:*

1 mg/day PO as monotherapy;
0.5–1 mg/day PO w/ levodopa.
ADJUST DOSE CYP1A2 inhibitors,
hepatic impairment
ADV EFF Arthralgia, dizziness, dyspepsia, dry mouth, headache, hypotension, **melanoma**, vertigo
INTERACTIONS Cyclobenzaprine,
CYP1A2 inhibitors (ciprofloxacin),
dextromethorphan, MAOIs, meperidine, methadone, mirtazapine, SSRIs,
St. John's wort, sympathomimetic
amines, TCAs, tramadol, tyramine-
rich food
NC/PT Obtain baseline LFTs, skin
evaluation. Continue other Parkinson
drugs. Use caution w/ pregnancy,
breast-feeding. Pt should avoid sun
exposure, tyramine-rich foods, St.
John's wort; take safety measures
w/ dizziness; tell all health care providers about prescribed/OTC drugs,
herbs being used (drug reacts
w/ many other drugs); report skin
changes, worsening of condition.

rasburicase (Elitek)
CLASS Enzyme
PREG/CONT C/NA

BBW Risk of anaphylaxis, hemolysis
(in pts w/ G6PD deficiency); screen
before tx), methemoglobinemia, uric
acid measurement alterations.
IND & DOSE Mgt of plasma uric
acid level in pts w/ leukemia, lymphoma, solid tumor malignancies
receiving anticancer tx expected to
result in tumor lysis. Adult: 0.15 or
0.2 mg/kg IV as single daily infusion
over 30 min for 5 days. Chemotherapy
should start 4–24 hr after first dose.
ADV EFF Abd pain, **anaphylaxis**,
anxiety, constipation, headache, **hemolysis**, n/v/d
NC/PT Screen for G6PD deficiency.
Monitor closely during infusion; stop
immediately if hypersensitivity reactions. Monitor CBC. Blood drawn to
monitor uric acid level must be col-
lected in prechilled, heparinized vials
and kept in ice-water bath; analysis

must be done within 4 hr. Give analgesics for headache. Pt should report
difficulty breathing, chest pain, rash.

raxibacumab (generic)
CLASS Monoclonal antibody
PREG/CONT B/NA

IND & DOSE Tx, px of inhalational
anthrax, w/ antibacterial drugs.
Adult, child over 50 kg: 40 mg/kg IV
over 2 hr, 15 min. Child over 15 kg–
50 kg: 60 mg/kg IV over 2 hr, 15 min.
Child 15 kg and less: 80 mg/kg IV over
2 hr, 15 min.
ADV EFF Extremity pain, infusion
reaction, pruritus, rash, somnolence
NC/PT TEACH Premedicate w/ diphenhydramine. Monitor for infusion
reaction; slow, interrupt infusion as
needed. Pt should report itching, difficulty breathing, rash.

regorafenib (Stivarga)
CLASS Antineoplastic, kinase
inhibitor
PREG/CONT D/NA

BBW Severe to fatal hepatotoxicity
reported; monitor LFTs before, during
tx.
IND & DOSE Tx of metastatic
colorectal cancer in pts previously
treated w/ other agents; tx of advanced, unresectable GI stomal tumors. Adult: 160 mg/day PO for first
21 days of 28-day cycle. Give
w/ low-fat breakfast.
ADV EFF Anorexia, **cardiac isch-
emia/ infarction, dermatologic toxicity**, diarrhea, dysphonia, **GI perfo-
ration/fistula, hepatotoxicity,
hypertension**, mucositis, **RPLS**,
weight loss, wound-healing complications
INTERACTIONS Grapefruit juice,
St. John's wort, strong CYP3A4 in-
ducers/inhibitors; avoid these combinations
NC/PT Monitor LFTs; arrange to
decrease dose or stop drug if

hepatotoxicity occurs. Monitor for skin reactions, bleeding, problems w/ wound healing. Not for use in pregnancy, breast-feeding. Stop drug at least 24 hr before scheduled surgery. Pt should take daily in a.m. w/ low-fat breakfast, report chest pain, severe GI pain, bleeding, urine/stool color changes.

DANGEROUS DRUG

repaglinide (Prandin)
CLASS Antidiabetic, meglitinide
PREG/CONT C/NA

IND & DOSE Adjunct to diet, exercise to lower blood glucose in pts w/ type 2 diabetes, as monotherapy or w/ other antidiabetics. *Adult:* 0.5–4 mg PO tid or qid 15–30 min (usually within 15 min) before meals; max, 16 mg/day.
ADJUST DOSE Hepatic, renal impairment
ADV EFF Diarrhea, headache, hypoglycemia, nausea, URI
INTERACTIONS Celery, coriander, dandelion root, fenugreek, garlic, gemfibrozil, ginseng, itraconazole, juniper berries
NC/PT Review complete diabetic teaching program. Pt should always take before meals (if meal is skipped or added, dose should be skipped or added appropriately); monitor serum glucose, continue exercise/diet program, report fever, unusual bleeding/bruising, frequent hypoglycemia.

ribavirin (Copegus, Rebetol, Ribasphere, Virazole)
CLASS Antiviral
PREG/CONT X/NA

BBW Inhaled form not for use in adults; testicular lesions, birth defects possible. Monotherapy not effective for tx of chronic hepatitis C; do not use alone for this indication. High risk of hemolytic anemia, which could lead to MI; do not use in significant,

unstable CV disease. Monitor respiratory status frequently; pulmonary deterioration, death have occurred during, shortly after tx w/ inhaled form. Risk of significant fetal defects; caution women to avoid pregnancy during tx (barrier contraceptives advised). Male partners of pregnant women should not take drug.
IND & DOSE Tx of hospitalized infants, children w/ severe RSV infection of lower respiratory tract. *Child:* Dilute aerosol powder to 20 mg/mL, deliver for 12–18 hr/day for at least 3 but not more than 7 days. Tx of chronic hepatitis C. *Adult over 75 kg:* Three 200-mg capsules PO in a.m., three 200-mg capsules PO in p.m. w/ *Intron A* 3 million international units subcut three times/wk, or w/ *Pegasys* 180 mcg/wk subcut for 24–48 wk. *Adult 75 kg or less:* Two 200-mg capsules PO in a.m., three 200-mg capsules PO in p.m. w/ *Intron A* 3 million international units subcut three times/wk, or w/ *Pegasys* 180 mcg/wk subcut for 24–48 wk. *Child:* 15 mg/kg/day PO in divided doses a.m. and p.m. Child 25–62 kg may use oral sol. Give w/ *Intron A* 3 million international units/m² subcut three times/wk.
ADJUST DOSE Anemia
ADV EFF Anemia, apnea, **cardiac arrest,** depression, deteriorating respiratory function, **hemolytic anemia,** nervousness, rash, **suicidality**
INTERACTIONS Antacids, nucleoside reverse transcriptase inhibitors
NC/PT Monitor CBC regularly. Review use, care of inhaler. Ensure pt on oral tx also taking other antivirals. Not for use in pregnancy (barrier contraceptives advised). Pt should report thoughts of suicide, chest pain, difficulty breathing.

rifabutin (Mycobutin)
CLASS Antibiotic
PREG/CONT B/NA

IND & DOSE Px, tx of disseminated *Mycobacterium avium* complex in pts

w/ advanced HIV infection. *Adult:*
300 mg/day PO. *Child:* 5 mg/kg/day PO.
ADV EFF Abd pain, anorexia, *Clostridium difficile* diarrhea, headache, nausea, rash, red to orange urine
INTERACTIONS Clarithromycin, delavirdine, indinavir, nelfinavir, oral contraceptives, ritonavir, saquinavir
NC/PT Negative TB test needed before starting tx. Not for use in pregnancy (barrier contraceptives advised), breast-feeding. Urine, body fluids may turn red to orange, staining fabric, contact lenses. Pt should report diarrhea, difficulty breathing.

rifampin (Rifadin)
CLASS Antibiotic, antituberculotic
PREG/CONT C/NA

IND & DOSE Tx of pulmonary TB.
Adult: 10 mg/kg/day PO or IV; max, 600 mg/day in single dose (w/ other antituberculotics). *Child:* 10–20 mg/kg/day PO or IV; max, 600 mg/day. Tx of *Neisseria meningitidis* carriers to eliminate meningococci from nasopharynx. *Adult:* 600 mg/day PO or IV for 4 consecutive days or 600 mg q 12 hr for 2 days. *Child over 1 mo:*
10 mg/kg PO or IV q 12 hr for 2 days; max, 600 mg/dose. *Child under 1 mo:*
5 mg/kg PO or IV q 12 hr for 2 days.
ADJUST DOSE Renal impairment
ADV EFF Acute renal failure, bone marrow suppression, discolored body fluids, dizziness, drowsiness, epigastric distress, fatigue, flulike sx, headache, heartburn, rash
INTERACTIONS Antiarrhythmics, benzodiazepine, buspirone, corticosteroids, cyclosporine, digoxin, doxycycline, fluoroquinolones, hormonal contraceptives, isoniazid, itraconazole, ketoconazole, methadone, metoprolol, nifedipine, oral anticoagulants, oral sulfonylureas, phenytoin, propranolol, quinidine, theophyllines, verapamil, zolpidem
NC/PT Monitor renal function, CBC, LFTs periodically. Body fluids will turn reddish orange. Pt should take once/

day on empty stomach 1 hr before or 2 hr after meals, take safety precautions w/ CNS effects, not wear soft contact lenses (may become permanently stained), report signs of infection, swelling, unusual bleeding/bruising.

rifapentine (Priftin)
CLASS Antibiotic, antituberculotic
PREG/CONT C/NA

IND & DOSE Tx of pulmonary TB.
Adult, child 12 and over: 600 mg PO twice wkly w/ interval of at least 72 hr between doses. Continue for 2 mo, then 600 mg/wk PO for 4 mo w/ other antituberculotics.
ADJUST DOSE Elderly pts
ADV EFF Diarrhea, dizziness, headache, hematuria, hyperuricemia, proteinuria, pyuria, reddish body fluids
INTERACTIONS Antiarrhythmics, benzodiazepine, buspirone, corticosteroids, cyclosporine, digoxin, doxycycline, fluoroquinolones, hormonal contraceptives, isoniazid, itraconazole, ketoconazole, methadone, metoprolol, nifedipine, oral anticoagulants, oral sulfonylureas, phenytoin, propranolol, protease inhibitors, quinidine, theophyllines, verapamil, zolpidem
NC/PT Always give w/ other antituberculotics. Body fluids will turn reddish orange. Not for use in pregnancy (barrier contraceptives advised). Pt should mark calendar for tx days, take once/day on empty stomach 1 hr before or 2 hr after meals (may become permanently stained), take safety precautions w/ CNS effects, report signs of infection, swelling, unusual bleeding/bruising.

rifaximin (Xifaxan)
CLASS Antibiotic, antidiarrheal
PREG/CONT C/NA

IND & DOSE Tx of traveler's diarrhea. *Adult, child 12 yr and older:*
200 mg PO tid for 3 days. To reduce

recurrence of hepatic encephalopathy in pts w/ advanced liver disease. *Adult:* 550 mg PO bid.
ADV EFF Diarrhea, dizziness, fever, flatulence, headache, **pseudomembranous colitis,** rash
NC/PT Do not use w/ diarrhea complicated by fever, blood in stool. Not for use in pregnancy, breast-feeding. Pt should swallow tablet whole and not cut, crush, or chew it; stop if diarrhea does not resolve or worsens in 48 hr; take safety precautions w/ dizziness; report bloody diarrhea, fever.

rilonacept (Arcalyst)
CLASS Anti-inflammatory, interleukin blocker
PREG/CONT C/NA

IND & DOSE Tx of cryopyrin-associated periodic syndromes, including familial cold autoinflammatory syndrome, Muckle-Wells syndrome. *Adult:* Loading dose, 320 mg as two 160-mg (2-mL) subcut injections at different sites; then once-wkly subcut injections of 160 mg (2 mL). *Child 12–17 yr:* Loading dose, 4.4 mg/kg subcut; max, 320 mg. May give in divided doses if needed. Then once-wkly injections of 2.2 mg/kg; max, 160 mg.
ADV EFF Injection-site reactions, lipid changes, **serious infections,** URI
INTERACTIONS Live vaccines, TNF blockers
NC/PT Stop if infection occurs. Use caution in pregnancy, breast-feeding. Teach proper administration, disposal of needles, syringes. Pt should rotate injection sites, report injection-site reactions, signs of infection.

rilpivirine (Edurant)
CLASS Antiviral, nonnucleoside reverse transcriptase inhibitor (NNRTI)
PREG/CONT B/NA

IND & DOSE Tx of HIV-1 infection in tx-naïve pts. *Adult:* 25 mg/day PO.

ADV EFF Body fat redistribution, depression, headache, immune reconstitution syndrome, insomnia, **prolonged QT interval,** rash, **suicidality**
INTERACTIONS Antacids, CYP3A4 inducers/inhibitors, drugs that decrease stomach acid, other NNRTIs, QT-prolonging drugs, St. John's wort
NC/PT Monitor viral load, response carefully. Ensure pt taking other antivirals. Not for use in pregnancy, breast-feeding. Body fat may redistribute to back, breasts, middle of body. Check pt drug list carefully; drug interacts w/ many drugs. Pt should report all drugs, herbs, OTC products used to health care provider; take once/day w/ meal; take precautions to prevent spread (drug not a cure); continue to take other antivirals; report signs of infection, thoughts of suicide.

riluzole (Rilutek)
CLASS Amyotrophic lateral sclerosis (ALS) drug
PREG/CONT C/NA

IND & DOSE Tx of ALS. *Adult:* 50 mg PO q 12 hr.
ADV EFF Abd pain, asthenia, anorexia, circumoral paresthesia, diarrhea, dizziness, **interstitial pneumonitis, liver injury, neutropenia,** somnolence, vertigo
INTERACTIONS Allopurinol, methyldopa, sulfasalazine, warfarin
NC/PT Monitor CBC, lung function, LFTs carefully. Protect from light. Use caution in pregnancy, breast-feeding. Slows disease progress; not a cure. Pt should take on empty stomach, use safety precautions w/ dizziness, report signs of infection, difficulty breathing.

rimantadine hydrochloride (Flumadine)
CLASS Antiviral
PREG/CONT C/NA

IND & DOSE Px of illness caused by influenza A virus. *Adult, child over*

10 yr: 100 mg/day PO bid. *Child 1–9 yr:* 5 mg/kg/day PO; max, 150 mg/dose. **Tx of illness caused by influenza A virus.** *Adult, child over 10 yr:* 100 mg/day PO as soon after exposure as possible, continuing for 7 days.

ADJUST DOSE Nursing home pts; hepatic, renal impairment

ADV EFF Ataxia, dizziness, dyspnea, **HF,** insomnia, light-headedness, mood changes, nausea

INTERACTIONS Acetaminophen, aspirin, cimetidine, intranasal influenza virus vaccine

NC/PT Pt should take full course of drug, take safety precautions for CNS effects, report swelling, severe mood changes.

riociguat (Adempas)
CLASS Cyclase stimulator, pulmonary hypertension drug
PREG/CONT X/NA

BBW Known teratogen. Serious to fatal birth defects; monthly negative pregnancy test required. Available by limited access program for women.

IND & DOSE Tx of thromboembolic pulmonary hypertension, idiopathic pulmonary hypertension. *Adult:* 1.5–2.5 mg PO tid.

ADJUST DOSE Severe renal, hepatic impairment (not recommended); smokers

ADJUST DOSE Anemia, bleeding, constipation, dizziness, dyspepsia, headache, hypotension, n/v/d, **pulmonary edema**

INTERACTIONS Antacids; CYP inhibitors; nitrates; P-glycoprotein, phosphodiesterase inhibitors

NC/PT Smokers may need higher doses. Monitor BP, respiratory status. Ensure negative pregnancy test, safety precautions w/ CNS effects. Pt should avoid pregnancy (during and for 1 mo after use), breast-feeding; monitor activity tolerance, re-

spiratory sx; take safety precautions; report worsening of sx, bleeding, severe n/v.

risedronate sodium (Actonel, Atelvia)
CLASS Bisphosphonate
PREG/CONT C/NA

IND & DOSE Tx, px of postmenopausal osteoporosis. *Adult:* 5 mg/day PO taken in upright position w/ 6–8 oz water at least 30 min before or after other beverage, food; may switch to 35-mg tablet PO once/wk, or 75 mg PO on 2 consecutive days each mo (total, 2 tablets/mo), or one 150-mg tablet PO per mo. **Tx, px of glucocorticoid osteoporosis.** *Adult:* 5 mg/day PO. **Tx of Paget disease.** *Adult:* 30 mg/day PO for 2 mo taken in upright position w/ 6–8 oz water at least 30 min before or after other beverage, food; may retreat after at least 2-mo posttreatment period if indicated. **To increase bone mass in men w/ osteoporosis.** *Adult:* 35 mg PO once/wk.

ADJUST DOSE Renal impairment
ADV EFF Anorexia, arthralgia, diarrhea, dizziness, dyspepsia, **esophageal rupture,** headache, increased bone pain, **osteonecrosis of jaw**

INTERACTIONS Aluminum, aspirin, calcium, magnesium

NC/PT Monitor serum calcium level. May increase risk of osteonecrosis of jaw; pts having invasive dental procedures should discuss risk. Give w/ full glass of plain (not mineral) water at least 30 min before or after other beverage, food, medication. Have pt remain in upright position for at least 30 min to decrease GI effects. Pt should swallow DR tablet whole and not cut, crush, or chew it; mark calendar if taking wkly; take supplemental calcium, vitamin D; report muscle twitching, difficulty swallowing, edema.

risperidone (Risperdal)

CLASS Antipsychotic, benzisoxazole
PREG/CONT C/NA

BBW Not for use in elderly pts w/ dementia; increased risk of CV mortality. Not approved for this use.

IND & DOSE Tx of schizophrenia. *Adult:* 1 mg PO bid or 2 mg PO once daily; target, 3 mg PO bid by third day. Range, 4–8 mg/day or 25 mg IM q 2 wk. Max, 50 mg IM q 2 wk. Delaying relapse time in long-term tx: 2–8 mg/day PO. *Child 13–17 yr:* 0.5 mg/day PO; target, 3 mg/day. **Tx of bipolar I disorder.** *Adult:* 25–50 mg IM q 2 wk. **Tx of bipolar mania.** *Adult:* 2–3 mg/day PO; range, 1–6 mg/day. *Child 10–17 yr:* 0.5 mg/day PO; target, 2.5 mg/day. **Irritability associated w/ autistic disorder.** *Child 5–17 yr:* 0.5 mg/day (20 kg or more), 0.25 mg/day PO (under 20 kg). After at least 4 days, may increase to 1 mg/day (20 kg or more), 0.5 mg/day (under 20 kg). Maintain dose for at least 14 days; then may increase in increments of 0.5 mg/day (20 kg or more), 0.25 mg/day (under 20 kg) at 2-wk intervals.

ADJUST DOSE Elderly pts; hepatic, renal impairment

ADV EFF Agitation, **arrhythmias,** anxiety, aggression, constipation, dizziness, drowsiness, headache, hyperglycemia, insomnia, n/v, **NMS,** photosensitivity

INTERACTIONS Alcohol, carbamazepine, clonidine, levodopa

NC/PT If restarting tx, follow initial dose guidelines, using extreme care due to increased risk of severe adverse effects w/ reexposure. Stop other antipsychotics before starting risperidone. Not for use in pregnancy. Pt should open blister units of orally disintegrating tablets individually (not push tablet through foil); use dry hands to remove tablet, immediately place on tongue but do not chew; mix oral sol in 3–4 oz water, coffee, orange juice, low-fat milk (not cola, tea); take safety precautions w/ CNS effects; avoid sun exposure; report signs of infection, palpitations, increased thirst/urination. Name confusion between *Risperdal* (risperidone) and *Requip* (ropinirole); use caution.

ritonavir (Norvir)

CLASS Antiviral
PREG/CONT B/NA

BBW Potentially large increase in serum conc, risk of serious arrhythmias, seizures, fatal reactions w/ alfuzosin, amiodarone, astemizole, bepridil, bupropion, clozapine, ergotamine, flecainide, meperidine, pimozide, piroxicam, propafenone, quinidine, rifabutin, terfenadine, voriconazole. Potentially large increase in serum conc of these sedatives/hypnotics: Alprazolam, clonazepam, diazepam, estazolam, flurazepam, midazolam, triazolam, zolpidem; extreme sedation, respiratory depression possible. Do not give ritonavir w/ any drugs listed above.

IND & DOSE Tx of HIV infection. *Adult:* 600 mg PO bid w/ food. *Child:* 250 mg/m² PO bid. Increase by 50 mg/m² bid at 2- to 3-day intervals to max 400 mg/m² PO bid. Max, 600 mg PO bid.

ADV EFF Abd pain, anorexia, anxiety, asthenia, dizziness, dysuria, n/v/d, peripheral/circumoral paresthesia

INTERACTIONS Grapefruit juice, QT-prolonging drugs, St. John's wort. See also *Black Box Warning* above.

NC/PT Carefully screen drug hx for potentially serious drug-drug interactions. Pt should store capsules, oral sol in refrigerator; avoid grapefruit juice, St. John's wort; use precautions to avoid spread (drug not a cure); report severe diarrhea, changes in drugs being taken, signs of infection. Name confusion between *Retrovir* (zidovudine) and ritonavir; use caution.

DANGEROUS DRUG
rituximab (Rituxan)

CLASS Antineoplastic, monoclonal antibody
PREG/CONT C/NA

BBW Fatal infusion reactions, severe cutaneous reactions, tumor lysis syndrome possible. Risk of reactivation of hepatitis B at drug initiation; screen for hepatitis B before use.

IND & DOSE Tx of lymphoma.
Adult: 375 mg/m² IV once wkly for four or eight doses. **To reduce s&sx of rheumatoid arthritis.** *Adult:* Two 1,000-mg IV infusions separated by 2 wk, w/ methotrexate. **Tx of chronic lymphocytic leukemia.** *Adult:* 375 mg/m² IV day before fludarabine/cyclophosphamide; then 500 mg/m² on day 1 of cycles 2–6 (q 28 days). **Tx of Wegener granulomatosis, microscopic polyangiitis.** *Adult:* 375 mg/m² IV once wkly for 4 wk, w/ glucocorticoids.

ADV EFF Bowel obstruction, bronchitis, cardiac arrhythmias, infusion reactions, **infections, hepatitis B reactivation, progressive multifocal leukoencephalopathy, tumor lysis syndrome,** URI

INTERACTIONS Live vaccines

NC/PT Premedicate w/ acetaminophen, diphenhydramine to decrease fever, chills associated w/ infusion. Protect from infection exposure. Monitor for hepatitis B reactivation; stop if viral hepatitis occurs. Use caution in pregnancy, breast-feeding. Pt should mark calendar of tx days, report severe abd pain, headache, signs of infection, urine/stool color changes.

rivaroxaban (Xarelto)

CLASS Anticoagulant, factor Xa inhibitor
PREG/CONT C/NA

BBW Risk of epidural, spinal hematomas w/ related neurologic impairment, possible paralysis if used in pts

receiving neuraxial anesthesia or undergoing spinal puncture. Carefully consider benefits/risks of neuraxial intervention in pts who are or will be anticoagulated. If rivaroxaban used, monitor frequently for neurologic impairment; be prepared for rapid tx if necessary. Stopping drug increases risk of thromboembolic events; if stopped for any reason other than pathological bleeding, start another anticoagulant.

IND & DOSE Px of DVT, which may lead to PE in pts undergoing knee, hip replacement; *Adult:* 10 mg/day PO. Start within 6–10 hr of surgery; continue for 12 days after knee replacement, 35 days after hip replacement, continuously for AF. **To reduce risk of stroke in pts w/ nonvalvular atrial fibrillation; to reduce risk of recurrent DVT, PE.** *Adult:* 20 mg/day PO w/ evening meal.

ADJUST DOSE Renal, hepatic impairment

ADV EFF Bleeding, dysuria, elevated liver enzymes, **hemorrhage,** rash

INTERACTIONS Aspirin, carbamazepine, clarithromycin, clopidogrel, erythromycin, ketoconazole, NSAIDs, phenytoin, platelet inhibitors, rifampin, ritonavir, St. John's wort, warfarin

NC/PT Monitor for bleeding. Do not stop abruptly (increased risk of stroke); taper when stopping, consider use of another anticoagulant. Not for use in pregnancy (contraceptives advised), breast-feeding. Pt should report all prescribed/OTC drugs, herbs being taken; take precautions to prevent injury; report stool color changes, unusual bleeding, dizziness.

rivastigmine tartrate (Exelon)

CLASS Alzheimer disease drug, cholinesterase inhibitor
PREG/CONT B/NA

IND & DOSE Tx of Alzheimer disease. *Adult:* 1.5 mg PO bid w/ food.

Range, 6–12 mg/day; max, 12 mg/day. Transdermal patch: one 4.6-mg/24 hr patch once/day; after 4 or more wk, may increase to one 9.5-mg/24 hr patch. **Tx of Parkinson dementia.** *Adult:* 3–12 mg/day PO bid in divided doses. Transdermal patch: one 4.6-mg/ 24 hr patch once/day; after 4 or more wk, may increase to one 9.5-mg/ 24 hr patch.
ADV EFF Abd pain, anorexia, ataxia, bradycardia, confusion, fatigue, insomnia, n/v/d
INTERACTIONS Anticholinergics, NSAIDs, other cholinesterase inhibitors, theophylline
NC/PT Establish baseline function before tx. Pt should take w/ food; mix sol w/ water, fruit juice, soda to improve compliance; apply patch to clean, dry skin (remove old patch before applying new one), rotate sites; take safety precautions w/ CNS effects; report diarrhea, changes in neurologic function.

rizatriptan (Maxalt)
CLASS Antimigraine, serotonin selective agonist
PREG/CONT C/NA

IND & DOSE Tx of acute migraine attacks. *Adult:* 5 or 10 mg PO at onset of headache; may repeat in 2 hr if needed. Max, 30 mg/day.
ADJUST DOSE Hepatic, renal impairment
ADV EFF Chest pain, dizziness, jaw pain, paresthesia, somnolence, throat pressure, vertigo, weakness
INTERACTIONS Ergots, MAOIs, propranolol
NC/PT Do not give within 14 days of MAOIs. For acute attack only, not px. Monitor BP in pts w/ known CAD. Not for use in pregnancy. Pt should place orally disintegrating tablet on tongue, then swallow; take safety measures w/ CNS effects; continue normal migraine relief measures; report chest pain, numbness/tingling.

roflumilast (Daliresp)
CLASS Phosphodiesterase-4 inhibitor
PREG/CONT C/NA

IND & DOSE To reduce exacerbation risk in severe COPD. *Adult:* 500 mcg/day PO.
ADJUST DOSE Hepatic impairment
ADV EFF Depression, diarrhea, dizziness, headache, insomnia, **suicidality**, weight loss
INTERACTIONS Carbamazepine, cimetidine, erythromycin, ethinyl estradiol, fluvoxamine, ketoconazole, phenobarbital, phenytoin, rifampin
NC/PT Not for acute bronchospasm. Monitor weight; if significant weight loss, stop drug. Not for use in pregnancy (contraceptives advised), breast-feeding. Pt should continue other COPD tx, report all drugs being taken, weight loss, thoughts of suicide.

romidepsin (Istodax)
CLASS Antineoplastic, histone deacetylase inhibitor
PREG/CONT D/NA

IND & DOSE Tx of pts w/ cutaneous, peripheral T-cell lymphoma who have received at least one prior systemic tx. *Adult:* 14 mg/m^2 IV over 4 hr on days 1, 8, 15 of 28-day cycle. Repeat q 28 days.
ADJUST DOSE Hepatic, severe renal impairment
ADV EFF Anemia, anorexia, **bone marrow suppression**, fatigue, infections, n/v/d, **QT prolongation, tumor lysis syndrome**
INTERACTIONS CYP3A4 inducers/ inhibitors. QT-prolonging drugs, warfarin
NC/PT Monitor CBC, LFTs, renal function. Obtain baseline, periodic ECG. Not for use in pregnancy (contraceptives advised), breast-feeding. Pt should mark calendar of tx days, avoid exposure to infection, report

signs of infection, unusual bleeding/bruising.

romiplostim (Nplate)

CLASS Thrombopoietin receptor agonist
PREG/CONT C/NA

IND & DOSE Tx of thrombocytopenia in pts w/ chronic immune thrombocytopenic purpura. *Adult:* 1 mcg/kg/wk subcut; adjust in increments of 1 mcg/kg to achieve platelet count of 50×10^9. Max, 10 mcg/kg/wk.
ADJUST DOSE Hepatic, severe renal impairment
ADV EFF Abd pain, arthralgia, dizziness, dyspepsia, headache, insomnia, myalgia, pain, paresthesia, **progression to acute myelogenous leukemia, severe thrombocytopenia, thrombotic events**
NC/PT Pt must be enrolled in *Nplate NEXUS* program; drug must be given by health care provider enrolled in program who will do blood test for platelet count before injection. Not for use in pregnancy, breast-feeding. Not for home administration. Pt should take safety precautions w/ dizziness, report difficulty breathing, numbness/tingling, leg pain.

ropinirole hydrochloride (Requip)

CLASS Antiparkinsonian, dopamine receptor agonist
PREG/CONT C/NA

IND & DOSE Tx of idiopathic Parkinson disease. *Adult:* 0.25 mg PO tid (1st wk); 0.5 mg PO tid (2nd wk); 0.75 mg PO tid (3rd wk); 1 mg PO tid (4th wk). May increase by 1.5 mg/day at 1-wk intervals to 9 mg/day, then by up to 3 mg/day at 1-wk intervals to max 24 mg/day. ER tablets: 2 mg/day PO. After 1–2 wk, may increase by 2 mg/day. Titrate w/ wkly increases of 2 mg/day to max 24 mg/day. If used w/ levodopa, decrease levodopa

gradually; average reduction, 31% w/ immediate-release ropinirole, 34% w/ ER form. Tx of restless legs syndrome. *Adult:* 0.25 mg/day PO 1–3 hr before bed. After 2 days, increase to 0.5 mg/day PO; after 1 wk, to 1 mg/day PO. Wk 3, increase to 1.5 mg/day; wk 4, 2 mg/day; wk 5, 2.5 mg/day; wk 6, 3 mg/day; wk 7, 4 mg/day PO.
ADJUST DOSE Elderly pts
ADV EFF Constipation, dizziness, hyperkinesia, hypokinesia, insomnia, nausea, orthostatic hypotension, somnolence, vision changes
INTERACTIONS Alcohol, ciprofloxacin, estrogens, levodopa, warfarin
NC/PT Withdraw gradually over 1 wk if stopping. Monitor orthostatic BP. Pt should swallow ER tablet whole and not cut, crush, or chew it; take w/ food; use safety precautions w/ CNS effects; change position slowly; report black tarry stools, hallucinations, falling asleep during daily activities. Name confusion between *Requip* (ropinirole) and *Risperdal* (risperidone); use caution.

rosiglitazone (Avandia)

CLASS Antidiabetic, thiazolidinedione
PREG/CONT C/NA

BBW Increased risk of HF, MI. Do not use in pts w/ known heart disease, symptomatic HF; monitor accordingly.
IND & DOSE As adjunct to diet, exercise to improve glycemic control in adults already on rosiglitazone and tolerating it well or who cannot achieve glycemic control w/ other antidiabetics. *Adult:* 4 mg PO daily; max, 8 mg/day.
ADJUST DOSE Hepatic impairment
ADV EFF Anemia, fluid retention, headache, **HF**, hypoglycemia, macular edema, **MI**, UTI, weight gain
INTERACTIONS CYP2C8 inducers/inhibitors, insulin
NC/PT Pt must enroll in limited-access program; not available in pharmacies.

Not for use in pregnancy, breast-feeding. Monitor weight; check for signs of HF. Ensure full diabetic teaching. Pt should continue diet, exercise program for diabetes; report weight gain of 3 or more lb/day, chest pain, swelling.

rosuvastatin calcium
(Crestor)

CLASS Antihyperlipidemic, statin
PREG/CONT X/NA

IND & DOSE Tx of hypercholesterolemia, mixed dyslipidemia, primary dysbetalipoproteinemia, hypertriglyceridemia; primary px of CAD; atherosclerosis. *Adult:* 5–40 mg/day PO; 10 mg/day PO if combined w/ other lipid-lowering drugs; 5 mg/day PO if combined w/ cyclosporine. Tx of heterozygous familial hypercholesterolemia. *Child 10–17 yr (girls must be at least 1 yr postmenarchal):* 5–20 mg/day PO.
ADJUST DOSE Renal impairment
ADV EFF Diarrhea, dizziness, flulike sx, headache, **liver failure, myopathy,** nausea, pharyngitis, **rhabdomyolysis,** rhinitis
INTERACTIONS Antacids, cyclosporine, gemfibrozil, lopinavir/ritonavir, warfarin
NC/PT Risk of increased adverse effects in Asian pts; initiate tx w/ 5 mg/day PO and adjust based on lipid levels, adverse effects. Obtain baseline lipid profile. Not for use in pregnancy (barrier contraceptives advised), breast-feeding. Pt should take at bedtime; have regular blood tests; continue diet, exercise program; take antacids at least 2 hr after rosuvastatin; report muscle pain w/ fever, unusual bleeding/bruising.

rotigotine (Neupro)

CLASS Antiparkinsonian, dopamine agonist
PREG/CONT C/NA

IND & DOSE Tx of s&sx of Parkinson's disease. *Adult:* 2 mg/24 hr

transdermal patch; range, 2–8 mg/24 hr patch. Tx of moderate to severe restless legs syndrome. *Adult:* 1 mg/24 hr transdermal patch; max, 3 mg/24 hr transdermal patch.
ADV EFF Anorexia, application-site reactions, dizziness, dyskinesia, edema, hallucinations, headache, hyperpyrexia, hypotension, insomnia, **melanoma,** n/v, orthostatic hypotension, severe allergic reaction
INTERACTIONS Antipsychotics, dopamine antagonists, metoclopramide
NC/PT Apply to clean, dry skin; press firmly for 30 sec. Rotate application sites; remove old patch before applying new one. Taper after long-term use. Remove patch before MRI. Not for use in pregnancy. Pt should not open patch until ready to apply; remove old patch before applying new one; rotate application sites; not stop suddenly; take safety precautions w/ CNS effects; report application-site reactions, skin reactions, difficulty breathing, fever, changes in behavior, dizziness.

rufinamide (Banzel)

CLASS Antiepileptic, sodium channel blocker
PREG/CONT C/NA

IND & DOSE Adjunct tx of seizures associated w/ Lennox-Gastaut syndrome. *Adult:* 400–800 mg/day PO in two equally divided doses; target, 3,200 mg/day PO in two equally divided doses. *Child 4 yr and older:* 10 mg/kg/day PO in two equally divided doses; target, 45 mg/kg/day or 3,200 mg/day.
ADJUST DOSE Hepatic, renal impairment
ADV EFF Ataxia, coordination disturbances, dizziness, fatigue, headache, nausea, **seizures, severe hypersensitivity reactions,** somnolence, **suicidality**
INTERACTIONS CYP450 inducers, hormonal contraceptives, valproate

NC/PT Withdraw gradually; do not stop abruptly. Stable for 90 days. Not for use in pregnancy (hormonal contraceptives may be ineffective; second contraceptive form advised), breast-feeding. Pt should take w/ food; swallow tablet whole and not cut, crush, or chew it; store suspension upright, measure using medical measuring device; take safety precautions w/ CNS effects; report difficulty breathing, rash, thoughts of suicide, mood changes.

ruxolitinib (Jakafi)
CLASS Kinase inhibitor
PREG/CONT C/NA

IND & DOSE Tx of intermediate, high-risk myelofibrosis. *Adult:* 20 mg PO bid; max, 25 mg bid.
ADJUST DOSE Hepatic, renal impairment
ADV EFF Anemia, bruising, dizziness, headache, **serious infections**, thrombocytopenia
INTERACTIONS CYP450 inducers/inhibitors
NC/PT Stop after 6 mo if no spleen reduction or sx improvement. Not for use in breast-feeding. Monitor for infection. Pt should take safety precautions w/ dizziness, report signs of infection, unusual bleeding.

sacrosidase (Sucraid)
CLASS Enzyme
PREG/CONT C/NA

IND & DOSE Oral replacement of genetically determined sucrase deficiency. *Adult, child over 15 kg:* 2 mL PO or 44 drops/meal or snack PO. *Adult, child 15 kg or less:* 1 mL or 22 drops/meal or snack PO.
ADV EFF Abd pain, constipation, dehydration, headache
NC/PT Do not use in known allergy to yeast. Must dilute w/ 60–120 mL water, milk, infant formula before giving. Do not dilute, consume w/ fruit juice. Refrigerate bottle; discard 4 wk after opening. Give cold or at room temp. Pt should report difficulty breathing, swelling of tongue/face.

saliva substitute
(Entertainer's Secret, Moi-Stir, MouthKote, Salivart)
CLASS Saliva substitute
PREG/CONT Unkn/NA

IND & DOSE Mgt of dry mouth, throat in xerostomia, hyposalivation. *Adult:* Spray for ½ second or apply to oral mucosa.
ADV EFF Excessive electrolyte absorption
NC/PT Monitor pt while eating; swallowing may be impaired and additional tx needed. Pt should swish around in mouth after application, report difficulty swallowing, headache, leg cramps.

salmeterol xinafoate
(Serevent Diskus)
CLASS Antiasthmatic, beta selective agonist
PREG/CONT C/NA

BBW Ensure drug not used for acute asthma or w/ worsening/deteriorating asthma; risk of death. Increased risk of asthma-related hospitalization when used in children, adolescents. When long-acting beta-agonist mimometic, inhaled corticosteroid needed, fixed-dose combination strongly recommended. Do not use for asthma unless combined w/ long-term asthma-control medication; risk of death. Use only as additional tx in pts not controlled by other medications.
IND & DOSE Maint tx for asthma, bronchospasm. *Adult, child 4 yr and over:* 1 inhalation (50 mcg) bid at 12-hr intervals. Px of exercise-induced asthma. *Adult, child 4 yr and older:* 1 inhalation 30 min or more before exertion. Long-term maint of bronchospasm w/ COPD. *Adult:* 1 inhalation (50 mcg) bid at 12-hr intervals.

ADV EFF Asthma-related deaths (risk higher in black pts), **bronchospasm,** headache, pain, palpitations, tachycardia, tremors
INTERACTIONS Beta blockers, diuretics, MAOIs, protease inhibitors, TCAs
NC/PT Arrange for periodic evaluation of respiratory condition. Not for tx of acute asthma attack. Review proper use of *Diskus.* Pt should never take drug alone for tx of asthma; take safety precautions w/ tremors; report irregular heartbeat, difficulty breathing, worsening of asthma.

salsalate (Amigesic, Argesic-SA, Disalcid, Marthritic, Salflex, Salsitab)
CLASS Analgesic, NSAID, salicylate
PREG/CONT C/NA

BBW Increased risk of GI bleeding, CV events; monitor accordingly.
IND & DOSE Relief of pain, sx of inflammatory conditions. *Adult:* 3,000 mg/day PO in divided doses.
ADV EFF Acute salicylate toxicity, anaphylactoid reactions to anaphylactic shock, bone marrow suppression, bronchospasm, constipation, **CV collapse,** dizziness, dyspepsia, GI pain, insomnia, **renal/respiratory failure**
INTERACTIONS Alcohol, antacids, carbonic anhydrase inhibitors, corticosteroids, insulin, probenecid, spironolactone, sulfonylureas, urine alkalinizers, valproic acid
NC/PT Pt should take w/ full glass of water; w/ food if GI upset. Continue other measures for relief of pain, inflammation; report ringing in ears, rapid, difficult breathing.

sapropterin dihydrochloride (Kuvan)
CLASS Coenzyme factor, phenylalanine reducer
PREG/CONT C/NA

IND & DOSE W/ diet to reduce blood phenylalanine level in hyperphenylalaninemia caused by tetrahydrobiopterin-in-responsive phenylketonuria. *Pt 4 yr and older:* 10 mg/kg/day PO. May adjust to 5–20 mg/kg/day based on blood phenylalanine level.
ADV EFF Abd pain, headache, n/v/d, pharyngolaryngeal pain
NC/PT Do not use w/ levodopa, ED drugs, drugs that inhibit folate metabolism. Must use w/ phenylalanine dietary restrictions. Protect from moisture; do not use if outdated. Dissolve tablets in water, apple juice; have pt drink within 15 min. Monitor phenylalanine level; adjust dose as needed. Pt should report severe headache, anorexia, fever.

saquinavir mesylate (Invirase)
CLASS Antiviral, protease inhibitor
PREG/CONT B/NA

BBW Capsules, tablets not interchangeable; use tablets only when combined w/ ritonavir. If saquinavir only protease inhibitor in regimen, use capsules.
IND & DOSE Tx of HIV infection. *Adult, child over 16 yr:* 1,000 mg PO bid w/ ritonavir 100 mg bid given together within 2 hr after meal. Or, w/ lopinavir 400 mg/ritonavir 100 mg PO bid (tablets). Or, 1,000 mg PO bid w/ ritonavir 400 mg/ritonavir 100 mg PO bid (capsules).
ADJUST DOSE Hepatic impairment
ADV EFF Asthenia, diarrhea, dizziness, dyspepsia, fat redistribution, GI pain, headache, nausea, **prolonged QT interval**

INTERACTIONS Antiarrhythmics, carbamazepine, clarithromycin, delavirdine, dexamethasone, ergots, grapefruit juice, indinavir, ketoconazole, midazolam, nelfinavir, nevirapine, phenobarbital, phenytoin, QT-prolonging drugs, rifabutin, rifampin, ritonavir, sildenafil, statins, triazolam, St. John's wort

NC/PT Store at room temp; use by expiration date. Give within 2 hr after full meal, always w/ other antivirals. Monitor for opportunistic infections. Pt should take precautions to prevent spread (drug not a cure), avoid grapefruit juice, St. John's wort; take safety precautions w/ dizziness, report severe headache, urine/stool color changes. Name confusion between saquinavir and *Sinequan*; use caution.

---

sargramostim (Leukine)
CLASS Colony-stimulating factor
PREG/CONT C/NA

IND & DOSE Myeloid reconstitution after autologous, allogeneic bone marrow transplantation. *Adult:* 250 mcg/m²/day for 21 days as 2-hr IV infusion starting 2–4 hr after autologous bone marrow infusion and not less than 24 hr after last dose of chemotherapy, radiation. Do not give until post-marrow infusion ANC less than 500 cells/mm³. Continue until ANC greater than 1,500 cells/mm³ for 3 consecutive days. **Bone marrow transplantation failure, engraftment delay.** *Adult:* 250 mcg/m²/day for 14 days as 2-hr IV infusion; may repeat after 7 days off tx if no engraftment. If still no engraftment, may give third dose of 500 mcg/m²/day for 14 days after another 7 days off tx. **Neutrophil recovery after chemotherapy in AML.** *Adult:* 250 mcg/m²/day IV over 4 hr starting about day 11 or 4 days after chemotherapy induction. **Mobilization of peripheral blood progenitor cells (PBPCs).** *Adult:* 250 mcg/m²/day IV over 24 hr or

subcut once daily; continue throughout harvesting. **Post-PBPC transplant.** *Adult:* 250 mcg/m²/day IV over 24 hr or subcut once daily starting immediately after PBPC infusion; continue until ANC greater than 1,500 cells/mm³ for 3 consecutive days.

ADV EFF Alopecia, bone pain, diarrhea, fever, **hemorrhage,** n/v/d

INTERACTIONS Corticosteroids, lithium

NC/PT Give no less than 24 hr after cytotoxic chemotherapy and within 2–4 hr of bone marrow infusion. Store in refrigerator; do not freeze/shake. Not for use in pregnancy (barrier contraceptives advised). Use powder within 6 hr of mixing. If using powder, use each vial for one dose; do not re-enter vial. Discard unused drug. Infuse over 2 hr. Do not use in-line membrane filter or mix w/ other drugs or in other diluent. Monitor CBC. Pt should cover head at temp extremes (hair loss possible), avoid exposure to infection, report fever, signs of infection, difficulty breathing.

DANGEROUS DRUG

saxagliptin (Onglyza)
CLASS Antidiabetic, DPP-4 inhibitor
PREG/CONT B/NA

IND & DOSE As adjunct to diet, exercise to improve glycemic control in type 2 diabetics. *Adult:* 2.5–5 mg/day PO without regard to meals.

ADJUST DOSE Renal impairment

ADV EFF Headache, hypoglycemia, URI, UTI

INTERACTIONS Atazanavir, celery, clarithromycin, coriander, dandelion root, fenugreek, garlic, ginseng, indinavir, itraconazole, juniper berries, ketoconazole, nefazodone, nelfinavir, ritonavir, saquinavir, telithromycin

NC/PT Monitor blood glucose, HbA1c, renal function before, periodically during tx. Ensure through diabetic teaching program. Pt may be switched to insulin during times of stress. Pt should continue diet, exercise program, other prescribed diabetes drugs; report all other prescribed/OTC drugs, herbs being taken (dose adjustment may be needed); report uncontrolled glucose levels, severe headache, signs of infection.

scopolamine hydrobromide
(Transderm-Scop)

CLASS Anticholinergic, antiemetic, anti–motion sickness drug, antiparkinsonian, belladonna alkaloid, parasympatholytic
PREG/CONT C/NA

IND & DOSE Tx of motion sickness. *Adult:* Apply 1 transdermal system to postauricular skin at least 4 hr before antiemetic effect needed or in evening before scheduled surgery; delivers scopolamine 1 mg over 3 days. May replace system q 3 days. **Obstetric amnesia, preoperative sedation.** *Adult:* 0.32–0.65 mg subcut or IM. May give IV after dilution in sterile water for injection. May repeat up to qid. *Child:* General guidelines, 0.006 mg/kg subcut, IM or IV; max, 0.3 mg. *3 yr–6 yr:* 0.2–0.3 mg IM or IV. *6 mo–3 yr:* 0.1–0.15 mg IM or IV. **Sedation, tranquilization.** *Adult:* 0.6 mg subcut or IM tid–qid. **Antiemetic.** *Adult:* 0.6–1 mg subcut. *Child:* 0.006 mg/kg subcut. **Refraction.** *Adult:* Instill 1–2 drops into eye(s) 1 hr before refracting. **Uveitis.** *Adult:* Instill 1–2 drops into eye(s) up to qid.
ADJUST DOSE Elderly pts
ADV EFF Anaphylaxis, blurred vision, constipation, decreased sweating, dizziness, drowsiness, dry mouth, nasal congestion, photophobia, pupil dilation, urinary hesitancy, urine retention
INTERACTIONS Alcohol, antidepressants, antihistamines, haloperidol, phenothiazines
NC/PT Ensure adequate hydration. Provide temp control to prevent hy-

perpyrexia. W/ transdermal system, have pt wash hands thoroughly after handling patch, dispose of patch properly to avoid contact w/ children/pets, remove old patch before applying new one, do not cut patch. Pt should empty bladder before each dose; avoid alcohol, hot environments; use laxative for constipation; take safety precautions w/ CNS effects; report severe dry mouth, difficulty breathing.

---

secobarbital sodium
(Seconal Sodium)

CLASS Antiepileptic, barbiturate, sedative-hypnotic
PREG/CONT D/C-II

IND & DOSE Intermittent use as sedative-hypnotic. *Adult:* 100 mg PO at bedtime for up to 2 wk. **Preop sedation.** *Adult:* 200–300 mg PO 1–2 hr before surgery. *Child:* 2–6 mg/kg PO 1–2 hr before surgery; max, 100 mg/dose.
ADJUST DOSE Elderly, debilitated pts; hepatic, renal impairment
ADV EFF Anaphylaxis, angioedema, agitation, anxiety, apnea, ataxia, bradycardia, confusion, constipation, dizziness, epigastric pain, hallucinations, hyperkinesia, hypotension, hypoventilation, insomnia, laryngospasm, n/v/d, psychiatric disturbances, respiratory depression, sleep disorders, somnolence, Stevens-Johnson syndrome, syncope
INTERACTIONS Alcohol, anticoagulants, antihistamines, corticosteroids, doxycycline, estrogens, hormonal contraceptives, hypnotics, metoprolol, metronidazole, oxyphenbutazone, phenylbutazone, propranolol, quinidine, sedatives, theophylline, verapamil
NC/PT Monitor blood levels, watch for anaphylaxis, angioedema w/ above interacting drugs. Not for use in pregnancy (barrier contraceptives advised), breast-feeding. Barbiturates

may produce irritability, excitability, inappropriate tearfulness, aggression in children; stay w/ children who receive preop sedation. Taper gradually after repeated use. Pt should avoid alcohol, take safety precautions, report difficulty breathing, swelling.

secretin (ChiRhoStim)
CLASS Diagnostic agent
PREG/CONT C/NA

IND & DOSE To stimulate pancreatic secretions to aid in dx of pancreatic exocrine dysfx, gastric secretions to aid in dx of gastrinoma. Adult: 0.2–0.4 mcg/kg IV over 1 min.
ADV EFF Abd pain, allergic reactions, flushing, n/v
INTERACTIONS Anticholinergics
NC/PT Monitor carefully during infusion for allergic reaction; have emergency equipment on hand. Do not use w/ acute pancreatitis. Pt should report severe abd pain, difficulty breathing.

selegiline hydrochloride
(Eldepryl, Emsam, Zelapar)
CLASS Antidepressant, antiparkinsonian, MAO type B inhibitor
PREG/CONT C/NA

BBW Increased risk of suicidality in children, adolescents, young adults; monitor accordingly.
IND & DOSE Mgt of pts w/ Parkinson disease whose response to levodopa/carbidopa has decreased. Adult: 10 mg/day PO in divided doses of 5 mg each at breakfast, lunch. After 2–3 days, attempt to reduce levodopa/carbidopa dose; reductions of 10%–30% typical. For orally disintegrating tablet, 1.25 mg/day PO in a.m. before breakfast. May increase after 6 wk to 2.5 mg/day; max, 10 mg/day. Tx of major depressive disorder. Adult, child over 12 yr: One patch (Emsam) daily to dry, intact skin on upper tor-

so, upper thigh, or outer surface of upper arm. Start w/ 6-mg/24 hr system; increase to max 12 mg/24 hr if needed, tolerated.
ADJUST DOSE Elderly pts
ADV EFF Abd pain, asthma, confusion, dizziness, dyskinesia, hallucinations, headache, light-headedness, local reactions to dermal patch, n/v, vivid dreams
INTERACTIONS Carbamazepine, fluoxetine, meperidine, methadone, opioid analgesics, oxcarbazepine, TCAs, tramadol, tyramine-rich foods
NC/PT Pt should place oral tablet on top of tongue, avoid food, beverage for 5 min; apply dermal patch to dry, intact skin on upper torso, upper thigh, or outer upper arm, replace q 24 hr (remove old patch before applying new one); continue other Parkinson disease drugs; take safety precautions w/ CNS effects; report all drugs being used (dose adjustments may be needed); report confusion, fainting, thoughts of suicide.

sertraline hydrochloride
(Zoloft)
CLASS Antidepressant, SSRI
PREG/CONT C (1st trimester); D (2nd, 3rd trimesters)/NA

BBW Increased risk of suicidality in children, adolescents, young adults; monitor accordingly.
IND & DOSE Tx of major depressive disorder, OCD. Adult: 50 mg PO once daily, a.m. or p.m.; may increase to max 200 mg/day. Child 13–17 yr: For OCD, 50 mg/day PO; max, 200 mg/day. Child 6–12 yr: For OCD, 25 mg/day PO; max, 200 mg/day. Tx of panic disorder, PTSD. Adult: 25–50 mg/day PO, up to max 200 mg/day. Tx of PMDD. Adult: 50 mg/day PO daily or just during luteal phase of menstrual cycle. Range, 50–150 mg/day. Tx of social anxiety disorder. Adult: 25 mg/day PO; range, 50–200 mg/day.
ADJUST DOSE Hepatic, renal impairment

ADV EFF Anxiety, diarrhea, dizziness, drowsiness, dry mouth, fatigue, headache, insomnia, nausea, nervousness, painful menstruation, rhinitis, **suicidality**, vision changes
INTERACTIONS Cimetidine, MAOIs, pimozide, St. John's wort
NC/PT Do not give within 14 days of MAOIs. Dilute oral concentrate in 4 oz water, ginger ale, lemon-lime soda, lemonade, orange juice only; give immediately after diluting. Not for use in pregnancy (barrier contraceptives advised). May take up to 4–6 wk to see depression improvement. Pt should take safety precautions w/ CNS effects, avoid St. John's wort, report difficulty breathing, thoughts of suicide.

sevelamer hydrochloride (Renagel)
CLASS Calcium-phosphate binder
PREG/CONT C/NA

IND & DOSE To reduce serum phosphorus level in hemodialysis pts w/ end-stage renal disease. *Adult:* 1–4 tablets PO w/ each meal based on serum phosphorus level; may increase by one tablet/meal to achieve desired serum phosphorus level.
ADV EFF Cough, diarrhea, dyspepsia, headache, hypotension, thrombosis, vomiting
NC/PT Do not use w/ hypophosphatemia or bowel obstruction. Pt should take other oral drugs at least 1 hr before or 3 hr after sevelamer; have blood tests regularly to monitor phosphorus level, report chest pain, difficulty breathing.

sildenafil citrate (Revatio, Viagra)
CLASS ED drug, phosphodiesterase inhibitor
PREG/CONT B/NA

IND & DOSE Tx of ED. *Adult:* 50 mg PO 1 hr before anticipated sexual activity; range, 25–100 mg PO. May take 30 min–4 hr before sexual activity. Limit use to once/day *(Viagra).* Tx of pulmonary arterial hypertension. *Adult:* 20 mg PO tid at least 4–6 hr apart without regard to food *(Revatio)*, or 10 mg by IV bolus tid *(Revatio).*
ADJUST DOSE Elderly pts; hepatic, renal impairment
ADV EFF Dyspepsia, flushing, headache, hearing/vision loss, hypotension, priapism
INTERACTIONS Alcohol, alpha adrenergic blockers, amlodipine, cimetidine, erythromycin, grapefruit juice, nitrates, protease inhibitors
NC/PT Ensure proper dx before tx. *Revatio* contraindicated in children 1–17 yr; deaths have been reported. Reserve IV use for pts unable to take orally. *Viagra* ineffective w/ absence of sexual stimulation. Pt should take appropriate measures to prevent STDs, report difficult urination, hearing/vision loss, erection lasting longer than 4 hr.

silodosin (Rapaflo)
CLASS Alpha blocker, BPH drug
PREG/CONT B/NA

IND & DOSE Tx of s&sx of BPH. *Adult:* 8 mg/day PO w/ meal.
ADJUST DOSE Hepatic, renal impairment
ADV EFF Abnormal/retrograde ejaculation, dizziness, headache, liver impairment, orthostatic hypotension, rash
INTERACTIONS Clarithromycin, cyclosporine, itraconazole, ketoconazole, other alpha blockers, ritonavir
NC/PT Rule out prostate cancer before tx. Pt undergoing cataract surgery at risk for intraop floppy iris syndrome; alert surgeon about drug use. Pt should take safety precautions for dizziness, orthostatic hypotension; report urine/stool color changes, worsening of sx.

simeprevir (Olysio)

CLASS Hepatitis C drug, protease inhibitor
PREG/CONT C/NA

IND & DOSE Tx of chronic hepatitis C, w/ other antiretrovirals. *Adult:* 150 mg/day PO w/ food; combined w/ peginterferon alfa and ribavirin for 12 wk, then peginterferon alfa and ribavirin for 24–36 wk.
ADV EFF Nausea, photosensitivity, rash
INTERACTIONS CYP3A inducers/inhibitor
NC/PT Ensure concurrent use of peginterferon alfa and ribavirin; not for monotherapy. Negative pregnancy test required monthly. Pt should swallow capsule whole, not cut, crush, or chew it; avoid pregnancy or fathering a child (two forms of contraception advised), breast-feeding, sun exposure; use precautions to avoid spread of disease; report rash, itching, severe nausea.

simethicone (Flatulex, Gas-X, Phazyme)

CLASS Antiflatulent
PREG/CONT C/NA

IND & DOSE Relief of sx of excess gas in digestive tract. *Adult:* 40–360 mg PO as needed after meals, at bedtime; max, 500 mg/day. *Child 2–12 yr, over 11 kg:* 40 mg PO as needed after meals, at bedtime. *Child under 2 yr:* 20 mg PO as needed after meals, at bedtime; max, 240 mg/day.
ADV EFF Constipation, diarrhea, flatulence
NC/PT Pt should shake drops thoroughly before each use; add drops to 30 mL cool water, infant formula, other liquid to ease administration to infants; let strips dissolve on tongue; chew chewable tablets thoroughly before swallowing; report extreme abd pain, vomiting.

simvastatin (Zocor)

CLASS Antihyperlipidemic, statin
PREG/CONT X/NA

IND & DOSE Tx of hyperlipidemia; px of coronary events. *Adult:* 10–20 mg PO, up to 40 mg, daily in evening. Range, 5–40 mg/day; max, 40 mg/day. Tx of familial hypercholesterolemia. *Adult:* 40 mg/day PO in evening. *Child 10–17 yr:* 10 mg/day PO in evening; range, 10–40 mg/day. Combination tx of CAD. *Adult:* Do not use w/ other statins. If used w/ fibrates, niacin, max of 10 mg/day. Give regular dose if used w/ bile acid sequestrants; give sequestrants at least 4 hr before simvastatin. If used w/ cyclosporine, start w/ 5 mg/day; max, 10 mg/day. If used w/ amiodarone, verapamil, max of 10 mg/day. If used w/ diltiazem, max of 10 mg/day.
ADJUST DOSE Renal impairment
ADV EFF Abd pain, acute renal failure, cramps, flatulence, headache, liver failure, n/v/d, rhabdomyolysis
INTERACTIONS Amiodarone, clarithromycin, cyclosporine, digoxin, diltiazem, erythromycin, fibrates, grapefruit juice, hepatotoxic drugs, HIV protease inhibitors, itraconazole, ketoconazole, nefazodone, niacin, verapamil, warfarin
NC/PT Ensure pt has tried cholesterol-lowering diet for 3–6 mo before starting tx. Avoid 80-mg dose because of increased risk of muscle injury, rhabdomyolysis; if pt already stable on 80 mg, monitor closely. Not for use in pregnancy (barrier contraceptives advised). Pt should continue diet, take in p.m., have blood tests regularly, avoid grapefruit juice, report urine/stool color changes, muscle pain/soreness.

sipuleucel-T (Provenge)

CLASS Cellular immunotherapy
PREG/CONT C/NA

IND & DOSE Tx of asymptomatic, minimally symptomatic metastatic

castrate-resistant prostate cancer. *Adult:* 50 million autologous CD54+ cells activated w/ PAP-GM-CSF suspended in 250 mL lactated Ringer's injection IV.

ADV EFF Acute infusion reactions, back pain, chills, fatigue, fever, headache, joint ache, nausea

INTERACTIONS Immunosuppressants

NC/PT Autologous use only. Leukapheresis will be done 3 days before infusion. Ensure pt identity. Premedicate w/ oral acetaminophen and antihistamine. Risk of acute infusion reactions; closely monitor pt during infusion. Universal precautions required. Pt should report difficulty breathing, signs of infection.

---

sirolimus (Rapamune)
CLASS Immunosuppressant
PREG/CONT C/NA

BBW Risk of increased susceptibility to infection; graft loss, hepatic artery thrombosis w/ liver transplant; bronchial anastomotic dehiscence in lung transplants.

IND & DOSE Px for organ rejection in renal transplant. *Adult, child 13 yr and older:* 40 kg or more: Loading dose of 6 mg PO as soon after transplant as possible, then 2 mg/day PO. Under 40 kg: Loading dose of 3 mg/m², then 1 mg/m²/day PO.

ADJUST DOSE Hepatic impairment
ADV EFF Abd pain, **anaphylaxis**, anemia, **angioedema**, arthralgia, delayed wound healing, edema, fever, headache, hypertension, **interstitial lung disease**, lipid profile changes, pain, skin cancer, thrombocytopenia

INTERACTIONS CYP3A4 inducers/inhibitors, grapefruit juice, live vaccines

NC/PT Always use w/ adrenal corticosteroids, cyclosporine. Monitor pulmonary function, LFTs, renal function. Not for use in pregnancy (contraceptives advised), breast-feeding. Pt should avoid grapefruit juice, sun

exposure; report difficulty breathing, swelling.

DANGEROUS DRUG

sitagliptin phosphate (Januvia)
CLASS Antidiabetic, DPP-4 inhibitor
PREG/CONT B/NA

IND & DOSE As adjunct to diet, exercise to improve glycemic control in type 2 diabetics. *Adult:* 100 mg/day PO.

ADJUST DOSE Renal impairment
ADV EFF Headache, hypoglycemia, URI, UTI

INTERACTIONS Atazanavir, celery, clarithromycin, coriander, dandelion root, fenugreek, garlic, ginseng, indinavir, itraconazole, juniper berries, ketoconazole, nefazodone, nelfinavir, ritonavir, saquinavir, telithromycin

NC/PT Monitor blood glucose, HbA₁c, renal function before, periodically during tx. Ensure thorough diabetic teaching program. Pt may be switched to insulin during times of stress. Pt should continue diet, exercise program, other prescribed diabetes drugs; report all other prescribed/OTC drugs, herbs being taken.

---

sodium bicarbonate (Bell/ans, Neut)
CLASS Antacid, electrolyte; systemic, urine alkalinizer
PREG/CONT C/NA

IND & DOSE Urine alkalinization. *Adult:* 3,900 mg PO, then 1,300–2,600 mg PO q 4 hr. *Child:* 84–840 mg/kg/day PO. Antacid. *Adult:* 300 mg–2 g PO daily–qid usually 1–3 hr after meals, at bedtime. Adjunct to advanced CV life support during CPR. *Adult:* Inject IV ever 300–500 mL of 5% sol or 200–300 mEq of 7.5% or 8.4% sol as rapidly as possible. Base further doses on subsequent blood gas values. Or,

1 mEq/kg dose, then repeat 0.5 mEq/kg q 10 min. *Child 2 yr and older:* 1 to 2 mEq/kg (1 mL/kg 8.4% sol) by slow IV. *Child under 2 yr:* 4.2% sol; max, 8 mEq/kg/day IV. **Severe metabolic acidosis.** *Adult, child:* Dose depends on blood carbon dioxide content, pH, pt's clinical condition. Usually, 90–180 mEq/L IV during first hr, then adjust PRN. **Less urgent metabolic acidosis.** *Adult, adolescent:* 5 mEq/kg as 4–8 hr IV infusion.
ADJUST DOSE Elderly pts, renal impairment
ADV EFF Local irritation, tissue necrosis at injection site, systemic alkalosis
INTERACTIONS Amphetamines, anorexiants, doxycycline, ephedrine, flecainide, lithium, methotrexate, quinidine, pseudoephedrine, salicylates, sulfonylureas, sympathomimetics, tetracyclines
NC/PT Monitor ABGs. Calculate base deficit when giving parenteral sodium bicarbonate. Give slowly. Do not attempt complete correction within first 24 hr; increased risk of systemic alkalosis. Monitor cardiac rhythm, potassium level. Pt should chew tablets thoroughly before swallowing, follow w/ full glass of water; avoid oral drug within 1–2 hr of other oral drugs; report pain at injection site, headache, tremors.

sodium ferric gluconate complex (Ferrlecit)
CLASS Iron product
PREG/CONT B/NA

IND & DOSE Tx of iron deficiency in pts undergoing long-term hemodialysis who are on erythropoietin.
Adult: Test dose: 2 mL diluted in 50 mL normal saline injection IV over 60 min. *Adult:* 10 mL diluted in 100 mL normal saline injection IV over 60 min. *Child 6 yr and over:* 0.12 mL/kg diluted in 25 mL normal saline by IV infusion over 1 hr for each dialysis session.

ADV EFF Cramps, dizziness, dyspnea, flushing, hypotension, **hypersensitivity reactions,** injection-site reactions, **iron overload,** n/v/d, pain
NC/PT Monitor iron level, BP. Most pts will initially need eight doses given at sequential dialysis sessions, then periodic use based on hematocrit. Do not mix w/ other drugs in sol. Have emergency equipment on hand for hypersensitivity reactions. Use caution in pregnancy, breast-feeding. Pt should take safety precautions w/ CNS effects, report difficulty breathing, pain at injection site.

sodium fluoride (Fluoritab, Flura, Karigel, Pharmaflur, Stop)
CLASS Mineral
PREG/CONT C/NA

IND & DOSE Px of dental caries.
Adult: 10 mL rinse once daily or wkly; swish around teeth, spit out. Or, apply thin ribbon to toothbrush or mouth tray for 1 min; brush, rinse, spit out. *Child:* Fluoride in drinking water over 0.6 ppm: No tx. Fluoride in drinking water 0.3–0.6 ppm: 6–16 yr, 0.5 mg/day PO; 3–6 yr, 0.25 mg/day PO. Fluoride in drinking water under 0.3 ppm: 6–16 yr, 1 mg/day PO; 3–6 yr, 0.5 mg/day PO; 6 mo–3 yr, 0.25 mg/day PO. *Child 6–12 yr:* 10 mL/day rinse; have pt swish around teeth for 1 min, spit out. Or, 4–6 drops gel on applicator. Have pt put applicator over teeth, bite down for 6 min, spit out excess gel.
ADV EFF Eczema, gastric distress, headache, rash, teeth staining, weakness
INTERACTIONS Dairy products
NC/PT Do not give within 1 hr of milk, dairy products. Pt may chew tablets, swallow whole, or add to drinking water, juice. Pt should brush, floss teeth before using rinse, then spit out fluid (should not swallow fluid, cream, gel, rinse); have regular dental exams; report increased salivation, diarrhea, seizures, teeth mottling.

sodium oxybate (Xyrem)

CLASS Anticataplectic, CNS depressant

PREG/CONT B/C-III

BBW Counsel pt that drug, also called GHB, is known for abuse. Pt will be asked to view educational program, agree to safety measures to ensure only pt has drug access, and agree to return for follow-up at least q 3 mo.

IND & DOSE Tx of excessive daytime sleepiness, cataplexy in pts w/ narcolepsy. Adult: 4.5 g/day PO divided into two equal doses of 2.25 g. Give at bedtime and again 2½–4 hr later. May increase no more often than q 1–2 wk to max 9 g/day in increments of 1.5 g/day (0.75 g/dose). Range, 6–9 g daily.

ADJUST DOSE Hepatic impairment

ADV EFF Dizziness, dyspepsia, flu-like sx, headache, n/v/d, pharyngitis, **respiratory depression**, somnolence, URI

INTERACTIONS Alcohol, CNS depressants

NC/PT Not for use in pregnancy. Dilute each dose w/ 60 mL water in child-resistant dosing cup. Give first dose of day when pt still in bed; should stay in bed after taking. Give second dose 2½–4 hr later, w/ pt sitting up in bed. After second dose, pt should lie in bed. Pt should take safety precautions w/ CNS effects; avoid eating for at least 2 hr before bed; keep drug secure; avoid alcohol; report difficulty breathing, confusion.

sodium phenylacetate/ sodium benzoate (Ammonul)

CLASS Ammonia reducer, urea substitute

PREG/CONT C/NA

IND & DOSE Adjunct tx in hyperammonemia, encephalopathy in pts w/ enzyme deficiencies associated w/ urea cycle. Adult, child: Over 20 kg, 55 mL/m². 0–20 kg, 2.5 mL/kg; Give IV through central line w/ arginine.

ADJUST DOSE Hepatic, renal impairment

ADV EFF Hyperglycemia, hyperventilation, hypokalemia, mental impairment, **injection-site reaction/necrosis, metabolic acidosis, neurotoxicity**, seizures

NC/PT Monitor plasma ammonia level. Not for use in pregnancy; use caution in breast-feeding. Ammonia level will be monitored; when normalized, dietary protein intake can be increased. Pt should report pain at injection site, numbness/tingling, rapid respirations.

sodium polystyrene sulfonate (Kalexate, Kayexalate, Kionex)

CLASS Potassium-removing resin

PREG/CONT C/NA

IND & DOSE Tx of hyperkalemia. Adult: 15–60 g/day PO best given as 15 g daily–qid. May give powder as suspension w/ water, syrup (20–100 mL). May introduce into stomach via NG tube. Or, 30–50 g by enema q 6 hr, retained for 30–60 min or as long as possible. Child: Give lower doses, using exchange ratio of 1 mEq potassium/g resin as basis for calculation.

ADV EFF Anorexia, constipation, gastric irritation, hypokalemia, n/v

INTERACTIONS Antacids

NC/PT Give resin through plastic stomach tube, or mixed w/ diet appropriate for renal failure. Give powder form in oral suspension w/ syrup base to increase palatability. Give enema after cleansing enema; help pt retain for at least 30 min. Monitor serum electrolytes; correct imbalances. If severe constipation, stop drug until function returns; do not use sorbitol, magnesium-containing laxatives.

Pt should report confusion, constipation, irregular heartbeat.

sofosbuvir (Sovaldi)

CLASS Hepatitis C drug, nucleoside analog inhibitor
PREG/CONT C/NA

IND & DOSE Tx of hepatitis C, w/ peginterferon alfa and ribavirin (genotype 1 or 4) or w/ ribavirin (genotypes 2 and 3). *Adult:* 400 mg PO w/ peginterferon and ribavirin for 12 wk (genotype 1 or 4); w/ ribavirin for 12 wk (genotype 2) or 24 wk (genotype 3).
ADJUST DOSE Hepatitis C virus/HIV coinfection, pts w/ hepatocellular carcinoma awaiting liver transplant
ADV EFF Anemia, fatigue, headache, insomnia, nausea
INTERACTIONS Rifampin, St. John's wort
NC/PT Ensure proper dx. Monthly negative pregnancy test required (use of barrier contraceptives advised for men and women during and for 6 mo after use). Drug is not a cure. Pt should eat small meals for nausea; take analgesic for headache; avoid St. John's wort; consult health care provider before stopping drug; take precautions to avoid spread of disease; report severe headache, color changes in urine/stool.

solifenacin succinate (VESIcare)

CLASS Muscarinic receptor antagonist, urinary antispasmodic
PREG/CONT C/NA

IND & DOSE Tx of overactive bladder. *Adult:* 5–10 mg/day PO swallowed whole w/ water.
ADJUST DOSE Moderate to severe hepatic impairment, severe renal impairment

ADV EFF Constipation, dizziness, dry eyes, dry mouth, **prolonged QT interval,** urine retention
INTERACTIONS CYP3A4 inhibitors, ketoconazole, potassium chloride, QT-prolonging drugs
NC/PT Arrange tx for underlying cause. Not for use in breast-feeding. Pt should empty bladder before each dose if urine retention an issue; swallow tablet whole and not cut, crush, or chew it; use sugarless lozenges for dry mouth, laxatives for constipation; take safety precautions w/ dizziness; report inability to void, fever, blurred vision.

somatropin (Genotropin, Humatrope, Norditropin, Nutropin, Omnitrope, Saizen, Serostim, Tev-Tropin, Zorbtive)

CLASS Hormone
PREG/CONT C; B (Genotropin, Omnitrope, Saizen, Serostim, Zorbtive)/NA

IND & DOSE (Adult) Tx of GH deficiency, replacement of endogenous GH in adults w/ GHD w/ multiple hormone deficiencies *(Genotropin, Humatrope, HumatroPen, Norditropin, Nutropin, Nutropin AQ, Omnitrope, Saizen). Genotropin, Omnitrope,* 0.04–0.08 mg/wk subcut divided into seven daily injections. *Humatrope, HumatroPen,* 0.006–0.0125 mg/day subcut. *Nutropin, Nutropin AQ,* Usual, 0.006 mg/kg/day subcut with max, 0.0125 mg/day (over 35 yr), 0.025 mg/kg/day (under 35 yr). *Norditropin,* 0.004–0.016 mg/kg/day subcut. *Saizen,* Up to 0.005 mg/kg/day subcut; may increase up to 0.01 mg/kg/day after 4 wk. **Tx of AIDS-wasting or cachexia.** *Serostim,* Over 55 kg: 6 mg/day subcut; 45–55 kg: 5 mg/day subcut; 35–45 kg: 4 mg/day subcut; under 35 kg: 0.1 mg/kg/day subcut. **Tx of short bowel syndrome in pts receiving specialized nutritional support** *(Zorbtive).* 0.1 mg/kg/day subcut for 4 wk; max, 8 mg/day.

IND & DOSE (Child) Tx of growth failure related to renal dysfx. 0.35 mg/kg/wk subcut divided into daily doses *(Nutropin, Nutropin AQ).* Tx of girls w/ Turner syndrome. 0.33 mg/kg/wk divided into six to seven subcut injections *(Genotropin).* Or, up to 0.375 mg/kg/wk subcut divided into equal doses six to seven times/wk *(Humatrope, HumatroPen).* Or, up to 0.067 mg/kg/day subcut *(Norditropin).* Or, up to 0.375 mg/kg/wk subcut divided into equal doses *(Nutropin, Nutropin AQ).* **Long-term tx of growth failure due to Prader-Willi syndrome.** 0.24 mg/kg/wk subcut divided into daily doses *(Genotropin).* **Small for gestational age.** 0.48 mg/kg/wk *(Genotropin).* **Tx of short stature, growth failure in short stature homeobox (SHOX)-containing gene deficiency.** 0.35 mg/kg/wk subcut *(Humatrope, HumatroPen).* **Tx of short stature in Noonan syndrome.** Up to 0.066 mg/kg/day subcut *(Norditropin).* **Long-term tx of idiopathic short stature when epiphyses not closed and diagnostic evaluation excludes other causes treatable by other means.** 0.47 mg/kg/wk subcut divided into six to seven doses *(Genotropin).* Or, 0.18–0.3 mg/kg/wk subcut or IM given in divided doses 3 time/wk *(Humatrope, HumatroPen).* Or, 0.3 mg/kg/wk subcut in divided doses *(Nutropin, Nutropin AQ).* **Long-term tx of growth failure due to lack of adequate endogenous GH secretion.** 0.18–0.3 mg/kg/wk subcut divided into daily doses given six to seven times/wk *(Accretropin).* Or, 0.18–0.3 mg/kg/wk subcut divided into doses six to seven 7 times/wk *(Humatrope, HumatroPen).* Or, 0.3 mg/kg/wk subcut in divided daily doses *(Nutropin, Nutropin AQ).* Or, 0.16–0.24 mg/kg/wk subcut divided into daily doses *(Genotropin).* Or, 0.16–0.24 mg/kg/wk subcut divided into daily doses *(Omnitrope).* Or, 0.06 mg/kg subcut, IM three times/wk *(Saizen).* Or, 0.024–0.034 mg/kg

subcut, six to seven times/wk *(Norditropin).* Or, up to 0.1 mg/kg subcut three times/wk *(Tev-Tropin).* **Tx of short stature w/ no catch-up growth by 2–4 yr.** 0.35 mg/kg/wk subcut injection divided into equal daily doses *(Humatrope, HumatroPen),* 0.024–0.034 mg/kg/wk subcut six to seven times/wk *(Norditropin).*

ADV EFF Development of GH antibodies, headache, hypothyroidism, insulin resistance, **leukemia,** pain, pain at injection site

INTERACTIONS CYP450 inducers/ inhibitors

NC/PT Arrange tests for glucose tolerance, thyroid function, growth hormone antibodies; tx as indicated. Rotate injection sites. Teach proper administration, disposal of needles, syringes. Pt should have frequent blood tests, report increased thirst/voiding, fatigue, cold intolerance.

DANGEROUS DRUG

sorafenib tosylate
(Nexavar)

CLASS Antineoplastic, kinase inhibitor
PREG/CONT D/NA

IND & DOSE Tx of advanced renal cell, hepatocellular carcinoma. *Adult:* 400 mg PO bid on empty stomach.

ADV EFF Alopecia, fatigue, **GI perforation, hand-foot syndrome, hemorrhage,** hypertension, **MI,** n/v/d, **QT prolongation,** skin reactions, weight loss, wound-healing complications

INTERACTIONS CYP3A4 inducers, grapefruit juice

NC/PT Obtain baseline, periodic ECG; monitor BP regularly. Not for use in pregnancy (contraceptives advised). Pt should take on empty stomach, avoid grapefruit juice, cover head at temp extremes (hair loss possible), report headache, rash, nonhealing wounds.

sotalol hydrochloride
(Betapace, Betapace AF, Sorine)

CLASS Antiarrhythmic, beta blocker

PREG/CONT B/NA

BBW Do not give for ventricular arrhythmias unless pt unresponsive to other antiarrhythmics and has life-threatening ventricular arrhythmia. Monitor response carefully; proarrhythmic effect can be pronounced. Do not initiate tx if baseline QT interval over 450 msec. If QT interval increases to 500 msec or more during tx, reduce dose, extend infusion time, or stop drug.

IND & DOSE Tx of life-threatening ventricular arrhythmias (Betapace); maint of sinus rhythm after atrial fibrillation (AF) conversion (Betapace AF). Adult: 80 mg PO bid. Adjust gradually, q 3 days, until appropriate response; may need 240–320 mg/day PO (Betapace); up to 120 mg bid PO (Betapace AF). Or, 75 mg IV over 5 hr bid; may increase in increments of 75 mg/day q 3 days. Range, 225–300 mg once or twice a day for ventricular arrhythmias; 112.5 mg once or twice a day IV for AF if oral not possible. Converting between oral, IV doses: 80 mg oral–75 mg IV; 120 mg oral–112.5 mg IV; 160 mg oral–150 mg IV. Child over 2 yr w/ normal renal function: 30 mg/m² tid PO. Max, 60 mg/m² tid.

ADJUST DOSE Elderly pts, renal impairment

ADV EFF Bronchospasm, cardiac arrhythmias, constipation, decreased exercise tolerance/libido, ED, flatulence, gastric pain, HF, laryngospasm, n/v/d, pulmonary edema, stroke

INTERACTIONS Antacids, aspirin, bismuth subsalicylate, clonidine, hormonal contraceptives, insulin, magnesium salicylate, NSAIDs, prazosin, QT-prolonging drugs, sulfinpyrazone

NC/PT Monitor QT interval. Switch from IV to oral as soon as possible. Do not stop abruptly; withdraw gradually. Pt should take on empty stomach, take safety precautions w/ dizziness, report difficulty breathing, confusion, edema, chest pain.

spironolactone
(Aldactone)

CLASS Aldosterone antagonist, potassium-sparing diuretic

PREG/CONT C; D (gestational hypertension)/NA

BBW Drug a tumerigen, w/ chronic toxicity in rats; avoid unnecessary use.

IND & DOSE Dx of hyperaldosteronism. Adult: Long test, 400 mg/day PO for 3–4 wk; correction of hypokalemia, hypertension presumptive evidence of primary hyperaldosteronism. Short test, 400 mg/day PO for 4 days. If serum potassium increases but decreases when drug stopped, presumptive dx can be made. Tx of edema. Adult: 100 mg/day PO; range, 25–200 mg/day. Tx of hypertension. Adult: 50–100 mg/day PO for at least 2 wk. Tx of hypokalemia. Adult: 25–100 mg/day PO. Tx of hyperaldosteronism. Adult: 100–400 mg/day PO in preparation for surgery. Tx of severe HF. Adult: 25–50 mg/day PO if potassium 5 mEq/L or less, creatinine 2.5 mg/dL or less.

ADV EFF Cramping, diarrhea, dizziness, drowsiness, gynecomastia, headache, hirsutism, hyperkalemia, voice deepening

INTERACTIONS ACE inhibitors, anticoagulants, antihypertensives, ganglionic blockers, licorice, potassium-rich diet, salicylates

NC/PT Monitor electrolytes periodically. Pt should avoid potassium-rich foods, excessive licorice intake; take safety precautions w/ dizziness; weigh self daily, report change of 3 lb or more/day; report swelling, muscle cramps/weakness.

stavudine (d4T) (Zerit)

CLASS Antiviral, nucleoside reverse transcriptase inhibitor
PREG/CONT C/NA

BBW Monitor closely for pancreatitis during tx; fatal, nonfatal pancreatitis has occurred. Monitor LFTs; lactic acidosis, severe hepatomegaly possible.
IND & DOSE Tx of HIV-1 infection. *Adult, child over 13 days:* 60 kg or more, 40 mg PO q 12 hr; 30—less than 60 kg, 30 mg PO q 12 hr; under 30 kg, 1 mg/kg/dose PO q 12 hr. *Child birth–13 days:* 0.5 mg/kg/dose PO q 12 hr.
ADJUST DOSE Renal impairment
ADV EFF Agranulocytopenia, asthenia, dizziness, fever, GI pain, headache, **hepatomegaly w/ steatosis, lactic acidosis,** n/v/d, **pancreatitis,** paresthesia
INTERACTIONS Didanosine, doxorubicin, ribavirin, zidovudine
NC/PT Monitor LFTs, pancreatic function, neurologic status before, q 2 wk during tx. Always give w/ other antivirals. Not for use in pregnancy (barrier contraceptives advised). Pt should take precautions to prevent spread (drug not a cure), avoid infections, take safety precautions w/ CNS effects, report numbness/tingling, severe headache, difficulty breathing.

streptomycin sulfate (generic)

CLASS Antibiotic
PREG/CONT D/NA

BBW Risk of severe neurotoxic, nephrotoxic reactions; monitor closely. Do not use w/ other neurotoxic, nephrotoxic drugs.
IND & DOSE Tx of subacute bacterial endocarditis, resistant TB. *Adult:* 15 mg/kg/day IM, or 25–30 mg/kg IM two or three times/wk. *Child:* 20–40 mg/kg/day IM or 25–30 mg/kg/IM two or three times/wk. **Tx of tularemia.** *Adult:* 1–2 g/day IM for 7–14 days. **Tx of plaque.** *Adult:* 2 g/day

IM in two divided doses for at least 10 days.
ADJUST DOSE Renal impairment
ADV EFF Dizziness, hearing loss, injection-site reactions, **renal toxicity, respiratory paralysis,** ringing in ears
INTERACTIONS Diuretics
NC/PT Monitor renal function regularly. Monitor injection sites. Teach appropriate administration, disposal of needles, syringes. Ensure pt with TB is also receiving other drugs. Not for use in pregnancy (barrier contraceptives advised), breast-feeding. Pt should take safety precautions w/ CNS effects, report difficulty breathing, dizziness, edema, hearing changes.

streptozocin (Zanosar)

CLASS Alkylating drug, antineoplastic
PREG/CONT D/NA

BBW Monitor for renal, liver toxicity. Special drug handling required.
IND & DOSE Tx of metastatic islet cell carcinoma of pancreas. *Adult:* 500 mg/m² IV for 5 consecutive days q 6 wk; or 1,000 mg/m² IV once/wk for 2 wk, then increase to 1,500 mg/m² IV each wk.
ADJUST DOSE Renal impairment
ADV EFF Bone marrow suppression, dizziness, drowsiness, glucose intolerance, n/v/d, **severe to fatal renal toxicity**
INTERACTIONS Doxorubicin
NC/PT Monitor LFTs, renal function closely. Handle drug as biohazard. Monitor CBC to determine dose. Give antiemetics for n/v. Not for use in pregnancy, breast-feeding. Pt should avoid exposure to infection, maintain nutrition, report unusual bleeding/bruising, increased thirst, swelling.

succimer (Chemet)

CLASS Antidote, chelate
PREG/CONT C/NA

IND & DOSE Tx of lead poisoning in child w/ blood level over 45 mcg/dL.

Child: 10 mg/kg or 350 mg/m² PO q 8 hr for 5 days; reduce to 10 mg/kg or 350 mg/m² PO q 12 hr for 2 wk (tx runs for 19 days).
ADV EFF Back pain, dizziness, drowsiness, flank pain, headache, n/v, rash, urination difficulties
INTERACTIONS EDTA
NC/PT Monitor serum lead level, transaminase levels before, q 2 wk during tx. Continue tx for full 19 days. Have pt swallow capsule whole; if unable to swallow capsule, open and sprinkle contents on soft food or give by spoon followed by fruit drink. Pt should maintain hydration, report difficulty breathing, tremors.

sucralfate (Carafate)
CLASS Antiulcer drug
PREG/CONT B/NA

IND & DOSE Tx, maint of duodenal, esophageal ulcers. *Adult:* 1 g PO qid on empty stomach for 4–8 wk; maint, 1 g PO bid.
ADV EFF Constipation, dizziness, dry mouth, gastric discomfort, rash, vertigo
INTERACTIONS Antacids, ciprofloxacin, digoxin, ketoconazole, levothyroxine, norfloxacin, penicillamine, phenytoin, quinidine, tetracycline, theophylline, warfarin
NC/PT Pt should take on empty stomach, 1 hr before or 2 hr after meals, and at bedtime; avoid antacids within 30 min of sucralfate; take safety precautions w/ CNS effects; use laxative for constipation; report severe gastric pain.

DANGEROUS DRUG
sufentanil citrate (Sufenta)
CLASS Opioid agonist analgesic
PREG/CONT C/C-II

IND & DOSE Adjunct to general anesthesia. *Adult:* Initially, 1–2 mcg/kg IV. Maint, 10–25 mcg; max, 1 mcg/kg/hr

of expected surgical time. **Anesthesia.** *Adult:* Initially, 8–30 mcg/kg IV; supplement w/ doses of 0.5–10 mcg/kg IV. Max, 30 mcg/kg for procedure. Give w/ oxygen, skeletal muscle relaxant. *Child 2–12 yr:* Initially, 10–25 mcg/kg IV; supplement w/ doses of 25–50 mcg IV. Give w/ oxygen, skeletal muscle relaxant. **Epidural analgesia.** *Adult:* 10–15 mcg via epidural administration w/ 10 mL bupivacaine 0.125%. May repeat twice at 1-hr or longer intervals (total, three doses).
ADV EFF Arrhythmias, bradycardia, bronchospasm, cardiac arrest, clamminess, confusion, constipation, dizziness, dry mouth, headache, floating feeling, **laryngospasm**, lethargy, light-headedness, n/v, sedation, **shock**, tachycardia, urinary hesitancy, urine retention, vertigo
INTERACTIONS Barbiturates beta blockers, calcium channel blockers, general anesthetics, grapefruit juice, hypnotics, opiate agonists, sedatives
NC/PT Protect vials from light. Provide opioid antagonist. Have equipment for assisted, controlled respiration on hand during parenteral administration. Give to breast-feeding women 4–6 hr before next feeding. Pt should avoid grapefruit juice, take safety precautions w/ CNS effects, report difficulty breathing, palpitations. Name confusion between sufentanil and fentanyl; use extreme caution.

sulfADIAZINE (generic)
CLASS Sulfonamide antibiotic
PREG/CONT C; D (labor & delivery)/NA

IND & DOSE Tx of acute infections caused by susceptible bacteria strains. *Adult:* 2–4 g PO, then 2–4 g/day PO in three to six divided doses. *Child over 2 mo:* 75 mg/kg PO, then 150 mg/kg/day PO in four to six divided doses; max 6 g/day **Tx of toxoplasmosis.** *Adult:* 1–1.5 g PO qid w/ pyrimethamine for 3–4 wk. *Child*

over 2 mo: 100–200 mg/kg/day PO w/ pyrimethamine for 3–4 wk. **Suppressive, maint tx in HIV pts.** *Adult:* 0.5–1 g PO q 6 hr w/ oral pyrimethamine, leucovorin. *Infant, child:* 85–120 mg/kg/day PO in two to four divided doses w/ oral pyrimethamine, leucovorin. *Adolescent:* 0.5–1 g PO q 6 hr w/ oral pyrimethamine, leucovorin. **Px of recurrent attacks of rheumatic fever.** *Adult:* Over 30 kg, 1 g/day PO. Under 30 kg, 0.5 g/day PO.
ADV EFF Abd pain, crystalluria, headache, hematuria, **hepatocellular necrosis,** n/v, photosensitivity, rash, **Stevens-Johnson syndrome**
INTERACTIONS Acetohexamide, chlorpropamide, cyclosporine, glyburide, glipizide, oral anticoagulants, phenytoin, tolbutamide, tolazamide
NC/PT Culture before tx. Pt should take on empty stomach 1 hr before or 2 hr after meals w/ full glass of water; drink 8 glasses of water/day; avoid sun exposure; take safety precautions w/ CNS effects; report bloody urine, ringing in ears, difficulty breathing. Name confusion between sulfadiazine and *Silvadene* (silver sulfadiazine); use caution.

sulfasalazine (Azulfidine)
CLASS Anti-inflammatory, antirheumatic, sulfonamide
PREG/CONT B/NA

IND & DOSE **Tx of ulcerative colitis.** *Adult:* 3–4 g/day PO in evenly divided doses. Maint, 2 g/day PO in evenly spaced doses (500 mg qid); max, 4 g/day. *Child 6 yr and over:* 40–60 mg/kg/24 hr PO in three to six divided doses. Maint, 30 mg/kg/ 24 hr PO in four equally divided doses; max, 2 g/day. **Tx of rheumatoid arthritis (RA).** *Adult:* 0.5–1 g/day PO (DR); may increase to 2 g daily in two evenly divided doses. **Tx of juvenile RA (polyarticular course).** *Child 6 yr and over:* 30–50 mg/kg/day PO in two evenly divided doses; max, 2 g/day.
ADV EFF Abd pain, **agranulocytosis, aplastic anemia,** crystalluria,

headache, hematuria, **hepatocellular necrosis,** n/v, paresthesia, photosensitivity, **Stevens-Johnson syndrome, thrombocytopenia**
INTERACTIONS Digoxin, folate
NC/PT Pt should take w/ meals; swallow DR tablet whole and not cut, crush, or chew it; drink 8 glasses of water/day; avoid sun exposure; take safety precautions w/ CNS effects; report difficulty breathing, bloody urine, rash.

sulindac (Clinoril)
CLASS NSAID
PREG/CONT B (1st, 2nd trimesters); D (3rd trimester)/NA

BBW Increased risk of CV events, GI bleeding; monitor accordingly. Contraindicated for periop pain in CABG surgery.
IND & DOSE **Tx of pain of rheumatoid arthritis, osteoarthritis, ankylosing spondylitis.** *Adult:* 150 mg PO bid. **Tx of acute painful shoulder, acute gouty arthritis.** *Adult:* 200 mg PO bid for 7–14 days (acute painful shoulder), 7 days (acute gouty arthritis).
ADJUST DOSE Hepatic, renal impairment
ADV EFF Anaphylactoid reactions to fatal anaphylactic shock, bone marrow suppression, constipation, dizziness, drowsiness, dyspepsia, edema, fatigue, GI pain, headache, insomnia, **HF,** n/v, vision disturbances
INTERACTIONS Beta blockers, diuretics, lithium
NC/PT Pt should take w/ food, milk if GI upset; take safety precautions w/ CNS effects, report swelling, difficulty breathing, black tarry stools.

sumatriptan succinate (Alsuma, Imitrex, Zecuity)
CLASS Antimigraine drug, triptan
PREG/CONT C/NA

IND & DOSE **Tx of acute migraine attacks.** *Adult:* 25, 50, or 100 mg PO;

may repeat in 2 hr or more. Max, 200 mg/day. Or, 6 mg subcut; may repeat in 1 hr. Max, 12 mg/24 hr. Or, 5, 10, or 20 mg into one nostril, or 10 mg divided into two doses (5 mg each), one in each nostril, repeated q 2 hr; max, 40 mg/24 hr. Battery-powered transdermal patch delivers 6.5 mg over 4 hr.

ADJUST DOSE Hepatic impairment
ADV EFF Altered BP, burning/tingling sensation, chest pain/pressure, dizziness, feeling of tightness, injection-site reactions, **shock**
INTERACTIONS Ergots, MAOIs, St. John's wort

NC/PT For tx, not px, of acute migraines. May repeat dose in 2 hr if needed. Teach proper administration of each form; disposal of needles, syringes for subcut use. Not for use in pregnancy (barrier contraceptives advised). Pt should continue migraine comfort measures, take safety precautions w/ CNS effects, avoid St. John's wort, report chest pain, swelling, numbness/tingling.

DANGEROUS DRUG

sunitinib (Sutent)
CLASS Antineoplastic, kinase inhibitor
PREG/CONT D/NA

BBW Risk of serious to fatal hepatotoxicity; monitor LFTs closely.
IND & DOSE Tx of GI stromal tumor, advanced renal cell carcinoma. *Adult:* 50 mg/day PO for 4 wk, then 2 wk of rest. Repeat cycle. **Tx of progressive neuroendocrine cancerous pancreatic tumors.** 37.5 mg/day PO continuously.
ADJUST DOSE Hepatic impairment
ADV EFF Abd pain, arthralgia, asthenia, anorexia, **cardiac toxicity,** constipation, cough, dyspnea, edema, fatigue, fever, **hemorrhage, hepatotoxicity, hypertension,** mucositis, n/v/d, **prolonged QT interval,** skin color changes, **thyroid dysfx**
INTERACTIONS CYP3A4 inducers/inhibitors, grapefruit juice

NC/PT Obtain baseline, periodic ECG, BP. Monitor LFTs. Not for use in pregnancy (barrier contraceptives advised), breast-feeding. Pt should mark calendar for tx days, take safety precaution w/ CNS effects, report unusual bleeding, palpitations, urine/stool color changes.

---

tacrolimus (Prograf, Protopic)
CLASS Immunosuppressant
PREG/CONT C/NA

BBW High risk of infection, lymphoma. Protect from infection; monitor closely. ER form not recommended for liver transplants; risk of death in female liver transplant pts.
IND & DOSE Px of rejection after kidney transplant. *Adult:* 0.2 mg/kg/day PO divided q 12 hr, or 0.03–0.05 mg/kg/day as continuous IV infusion. Or, 0.1 mg/kg/day PO ER capsule preop, 0.2 mg/kg/day PO ER capsule postop; if using basiliximab, 0.15 mg/kg/day PO ER capsule. **Px of rejection after liver transplant.** *Adult:* 0.10–0.15 mg/kg/day PO divided q 12 hr; give initial dose no sooner than 6 hr after transplant. Or, 0.03–0.05 mg/kg/day as continuous IV infusion. *Child:* 0.15–0.20 mg/kg/day PO, or 0.03–0.05 mg/kg/day IV infusion. **Px of rejection after heart transplant.** *Adult:* 0.075 mg/kg/day PO or IV in two divided doses q 12 hr; give first dose no sooner than 6 hr after transplant. **Tx of atopic dermatitis.** *Adult:* Apply thin layer 0.03% or 0.1% ointment to affected area bid; rub in gently, completely. *Child 2–15 yr:* Apply thin layer 0.03% ointment bid.
ADJUST DOSE Hepatic, renal impairment
ADV EFF Abd pain, **anaphylaxis,** constipation, diarrhea, fever, headache, **hepatotoxicity, infections,** renal impairment

INTERACTIONS Calcium channel blockers, carbamazepine, cimetidine, clarithromycin, cyclosporine, erythromycin, grapefruit juice, live vaccines, metoclopramide, nicardipine, phenobarbital, phenytoin, rifamycins, statins, St. John's wort
NC/PT Monitor LFTs, serum tacrolimus. Use IV route only if PO not possible; switch to PO as soon as possible. Not for use in pregnancy. Pt should avoid exposure to sunlight (topical form), infection; avoid grapefruit juice, St. John's wort, live vaccines; report unusual bleeding, signs of infection.

---

tadalafil (Adcirca, Cialis)
CLASS Impotence drug, phosphodiesterase-5 inhibitor
PREG/CONT B/NA

IND & DOSE Tx of ED, BPH w/ ED (*Cialis*). *Adult:* 10 mg PO before anticipated sexual activity; range, 5–20 mg PO. Limit use to once/day. Or, 2.5–5 mg/day PO w/out regard to timing of sexual activity. Tx of pulmonary arterial hypertension (*Adcirca*). 40 mg/day PO.
ADJUST DOSE Hepatic, renal impairment; tx with CYP3A4 inhibitors
ADV EFF Diarrhea, dizziness, dyspepsia, dry mouth, flulike symptoms, flushing, headache, **MI**, priapism, **Stevens-Johnson syndrome**
INTERACTIONS Alcohol, alpha blockers, erythromycin, grapefruit juice, indinavir, itraconazole, ketoconazole, nitrates, rifampin, ritonavir
NC/PT Ensure proper dx. For ED, does not protect against STDs, will not work in absence of sexual stimulation. Pt should not use w/ nitrates, antihypertensives, grapefruit juice, alcohol; report vision changes, loss of vision, erection lasting more than 4 hr, sudden hearing loss.

---

talc, USP (Sterile Talc Powder)
CLASS Sclerosing drug
PREG/CONT B/NA

IND & DOSE To decrease recurrence of malignant pleural effusion. *Adult:* 5 g in 50–100 mL sodium chloride injection injected into chest tube after pleural fluid drained; clamp chest tube, have pt change positions for 2 hr; unclamp chest tube, continue external suction.
ADV EFF Acute pneumonitis, dyspnea, hypotension, localized bleeding, **MI**, **RDS**, tachycardia
NC/PT Ensure proper chest tube placement, pt positioning, draining. Pt should report difficulty breathing, chest pain.

---

taliglucerase alfa (Elelyso)
CLASS Enzyme
PREG/CONT B/NA

IND & DOSE Long-term enzyme replacement tx for adult w/ type 1 Gaucher disease. *Adult:* 60 units/kg IV q other wk as 60–120 min infusion.
ADV EFF Anaphylaxis, arthralgia, back pain, headache, influenza, **infusion reaction**, pain, pharyngitis, throat infection, URI
NC/PT Give IV only. Monitor for infusion reactions; decrease infusion rate, consider use of antipyretics, antihistamines. Pt should mark calendar for infusion dates; report difficulty breathing, fever, chest/back pain, rash.

DANGEROUS DRUG

tamoxifen citrate (Soltamox)
CLASS Antiestrogen, antineoplastic
PREG/CONT D/NA

BBW Alert women w/ ductal carcinoma in situ (DCIS) and those at high risk for breast cancer of risks of serious to potentially fatal drug effects, including stroke, embolic events, uterine malignancies; discuss benefits/risks.

IND & DOSE Tx of metastatic breast cancer. *Adult:* 20–40 mg/day PO for 5 yr. Give doses of more than 20 mg/day in divided doses, a.m. and p.m. **To reduce breast cancer incidence in high-risk women; tx of DCIS.** *Adult:* 20 mg/day PO for 5 yr.

ADV EFF Corneal changes, depression, dizziness, **DVT**, edema, hot flashes, n/v, **PE**, rash, **stroke**, vaginal bleeding

INTERACTIONS Bromocriptine, cytotoxic agents, grapefruit juice, oral anticoagulants

NC/PT Monitor CBC periodically. Not for use in pregnancy (barrier contraceptives advised). Pt should have regular gynecologic exams, take safety precautions w/ CNS effects, report leg pain/swelling, chest pain, difficulty breathing.

tamsulosin hydrochloride (Flomax)
CLASS Alpha-adrenergic blocker, BPH drug
PREG/CONT B/NA

IND & DOSE Tx of s&sx of BPH. *Adult:* 0.4–0.8 mg PO daily 30 min after same meal each day.

ADV EFF Abnormal ejaculation, dizziness, headache, insomnia, orthostatic hypotension, somnolence

INTERACTIONS Alpha-adrenergic antagonists, cimetidine, saw palmetto, sildenafil, tadalafil, vardenafil

NC/PT Ensure accurate dx. Alert surgeon; increased risk of intraop floppy iris syndrome w/ cataract surgery. Pt should swallow capsule whole and not cut, crush, or chew it; change position slowly to avoid dizziness; not take w/ ED drugs; take safety precautions w/ CNS effects; avoid

saw palmetto; report fainting, worsening of sx. Name confusion between *Flomax* (tamsulosin) and *Fosamax* (alendronate); use caution.

tapentadol (Nucynta, Nucynta ER)
CLASS Norepinephrine reuptake inhibitor, opioid receptor agonist
PREG/CONT C/C-II

BBW Risk of abuse potention; limit use w/ hx of addiction. Risk of fatal respiratory depression, highest at start and w/ dose changes; monitor accordingly. Accidental ingestion of ER form can cause fatal overdose in child; secure drug. Risk of fatally high tapentadol level w/ alcohol; pt should avoid alcohol, all medications containing alcohol.

IND & DOSE Relief of moderate to severe pain. *Adult:* 50–100 mg PO q 4–6 hr. **mgt of moderate to severe chronic pain when round-the-clock opioid use needed (ER form);.** *Adult:* 100–250 mg PO bid. Reduce initial dose to 50 mg in analgesic-naïve pt; max, 500 mg/day. **Relief of pain of diabetic peripheral neuropathy (***Nucynta ER***).** *Adult:* 50 mg PO bid.

ADJUST DOSE Elderly, debilitated pts; hepatic impairment

ADV EFF Dizziness, drowsiness, headache, n/v, respiratory depression

INTERACTIONS Alcohol, general anesthetics, hypnotics, MAOIs, opioids, phenothiazines, sedatives, St. John's wort, SSRIs, TCAs, triptans

NC/PT Assess pain before, periodically during tx. Safety precautions needed w/ CNS effects. Do not give within 14 days of MAOIs. Pt should avoid alcohol, St. John's wort; if breast-feeding, take at least 3–4 hr before next feeding; take safety precautions w/ CNS effects; report difficulty breathing, rash.

tasimelteon (Hetlioz)
CLASS Melatonin receptor agonist
PREG/CONT C/NA

IND & DOSE Tx of non-24 hr-sleep-wake disorder in totally blind pts.
Adult: 20 mg before bedtime at same time each night.

ADJUST DOSE Severe hepatic impairment, smokers
ADV EFF Elevated alanine aminotransferase, headache, nightmares, somnolence, URI, UTI
INTERACTIONS Fluvoxamine, ketoconazole, rifampin
NC/PT Monitor LFTs. Pt should swallow capsule whole, not cut, crush, or chew it; avoid pregnancy, breast-feeding; limit activities after taking drug; take safety measures w/ somnolence; report changes in behavior, severe somnolence.

teduglutide (Gattex)
CLASS Glucagon-like peptide-2
PREG/CONT B/NA

IND & DOSE Tx of adults w/ short bowel syndrome who are dependent on parenteral support *Adult:* 0.05 mg/kg subcut.

ADJUST DOSE Renal impairment
ADV EFF Abd pain/distention, biliary and pancreatic disease, fluid overload, headache, intestinal obstruction, neoplastic growth, n/v
INTERACTIONS Oral drugs
NC/PT Subcut use only. Single-use vial; discard within 3 hr of reconstitution. Ensure complete colonoscopy, polyp removal before tx and at least q 5 yr. Rotate injection sites. Monitor for fluid overload; support as needed. Oral drugs may not be absorbed; monitor pt, consider need for oral drug dosage adjustment. Monitor pancreatic function. Pt should learn preparation of subcut injection, disposal of syringes, needles; rotate injection sites; schedule periodic blood tests; report severe abd pain, chest pain, swelling in extremities, severe epigastric pain, difficulty swallowing.

telaprevir (Incivek)
CLASS Antiviral, protease inhibitor
PREG/CONT B/NA

BBW Risk of serious to fatal skin reactions; monitor accordingly.
IND & DOSE Tx of chronic hepatitis C genotype 1 infection. *Adult:* 750 mg PO tid at 7- to 9-hr intervals w/ food; must give w/ ribavirin, peginterferon alfa.

ADJUST DOSE Hepatic impairment
ADV EFF Anemia, anal pruritus, anorectal discomfort, fatigue, hemorrhoids, rash, **serious skin reactions**
INTERACTIONS Alprazolam, atazanavir, atorvastatin, cyclosporine, darunavir, digoxin, efavirenz, estrogens, fosamprenavir, ketoconazole, lopinavir, methadone, midazolam, tacrolimus, zolpidem
NC/PT Ensure negative pregnancy test before tx; men, women should use two forms of contraceptives during, for 6 mo after tx. Must give w/ ribavirin, peginterferon alfa. Monitor CBC. Pt should allow 7–9 hr between doses, report rash, increasing fatigue.

telavancin (Vibativ)
CLASS Antibiotic, lipoglycopeptide
PREG/CONT C/NA

BBW Fetal risk; women of childbearing age should have serum pregnancy test before start of tx. Avoid use in pregnancy; advise contraceptive use.
IND & DOSE Tx of complicated skin, skin-structure infections caused by susceptible strains of gram-positive organisms. Tx of hospital-acquired and ventilator-assisted pneumonia caused by *Staphylococcus aureus* when other tx not suitable. *Adult:* 10 mg/kg IV infused over 60 min once q 24 hr for 7–14 days.

ADJUST DOSE Renal impairment
ADV EFF Bleeding, *Clostridium difficile* diarrhea, dizziness, foamy urine, **nephrotoxicity,** n/v, **QT prolongation,** red man syndrome (w/ rapid infusion), taste disturbance
INTERACTIONS Nephrotoxic drugs, QT-prolonging drugs
NC/PT Culture before tx. Infuse over at least 60 min. Monitor clotting time, renal function periodically. Not for use in pregnancy (contraceptives advised), breast-feeding. Negative pregnancy test needed before tx. Urine may become foamy. Pt should take safety precautions w/ CNS effects, report fever, unusual bleeding, irregular heartbeat.

---

telbivudine (Tyzeka)
CLASS Antiviral, nucleoside
PREG/CONT B/NA

BBW Monitor for myopathy, severe hepatic failure w/ steatosis, hepatitis B exacerbation w/ drug discontinuation.
IND & DOSE Tx of chronic hepatitis B. *Adult, child over 16 yr:* 600 mg/day PO w/ or without food.
ADJUST DOSE Renal impairment
ADV EFF Abd pain, arthralgia, back pain, cough, diarrhea, dyspepsia, headache, **hepatitis B exacerbation, hepatomegaly w/ steatosis,** insomnia, **myopathy, nephrotoxicity, peripheral neuropathy**
INTERACTIONS Nephrotoxic drugs, peginterferon alfa-2a
NC/PT Monitor LFTs, renal function. Not for use in pregnancy (contraceptives advised), breast-feeding. Pt should take safety precautions w/ CNS effects, report unusual bleeding, urine/stool color changes, numbness/tingling.

---

telithromycin (Ketek)
CLASS Ketolide antibiotic
PREG/CONT C/NA

BBW Contraindicated w/ myasthenia gravis; life-threatening respiratory failure possible.

IND & DOSE Tx of mild to moderately severe community-acquired pneumonia caused by susceptible strains. *Adult:* 800 mg/day PO for 7–10 days.
ADJUST DOSE Renal impairment
ADV EFF Anaphylaxis, diarrhea, dizziness, headache, **hepatic impairment,** n/v, **pseudomembranous colitis,** superinfections, visual disturbances
INTERACTIONS Serious reactions w/ atorvastatin, lovastatin, midazolam, pimozide, simvastatin; avoid these combinations. Also, carbamazepine, digoxin, metoprolol, phenobarbital, phenytoin, rifampin, theophylline.
NC/PT Culture before tx. Monitor LFTs. Treat superinfections. Pt should swallow tablet whole and not cut, crush, or chew it; take safety precautions w/ dizziness; avoid quickly looking between distant and nearby objects (if visual difficulties); report bloody diarrhea, difficulty breathing, unusual bleeding.

---

telmisartan (Micardis)
CLASS Antihypertensive, ARB
PREG/CONT D/NA

BBW Rule out pregnancy before tx. Suggest barrier contraceptives during tx; fetal injury, deaths have occurred.
IND & DOSE Tx of hypertension. *Adult:* 40 mg/day PO. Range, 20–80 mg/day; max, 80 mg/day. **To reduce CV risk in high-risk pts unable to** take ACE inhibitors. *Adult:* 80 mg/day PO.
ADV EFF Dermatitis, dizziness, flatulence, gastritis, headache, hypotension, light-headedness, palpitations, rash
INTERACTIONS Digoxin, potassium-sparing diuretics
NC/PT Monitor BP carefully. Alert surgeon; volume replacement may be needed postop. Not for use in pregnancy (contraceptives advised), breast-feeding. Pt should take safety

precautions w/ CNS effects, report fever, severe dizziness.

temazepam (Restoril)
CLASS Benzodiazepine, sedative-hypnotic
PREG/CONT X/C-IV

BBW Taper dosage gradually after long-term use; risk of refractory seizures.

IND & DOSE Short-term tx of insomnia. *Adult:* 15–30 mg PO before bedtime for 7-10 days; 7.5 mg may be sufficient for some pts.

ADJUST DOSE Elderly, debilitated pts

ADV EFF Anaphylaxis, **angioedema**, bradycardia, confusion, constipation, **CV collapse**, diarrhea, drowsiness, drug dependence, fatigue, hiccups, nervousness, tachycardia, urticaria

INTERACTIONS Alcohol, aminophylline, CNS depressants, dyphylline, theophylline

NC/PT Not for use in pregnancy (contraceptives advised). Pt should take for no longer than 7–10 days, avoid alcohol, take safety precautions w/ CNS effects, report difficulty breathing, face/eye swelling, continued sleep disorders.

DANGEROUS DRUG
temozolomide (Temodar)
CLASS Antineoplastic
PREG/CONT D/NA

IND & DOSE Tx of refractory astrocytoma. *Adult:* 150 mg/m²/day PO or IV for 5 consecutive days for 28-day tx cycle. Tx of glioblastoma multiforme. *Adult:* 75 mg/m²/day PO or IV for 42 days w/ focal radiation therapy; then six cycles: Cycle 1, 150 mg/m²/day PO, IV for 5 days then 23 days rest; cycles 2–6, 200 mg/m²/day PO or IV for 5 days then 23 days rest.

ADJUST DOSE Elderly pts; hepatic, renal impairment

ADV EFF Amnesia, **bone marrow suppression, cancer,** constipation, dizziness, headache, insomnia, n/v/d, **PCP,** rash, seizures

INTERACTIONS Valproic acid

NC/PT Monitor CBC before each dose; adjustment may be needed. Not for use in pregnancy (contraceptives advised), breast-feeding. Pt should take safety precautions w/ CNS effects, avoid exposure to infection, report unusual bleeding, difficulty breathing.

DANGEROUS DRUG
temsirolimus (Torisel)
CLASS Antineoplastic, kinase inhibitor
PREG/CONT D/NA

IND & DOSE Tx of advanced renal cell carcinoma. *Adult:* 25 mg/wk IV infused over 30–60 min; give 30 min after giving prophylactic diphenhydramine 25–50 mg IV.

ADJUST DOSE Elderly pts, hepatic impairment

ADV EFF Abd pain, alopecia, body aches, **bowel perforation,** confusion, constipation, drowsiness, **hepatic impairment, hyperglycemia, hypersensitivity/infusion reactions, interstitial pneumonitis, nephrotoxicity,** n/v/d, painful urination, rash, wound-healing problems

INTERACTIONS CYP3A4 inducers/inhibitors, grapefruit juice, live vaccines, St. John's wort

NC/PT Monitor LFTs, renal/respiratory function. Premedicate to decrease infusion reaction risk. Not for use in pregnancy (barrier contraceptives advised), breast-feeding. Pt should mark calendar of tx days; cover head at temp extremes (hair loss possible); take safety precautions w/ CNS effects; avoid St. John's wort, grapefruit juice; report difficulty breathing, severe abd pain, urine/stool color changes.

DANGEROUS DRUG

tenecteplase (TNKase)

CLASS Thrombolytic enzyme
PREG/CONT C/NA

BBW Arrange to stop concurrent heparin, tenecteplase if serious bleeding occurs.

IND & DOSE To reduce mortality associated w/ acute MI. *Adult:* Initiate tx as soon as possible after onset of acute MI. Give as IV bolus over 5 sec. Dose based on weight (max, 50 mg/dose): 90 kg or more, 50 mg; 80–89 kg, 45 mg; 70–79 kg, 40 mg; 60–69 kg, 35 mg; under 60 kg, 30 mg.

ADJUST DOSE Elderly pts
ADV EFF Bleeding, cardiac arrhythmias, **MI,** rash, urticaria
INTERACTIONS Aminocaproic acid, anticoagulants, aspirin, clopidogrel, dipyridamole, heparin, ticlopidine
NC/PT Can only give IV under close supervision. Do not add other drugs to infusion sol. Stop current heparin tx. Apply pressure to all dressings. Avoid invasive procedures. Monitor coagulation studies; watch for signs of bleeding. Pt should report blood in urine, bleeding, chest pain, difficulty breathing.

---

tenofovir disoproxil fumarate (Viread)

CLASS Antiviral, nucleoside reverse transcriptase inhibitor
PREG/CONT B/NA

BBW Risk of lactic acidosis, severe hepatotoxicity; monitor hepatic function closely. Severe hepatitis B exacerbation has occurred when anti–hepatitis B tx stopped; monitor for several mo if drug discontinued.

IND & DOSE Tx of HIV-1 infection. *Adult, child 12 yr and older, 35 kg or more:* 300 mg/day PO. *Child 2–11 yr:* 8 mg/kg/day PO. **Tx of chronic hepatitis B.** *Adult, child 12 yr and older, 35 kg or more:* 300 mg/day PO.

ADJUST DOSE Renal impairment
ADV EFF Asthenia, body fat redistribution, headache, **lactic acidosis,** n/v/d, **severe hepatomegaly w/ steatosis**
INTERACTIONS Atazanavir, didanosine, lopinavir, ritonavir
NC/PT Always give w/ other antivirals. Monitor LFTs, renal function regularly; stop at first sign of lactic acidosis. Not for use in pregnancy, breast-feeding. Body fat may redistribute to back, middle, chest. Pt should take precautions to avoid disease spread (drug not a cure); avoid exposure to infections, report urine/stool color changes, rapid respirations.

---

terazosin hydrochloride (Hytrin)

CLASS Alpha blocker, antihypertensive, BPH drug
PREG/CONT C/NA

BBW Give first dose just before bed to lessen likelihood of first-dose syncope due to orthostatic hypotension.

IND & DOSE Tx of hypertension. *Adult:* 1 mg PO at bedtime. Slowly increase to achieve desired BP response. Usual range, 1–5 mg PO daily. **Tx of BPH.** *Adult:* 1 mg PO at bedtime. Increase to 2, 5, or 10 mg PO daily. May need 10 mg/day for 4–6 wk to assess benefit.

ADV EFF Allergic anaphylaxis, blurred vision, dizziness, drowsiness, dyspnea, headache, nasal congestion, n/v, orthostatic hypotension, palpitations, priapism, sinusitis
INTERACTIONS ED drugs
NC/PT If not taken for several days, restart w/ initial dose. Always start first dose at bedtime to lessen likelihood of syncope; have pt lie down if syncope occurs. Pt should take safety precautions w/ CNS effects, use caution w/ ED drugs, report fainting, dizziness.

terbinafine hydrochloride (Lamisil)

CLASS Allylamine, antifungal
PREG/CONT B/NA

BBW Monitor regularly for s&sx of hepatic impairment; liver failure possible.

IND & DOSE Tx of onychomycosis of fingernail, toenail. *Adult:* 250 mg/day PO for 6 wk (fingernail), 12 wk (toenail). Tx of tinea capitis. *Adult:* 250 mg/day PO for 6 wk. *Child 4 yr and over:* Over 35 kg, 250 mg/day PO for 6 wk; 25–35 kg, 187.5 mg/day PO for 6 wk; under 25 kg, 125 mg/day PO for 6 wk. Tx of athlete's foot. *Adult, child:* Apply topically between toes bid for 1 wk. Tx of ring worm, jock itch. *Adult, child:* Apply topically once daily for 1 wk.

ADV EFF Abd pain, dyspepsia, headache, **hepatic failure**, nausea, pruritus, rash

INTERACTIONS Cimetidine, cyclosporine, dextromethorphan, rifampin
NC/PT Culture before tx. Monitor LFTs regularly. Not for use in pregnancy, breast-feeding. Pt should sprinkle oral granules on spoonful of nonacidic food such as mashed potatoes, swallow entire spoonful without chewing; take analgesics for headache; report urine/stool color changes, unusual bleeding, rash. Name confusion w/ *Lamisil* (terbinafine), *Lamictal* (lamotrigine), *Lamisil AF* (tolnaftate), *Lamisil AT* (terbinafine); use caution.

terbutaline sulfate (generic)

CLASS Antiasthmatic, beta selective agonist, bronchodilator, sympathomimetic
PREG/CONT B/NA

BBW Do not use injectable form in pregnant women for px, prolonged tx (beyond 48–72 hr) of preterm labor in hospital or outpt setting; risk of serious maternal heart problems, death.

IND & DOSE Px, tx of bronchial asthma, reversible bronchospasm. *Adult, child over 15 yr:* 2.5–5 mg PO tid at 6-hr intervals during waking hours; max, 15 mg/day. Or, 0.25 mg subcut into lateral deltoid area. If no significant improvement in 15–30 min, give another 0.25-mg dose. Max, 0.5 mg/4 hr. *Child 12–15 yr:* 2.5 mg PO tid; max, 7.5 mg/24 hr.

ADJUST DOSE Elderly pts
ADV EFF Anxiety, apprehension, **bronchospasm**, cardiac arrhythmias, cough, fear, nausea, palpitations, **pulmonary edema**, **respiratory difficulties**, restlessness, sweating
INTERACTIONS Diuretics, halogenated hydrocarbons, MAOIs, sympathomimetics, TCAs, theophylline
NC/PT Due to similar packaging, terbutaline injection confused w/ *Methergine* injection (methylergonovine maleate); use extreme caution. Have beta blocker on hand for arrhythmias, respiratory distress. Pt should take safety precautions w/ CNS effects, report chest pain, difficulty breathing, irregular heartbeat, failure to respond to usual dose.

teriflunomide (Aubagio)

CLASS MS drug, pyrimidine synthesis inhibitor
PREG/CONT X/NA

BBW Risk of severe hepatotoxicity; monitor LFTs before tx and at least monthly for 6 mo. Risk of major birth defects. Contraindicated in pregnancy; contraceptives required.

IND & DOSE Tx of relapsing MS. *Adult:* 7 or 14 mg/day PO.

ADJUST DOSE Severe hepatic impairment
ADV EFF Alopecia, **BP changes**, hyperkalemia, influenza, **neutropenia**, n/v, paresthesia, **peripheral neuropathy**, **renal failure**, **severe skin reactions**
INTERACTIONS Alosetron, duloxetine, hormonal contraceptives,

paclitaxel, pioglitazone, repaglinide, rosiglitazone, theophylline, tizanidine, warfarin

NC/PT Do not begin tx if acute infection; monitor for s&sx of infection, changes in potassium levels, BP changes, peripheral neuropathy, skin reactions. Monitor LFTs before, during tx. Not for use in pregnancy (contraceptives required), breast-feeding; advise pt of risk of fetal harm. Pt should take once daily; avoid exposure to infection; report urine/stool color changes, extreme fatigue, fever, infection, skin reactions, muscle cramping, numbness/tingling.

---

teriparatide (Forteo)
CLASS Calcium regulator, parathyroid hormone
PREG/CONT C/NA

BBW Increased risk of osteosarcoma in rats; do not use in pts w/ increased risk of osteosarcoma (Paget disease, unexplained alkaline phosphatase elevations, open epiphyses, prior external beam, implant radiation involving skeleton). Not recommended for bone disease other than osteoporosis.

IND & DOSE Tx of postmenopausal women w/ osteoporosis, glucocorticoid-related osteoporosis, hypogonadal osteoporosis in men. *Adult:* 20 mcg/day subcut in thigh or abd wall for no more than 2 yr.

ADV EFF Arthralgia, hypercalcemia, nausea, orthostatic hypotension, pain, urolithiasis

INTERACTIONS Digoxin

NC/PT Do not use in pts at risk for osteoporosis; use for no more than 2 yr. Monitor serum calcium. Not for use in pregnancy, breast-feeding. Teach proper administration, disposal of needles, delivery device. Pt should rotate injection sites, have blood tests to monitor calcium level, change positions slowly after injection, report constipation, muscle weakness.

---

tesamorelin (Egrifta)
CLASS GHRF analogue
PREG/CONT X/NA

IND & DOSE To reduce excess abd fat in HIV-infected pts w/ lipodystrophy related to antiviral use. *Adult:* 2 mg/day subcut.

ADV EFF Acute illness, arthralgia, cancer, edema, fluid retention, glucose intolerance, hypersensitivity reactions, injection-site reactions

INTERACTIONS Anticonvulsants, corticosteroids, cyclosporine, estrogen, progesterone, testosterone

NC/PT Monitor blood glucose. Arrange for cancer screening. Teach proper administration, disposal of needles, syringes. Not for use in pregnancy, breast-feeding. Pt should rotate injection sites, report signs of infection, injection-site reaction, increased thirst.

---

testosterone (Androderm, AndroGel, Axiron, Delatestryl, Fortesta, Striant, Testim, Testopel)
CLASS Androgen, hormone
PREG/CONT X/C-III

BBW Risk of toxic effects (enlarged genitalia, greater-than-normal bone age) in children exposed to pt using transdermal form (AndroGel, Testim). Pt should wash hands after applying, cover treated area w/ clothing to reduce exposure.

IND & DOSE Replacement tx in hypogonadism. *Adult:* 50–400 mg (cypionate, enanthate) IM q 2–4 wk, or 150–450 mg (enanthate pellets) implanted subcut q 3–6 mo. Or, initially 5-mg/day system (patch) applied to nonscrotal skin; then 2.5-mg/day system (Androderm). Or, 5 mg/day AndroGel, Testim (preferably in a.m.) applied to clean, dry, intact skin of shoulders, upper arms, or abdomen. Or, 4 actuations (40 mg) Fortesta applied to inner thighs in a.m. Or,

1 pump actuation (30 mg) *Axiron* to each axilla once/day. Or, 2 actuations (40.5 mg) *AndroGel* 1.62% once daily in a.m. to shoulders or upper arms. Or, 1 buccal system (30 mg) *(Striant)* to gum region bid (a.m. and p.m.). Rotate sites; usual position is above incisor on either side of mouth. **Tx of males w/ delayed puberty.** *Adult:* 50–200 mg enanthate IM q 2–4 wk for 4–6 mo, or 150 mg pellets subcut q 3–6 mo. **Tx of carcinoma of breast, metastatic mammary cancer.** *Adult:* 200–400 mg IM enanthate q 2–4 wk.
ADV EFF Androgenic effects, chills, dizziness, fatigue, fluid retention, headache, **hepatocellular carcinoma**, hypoestrogenic effects, leukopenia, polycythemia, rash
INTERACTIONS Grapefruit juice, metronidazole
NC/PT Monitor blood glucose, serum calcium, LFTs, serum electrolytes, lipids. Review proper administration of each delivery form; sprays not interchangeable. Women using drug should avoid pregnancy. Pt should mark calendar of tx days; remove old transdermal patch before applying new one; cover topical gel application sites if in contact w/ children; avoid grapefruit juice; report swelling, urine/stool color changes, unusual bleeding/bruising.

tetrabenazine (Xenazine)
CLASS Anti-chorea drug, monoamine depletor
PREG/CONT C/NA

BBW Increased risk of depression, suicidality; monitor accordingly.
IND & DOSE **Tx of chorea associated w/ Huntington disease.** *Adult:* 12.5 mg/day PO in a.m. After 1 wk, increase to 12.5 mg PO bid; max, 100 mg/day in divided doses.
ADV EFF Akathisia, anxiety, confusion, depression, fatigue, insomnia, nausea, Parkinson-like sx, **QT prolongation**, sedation, URI

INTERACTIONS Alcohol, antiarrhythmics, antipsychotics, dopamine agonists, fluoxetine, MAOIs, paroxetine, quinidine
NC/PT Obtain baseline of chorea sx. Do not give within 14 days of MAOIs. Not for use in pregnancy (contraceptives advised), breast-feeding. Pt should take safety measures w/ CNS effects, avoid alcohol; report tremors, behavior changes, thoughts of suicide.

tetracycline hydrochloride (generic)
CLASS Antibiotic
PREG/CONT D/NA

IND & DOSE **Tx of infections caused by susceptible bacteria.** *Adult:* 1–2 g/day PO in two to four equal doses; max, 500 mg PO qid. *Child over 8 yr:* 25–50 mg/kg/day PO in four equal doses. **Tx of brucellosis.** *Adult:* 500 mg PO qid for 3 wk w/ 1 g streptomycin IM bid first wk and daily second wk. **Tx of syphilis.** *Adult:* 30–40 g PO in divided doses over 10–15 days *(Sumycin)*; 500 mg PO qid for 15–30 days (all others). **Tx of uncomplicated gonorrhea.** *Adult:* 500 mg PO q 6 hr for 7 days. **Tx of gonococcal urethritis.** *Adult:* 500 mg PO q 4–6 hr for 4–6 days. **Tx of uncomplicated urethral, endocervical, rectal infections w/ *Chlamydia trachomatis.*** *Adult:* 500 mg PO qid for at least 7 days. **Tx of severe acne.** *Adult:* 1 g/day PO in divided doses; then 125–500 mg/day.
ADV EFF **Anaphylaxis; bone marrow suppression;** discoloring, inadequate calcification of primary teeth of fetus if used by pregnant women, of permanent teeth if used during dental development; **hepatic impairment;** phototoxic reactions; superinfections
INTERACTIONS Aluminum, bismuth, calcium salts; charcoal; dairy products; food; hormonal contraceptives; iron, magnesium salts; penicillins; urinary alkalinizers; zinc salts
NC/PT Culture before tx. Arrange tx of superinfections. Not for use in

pregnancy (hormonal contraceptives may be ineffective; barrier contraceptives advised). Pt should take on empty stomach 1 hr before or 2 hr after meals; do not use outdated drugs; report rash, urine/stool color changes.

tetrahydrozoline hydrochloride (Murine Plus, Opticlear, Optigene 3, Tyzine, Visine)

CLASS Alpha agonist; decongestant; ophthalmic vasoconstrictor, mydriatic
PREG/CONT C/NA

IND & DOSE Relief of nasal, naso-pharyngeal mucosal congestion. *Adult, child 6 yr and older:* 2–4 drops 0.1% sol in each nostril three to four times/day; or 3–4 sprays in each nostril q 4 hr as needed. Not more often than q 3 hr. *Child 2–6 yr:* 2–3 drops 0.05% sol in each nostril q 4–6 hr as needed Not more often than q 3 hr. **Temporary relief of eye redness, burning, irritation.** *Adult:* 1–2 drops into eye(s) up to qid.

ADV EFF Anxiety, **CV collapse w/ hypotension,** dizziness, drowsiness, headache, light-headedness, pallor, rebound congestion, restlessness, tenseness

INTERACTIONS Methyldopa, MAO-Is, reserpine, TCAs, urine acidifiers/ alkalinizers

NC/PT Monitor BP in pt w/ CAD. Review proper administration. Rebound congestion may occur when drug stopped. Pt should remove contact lenses before using drops, drink plenty of fluids, use humidifier for at least 72 hr, take safety precautions w/ CNS effects, report blurred vision, fainting.

thalidomide (Thalomid)

CLASS Immunomodulator
PREG/CONT X/NA

BBW Associated w/ severe birth defects. Women must have pregnancy

test, signed consent to use birth control to avoid pregnancy during tx (STEPS program). Significant risk of venous thromboembolic events when used in multiple myeloma; monitor accordingly.

IND & DOSE Tx of erythema nodosum leprosum. *Adult* 100–300 mg/day PO at bedtime for at least 2 wk. Taper in decrements of 50 mg q 2–4 wk. **Tx of newly diagnosed multiple myeloma.** *Adult:* 200 mg/day PO w/ dexamethasone.

ADV EFF Agitation, anorexia, anxiety, bradycardia, dizziness, dry skin, dyspnea, headache, nausea, **neutropenia,** orthostatic hypotension, peripheral neuropathy, rash, somnolence, **Stevens-Johnson syndrome,** tumor lysis syndrome

INTERACTIONS Alcohol, CNS depressants, hormonal contraceptives
NC/PT Rule out pregnancy; ensure pt has read, agreed to contraceptive use. Monitor BP, WBC count. Not for use in breast-feeding. Pt should take safety precautions w/ CNS effects, avoid exposure to infection, report dizziness, rash, signs of infection.

theophylline (Elixophyllin, Theo-24, Theochron)

CLASS Bronchodilator, xanthine
PREG/CONT C/NA

IND & DOSE Sx relief or px of bronchial asthma, reversible bronchospasm. *Note:* For dosages for specific populations, see manufacturer's details. *Adult, child over 45 kg:* 300–600 mg/day PO, or 0.4 mg/kg/hr IV. *Child under 45 kg:* Total dose in mg = [(0.2 × age in wk) + 5] × body wt in kg PO/day in four equal doses. Or, 0.7 – 0.8 mg/kg/hr IV (1 – 1.5 mg/kg/12 hr IV for neonate).

ADV EFF Anorexia, **death,** dizziness, headache, insomnia, irritability, **life-threatening ventricular arrhythmias,** n/v, restlessness, **seizures**

INTERACTIONS Barbiturates, benzodiazepines, beta blockers, charcoal, cigarette smoking, cimetidine, ciprofloxacin, erythromycin, halothane, hormonal contraceptives, NMJ blockers, norfloxacin, ofloxacin, phenytoins, rifampin, ranitidine, St. John's wort, ticlopidine, thioamides, thyroid hormones **NC/PT** Maintain serum level in therapeutic range (5–15 mcg/mL); adverse effects related to serum level. Do not add in sol w/ other drugs. Not for use in pregnancy (barrier contraceptives advised). Pt should take ER form on empty stomach 1 hr before or 2 hr after meals, do not cut, crush or chew it; limit caffeine intake; avoid St. John's wort; report smoking changes (dose adjustment needed); take safety precautions w/ CNS effects; report irregular heartbeat, severe GI pain.

DANGEROUS DRUG

thioguanine (Tabloid)
CLASS Antimetabolite, antineoplastic
PREG/CONT D/NA

IND & DOSE Remission induction, consolidation, maint tx of acute nonlymphocytic leukemias. *Adult, child 3 yr and over:* 2 mg/kg/day PO for 4 wk. If no clinical improvement, no toxic effects, increase to 3 mg/kg/day PO.
ADV EFF Anorexia, bone marrow suppression, hepatotoxicity, hyperuricemia, n/v, stomatitis, weakness
NC/PT Monitor CBC (dose adjustment may be needed), LFTs. Not for use in pregnancy (contraceptives advised). Pt should drink 8–10 glasses of fluid/day; avoid exposure to infection; have regular blood tests; perform mouth care for mouth sores; report signs of infection, urine/stool color changes, swelling.

DANGEROUS DRUG

thiotepa (Thioplex)
CLASS Alkylating agent, antineoplastic
PREG/CONT D/NA

IND & DOSE Tx of adenocarcinoma of breast, ovary. *Adult:* 0.3–0.4 mg/kg

IV at 1- to 4-wk intervals. Or, diluted in sterile water to conc of 10 mg/mL, then 0.6–0.8 mg/kg injected directly into tumor after local anesthetic injected through same needle. Maint, 0.6–0.8 mg/kg IV q 1–4 wk. Or, 0.6–0.8 mg/kg intracavity q 1–4 wk through same tube used to remove fluid from bladder. **Superficial papillary carcinoma of urinary bladder.** *Adult:* Dehydrate pt for 8–12 hr before tx. Instill 30–60 mg in 60 mL normal saline injection into bladder by catheter. Have pt retain for 2 hr. If pt unable to retain 60 mL, give in 30 mL. Repeat once/wk for 4 wk.
ADV EFF Amenorrhea, bone marrow suppression, dizziness, fever, headache, n/v, skin reactions
NC/PT Monitor CBC; dose adjustment may be needed. IV sol should be clear w/out solutes. Not for use in pregnancy. Pt should mark calendar of tx days, avoid exposure to infections, take safety precautions w/ dizziness, report unusual bleeding, signs of infection, rash.

---

thiothixene (Navane)
CLASS Antipsychotic, dopaminergic blocker, thioxanthene
PREG/CONT C/NA

BBW Increased risk of death if antipsychotics used to treat elderly pts w/ dementia-related psychosis; not approved for this use.
IND & DOSE Mgt of schizophrenia. *Adult, child over 12 yr:* 2 mg PO tid (mild conditions), 5 mg bid (more severe conditions). Range, 20–30 mg/day; max, 60 mg/day.
ADJUST DOSE Elderly, debilitated pts
ADV EFF Aplastic anemia, autonomic disturbances, blurred vision, bronchospasm, drowsiness, dry mouth, extrapyramidal effects, gynecomastia, HF, laryngospasm, nonthrombocytopenic purpura, pancytopenia, photophobia, pink to red-brown urine, refractory arrhythmias

INTERACTIONS Alcohol, antihypertensives, carbamazepine
NC/PT Monitor renal function, CBC. Urine will turn pink to red-brown. Pt should avoid sun exposure, take safety precautions w/ CNS effects, maintain fluid intake, report signs of infection, unusual bleeding, difficulty breathing. Name confusion between *Navane* (thiothixene) and *Norvasc* (amlodipine); use caution.

thyroid, desiccated
(Armour Thyroid, Nature Thyroid, Thyroid USP, Westhroid)
CLASS Thyroid hormone
PREG/CONT A/NA

BBW Do not use to treat obesity. Large doses in euthyroid pts may produce serious to life-threatening s&sx of toxicity.

IND & DOSE Tx of hypothyroidism. *Adult:* 30 mg/day PO, increased by 15 mg/day q 2–3 wk. Usual main, 60–120 mg PO daily. *Child:* Over 12 yr, 90 mg/day PO; 6–12 yr, 60–90 mg/day PO; 1–5 yr, 45–60 mg/day PO; 6–12 mo, 30–45 mg/day PO; 0–6 mo, 7.5–30 mg/day PO.
ADJUST DOSE Elderly pts, long-standing heart disease
ADV EFF Cardiac arrest, hyperthyroidism, n/v/d, skin reactions
INTERACTIONS Antacids, cholestyramine, digoxin, theophylline, warfarin
NC/PT Monitor thyroid function to establish dose, then at least yearly. Pt should wear medical ID, report headache, palpitations, heat/cold intolerance.

tiagabine hydrochloride
(Gabitril Filmtabs)
CLASS Antiepileptic
PREG/CONT C/NA

BBW Increased risk of suicidal ideation; monitor accordingly.

IND & DOSE Adjunctive tx in partial seizures. *Adult:* 4 mg/day PO for 1 wk; may increase by 4–8 mg/wk until desired response. Usual maint, 32–56 mg daily; max, 56 mg/day in two to four divided doses. *Child 12–18 yr:* 4 mg/day PO for 1 wk; may increase to 8 mg/day in two divided doses for 1 wk, then by 4–8 mg/wk. Max, 32 mg/day in two to four divided doses.
ADV EFF Asthenia, dizziness, GI upset, incontinence, eye changes, **potentially serious rash**, somnolence
INTERACTIONS Alcohol, carbamazepine, CNS depressants, phenobarbital, phenytoin, primidone, valproate
NC/PT Taper when stopping. Not for use in pregnancy (contraceptives advised). Pt should not stop suddenly; take w/ food; avoid alcohol, sleeping pills; wear medical ID; take safety precautions w/ dizziness, vision changes; report rash, thoughts of suicide, vision changes.

ticagrelor (Brilinta)
CLASS Antiplatelet
PREG/CONT C/NA

BBW Significant to fatal bleeding possible; do not use w/ active bleeding, CABG planned within 5 days, surgery. Maint aspirin doses above 100 mg reduce effectiveness; maintain aspirin dose at 75–100 mg/day.
IND & DOSE To reduce rate of thrombotic CV events in pts w/ acute coronary syndrome. *Adult:* Loading dose, 180 mg PO; then 90 mg PO bid w/ 325 mg PO aspirin as loading dose, then maint aspirin dose of 75–100 mg/day PO.
ADV EFF Bleeding, dyspnea
INTERACTIONS Potent CYP3A4 inducers (carbamazepine, dexamethasone, phenobarbital, phenytoin, rifampin), potent CYP3A4 inhibitors (atazanavir, clarithromycin, indinavir, itraconazole, ketoconazole, nefazodone, nelfinavir, ritonavir, saquinavir, telithromycin, voriconazole); avoid these combinations. Digoxin, drugs affecting coagulation, lovastatin, simvastatin

NC/PT Continually monitor for s&sx of bleeding. Ensure concurrent use of 75–100 mg aspirin; do not stop drug except for pathological bleeding. Increased risk of CV events; if drug must be stopped, start another anticoagulant. Assess pt w/ dyspnea for potential underlying cause. Not for use in pregnancy (barrier contraceptive advised), breast-feeding. Pt should take drug exactly as prescribed w/ prescribed dose of aspirin; not increase doses; not stop drug suddenly; report other drugs or herbs being used (many reactions possible; bleeding time may be prolonged), excessive bleeding, difficulty breathing, chest pain, numbness/tingling.

ticlopidine hydrochloride (Ticlid)
CLASS Antiplatelet
PREG/CONT B/NA

BBW Monitor WBC count before, frequently while starting tx; if neutropenia present, stop drug immediately.
IND & DOSE To reduce thrombotic stroke risk in pts who have experienced stroke precursors; px of acute stent thrombosis in coronary arteries. *Adult:* 250 mg PO bid w/ food.
ADV EFF Abd pain, **bleeding**, dizziness, **neutropenia**, n/v/d, pain, rash
INTERACTIONS Antacids, aspirin, cimetidine, digoxin, NSAIDs, theophylline
NC/PT Mark chart to alert all health care providers of use. Monitor WBC; watch for signs of bleeding. Pt should take w/ meals, report unusual bleeding/bruising, signs of infection.

tigecycline (Tygacil)
CLASS Glycylcycline antibiotic
PREG/CONT D/NA

IND & DOSE Tx of complicated skin, skin-structure infections; community-acquired pneumonia; intra-abdominal infections caused by sus-

ceptible bacteria strains. *Adult:* 100 mg IV, then 50 mg IV q 12 hr for 5–14 days; infuse over 30–60 min.
ADJUST DOSE Severe hepatic impairment
ADV EFF Cough, dizziness, dyspnea, headache, n/v/d, photosensitivity, **pseudomembranous colitis**, superinfections
INTERACTIONS Oral contraceptives, warfarin
NC/PT Culture before tx. Not for use in pregnancy, breast-feeding. Pt should avoid sun exposure, report bloody diarrhea, rash, pain at injection site.

tiludronate disodium (Skelid)
CLASS Bisphosphonate
PREG/CONT D/NA

IND & DOSE Tx of Paget disease. *Adult:* 400 mg/day PO for 3 mo w/ 6–8 oz plain water at least 2 hr before food or other beverage.
ADJUST DOSE Severe hepatic impairment
ADV EFF Dyspepsia, flulike sx, headache, hypocalcemia, n/v/d
INTERACTIONS Antacids, aspirin, calcium, indomethacin
NC/PT Monitor serum calcium. Not for use in pregnancy. Allow 3-mo rest period if retreatment needed. Pt should take w/ full glass of water, stay upright for 30 min after taking; not take within 2 hr of food, other oral drug; maintain calcium, vitamin D intake; report difficulty swallowing, muscle tremors.

timolol maleate (Betimol, Blocadren, Istalol, Timoptic)
CLASS Antiglaucoma, antihypertensive, beta blocker
PREG/CONT C/NA

BBW Do not stop abruptly after long-term tx (hypersensitivity to catecholamines possible, causing angina

exacerbation, MI, ventricular arrhythmias). Taper gradually over 2 wk w/monitoring.
IND & DOSE Tx of hypertension. **Adult:** 10 mg bid PO; max, 60 mg/day in two divided doses. Usual range, 20–40 mg/day in two divided doses. Px of reinfarction in MI. 10 mg PO bid within 1–4 wk of infarction. Px of migraine. **Adult:** 10 mg PO bid; during maint, may give 20 mg/day as single dose. To reduce IOP in chronic open-angle glaucoma. 1 drop 0.25% sol bid into affected eye(s); adjust based on response to 1 drop 0.5% sol bid or 1 drop 0.25% sol daily. Or, 1 drop in affected eye(s) each morning (Istalol).
ADV EFF Arrhythmias, **bronchospasm**, constipation, decreased exercise tolerance, dizziness, ED, flatulence, gastric pain, **HF**, hyperglycemia, **laryngospasm**, n/v/d, ocular irritation w/ eyedrops, **PE**, **stroke**
INTERACTIONS Antacids, aspirin, calcium, indomethacin
NC/PT Alert surgeon if surgery required. Do not stop abruptly; must be tapered. Teach proper eyedrop administration. Pt should take safety precautions w/ dizziness; report difficulty breathing, swelling, numbness/tingling.

tinidazole (Tindamax)
CLASS Antiprotozoal
PREG/CONT C/NA

BBW Avoid use unless clearly needed; carcinogenic in lab animals.
IND & DOSE Tx of trichomoniasis, giardiasis. **Adult:** Single dose of 2 g PO w/ food. **Child over 3 yr:** For giardiasis, single dose of 50 mg/kg PO (up to 2 g) w/ food. Tx of amebiasis. **Adult:** 2 g/day PO for 3 days w/ food. **Child over 3 yr:** 50 mg/kg/day PO (up to 2 g/day) for 3 days w/ food. For giardiasis, Tx of amebic liver abscess. **Adult:** 2 g/day PO for 3–5 days

w/ food. **Child over 3 yr:** 50 mg/kg/day PO (up to 2 g/day) for 3–5 days w/ food.
ADV EFF Anorexia, dizziness, drowsiness, metallic taste, neutropenia, **seizures**, **severe hypersensitivity reactions**, superinfections, weakness
INTERACTIONS Alcohol, cholestyramine, cimetidine, cyclosporine, disulfiram, 5-FU, ketoconazole, lithium, oral anticoagulants, oxytetracycline, phenytoin, tacrolimus
NC/PT Give w/ food. Ensure proper hygiene, tx of superinfections. Urine may become very dark. Pt should take safety precautions w/ dizziness; avoid alcohol during, for 3 days after tx; report vaginal itching, white patches in mouth, difficulty breathing.

tiopronin (Thiola)
CLASS Thiol compound
PREG/CONT C/NA

IND & DOSE Px of cystine kidney stone formation in severe homozygous cystinuria. **Adult:** 800 mg/day PO; increase to 1,000 mg/day in divided doses on empty stomach. **Child 9 yr and over:** 15 mg/kg/day PO on empty stomach; adjust based on urine cystine level.
ADV EFF **Hepatotoxicity**, nephrotoxicity, n/v/d, rash, skin/taste changes
NC/PT Monitor cystine at 1 mo, then q 3 mo. Not for use in breast-feeding. Pt should drink fluids liberally (to 3 L/day), report urine/stool color changes, rash.

tiotropium bromide (Spiriva)
CLASS Anticholinergic, bronchodilator
PREG/CONT C/NA

IND & DOSE Long-term once-daily maint tx of bronchospasm. **Adult:** 2 inhalations/day of contents of one capsule using HandiHaler device.

ADV EFF Abd pain, blurred vision, constipation, dry mouth, epistaxis, glaucoma, rash, urine retention
INTERACTIONS Anticholinergics
NC/PT Evaluate for glaucoma; stop drug if increased IOP. Not for use in acute attacks. Review proper use of *HandiHaler* device. Pt should empty bladder before each dose, use sugarless lozenges for dry mouth, report eye pain, vision changes.

tipranavir (Aptivus)
CLASS Antiviral, protease inhibitor
PREG/CONT C/NA

BBW Increased risk of hepatotoxicity in pts w/ hepatitis; assess liver function before, periodically during tx. Giving w/ ritonavir has caused nonfatal, fatal intracranial hemorrhage; monitor results.
IND & DOSE Tx of HIV infection.
Adult: 500 mg/day PO w/ ritonavir 200 mg, w/ food. *Child 2–18 yr:* 14 mg/kg w/ ritonavir 6 mg/kg PO bid (375 mg/m² w/ ritonavir 150 mg/m² PO bid). Max, 500 mg bid w/ ritonavir 200 mg bid, w/ food.
ADV EFF Abd pain, cough, depression, fever, flulike sx, headache, **hepatomegaly and steatosis**, n/v/d, **potentially fatal liver impairment**
INTERACTIONS Amprenavir, atorvastatin, calcium channel blockers, cyclosporine, desipramine, didanosine, disulfiram, hormonal contraceptives, itraconazole, ketoconazole, lopinavir, meperidine, methadone, metronidazole, oral antidiabetics, saquinavir, sildenafil, sirolimus, SSRIs, St. John's wort, tacrolimus, tadalafil, vardenafil, voriconazole, warfarin. Contraindicated w/ amiodarone, dihydroergotamine, ergotamine, flecainide, lovastatin, methylergonovine, midazolam, pimozide, propafenone, quinidine, rifampin, simvastatin, triazolam.
NC/PT Ensure pt also taking ritonavir. Review drug hx before tx; multiple interactions possible. Monitor LFTs. Not

for use in pregnancy, breast-feeding. Pt should take w/ food; swallow capsule whole and not cut, crush, or chew it; store capsules in refrigerator (do not refrigerate sol); not use after expiration date; use precautions to prevent spread (drug not a cure); avoid exposure to infection, St. John's wort; report general malaise, urine/stool color changes, yellowing of skin/eyes.

tirofiban hydrochloride (Aggrastat)
CLASS Antiplatelet
PREG/CONT B/NA

IND & DOSE Tx of acute coronary syndromes, w/ heparin; px of cardiac ischemic complications in percutaneous coronary intervention.
Adult: 0.4 mcg/kg/min IV infusion over 30 min; continue at rate of 0.1 mcg/kg/min.
ADJUST DOSE Renal impairment
ADV EFF Bleeding, bradycardia, dizziness, flushing, hypotension, syncope
INTERACTIONS Antiplatelets, aspirin, chamomile, don quai, feverfew, garlic, ginger, ginkgo, ginseng, grape seed extract, green leaf tea, heparin, horse chestnut seed, NSAIDs, turmeric, warfarin
NC/PT Obtain baseline, periodic CBC, PT, aPTT, active clotting time. Maintain aPTT between 50 and 70 sec, and active clotting time between 300 and 350 sec. Avoid noncompressible IV access sites to prevent excessive, uncontrollable bleeding. Pt should report light-headedness, palpitations, pain at injection site. Name confusion between *Aggrastat* (tirofiban) and argatroban; use caution.

tizanidine (Zanaflex)
CLASS Alpha agonist, antispasmodic
PREG/CONT C/NA

IND & DOSE Acute, intermittent mgt of increased muscle tone

associated w/ spasticity. *Adult:*
4 mg/day PO, increased in 2- to 4-mg
increments as needed over 2–4 wk.
Maint, 8 mg PO q 6–8 hr; max,
36 mg/day in divided doses.
ADJUST DOSE Hepatic, renal impairment
ADV EFF Asthenia, constipation,
dizziness, drowsiness, dry mouth, **QT
prolongation,** sedation
INTERACTIONS Alcohol, baclofen,
CNS depressants, hormonal contraceptives, other alpha$_2$-adrenergic agonists
NC/PT Continue all supportive measures for neurologically damaged pt.
Pt should take around the clock for
best results, use sugarless lozenges
for dry mouth, avoid alcohol, take
safety precautions w/ CNS effects,
know that hormonal contraceptives
may be ineffective; report vision
changes, difficulty swallowing, fainting.

tobramycin sulfate
(TOBI, Tobrex Ophthalmic)
CLASS Alpha agonist,
antispasmodic
PREG/CONT D (injection,
inhalation); B (ophthalmic)/NA

BBW Injection may cause serious
ototoxicity, nephrotoxicity, neurotoxicity. Monitor closely for changes in
renal, CNS function.
IND & DOSE **Tx of serious infections caused by susceptible bacteria
strains.** *Adult:* 3 mg/kg/day IM or IV
in three equal doses q 8 hr; max,
5 mg/kg/day. *Child over 1 wk:*
6–7.5 mg/kg/day IM or IV in three to
four equally divided doses. *Premature
infants, neonates 1 wk or younger:* Up
to 4 mg/kg/day IM or IV in two equal
doses q 12 hr. **Mgt of cystic fibrosis
pts w/** *Pseudomonas aeruginosa.*
Adult, child 6 yr and older: 300 mg bid
by nebulizer inhaled over 10–15 min.
Give in 28-day cycles: 28 days on,
28 days rest. **Tx of superficial ocular
infections due to susceptible organ-**

ism strains. *Adult, child 6 yr and older:* 1–2 drops into conjunctival sac of
affected eye(s) q 4 hr, 2 drops/hr in
severe infections. Or, ½ inch ribbon
bid–tid.
ADJUST DOSE Elderly pts, renal
impairment
ADV EFF Anorexia, leukemoid reaction, palpitations, ototoxicity, **nephrotoxicity,** numbness/tingling, n/v/d,
purpura, rash, superinfections, vestibular paralysis
INTERACTIONS Aminoglycosides,
beta-lactam antibiotics, cephalosporins, NMJ blockers, penicillin, succinylcholine
NC/PT Culture before tx. Limit tx duration to 7–14 days to decrease toxic
reactions. Do not mix in sol w/ other
drugs. Review proper administration
of eyedrops, nebulizer. Pt should
mark calendar of tx days; store in refrigerator, protected from light; drink
8–10 glasses of fluid/day; take safety
precautions w/ CNS effects; report
hearing changes, dizziness, pain at
injection site.

tocilizumab (Actemra)
CLASS Antirheumatic,
interleukin-6 receptor inhibitor
PREG/CONT C/NA

BBW Serious to life-threatening infections possible, including TB and
bacterial, invasive fungal, viral, opportunistic infections. Perform TB
test before tx. Interrupt tx if serious
infection occurs; monitor for TB s&sx
during tx.
IND & DOSE **Tx of moderately to
severely active rheumatoid arthritis.** *Adult:* 4 mg/kg by IV infusion
over 1 hr, then increase to 8 mg/kg
based on clinical response; may repeat once q 4 wk; max, 800 mg/infusion. **Tx of active systemic juvenile
arthritis/Still disease (systemic idiopathic juvenile arthritis).** *Child
2 yr and over:* 30 kg or more, 8 mg/kg
IV q 2 wk; under 30 kg, 12 mg/kg IV
q 2 wk.

ADV EFF Anaphylaxis, dizziness, hypertension, increased liver enzymes, nasopharyngitis, **potentially serious infections**, URI
INTERACTIONS Anti-CD20 monoclonal antibodies, cyclosporine, interleukin receptor antagonists, live vaccines, omeprazole, statins, TNF antagonists, warfarin
NC/PT Do not mix in sol w/ other drugs. Monitor CBC, LFTs, lipids carefully. Not for use in pregnancy, breast-feeding. Pt should consider other drugs for arthritis; avoid live vaccines, exposure to infection; report signs of infection, difficulty breathing, easy bruising/bleeding.

tofacitinib (Xeljanz)
CLASS Antirheumatic, kinase inhibitor
PREG/CONT C/NA

BBW Risk of serious to fatal infections, including TB; test for TB before tx; do not give w/ active infections. Risk of lymphoma, other malignancies.
IND & DOSE Tx of adults w/ moderately to severely active rheumatoid arthritis intolerant to other therapies. Adult: 5 mg PO bid.
ADJUST DOSE Hepatic, renal impairment
ADV EFF Diarrhea, GI perforation, headache, **lymphoma, serious to fatal infections**, URI
INTERACTIONS Fluconazole, ketoconazole, rifampin, vaccines
NC/PT Screen for TB, active infection before tx; monitor for s&sx of infection. Monitor for lymphoma, other malignancies. May combine w/ other antirheumatics. Not for use in pregnancy. Pt should take as directed bid; avoid exposure to infections; avoid vaccines; report severe GI pain, fever, s&sx of infection.

TOLAZamide (generic)
CLASS Antidiabetic, sulfonylurea
PREG/CONT C/NA

BBW Increased risk of CV mortality; monitor accordingly.
IND & DOSE Adjunct to diet, exercise to control blood glucose in pts w/ type 2 diabetes; w/ insulin to control blood glucose in select pts with type 1 diabetes. Adult: 100–250 mg/day PO; max, 1 g/day.
ADJUST DOSE Elderly pts
ADV EFF Bone marrow suppression, dizziness, fatigue, heartburn, hypoglycemia, rash, vertigo
INTERACTIONS Beta-adrenergic blockers, calcium channel blockers, chloramphenicol, corticosteroids, coumarins, estrogens, isoniazid, MAOIs, miconazole, nicotinic acid, oral contraceptives, phenothiazines, phenytoin, probenecid, salicylates, sulfonamides, sympathomimetics, thyroid products
NC/PT Review complete diabetic teaching program. Pt should take in a.m. w/ breakfast (do not take if not eating that day); continue diet, exercise program; avoid exposure to infection; report uncontrolled blood glucose, dizziness.

TOLBUTamide (Orinase)
CLASS Antidiabetic, sulfonylurea
PREG/CONT C/NA

BBW Increased risk of CV mortality; monitor accordingly.
IND & DOSE Adjunct to diet, exercise to control blood glucose in pts w/ type 2 diabetes; w/ insulin to control blood glucose in select pts with type 1 diabetes. Adult: 1–2 g/day PO in a.m. before breakfast. Maint, 0.25–3 g/day PO; max, 3 g/day.
Dx of pancreatic islet cell adenoma. Adult: 20 mL IV infused over 2–3 min.
ADJUST DOSE Elderly pts

ADV EFF Bone marrow suppression, dizziness, fatigue, heartburn, hypoglycemia, rash, vertigo
INTERACTIONS Beta-adrenergic blockers, calcium channel blockers, chloramphenicol, corticosteroids, coumarins, estrogens, isoniazid, MAOIs, miconazole, nicotinic acid, oral contraceptives, phenothiazines, phenytoin, probenecid, salicylates, sulfonamides, sympathomimetics, thyroid products
NC/PT Review complete diabetic teaching program. Pt may be switched to insulin during high stress. Pt should take in a.m. w/ breakfast (do not take if not eating that day); continue diet, exercise program; avoid exposure to infection; report uncontrolled blood glucose, dizziness.

tolcapone (Tasmar)
CLASS Antiparkinsonian, COMT inhibitor
PREG/CONT C/NA

BBW Risk of potentially fatal acute fulminant liver failure. Monitor LFTs before, q 2 wk during tx; discontinue if signs of liver damage. Use for pts no longer responding to other therapies.
IND & DOSE Adjunct w/ levodopa/carbidopa in tx of s&sx of idiopathic Parkinson disease. *Adult:* 100 mg PO tid; max, 600 mg.
ADJUST DOSE Hepatic, renal impairment
ADV EFF Confusion; constipation; disorientation; dry mouth; **fulminant, possibly fatal liver failure;** hallucinations; hypotension; light-headedness; n/v, rash, weakness
INTERACTIONS MAOIs
NC/PT Monitor LFTs before, q 2 wk during tx. Always give w/ levodopa/carbidopa. Do not give within 14 days of MAOIs. Taper over 2 wk when stopping. Not for use in pregnancy, breast-feeding. Pt should take w/ meals, use sugarless lozenges for dry mouth, take safety precautions w/ CNS effects, use laxative for

constipation, report urine/stool color changes, fever.

tolmetin sodium
(generic)
CLASS NSAID
PREG/CONT C (1st, 2nd trimesters); D (3rd trimester)/NA

BBW Increased risk of CV events, GI bleeding; monitor accordingly. Not for use for periop pain in CABG surgery.
IND & DOSE Tx of acute flares; long-term mgt of rheumatoid arthritis (RA), osteoarthritis. *Adult:* 400 mg PO tid (1,200 mg/day) preferably including dose on arising and at bedtime. Maint, 600–1,800 mg/day in three to four divided doses for RA, 600–1,600 mg/day in three to four divided doses for osteoarthritis. Tx of juvenile RA. *Child 2 yr and older:* 20 mg/kg/day PO in three to four divided doses. Usual dose, 15–30 mg/kg/day max, 30 mg/kg/day.
ADV EFF Anaphylactoid reactions to fatal anaphylactic shock, bone marrow suppression, bronchospasm, diarrhea, dizziness, dyspepsia, dysuria, GI pain, headache, insomnia, rash, somnolence, vision problems
NC/PT Pt should take w/ milk if GI upset a problem, have periodic eye exams, take safety precautions w/ CNS effects, report signs of infection, difficulty breathing, unusual bleeding.

tolterodine tartrate
(Detrol)
CLASS Antimuscarinic
PREG/CONT C/NA

IND & DOSE Tx of overactive bladder. *Adult:* 1–2 mg PO bid. ER form, 2–4 mg/day PO.
ADJUST DOSE Hepatic, renal impairment
ADV EFF Blurred vision, constipation, dizziness, dry mouth, dyspepsia, n/v, vision changes, weight gain

INTERACTIONS CYP2D6, CYP3A4 inhibitors
NC/PT Pt should swallow capsule whole and not cut, crush, or chew it; use sugarless lozenges for dry mouth; take laxative for constipation, safety precautions w/ CNS effects; report rash, difficulty breathing, palpitations.

tolvaptan (Samsca)
CLASS Selective vasopressin receptor antagonist
PREG/CONT C/NA

BBW Initiate tx in hospital setting, w/ close supervision of sodium, volume. Not for use when rapid correction of hyponatremia needed.
IND & DOSE Tx of clinically significant hypervolemic, euvolemic hyponatremia. *Adult:* 15 mg PO daily; may increase after at least 24 hr to max 60 mg/day.
ADV EFF Asthenia, constipation, dehydration, dry mouth, hyperglycemia, polyuria, **serious liver toxicity,** thirst
INTERACTIONS CYP3A inducers/inhibitors
NC/PT Do not use w/ hypertonic saline sol. Monitor serum electrolytes. Not for use in emergency situation, pregnancy, breast-feeding. Pt should report severe constipation, increasing thirst, fainting.

topiramate (Topamax, Topiragen)
CLASS Antiepileptic, antimigraine
PREG/CONT D/NA

BBW Increased risk of suicidality; monitor accordingly. Reduce dose, stop, or substitute other antiepileptic gradually; stopping abruptly may precipitate status epilepticus.
IND & DOSE Px of migraines: *Adult, child 17 yr and older:* 25 mg PO in p.m. for 1 wk; wk 2, 25 mg PO bid a.m. and p.m.; wk 3, 25 mg PO in a.m., 50 mg PO in p.m.; wk 4, 50 mg PO a.m. and

p.m. **Tx of seizure disorders.** *Adult, child 17 yr and older:* 200–400 m/day PO in two divided doses. *Child 10 yr and older:* 25 mg PO bid, titrating to maint dose of 200 mg PO bid over 6 wk. wk 1, 25 mg bid; wk 2, 50 mg bid; wk 3, 75 mg bid; wk 4, 100 mg bid; wk 5, 150 mg bid; wk 6, 200 mg bid. Or ER form, 25 mg PO at bedtime, range 1–3 mg/kg for first week; titrate at 1- to 2-wk intervals by 1- to 3-mg/kg increments to 5–9 mg/kg/day PO. *Child 2–16 yr:* 5–9 mg/kg/day PO in two divided doses. Start tx at nightly dose of 25 mg (or less, based on 1–3 mg/kg/day) for first wk. May titrate up by increments of 1–3 mg/kg/day (in two divided doses) at 1- to 2-wk intervals.
ADJUST DOSE Hepatic, renal impairment
ADV EFF Ataxia, dizziness, dysmenorrhea, dyspepsia, fatigue, nausea, nystagmus, paresthesia, renal stones, somnolence, URI
INTERACTIONS Alcohol, carbamazepine, carbonic anhydrase inhibitors, CNS depressants, hormonal contraceptives, phenytoin, valproic acid
NC/PT Taper if stopping. Not for use in pregnancy (may make hormonal contraceptives ineffective; barrier contraceptives advised). Pt should not cut, crush, or chew tablets (bitter taste); may swallow sprinkle capsule whole or sprinkle contents on soft food, swallow immediately; should avoid alcohol; take safety precautions w/ CNS effects; report vision changes, flank pain, thoughts of suicide. Name confusion between *Topamax* and *Toprol-XL* (metoprolol); use caution.

DANGEROUS DRUG

topotecan hydrochloride (Hycamtin)
CLASS Antineoplastic
PREG/CONT D/NA

BBW Monitor bone marrow carefully; do not give dose until bone marrow responsive.

IND & DOSE Tx of metastatic ovarian cancer, small-cell lung cancer. *Adult:* 1.5 mg/m²/day IV over 30 min for 5 days, starting on day 1 of 21-day course. Minimum four courses recommended. **Tx of persistent cervical cancer.** *Adult:* 0.75 mg/m² by IV infusion over 30 min on days 1, 2, 3 followed by cisplatin on day 1. Repeat q 21 days.

ADJUST DOSE Hepatic, renal impairment

ADV EFF Alopecia, **bone marrow suppression,** constipation, fever, infections, **interstitial pneumonitis,** n/v/d, pain

INTERACTIONS Cytotoxic drugs

NC/PT Monitor CBC; dose adjustment may be needed. Not for use in pregnancy (barrier contraceptives advised), breast-feeding. Pt should mark calendar of tx days, cover head at temp extremes (hair loss possible), avoid exposure to infection, take analgesics for pain, report difficulty breathing, unusual bleeding, signs of infection.

DANGEROUS DRUG

toremifene citrate (Fareston)
CLASS Antineoplastic, estrogen receptor modulator
PREG/CONT D/NA

BBW Risk of prolonged QT interval. Obtain baseline, periodic ECG; avoid concurrent use of other QT-prolonging drugs.

IND & DOSE Tx of advanced breast cancer in postmenopausal women. *Adult:* 60 mg PO daily; continue until disease progression.

ADV EFF Depression, dizziness, headache, hot flashes, n/v, **prolonged QT interval,** rash, vaginal discharge

INTERACTIONS Oral anticoagulants, other drugs that decrease calcium excretion, QT-prolonging drugs

NC/PT Obtain baseline ECG; monitor periodically during tx. Not for use in pregnancy (barrier contraceptives advised). Pt should take safety precautions w/ dizziness, report palpitations, vision changes.

---

torsemide (Demadex)
CLASS Loop diuretic, sulfonamide
PREG/CONT B/NA

IND & DOSE Tx of edema associated w/ HF. *Adult:* 10–20 mg/day PO or IV; max, 200 mg/day. **Tx of edema associated w/ chronic renal failure.** *Adult:* 20 mg/day PO or IV; max, 200 mg/day. **Tx of edema associated w/ hepatic failure.** *Adult:* 5–10 mg/day PO or IV; max, 40 mg/day. **Tx of hypertension.** *Adult:* 5 mg/day PO.

ADV EFF Anorexia, asterixis, dizziness, drowsiness, headache, hypokalemia, nocturia, n/v/d, orthostatic hypotension, ototoxicity, pain, phlebitis at injection site, polyuria

INTERACTIONS Aminoglycoside antibiotics, cisplatin, digoxin, ethacrynic acid, NSAIDs

NC/PT Monitor serum electrolytes. Pt should take early in day to prevent sleep disruption; weigh self daily, report changes of more than 3 lb/day; take safety precautions w/ CNS effects; report swelling, hearing loss, muscle cramps/weakness.

DANGEROUS DRUG

tositumomab and iodine I-131 tositumomab (Bexxar)
CLASS Antineoplastic, monoclonal antibody
PREG/CONT X/NA

BBW Risk of severe, prolonged cytopenia. Hypersensitivity reactions, including anaphylaxis, have occurred.

IND & DOSE Tx of CD20-positive, follicular non-Hodgkin lymphoma. *Adult:* 450 mg tositumomab IV in 50 mL normal saline over 60 min, 5 mCi I-131 w/ 35 mg tositumomab in 30 mL normal saline IV over 20 min;

then repeat as therapeutic step, adjusting I-131 dose per pt response.
ADV EFF Anorexia, asthenia, **cancer development,** fever, headache, hypothyroidism, n/v/d, **severe cytopenia**
NC/PT Radioactive; use special handling precautions. Rule out pregnancy; not for use in pregnancy (two types of contraceptives advised), breast-feeding. Monitor CBC, renal function. Discuss limiting exposure to family; will take about 12 days to clear body. Pt should report signs of infection, unusual bleeding.

DANGEROUS DRUG

tramadol hydrochloride (ConZip, Rybix ODT, Ryzolt, Ultram)
CLASS Opioid analgesic
PREG/CONT C/NA

IND & DOSE Relief of moderate to moderately severe pain.
Adult: 50–100 mg PO q 4–6 hr; max, 400 mg/day. For chronic pain, 25 mg/day PO in a.m.; titrate in 25-mg increments q 3 days to 100 mg/day. Then, increase in 50-mg increments q 3 days to 200 mg/day. After titration, 50–100 mg q 4–6 hr PO; max, 400 mg/day. Or, 100-mg PO ER tablet once daily, titrated by 100-mg increments q 5 days; max, 300 mg/day. For orally disintegrating tablets, max, 200 mg/day PO.
ADJUST DOSE Elderly pts; hepatic, renal impairment
ADV EFF Anaphylactoid reactions, constipation, dizziness, headache, hypotension, n/v, sedation, **seizures, suicidality,** sweating, vertigo
INTERACTIONS Alcohol, carbamazepine, CNS depressants, MAOIs, SSRIs
NC/PT Control environment; use other measures to relieve pain. Limit use w/ hx of addiction. Pt should swallow ER tablet whole and not cut, crush, or chew it; dissolve orally disintegrating tablets in mouth, then

swallow w/ water; take safety precautions w/ CNS effects; report thoughts of suicide.

---

trametinib (Mekinist)
CLASS Antineoplastic, kinase inhibitor
PREG/CONT D/NA

IND & DOSE Tx of unresectable or metastatic melanoma with BRAF V600E or V600K mutations. *Adult:* 2 mg/day PO 1 hr before or 2 hr after meal.
ADJUST DOSE Severe renal, hepatic impairment
ADV EFF **Cardiomyopathy,** diarrhea, **interstitial lung disease,** lymphedema, **retinal pigment epithelial detachment, retinal vein occlusion, serious skin toxicity**
NC/PT Ensure regular ophthalmic exams. Evaluate left ventricular ejection fraction before and every 2 mo during tx. Evaluate lung function; stop drug if sx of interstitial pneumonitis. Watch for rash, skin toxicity; stop drug if grade 2–4 rash does not improve with 3-wk interruption. Pt should take drug 1 hr before or 2 hr after meal; avoid pregnancy, breast-feeding; know frequent testing and follow-up will be needed; be aware drug could impair fertility; report difficulty breathing, extreme fatigue, swelling of extremities, rash, vision changes.

---

trandolapril (Mavik)
CLASS ACE inhibitor, antihypertensive
PREG/CONT D/NA

BBW Rule out pregnancy before tx; advise use of barrier contraceptives. Fetal injury, death has occurred when used in second, third trimester.
IND & DOSE Tx of hypertension. *Adult:* African-American pts: 2 mg/day PO. All other pts: 1 mg/day PO. Maint, 2–4 mg/day; max, 8 mg/day. **Tx of HF post-MI.** *Adult:* 1 mg/day PO; may

start 3–5 days after MI. Adjust to target 4 mg/day.
ADJUST DOSE Hepatic, renal impairment
ADV EFF Cough, diarrhea, dizziness, headache, **hypersensitivity reactions, MI**, renal impairment, tachycardia
INTERACTIONS Diuretics, lithium, potassium supplements
NC/PT If pt on diuretic, stop diuretic 2–3 days before starting trandolapril; resume diuretic only if BP not controlled. If diuretic cannot be stopped, start at 0.5 mg PO daily; adjust upward as needed. Alert surgeon; volume replacement may be needed postop. Not for use in pregnancy (barrier contraceptives advised). Pt should use care in situations that could lead to BP drop; take safety precautions w/ CNS effects; report difficulty breathing, swelling of lips/face, chest pain.

tranexamic acid
(Lysteda)
CLASS Antifibrinolytic
PREG/CONT B/NA

IND & DOSE Tx of cyclic heavy menstrual bleeding. *Adult:* 1,300 mg PO tid for max 5 days during monthly menstruation.
ADJUST DOSE Hepatic, renal impairment
ADV EFF Abd pain, **anaphylactic shock, anaphylactoid reactions,** arthralgia, back pain, fatigue, headache, n/v/d, **thromboembolic events,** visual disturbances
INTERACTIONS Hormonal contraceptives, TPAs
NC/PT Obtain baseline, periodic evaluation of bleeding. Not for use in pregnancy (hormonal contraceptives may increase thromboembolic event risk; barrier contraceptives advised). Pt should report difficulty breathing, leg pain/swelling, severe headache, vision changes.

tranylcypromine sulfate
(Parnate)
CLASS Antidepressant, MAOI
PREG/CONT C/NA

BBW Limit amount available to suicidal pts. Possible increased risk of suicidality in children, adolescents, young adults; monitor accordingly.
IND & DOSE Tx of major depressive disorder. *Adult:* 30 mg/day PO in divided doses. If no improvement within 2–3 wk, increase in 10-mg/day increments q 1–3 wk. Max, 60 mg/day.
ADJUST DOSE Elderly pts
ADV EFF Abd pain, anorexia, blurred vision, confusion, constipation, dizziness, drowsiness, dry mouth, headache, hyperreflexia, **hypertensive crises,** hypomania, hypotension, insomnia, jitteriness, **liver toxicity,** n/v/d, orthostatic hypotension, photosensitivity, suicidal thoughts, twitching, vertigo
INTERACTIONS Alcohol, amphetamines, antidiabetics, beta blockers, bupropion, buspirone, general anesthetics, meperidine, SSRIs, sympathomimetics, TCAs, thiazides, tyramine-containing foods
NC/PT Have phentolamine, another alpha-adrenergic blocker on hand for hypertensive crisis. Do not use within 14 days of MAOIs, within 10 days of buspirone, bupropion. Monitor LFTs, BP regularly. Pt should avoid diet high in tyramine-containing foods during, for 2 wk after tx; avoid alcohol, OTC appetite suppressants; take safety precautions w/ CNS effects; change position slowly w/ orthostatic hypotension; report rash, urine/stool color changes, thoughts of suicide.

DANGEROUS DRUG

trastuzumab (Herceptin)

CLASS Antineoplastic, monoclonal antibody (anti-HER2)
PREG/CONT D/NA

BBW Monitor pt during infusion; provide comfort measures, analgesics as appropriate for infusion reaction. Monitor cardiac status, especially if pt receiving chemotherapy; do not give w/ anthracycline chemotherapy. Have emergency equipment on hand for cardiotoxicity; cardiomyopathy possible. Monitor for possibly severe pulmonary toxicity, especially within 24 hours of infusion. Stop if s&sx of respiratory involvement. Embryotoxic; ensure pt is not pregnancy before tx (advise use of contraceptive measures).

IND & DOSE Tx of metastatic HER2 overexpressing breast cancer. *Adult:* 4 mg/kg IV once by IV infusion over 90 min. Maint, 2 mg/kg/wk IV over at least 30 min as tolerated; max, 500 mg/dose. **Adjunct tx of HER2-overexpressing breast cancer.** *Adult:* After completion of doxorubicin, cyclophosphamide tx, give wkly for 52 wk. Initially, 4 mg/kg by IV infusion over 90 min; maint, 2 mg/kg/wk by IV infusion over 30 min. Or, initially, 8 mg/kg by IV infusion over 90 min; then 6 mg/kg by IV infusion over 30–90 min q 3 wk. During first 12 wk, give w/ paclitaxel. **Tx of metastatic gastric cancer.** *Adult:* 8 mg/kg IV over 90 min; then 6 mg/kg IV over 30 min q 3 wk until disease progression.

ADV EFF Abd pain, anemia, diarrhea, fever, infections, injection-site reactions, leukopenia, paresthesia, **pulmonary toxicity, serious cardiac toxicity**
NC/PT Do not mix w/ other drug sols or add other drugs to IV line. Monitor cardiac status; have emergency equipment on hand. Monitor respiratory status. Pt should mark calendar of tx days; avoid exposure to infection; avoid pregnancy (contraceptive

measures advised); report chest pain, difficulty breathing, pain at injection site.

trazodone hydrochloride (Oleptro)

CLASS Antidepressant
PREG/CONT C/NA

BBW Increased risk of suicidality; limit quantities in depressed, suicidal pts.

IND & DOSE Tx of depression. *Adult:* 150 mg/day PO in divided doses; max, 400 mg/day PO in divided doses. ER tablets *(Oleptro)*, 150 mg/day PO; max, 375 mg/day. For severe depression, max, 600 mg/day PO.
ADJUST DOSE Elderly pts
ADV EFF Blurred vision, constipation, dizziness, **NMS**, orthostatic hypotension, sedation, withdrawal syndrome
INTERACTIONS Alcohol, aspirin, CNS depressants, CYP3A4 inducers/inhibitors, digoxin, MAOIs, NSAIDS, phenytoin, SSRIs, St. John's wort
NC/PT Do not give within 14 days of MAOIs. Taper when stopping; do not stop abruptly. Use caution in pregnancy, breast-feeding. Pt should take safety precautions w/ CNS effects, report fever, severe constipation, thoughts of suicide.

treprostinil sodium (Remodulin, Tyvaso)

CLASS Endothelin receptor antagonist, vasodilator
PREG/CONT B/NA

IND & DOSE Tx of pulmonary arterial hypertension. *Adult:* 1.25 ng/kg/min subcut infusion. Increase rate in increments of no more than 1.25 ng/kg/min wkly for first 4 wk, then by 2.5 ng/kg/min wkly. Max, 40 ng/kg/min or 3 breaths (18 mcg), using *Tyvaso* Inhalation System, per tx session; 4 sessions/day, approximately 4 hr apart during waking hours. Increase by additional

3 breaths/session at 1- to 2-wk intervals if needed, tolerated. Maint, 9 breaths (54 mcg)/session.

ADJUST DOSE Hepatic impairment
ADV EFF Edema, headache, infusion-site reaction, jaw pain, n/d, rash
INTERACTIONS Anticoagulants, antihypertensives, antiplatelets
NC/PT See manufacturer's instructions if switching from epoprostenol *(Flolan)*. Obtain baseline pulmonary status, exercise tolerance. Not for use in pregnancy (barrier contraceptives advised). Taper slowly when stopping. Evaluate subcut infusion site wkly; give analgesics for headache. Teach proper care, use of continuous subcut infusion; if using inhalation, review proper use. Pt should continue usual tx procedures, report swelling, injection site pain/swelling, worsening condition.

DANGEROUS DRUG

tretinoin (Atralin, Avita, Renova, Retin-A, Tretin-X)
CLASS Antineoplastic, retinoid
PREG/CONT D/NA

BBW Rule out pregnancy before tx; arrange for pregnancy test within 2 wk of starting tx. Advise use of two forms of contraception during tx, for 1 mo after tx ends. Should only be used under supervision of experienced practitioner or in institution experienced w/ its use. Risk of rapid leukocytosis (40% of pts); notify physician immediately if this occurs. Stop drug, notify physician if LFTs over five times upper limit of normal, pulmonary infiltrates appear, or pt has difficulty breathing; serious side effects possible. Monitor for retinoic acid-APL syndrome (fever, dyspnea, acute respiratory distress, weight gain, pulmonary infiltrates, pleural/pericardial effusion, multiorgan failure); endotracheal intubation, mechanical ventilation may be needed.
IND & DOSE To induce remission in acute promyelocytic leukemia

(APL). *Adult, child 1 yr and over:* 45 mg/m²/day PO in two evenly divided doses until complete remission; stop tx 30 days after complete remission obtained or after 90 days, whichever first. **Topical tx of acne vulgaris; mitigation of wrinkles; mottled hyperpigmentation.** *Adult, child 1 yr and over:* Apply once/day before bedtime. Cover entire affected area lightly, avoiding mucous membranes.

ADV EFF Cardiac arrest, dry skin, earache, fever, GI bleeding, headache, lipid changes, **MI,** n/v, **pseudotumor cerebri, rapid/evolving leukocytosis,** rash, sweating, visual disturbances.
INTERACTIONS Hydroxyurea, keratolytic agents, ketoconazole, tetracyclines
NC/PT Monitor LFTs, lipids, vision. Not for use in pregnancy (two forms of contraceptives, during and for 1 mo after tx, advised). Pt cannot donate blood during tx. Pt should not cut, crush oral capsule; have frequent blood tests; avoid products containing vitamin D; take safety precautions w/ CNS effects; use sugarless lozenges w/ dry mouth; report severe/bloody diarrhea, difficulty breathing, thoughts of suicide.

---

triamcinolone acetonide (Kenalog, Nasacort), **triamcinolone diacetate, triamcinolone hexacetonide** (Aristospan)
CLASS Corticosteroid
PREG/CONT C/NA

IND & DOSE Hypercalcemia of cancer; mgt of various inflammatory disorders; tx of idiopathic thrombocytopenic purpura. *Adult:* Individualize dose, depending on condition severity, pt response. Give daily dose before 9 a.m. to minimize adrenal suppression. If long-term tx needed, consider alternate-day tx. After long-term tx, withdraw slowly to avoid adrenal insufficiency. Range, 2.5–100 mg/day IM. *Child:* Individualize dose based on response, not formulae; monitor growth. **Maint, tx of bronchial asthma.** *Adult, child 6–12 yr:* 200 mcg inhalant released w/ each actuation delivers about 100 mcg. Two inhalations tid–qid; max, 16 inhalations/day. **Tx of seasonal, perennial allergic rhinitis.** *Adult:* 2 sprays (220 mcg total dose) in each nostril daily; max, 4 sprays/day. *Child 6–12 yr:* 1 spray in each nostril once/day (100–110 mcg dose); max, 2 sprays/nostril/day. **Intra-articular relief of inflammatory conditions.** *Adult, child:* Acetonide, 2.5–15 mg intra-articular. Diacetate, 5–40 mg intra-articular, 5–48 mg intralesional; max, 12.5 mg/injection site, 25 mg/lesion. Hexacetonide, 2–20 mg intra-articular; up to 0.5 mg/square inch of affected area intralesional. **Relief of inflammatory, pruritic s&sx of dermatoses.** *Adult, child:* Apply sparingly to affected area bid–qid. **Tx of oral lesions.** *Adult:* Press small dab (1/4 inch) to each lesion until thin film develops, two to three times/day after meals.

ADV EFF Headache, increased appetite, immunosuppression, impaired wound healing, infections, menstrual changes, osteoporosis, sodium/fluid retention, vertigo, weight gain

INTERACTIONS Barbiturates, edrophonium, neostigmine, oral antidiabetics, phenytoin, pyridostigmine, rifampin, salicylates

NC/PT Not for acute asthmatic attack. Give in a.m. to mimic normal levels. Taper when stopping after long-term tx. Do not use occlusive dressings w/ topical form. Review proper administration. Pt should avoid exposure to infection, joint overuse after intra-articular injection; keep topical forms away from eyes; report swelling, signs of infection, worsening of condition.

triamterene (Dyrenium)
CLASS Potassium-sparing diuretic
PREG/CONT C/NA

BBW Risk of hyperkalemia (possibly fatal), more likely w/ diabetics, elderly/severely ill pts; monitor potassium carefully.

IND & DOSE Tx of edema associated w/ systemic conditions. *Adult:* 100 mg PO bid; max, 300 mg/day. **Tx of hypertension.** *Adult:* 25 mg/day PO; usual dose, 50–100 mg/day.

ADV EFF Abd pain, anorexia, dizziness, drowsiness, dry mouth, **hyperkalemia,** n/v/d, rash, renal stones

INTERACTIONS Amantadine, lithium, potassium supplements

NC/PT Pt should take in a.m. to decrease sleep interruption, w/ food if GI upset; weigh self regularly, report change of 3 lb/day; take safety precautions w/ CNS effects; avoid foods high in potassium; report swelling, difficulty breathing, flank pain, muscle cramps, tremors.

triazolam (Halcion)
CLASS Benzodiazepine, sedative-hypnotic
PREG/CONT X/C-IV

IND & DOSE Tx of insomnia. *Adult:* 0.125–0.25 mg PO before retiring. May increase to max 0.5 mg. Limit use to 7–10 days.

ADJUST DOSE Elderly, debilitated pts

ADV EFF Anaphylaxis, angioedema, bradycardia, confusion, constipation, **CV collapse,** diarrhea, drowsiness, drug dependence, fatigue, hiccups, nervousness, tachycardia, urticaria

INTERACTIONS Alcohol, aminophylline, cimetidine, CNS depressants, disulfiram, dyphylline, grapefruit juice, hormonal contraceptives, itraconazole, ketoconazole, omeprazole, theophylline

NC/PT Taper gradually after long-term use. Monitor renal function, CBC periodically. Not for use in pregnancy (barrier contraceptives advised). Pt should avoid grapefruit juice, alcohol; take safety measures w/ CNS effects; report difficulty breathing, swelling of face/eyes, continued sleep disorders.

---

trientine hydrochloride
(Syprine)
CLASS Chelate
PREG/CONT C/NA

IND & DOSE Tx of pts w/ Wilson disease intolerant of penicillamine. *Adult:* 750–1,250 mg/day PO in divided doses; max, 2 g/day. *Child:* 500–750 mg/day PO; max, 1,500 mg/day.
ADV EFF Abd pain, anorexia, epigastric pain, **hypersensitivity reactions**, iron deficiency, muscle spasm, myasthenia gravis, rash, rhabdomyolysis, SLE, weakness
NC/PT Pt should take on empty stomach 1 hr before, 2 hr after meals; swallow capsule whole and not cut, crush, or chew it; monitor temp nightly for first mo of tx; space iron supplement at least 2 hr apart from trientine; report fever, muscle weakness/pain, difficulty breathing.

---

trihexyphenidyl hydrochloride (generic)
CLASS Antiparkinsonian (anticholinergic type)
PREG/CONT C/NA

BBW Stop or decrease dosage if dry mouth interferes with swallowing, speaking.
IND & DOSE Adjunct in tx of parkinsonism. *Adult:* 1 mg PO first day. Increase by 2-mg increments at 3- to 5-day intervals until total of 6–10 mg/day. Postencephalitic pts may need 12–15 mg/day. W/ levodopa:

Adjust based on response; usual, 3–6 mg/day PO. **Tx of drug-induced extrapyramidal sx.** *Adult:* 1 mg PO. May need to temporarily reduce tranquilizer dose to expedite control of extrapyramidal sx. Usual dose, 5–15 mg/day.
ADJUST DOSE Elderly pts
ADV EFF Blurred vision, confusion, constipation, decreased sweating, delusions, disorientation, dizziness, drowsiness, dry mouth, flushing, light-headedness, urine retention
INTERACTIONS Haloperidol, phenothiazines
NC/PT Pt should empty bladder before each dose; use caution in hot weather (decreased sweating can lead to heat stroke); use sugarless lozenges for dry mouth; take safety precautions w/ CNS effects; report eye pain, rash, rapid heartbeat, difficulty swallowing/speaking.

---

trimethobenzamide hydrochloride (Tigan)
CLASS Antiemetic (anticholinergic)
PREG/CONT C/NA

IND & DOSE Control of postop n/v, nausea associated w/ gastroenteritis. *Adult:* 300 mg PO tid–qid, or 200 mg IM tid–qid.
ADJUST DOSE Elderly pts
ADV EFF Blurred vision, dizziness, drowsiness, headache, hypotension, pain/swelling at injection site
NC/PT Ensure adequate hydration. Pt should avoid alcohol (sedation possible), take safety precautions w/ CNS effects, report unusual bleeding, visual disturbances, pain at injection site.

---

trimethoprim (Primsol, Trimpex)
CLASS Antibiotic
PREG/CONT C/NA

IND & DOSE Uncomplicated UTIs caused by susceptible bacteria

strains. *Adult, child 12 yr and older:* 100 mg PO q 12 hr or 200 mg PO q 24 hr for 10–14 days. **Tx of otitis media.** *Child under 12 yr:* 10 mg/kg/day PO in divided doses q 12 hr for 10 days.
ADJUST DOSE Elderly pts, renal impairment
ADV EFF Bone marrow suppression, epigastric distress, exfoliative dermatitis, **hepatic impairment**, pruritus, rash
INTERACTIONS Phenytoin
NC/PT Culture before tx. Protect drug from light. Monitor CBC. Pt should take full course, avoid exposure to infection, report unusual bleeding, signs of infection, rash.

trimipramine maleate
(Surmontil)
CLASS TCA
PREG/CONT C/NA

BBW Limit access in depressed, potentially suicidal pts. Monitor for suicidal ideation, especially when beginning tx, changing doses. High risk of suicidality in children, adolescents, young adults.
IND & DOSE **Relief of sx of depression.** *Adult:* Inpts, 100 mg/day PO in divided doses. Gradually increase to 200 mg/day as needed; max, 250–300 mg/day. Outpts, 75 mg/day PO in divided doses. May increase to 150 mg/day; max, 200 mg/day. *Child 12 yr and older:* 50 mg/day PO w/ gradual increases up to 100 mg/day.
ADJUST DOSE Elderly pts
ADV EFF Anticholinergic effects, bone marrow suppression, constipation, dry mouth, extrapyramidal effects, **MI**, orthostatic hypotension, photosensitivity, rash, **stroke**
INTERACTIONS Alcohol, cimetidine, clarithromycin, clonidine, fluoroquinolones, fluoxetine, MAOIs, ranitidine, sympathomimetics, tramadol

NC/PT Monitor CBC periodically. Not for use in pregnancy (contraceptives advised). Pt should not stop suddenly; avoid sun exposure, alcohol; take safety precautions w/ CNS effects; use sugarless lozenges for dry mouth; report thoughts of suicide, excessive sedation.

DANGEROUS DRUG
triptorelin pamoate
(Trelstar)
CLASS Antineoplastic, LHRH analogue
PREG/CONT X/NA

IND & DOSE **Palliative tx of advanced prostate cancer.** *Adult:* 3.75-mg depot injection IM once monthly into buttock, or 11.25-mg injection IM q 12 wk into buttock, or 22.5 mg IM q 24 wk into buttock.
ADV EFF Anaphylaxis, angioedema, bone pain, decreased erection, headache, **HF**, hot flashes, injection-site pain, insomnia, sexual dysfx, urinary tract sx
INTERACTIONS Antipsychotics, metoclopramide
NC/PT Monitor testosterone, PSA before, periodically during tx. Not for use in pregnancy. Pt should mark calendar for injection days; use comfort measures for hot flashes, pain; report swelling, difficulty breathing, signs of infection at injection sites.

---

trospium chloride
(Sanctura)
CLASS Antimuscarinic, antispasmodic
PREG/CONT C/NA

IND & DOSE **Tx of s&sx of overactive bladder.** *Adult under 75 yr:* 20 mg PO bid on empty stomach, at least 1 hr before meals. Or, 60 mg ER tablet PO once/day. *Adult over 75 yr:* Monitor pt response; adjust down to 20 mg/day.

ADJUST DOSE Renal impairment
ADV EFF Constipation, decreased sweating, dizziness, drowsiness, dry mouth, fatigue, headache, urine retention
INTERACTIONS Digoxin, metformin, morphine, other anticholinergics, procainamide, pancuronium, tenofovir, vancomycin
NC/PT Pt should empty bladder before each dose; take on empty stomach 1 hr before, 2 hr after food; not cut, crush, or chew ER tablet; use sugarless lozenges, mouth care for dry mouth; maintain hydration; use caution in hot environments (decreased sweating could lead to heat stroke); take safety precautions w/ CNS effects; report inability to urinate, fever.

urofollitropin (Bravelle)
CLASS Fertility drug
PREG/CONT X/NA

IND & DOSE Stimulation of follicle development, ovulation. *Adults who have received gonadotropin-releasing hormone agonist, antagonist suppression:* 150 units/day subcut or IM for first 5 days. Subsequent dosing should not exceed 75–150 units/adjustment. Max, 450 units/day. Tx beyond 12 days not recommended. If pt response appropriate, give HCG 5,000–10,000 units 1 day after last *Bravelle* dose.
ADV EFF Multiple births, nausea, ovarian cyst, **ovarian hyperstimulation, pulmonary/vascular complications,** URI
NC/PT Ensure uterine health. Alert pt to risk of multiple births. Monitor regularly; monitor for thrombotic events. Teach proper administration, disposal of needles, syringes.

ursodiol (Actigall, URSO)
CLASS Gallstone-solubilizing drug
PREG/CONT B/NA

IND & DOSE **Gallstone solubilization.** *Adult:* 8–10 mg/kg/day PO in two to three divided doses. **Px of gallstones w/ rapid weight loss.** *Adult:* 300 mg PO bid or 8–10 mg/kg/day PO in two to three divided doses. **Tx of biliary cirrhosis.** *Adult:* 13–15 mg/kg/day PO in two to four divided doses w/ food.
ADV EFF Abd pain, cramps, diarrhea, epigastric distress, fatigue, headache, rash
INTERACTIONS Antacids, bile-acid sequestrants
NC/PT Drug not a cure; gallstones may recur. Schedule periodic oral cholecystograms or ultrasonograms to evaluate effectiveness at 6-mo intervals until resolution, then every 3 mo to monitor stone formation. Monitor LFTs periodically. Pt should avoid antacids, report yellowing of skin/eyes, gallstone attacks.

ustekinumab (Stelara)
CLASS Monoclonal antibody
PREG/CONT B/NA

IND & DOSE **Tx of mild to moderate plaque psoriasis.** *Adult:* Over 100 kg, 90 mg subcut, then 90 mg in 4 wk, then q 12 wk. 100 kg or less, 45 mg subcut, then 45 mg in 4 wk, then q 12 wk.
ADV EFF Fatigue, headache, **malignancies, serious infections,** URI
INTERACTIONS Immunosuppressants, live vaccines, phototherapy
NC/PT Not for use in pregnancy, breast-feeding. Ensure appropriate cancer screening. Pt should mark calendar of injection days, avoid live vaccines, report signs of infection, worsening of condition.

valacyclovir hydrochloride (Valtrex)

CLASS Antiviral
PREG/CONT B/NA

IND & DOSE Tx of herpes zoster.
Adult: 1 g PO tid for 7 days; most effective if started within 48 hr of sx onset (rash). **Tx of genital herpes.** *Adult:* 1 g PO bid for 7–10 days for initial episode. **Episodic tx of recurrent genital herpes.** *Adult:* 500 mg PO bid for 3 days, or 1 g/day for 5 days. **To suppress recurrent episodes of genital herpes.** *Adult:* 1 g/day PO; pts w/ hx of less than nine episodes in 1 yr may respond to 500 mg PO once daily. **To suppress recurrent episodes of genital herpes in pts w/ HIV.** 500 mg PO bid for 5–10 days. **To reduce risk of herpes zoster transmission.** *Adult:* 500 mg/day PO for source partner. For HIV-positive pts, 500 mg PO bid. **Tx of cold sores.** *Adult, child 12 yr and over:* 2 g PO bid for 1 day, 12 hr apart. **Tx of chickenpox.** *Child 2–18 yr:* 20 mg/kg PO tid for 5 days; max, 1 g tid.
ADJUST DOSE Renal impairment
ADV EFF Abd pain, **acute renal failure,** dizziness, headache, n/v/d, rash
INTERACTIONS Cimetidine, probenecid
NC/PT Begin tx within 48–72 hr of onset of shingles sx or within 24 hr of onset of chickenpox rash. Pt should take full course of tx; avoid contact w/ lesions; avoid intercourse when lesions present; take analgesics for headache; report severe diarrhea, worsening of condition. Name confusion between *Valtrex* (valacyclovir) and *Valcyte* (valganciclovir); use caution.

valganciclovir hydrochloride (Valcyte)

CLASS Antiviral
PREG/CONT C/NA

BBW Arrange for CBC before tx, at least wkly thereafter. Arrange for reduced dose if WBC, platelet counts fall.

Toxicity includes granulocytopenia, anemia, thrombocytopenia. Advise pt drug has caused cancer, fetal damage in animals and that risk possible in humans.
IND & DOSE Tx of cytomegalovirus (CMV) infection. *Adult:* 900 mg PO bid for 21 days; maint, 900 mg/day PO. **Px of CMV infection in high-risk kidney, pancreas, kidney, heart transplant.** *Adult:* 900 mg/day PO initiated within 10 days of transplant, continued for 100 days after transplant. *Child 4 mo–16 yr:* Dose in mg = $7 \times BSA \times CrCl$ PO. Max, 900 mg/day. May use oral sol, tablets.
ADJUST DOSE Renal impairment
ADV EFF Anemia, **bone marrow suppression,** confusion, dizziness, drowsiness, fever, headache, insomnia, n/v/d
INTERACTIONS Cytotoxic drugs, didanosine, imipenem/cilastatin, probenecid, zidovudine
NC/PT Cannot be substituted for ganciclovir capsules on one-to-one basis. Monitor CBC. Precautions needed for disposal of nucleoside analogues; consult pharmacy for proper disposal of unused tablets. Not for use in pregnancy; men, women should use barrier contraceptives during, for 90 days after tx. Avoid handling broken tablets. Pt should not cut, crush, or chew tablets; drink 2–3 L water/day; have frequent blood tests, eye exams to evaluate progress; take safety precautions w/ CNS effects; avoid exposure to infection; report bruising/bleeding, signs of infection. Name confusion between *Valcyte* (valganciclovir) and *Valtrex* (valacyclovir); use caution.

valproic acid (Stavzor), sodium valproate (Depakene, Depacon), divalproex sodium (Depakote, Divalproex)

CLASS Antiepileptic
PREG/CONT D, X (migraine prophylaxis)/NA

BBW Increased risk of suicidal ideation, suicidality; monitor accordingly. Arrange for frequent LFTs; stop drug immediately w/ suspected, apparent significant hepatic impairment. Continue LFTs to determine if hepatic impairment progresses despite discontinuation. Arrange for counseling for women of childbearing age who wish to become pregnant; drug may be teratogenic. Not recommended for women of childbearing age; risk of lower cognitive test scores in children when drug taken during pregnancy compared to other anticonvulsants. Stop drug at any sign of pancreatitis; life-threatening pancreatitis has occurred.

IND & DOSE Tx of simple, complex absence seizures. *Adult:* 10–15 mg/kg/day PO, increasing at 1-wk intervals by 5–10 mg/kg/day until seizures controlled or side effects preclude further increases; max, 60 mg/kg/day PO. If total dose exceeds 250 mg/day, give in divided doses. *Child 10 yr and older:* 10–15 mg/kg/day PO. Tx of acute mania, bipolar disorder. *Adult:* 25 mg/kg/day PO. Increase rapidly to achieve lowest therapeutic dose. Max, 60 mg/kg/day PO (*Depakote ER* only). Tx of bipolar mania: *Adult:* 750 mg/day PO in divided doses; max, 60 mg/kg/day (*Divalproex* DR only). Px of migraine. *Adult:* 250 mg/day PO bid; up to 1,000 mg/day has been used (*Divalproex* DR, *Stavzor*); 500 mg/day ER tablet.

ADV EFF Bone marrow suppression, dizziness, **hepatic failure**, indigestion, **life-threatening pancreatitis**, n/v/d, rash

INTERACTIONS Alcohol, carbamazepine, charcoal, cimetidine, chlorpromazine, CNS depressants, diazepam, erythromycin, ethosuximide, felbamate, lamotrigine, phenobarbital, phenytoin, primidone, rifampin, salicylates, zidovudine

NC/PT Taper when stopping. Monitor CBC, LFTs, therapeutic serum level (usually 50–100 mcg/mL). Not for use in pregnancy (barrier contraceptives advised). May open *Depakote* Sprinkle tablets and sprinkle on applesauce, pudding. Pt should swallow tablet/capsule whole and not chew it; avoid alcohol, OTC sleeping pills; have frequent blood tests; wear medical ID; take

safety precautions w/ CNS effects; avoid injury, exposure to infection; report bleeding, stool color changes, thoughts of suicide. Confusion between DR *Depakote* and *Depakote* ER. Dosage very different; serious adverse effects possible; use extreme caution.

valsartan (Diovan)
CLASS Antihypertensive, ARB
PREG/CONT D/NA

BBW Rule out pregnancy before starting tx. Suggest barrier contraceptives during tx; fetal injury, deaths have occurred.

IND & DOSE Tx of hypertension. *Adult:* 80 mg PO; range, 80–320 mg/day. *Child 6–16 yr:* 1.3 mg/kg/day PO (max, 40 mg). Target, 1.3–2.7 mg/kg/day PO (40–160 mg/day). Tx of HF. *Adult:* 40 mg PO bid; titrate to 80 mg and 160 mg bid, to highest dose tolerated by pt. Max, 320 mg/day. Tx of post-MI left ventricular dysfx. *Adult:* Start as early as 12 hr post-MI; 20 mg PO bid. May increase after 7 days to 40 mg PO bid. Titrate to 160 mg PO bid if tolerated.

ADJUST DOSE Hepatic, renal impairment

ADV EFF Abd pain, cough, dizziness, headache, hypotension, n/v/d, URI

NC/PT Alert surgeon; volume replacement may be needed postop. Do not stop abruptly. Not for use in pregnancy (barrier contraceptives advised), breast-feeding. Pt should take safety precautions w/ CNS effects, use caution in situations that can lead to BP drop; report chills, pregnancy.

vancomycin hydrochloride (Vancocin)
CLASS Antibiotic
PREG/CONT C; B (pulvules)/NA

BBW Pt at risk for development of multiple drug-resistant organisms; ensure appropriate use.

IND & DOSE Tx of severe to life-threatening infections caused by susceptible bacteria strains and unresponsive to other antibiotics. *Adult:* 500 mg–2 g/day PO in three to four divided doses for 7–10 days. Or, 500 mg IV q 6 hr or 1 g IV q 12 hr. *Child:* 40 mg/kg/day IV in three to four divided doses for 7–10 days. Or, 10 mg/kg/dose IV q 6 hr. Max, 2 g/day. *Premature, full-term neonate:* Use w/ caution because of incompletely developed renal function. Initially, 15 mg/kg IV, then 10 mg/kg q 12 hr in first wk of life, then q 8 hr up to age 1 mo. Tx of pseudomembranous colitis due to *Clostridium difficile. Adult:* 500 mg–2 g/day PO in three to four divided doses for 7–10 days, or 125 mg PO tid–qid. *Child:* 40 mg/kg/day PO in four divided doses for 7–10 days. Max, 2 g/day.

ADJUST DOSE Elderly pts, renal failure

ADV EFF Fever, hypotension, nausea, **nephrotoxicity**, ototoxicity, paresthesia, "red man syndrome," superinfections, rash

INTERACTIONS Aminoglycosides, amphotericin B, atracurium, bacitracin, cisplatin, pancuronium, tubocurarine, vecuronium

NC/PT Culture before tx. Monitor for red man syndrome during IV infusion. Monitor renal function. Monitor for safe serum level (conc of 60–80 mcg/mL toxic). Pt should take full course; perform hygiene measures to avoid possible infections of mouth, vagina; report ringing in ears, hearing loss, swelling.

vardenafil hydrochloride (Levitra, Staxyn)
CLASS ED drug, phosphodiesterase type 5 inhibitor
PREG/CONT B/NA

IND & DOSE Tx of ED. *Adult:* 5–10 mg PO 1 hr before anticipated sexual activity; range, 5–20 mg PO. Limit use to once/day.

ADJUST DOSE Elderly pts, hepatic impairment

ADV EFF Abnormal ejaculation, angina, dyspnea, flushing, GERD, headache, hearing loss, hypotension, rhinitis, vision changes/loss

INTERACTIONS Alpha blockers, erythromycin, indinavir, itraconazole, ketoconazole, nitrates, ritonavir

NC/PT Ensure dx. Drug not effective without sexual stimulation. Does not protect against STDs. Pt should avoid nitrates, alpha blocker antihypertensives; stop drug, immediately report loss of vision/hearing; report difficult urination, erection lasting longer than 4 hr, fainting.

varenicline tartrate (Chantix)
CLASS Nicotine receptor antagonist, smoking deterrent
PREG/CONT C/NA

BBW Risk of serious mental health events, including changes in behavior, depressed mood, hostility, suicidal thoughts; monitor accordingly. Higher risk of MI, stroke, death compared with placebo; use w/ caution.

IND & DOSE Aid to smoking cessation tx. *Adult:* Pt should pick date to stop smoking, begin tx 1 wk before that date. Or, pt can begin drug, quit smoking between days 8 and 35 of tx. days 1–3, 0.5 mg PO daily; days 4–7, 0.5 mg PO bid; day 8 until end of tx, 1 mg PO bid.

ADJUST DOSE Severe renal impairment

ADV EFF Abd pain, abnormal dreams, constipation, fatigue, flatulence, headache, insomnia, **MI**, nausea, rhinorrhea, **stroke**, **suicidality**

INTERACTIONS Cimetidine, nicotine transdermal systems

NC/PT Ensure comprehensive tx program. Not for use in pregnancy, breast-feeding; Tx should last 12 wk; pt who successfully quits smoking in that time may benefit from another 12 wk to increase likelihood of long-term abstinence. Use caution w/ known CAD. Pt should take after eating w/ full glass of water; follow dosing protocol closely; if relapse occurs, discuss w/ prescribe; report failure to quit smoking, behavioral changes, thoughts of suicide, chest pain.

velaglucerase (VPRIV)

CLASS Lysosomal enzyme
PREG/CONT B/NA

IND & DOSE Long-term replacement tx for type 1 Gaucher disease. *Adult, child:* 60 units/kg as 60-min IV infusion q 2 wk.
ADV EFF Abd pain, back pain, dizziness, headache, **hypersensitivity/infusion reactions**, joint pain, nausea, URI
NC/PT May use antihistamines, corticosteroids to alleviate infusion reactions. Pt should mark calendar for infusion days, report difficulty breathing, pain at injection site.

vemurafenib (Zelboraf)

CLASS Antineoplastic, kinase inhibitor
PREG/CONT B/NA

IND & DOSE Tx of pts w/ unresectable, metastatic melanoma w/ BRAF mutation as detected by approved BRAF test. *Adult:* 960 mg PO bid approximately 12 hr apart.
ADV EFF Alopecia, arthralgia, **cutaneous squamous cell carcinoma**, fatigue, **liver toxicity**, nausea, **new malignant melanomas**, photosensitivity, pruritus, **QT prolongation, serious hypersensitivity reactions, serious ophthalmologic toxicity**, skin papilloma, **Stevens-Johnson syndrome**
INTERACTIONS CYP substrates, warfarin
NC/PT BRAF confirmation test required before use to ensure appropriate drug selection. Obtain baseline

ECG; periodically monitor QT interval. Monitor skin, eye reactions. Not for use in pregnancy, breast-feeding. Pt should cover head at temp extremes (hair loss possible); avoid sun exposure, report rash, difficulty breathing, urine/stool color changes, vision changes.

venlafaxine hydrochloride (Effexor XR)

CLASS Antidepressant, anxiolytic
PREG/CONT C/NA

BBW Monitor pts for suicidal ideation, especially when starting tx, changing dose; high risk in children, adolescents, young adults.
IND & DOSE Tx of depression. *Adult:* 75 mg/day PO in two to three divided doses (or once/day, ER capsule). Increase at intervals of no less than 4 days up to 225 mg/day to achieve desired effect; max, 375 mg/day in three divided doses. Tx of generalized anxiety disorder/social anxiety. *Adult:* 75–225 mg/day ER form PO. Tx of panic disorder. *Adult:* 37.5 mg/day PO for 7 days, then 75 mg/day for 7 days, then 75 mg/day wkly. Max, 225 mg/day (ER only).
ADJUST DOSE Hepatic, renal impairment
ADV EFF Abnormal ejaculation, asthenia, anorexia, constipation, dizziness, dry mouth, headache, insomnia, nausea, nervousness, somnolence, sweating, **suicidality**
INTERACTIONS Alcohol, MAOIs, St. John's wort, trazodone
NC/PT To transfer to, from MAOI: Allow at least 14 days to elapse from stopping MAOI to starting venlafaxine; allow at least 7 days to elapse from stopping venlafaxine to starting MAOI. Not for use in pregnancy. Pt should swallow ER capsule whole and not cut, crush, or chew it; take w/ food; avoid alcohol, St. John's wort; take safety precautions w/ CNS

effects; use sugarless lozenges w/ dry mouth; report rash, thoughts of suicide.

DANGEROUS DRUG

verapamil hydrochloride (Calan, Verelan)

CLASS Antianginal, antihypertensive, calcium channel blocker

PREG/CONT C/NA

BBW Monitor pt carefully during drug titration; dosage may be increased more rapidly w/ hospitalized, monitored pts.

IND & DOSE Tx of angina.
Adult: 80–120 mg PO tid. Maint, 240–480 mg/day. **Tx of arrhythmias.**
Adult: 240–480 mg/day PO in divided doses. Or, 120–240 mg/day PO in a.m. ER capsules; max, 480 mg/day. Or, 120–180 mg/day PO in a.m. ER or SR tablets. Or, 5–10 mg IV over 2 min; may repeat dose of 10 mg 30 min after first dose if initial response inadequate. In digitalized pts, 240–320 mg/ day PO. *Child 1–15 yr:* 0.1–0.3 mg/kg IV over 2 min; max, 5 mg. Repeat dose 30 min after initial dose if response inadequate. Max for repeat dose, 10 mg. *Child 1 yr and younger:* 0.1–0.2 mg/kg IV over 2 min. **Tx of hypertension.** *Adult:* 40–80 mg PO tid.

ADJUST DOSE Elderly pts, renal impairment

ADV EFF Cardiac arrhythmias, constipation, dizziness, edema, headache, hypotension, nausea

INTERACTIONS Antihypertensives, beta blockers, calcium, carbamazepine, digoxin, grapefruit juice, prazosin, quinidine, rifampin, verapamil

NC/PT When pt stabilized, may switch to ER capsules (max, 480 mg/day), ER tablets (max, 240 mg q 12 hr), SR forms (max, 480 mg in a.m.). Protect IV sol from light. Monitor BP, cardiac rhythm closely. Pt should swallow ER, SR forms whole and not cut, crush, or chew them; take safety precautions w/ dizziness; avoid grapefruit juice; report swelling, difficulty breathing.

---

verteporfin (Visudyne)

CLASS Ophthalmic drug

PREG/CONT C/NA

IND & DOSE Tx of age-related macular degeneration, pathologic myopia, ocular histoplasmosis. *Adult:* 6 mg/m^2 diluted in D$_5$W to total 30 mL IV into free-flowing IV over 10 min at 3 mL/min using inline filter, syringe pump.

ADJUST DOSE Hepatic impairment

ADV EFF Dizziness, headache, injection-site reactions, malaise, photosensitivity, pruritus, rash, visual disturbances

NC/PT Laser light tx should begin within 15 min of starting IV; may repeat in 3 mo if needed. Not for use in breast-feeding. Protect pt from exposure to bright light for at least 5 days after tx. Pt should report vision changes, eye pain, injection-site pain/swelling.

---

vigabatrin (Sabril)

CLASS Antiepileptic, GABAase inhibitor

PREG/CONT C/NA

BBW Available only through restricted distribution program. Causes progressive, permanent, bilateral vision loss. Monitor vision; stopping drug may not stop vision loss. Increased risk of suicidality; monitor accordingly.

IND & DOSE Adjunct tx of refractory complex seizures *Adult:* 500 mg PO bid; increase slowly to max 1.5 mg PO bid.

ADJUST DOSE Renal impairment

ADV EFF Abnormal coordination, anemia, arthralgia, confusion, edema, fatigue, nystagmus, **permanent**

vision loss, somnolence, **suicidality,** tremor, weight gain

NC/PT Available only through limited access. Taper gradually to avoid withdrawal effect. Monitor vision; permanent vision loss possible. Give w/ other antiepileptics. Nor for use in pregnancy, breast-feeding. Pt should take precautions w/ CNS effects, report changes in vision, thoughts of suicide, extreme fatigue, weight gain.

vilazodone hydrochloride (Viibryd)
CLASS SSRI
PREG/CONT C/NA

BBW High risk of suicidality in children, adolescents, young adults. Establish suicide precautions for severely depressed pts, limit quantity of drug dispensed. Vilazodone not approved for use in children.

IND & DOSE Tx of major depressive disorder. *Adult:* 10 mg/day PO for 7 days, then 20 mg/day PO for 7 days; maint, 40 mg/day PO.

ADV EFF Dizziness, dry mouth, insomnia, n/v/d, **NMS,** paresthesia, **seizures**

INTERACTIONS Alcohol, aspirin, diltiazem, ketoconazole, MAOIs, NSAIDs, serotonergic drugs, St. John's wort, warfarin

NC/PT Therapeutic effects may not occur for 4 wk. Taper when stopping. Not for use in pregnancy, breast-feeding. Pt should take w/ food in a.m.; avoid alcohol, NSAIDs, St. John's wort; take safety precautions w/ CNS effects; report seizures, thoughts of suicide.

DANGEROUS DRUG
vinBLAStine sulfate
(generic)
CLASS Antineoplastic, mitotic inhibitor
PREG/CONT D/NA

BBW Do not give IM, subcut due to severe local reaction, tissue necro-

sis. Fatal if given intrathecally; use extreme caution. Watch for irritation, infiltration; extravasation causes tissue damage, necrosis. If it occurs, stop injection immediately; give remainder of dose in another vein. Arrange for hyaluronidase injection into local area, after which apply moderate heat to disperse drug, minimize pain.

IND & DOSE Palliative tx of lymphocytic/histiocytic lymphoma, generalized Hodgkin lymphoma (stages III, IV), mycosis fungoides, advanced testicular carcinoma, Kaposi sarcoma, Letterer-Siwe disease; tx of choriocarcinoma, breast cancer, Hodgkin lymphoma, advanced testicular germinal-cell cancers. *Adult:* Initially, 3.7 mg/m² as single IV dose, followed at wkly intervals by increasing doses at 1.8-mg/m² increments; use these increments until max 18.5 mg/m² reached. When WBC count 3,000/mm³, use one increment smaller for wkly maint. Do not give another dose until WBC count is 4,000/mm³ even if 7 days have passed. *Child:* 2.5 mg/m² as single IV dose, followed at wkly intervals by increasing doses at 1.25-mg/m² increments. Max, 12.5 mg/m²/dose.

ADJUST DOSE Hepatic impairment

ADV EFF Alopecia, anorexia, **bone marrow suppression,** cellulitis at injection site, headache, n/v/d, paresthesia, weakness

INTERACTIONS Erythromycin, grapefruit juice, phenytoins

NC/PT Do not give IM, subcut. Monitor CBC closely. Give antiemetic for severe n/v. Not for use in pregnancy. Pt should mark calendar of tx days; take safety precautions w/ CNS effects; cover head at temp extremes (hair loss possible); avoid exposure to infection, injury; avoid grapefruit juice; report pain at injection site, signs of infection, bleeding. Name confusion between vinblastine and vincristine; use caution.

DANGEROUS DRUG

vinCRIStine sulfate
(Marqibo)

CLASS Antineoplastic, mitotic inhibitor

PREG/CONT D/NA

BBW Do not give IM, subcut due to severe local reaction, tissue necrosis. Fatal if given intrathecally; use extreme caution. Watch for irritation, infiltration; extravasation causes tissue damage, necrosis. If it occurs, stop injection immediately; give remainder of dose in another vein. Arrange for hyaluronidase injection into local area, after which apply moderate heat to disperse drug, minimize pain.

IND & DOSE Tx of acute leukemia, Hodgkin lymphoma, non-Hodgkin lymphoma, rhabdomyosarcoma, neuroblastoma, Wilms tumor.
Adult: 1.4 mg/m^2 IV at wkly intervals. *Child over 10 kg or BSA over 1 m^2:* 1–2 mg/m^2/wk IV. Max, 2 mg/dose. *Child under 10 kg or BSA under 1 m^2:* 0.05 mg/kg/wk IV. Tx of adults with Philadelphia chromosome–negative acute ALL who have relapsed after other tx. *Adult:* 2.25 mg/m^2 IV over 1 hr q 7 days *(Marqibo)*.

ADJUST DOSE Elderly pts, hepatic impairment

ADV EFF Alopecia, ataxia, constipation, cranial nerve manifestations, **death**, neuritic pain, paresthesia, photosensitivity, renal impairment, weight loss

INTERACTIONS Digoxin, grapefruit juice, L-asparaginase

NC/PT Do not give IM, subcut. Monitor renal function. Not for use in pregnancy. Pt should use laxative for constipation, take safety precautions w/ CNS effects, cover head at temp extremes (hair loss possible), avoid sun exposure, report pain at injection site, swelling, severe constipation. Name confusion between vinblastine and vincristine; use caution.

DANGEROUS DRUG

vinorelbine tartrate
(Navelbine)

CLASS Antineoplastic, mitotic inhibitor

PREG/CONT D/NA

BBW Do not give IM, subcut due to severe local reaction, tissue necrosis. Fatal if given intrathecally; use extreme caution. Watch for irritation, infiltration; extravasation can cause tissue damage, necrosis. If it occurs, stop injection immediately; arrange for hyaluronidase injection into local area, after which apply moderate heat to disperse drug, minimize pain. Check CBC before each dose; severe granulocytosis possible. Adjust, delay dose as appropriate.

IND & DOSE First-line tx of ambulatory pts w/ unresectable advanced non-small-cell lung cancer; tx of stage IV non-small-cell lung cancer. *Adult:* 30 mg/m^2 as single IV dose; repeat once/wk until disease progresses or toxicity limits use. Tx of stage III, IV non-small-cell lung cancer, w/ cisplatin.
Adult: 25 mg/m^2 IV w/ cisplatin 100 mg/m^2 q 4 wk, or 30 mg/m^2 w/ cisplatin 120 mg/m^2 on days 1 and 29, then q 6 wk.

ADJUST DOSE Hepatic impairment

ADV EFF Alopecia, anorexia, headache, hepatic impairment, **severe bone marrow suppression**, paresthesia, vesiculation of GI tract

INTERACTIONS Cisplatin, mitomycin, paclitaxel

NC/PT Check CBC before each dose; adjustment may be needed. Give antiemetic if needed. Not for use in pregnancy (contraceptives advised). Pt should mark calendar of tx days; cover head at temp extremes (hair loss possible); take safety precautions w/ CNS effects; avoid exposure to infection, injury; report pain at injection site, unusual bleeding, signs of infection.

vismodegib (Erivedge)

CLASS Antineoplastic, hedgehog pathway inhibitor
PREG/CONT D/NA

BBW Risk of embryo-fetal death, severe birth defects; men, women advised to use barrier contraceptives.

IND & DOSE Tx of pts w/ metastatic or locally advanced basal cell carcinoma not candidates for surgery or radiation. *Adult:* 150 mg/day PO.

ADV EFF Alopecia, anorexia, arthralgia, constipation, fatigue, muscle spasms, n/v/d

NC/PT Rule out pregnancy before tx; advise men, women to use barrier contraceptives (due to risk of fetal toxicity). Not for use in breast-feeding. Advise pt not to donate blood. Pt should take as directed; not donate blood during and for 7 mo after tx; know that hair loss possible; report weight loss, severe GI complaints.

voriconazole (Vfend)

CLASS Triazole antifungal
PREG/CONT D/NA

IND & DOSE Tx of invasive aspergillosis, serious infections caused by susceptible fungi strains; candidemia in nonneutropenic pts w/ disseminated skin infections and abd, kidney, bladder wall, and wound infections. *Adult:* Loading dose, 6 mg/kg IV q 12 hr for two doses, then 3–4 mg/ kg IV q 12 hr or 200 mg PO q 12 hr. Switch to PO as soon as possible. 40 kg or more, 200 mg PO q 12 hr; may increase to 300 mg PO q 12 hr if needed. Under 40 kg, 100 mg PO q 12 hr; may increase to 150 mg PO q 12 hr if needed. Tx of esophageal candidiasis. *Adult:* 200–300 mg PO q 12 hr (100–150 mg PO q 12 hr if under 40 kg) for 14 days or for at least 7 days after sx resolution.

ADV EFF Anaphylactic reaction, BP changes, dizziness, headache, **hepatotoxicity,** n/v/d, photosensitivity, QT prolongation, rash, **Stevens-Johnson syndrome,** visual disturbances

INTERACTIONS Benzodiazepine, calcium channel blockers, cyclosporine, omeprazole, oral anticoagulants, phenytoin, protease inhibitors, statins, St. John's wort, sulfonylureas, tacrolimus, vinblastine, vincristine, warfarin. Do not use w/ carbamazepine, ergot alkaloids, mephobarbital, phenobarbital, pimozide, quinidine, rifabutin, rifampin, sirolimus.

NC/PT Obtain baseline ECG, LFTs before, periodically during tx. Review drug list carefully; many interactions possible. Not for use in pregnancy (contraceptives advised). Pt should take oral drug on empty stomach 1 hr before or 2 hr after meals; avoid sun exposure, St. John's wort; report all drugs/herbs being used, vision changes, urine/stool color changes.

vorinostat (Zolinza)

CLASS Antineoplastic, histone deacetylase inhibitor
PREG/CONT D/NA

BBW Monitor for bleeding, excessive n/v, thromboembolic events.

IND & DOSE Tx of cutaneous manifestations in cutaneous T-cell lymphoma. *Adult:* 400 mg/day PO w/ food; continue until disease progression or unacceptable toxicity.

ADJUST DOSE Hepatic impairment

ADV EFF Anorexia, dehydration, dizziness, **GI bleeding,** hyperglycemia, n/v/d, **thromboembolic events**

INTERACTIONS Warfarin

NC/PT Monitor CBC, electrolytes, serum blood glucose. Give antiemetics if needed. Encourage fluid intake of 2 L/day to prevent dehydration. Not for use in pregnancy (barrier contraceptives advised), breast-feeding. Pt should take safety precaution w/ dizziness, use caution in hot environments, maintain hydration, report bloody diarrhea, numbness/tingling, chest pain, difficulty breathing.

vortioxetine (Brintellix)

CLASS Antidepressant, SSRI
PREG/CONT C/N/A

BBW Increased risk of suicidality in children, adolescents, young adults, severely depressed pts. Limit quantity; monitor pt.

IND & DOSE Tx of major depressive disorder. *Adult:* 10 mg/day PO. Increase to 20 mg/day PO as tolerated.

ADV EFF Abnormal dreams, activation of mania, constipation, dizziness, dry mouth, hyponatremia, n/v/d, pruritus, serotonin syndrome, **suicidality**
INTERACTIONS Antihypertensives, aprepitant, aspirin, bupropion, carbamazepine, fluoxetine, linezolid, MAOIs, methylene blue (IV), NSAIDs, opioids, paroxetine, phenytoin, quinidine, rifampin, SSRIs, St. John's wort

NC/PT Monitor for hyponatremia, activation of mania. Taper when discontinuing. Pt should take in a.m.; not stop suddenly; avoid pregnancy, breast-feeding, St. John's wort; take safety precautions w/ CNS effects; eat small, frequent meals for GI upset; report rash, mania, severe n/v, thoughts of suicide.

DANGEROUS DRUG

warfarin sodium (Coumadin, Jantoven)

CLASS Coumarin derivative, oral anticoagulant
PREG/CONT X/N/A

BBW Evaluate pt regularly for signs of blood loss (petechiae, bleeding gums, bruises, dark stools, dark urine). Maintain INR of 2–3, 3–4.5 w/ mechanical prosthetic valves or recurrent systemic emboli; risk of serious to fatal bleeding.

IND & DOSE Tx, px of PE, venous thrombosis; tx of thromboembolic complications of atrial fibrillation; px of systemic embolization after acute MI. *Adult:* 2–5 mg/day PO or IV. Adjust according to PT response. Maint, 2–10 mg/day PO based on INR.
ADJUST DOSE Elderly pts
ADV EFF Alopecia, dermatitis, **hemorrhage**, n/v/d, priapism, red-orange urine
INTERACTIONS Acetaminophen, alcohol, allopurinol, amiodarone, androgens, angelica, azole antifungals, barbiturates, carbamazepine, cat's claw, cefazolin, cefotetan, cefoxitin, ceftriaxone, chamomile, chloramphenicol, cholestyramine, chondroitin, cimetidine, clofibrate, co-trimoxazole, danazol, disulfiram, erythromycin, famotidine, feverfew, fish oil, fluvastatin, garlic, ginkgo, glucagon, goldenseal, grape seed extract, green leaf tea, griseofulvin, horse chestnut seed, lovastatin, meclofenamate, mefenamic acid, methimazole, metronidazole, nalidixic acid, nizatidine, NSAIDs, phenytoin, propylthiouracil, psyllium, quinidine, quinine, quinolones, ranitidine, rifampin, simvastatin, sulfinpyrazone, thyroid drugs, turmeric, vitamins E, K
NC/PT Genetic testing can help determine reasonable dose. Decreased clearance w/ CYP2C9*2, CYP2C9*3 variant alleles. Monitor blood clotting; target, INR of 2–3. IV use reserved for situations in which oral warfarin not feasible. Have vitamin K and/or prothrombin complex concentrate on hand for overdose. Check pt's drug regimen closely; many interactions possible. Carefully add, remove drugs from regimen; dose adjustment may be needed. Not for use in pregnancy (contraceptives advised). Urine may turn red-orange. Pt should not start, stop any drug, herb without consulting health care provider (dose adjustments may be needed); have regular blood tests; avoid injury.

zafirlukast (Accolate)

CLASS Antiasthmatic, leukotriene receptor antagonist
PREG/CONT B/NA

IND & DOSE Px, long-term tx of bronchial asthma. *Adult, child 12 yr and over:* 20 mg PO bid on empty stomach 1 hr before or 2 hr after meals. *Child 5–11 yr:* 10 mg PO bid on empty stomach.
ADV EFF Headache, **Churg-Strauss syndrome**, dizziness, n/v/d
INTERACTIONS Calcium channel blockers, corticosteroids, cyclosporine, erythromycin, theophylline, warfarin
NC/PT Not for acute asthma attack. Pt should take on empty stomach q day, consult health care provider before using OTC products, take safety precautions w/ dizziness; report severe headache, fever, increased acute asthma attacks.

zaleplon (Sonata)

CLASS Sedative-hypnotic (nonbenzodiazepine)
PREG/CONT C/C-IV

IND & DOSE Short-term tx of insomnia. *Adult:* 10 mg PO at bedtime. Pt must remain in bed for 4 hr after taking. Max, 20 mg/day.
ADJUST DOSE Elderly, debilitated pts; hepatic impairment
ADV EFF Anaphylaxis, angioedema, depression, dizziness, drowsiness, headache, short-term memory impairment, sleep disorders
INTERACTIONS Alcohol, CNS depressants, cimetidine, CYP3A4 inhibitors, rifampin
NC/PT Rule out medical causes for insomnia; institute sleep hygiene protocol. Pt will feel drug's effects for 4 hr; after 4 hr, pt may safely become active again. Pt should take dose immediately before bedtime; avoid alcohol, OTC sleeping aids; take safety precautions w/ CNS effects; report

difficulty breathing, swelling, sleep-related behaviors.

zanamivir (Relenza)

CLASS Antiviral, neuraminidase inhibitor
PREG/CONT C/NA

IND & DOSE Tx of uncomplicated acute illness due to influenza virus. *Adult, child 7 yr and over:* 2 inhalations (one 5-mg blister/inhalation administered w/ *Diskhaler*, for total 10 mg) bid at 12-hr intervals for 5 days. Should start within 2 days of onset of flu sx; give two doses on first tx day, at least 2 hr apart; separate subsequent doses by 12 hr. Px of influenza. *Adult, child 5 yr and over:* Two inhalations (10 mg)/day for 28 days w/ community outbreak, 10 days for household exposure.
ADV EFF Anorexia, **bronchospasm**, cough, diarrhea, dizziness, headache, nausea, **serious respiratory effects**
NC/PT Caution COPD, asthma pts of bronchospasm risk; pt should have fast-acting bronchodilator on hand. Review proper use of *Diskhaler* delivery system. Pt should take full course; if using bronchodilator, use before this drug; take safety precautions w/ dizziness; report worsening of sx.

ziconotide (Prialt)

CLASS Analgesic, N-type calcium channel blocker
PREG/CONT C/NA

BBW Severe neuropsychiatric reactions, neurologic impairment; monitor pt closely. Do not use w/ hx of psychosis.
IND & DOSE Mgt of severe chronic pain in pts who need intrathecal tx. *Adult:* 2.4 mcg/day by continuous intrathecal pump; may titrate to max 19.2 mcg/day (0.8 mcg/hr).
ADV EFF Confusion, dizziness, meningitis, nausea, **neurologic**

impairment, nystagmus, **psychotic behavior**

NC/PT Teach pt proper care of pump, injection site. Not for use in pregnancy, breast-feeding. Pt should take safety precautions w/ CNS effects, report changes in mood/behavior, muscle pain/weakness, rash.

zidovudine (Retrovir)
CLASS Antiviral
PREG/CONT C/NA

BBW Monitor hematologic indices q 2 wk; hematologic toxicity has occurred. Monitor LFTs; lactic acidosis w/ severe hepatomegaly possible. Increased risk of symptomatic myopathy; monitor accordingly.

IND & DOSE Tx of HIV, w/ other antiretrovirals. Adult, child over 12 yr: 600 mg/day PO in divided doses as either 200 mg tid or 300 mg bid. Monitor hematologic indices q 2 wk. If significant anemia (Hgb under 7.5 g/dL, reduction over 25%) or granulocyte reduction over 50% below baseline occurs, dose interruption necessary until evidence of bone marrow recovery. Or, 1 mg/kg five to six times/day IV infused over 1 hr. Child 6 wk–12 yr: 30 kg and over, 600 mg/day PO in two to three divided doses. 9 to under 30 kg, 18 mg/kg/day PO in two to three divided doses. 4 to under 9 kg, 24 mg/kg/day PO in two to three divided doses. Infant born to HIV-infected mother: 2 mg/kg PO q 6 hr starting within 12 hr of birth to 6 wk of age, or 1.5 mg/kg IV over 30 min q 6 hr until able to take oral form. **Px of maternal-fetal transmission.** Adult: 100 mg PO five times/day until start of labor.

ADV EFF Agranulocytosis, anorexia, asthenia, diarrhea, flulike sx, GI pain, headache, nausea, rash

INTERACTIONS Acyclovir, bone marrow suppressants, cyclosporine, cytotoxic drugs, ganciclovir, interferon alfa, methadone, nephrotoxic drugs, phenytoin, probenecid, St. John's wort

NC/PT Do not infuse IV w/ blood product. Pt should take drug around the clock; take precautions to prevent transmission (drug not a cure); avoid exposure to infection, St. John's wort; take w/ other antivirals; report signs of infection, difficulty breathing, severe headache. Name confusion between *Retrovir* (zidovudine) and ritonavir; use caution.

zileuton (Zyflo)
CLASS Antiasthmatic
leukotriene synthesis inhibitor
PREG/CONT C/NA

IND & DOSE Px, long-term tx of asthma. Adult, child 12 yr and over: CR tablets, 1,200 mg (2 tablets) PO bid within 1 hr a.m., p.m. meals for total daily dose of 2,400 mg. Tablets, 600 mg PO qid for total daily dose of 2,400 mg.

ADJUST DOSE Hepatic impairment

ADV EFF Diarrhea, dizziness, headache, **liver enzyme elevations,** neuropsychiatric events, pain, rash

INTERACTIONS Propranolol, theophylline, warfarin

NC/PT Not for acute asthma attack. Monitor LFTs, mood, behavior. Pt should take daily; take CR tablets on empty stomach 1 hr before or 2 hr after meals; swallow tablet whole and not cut, crush, or chew it; take safety precaution w/ CNS effects; report acute asthma attacks, urine/stool color changes, rash.

ziprasidone (Geodon)
CLASS Atypical antipsychotic,
benzisoxazole
PREG/CONT C/NA

BBW Increased risk of death if used in elderly pts w/ dementia-related psychosis. Do not use in these pts; not approved for this use.

IND & DOSE Tx of schizophrenia. Adult: Initially, 20 mg PO bid w/ food; range, 20–100 mg PO bid. **Rapid**

control of agitated behavior. *Adult:* 10–20 mg IM; may repeat 10-mg doses q 2 hr; may repeat 20-mg doses in 4 hr. Max, 40 mg/day. Tx of bipolar mania. *Adult:* 40 mg PO bid w/ food. May increase to 60–80 mg PO bid w/ food. ADV EFF Arrhythmias, constipation, drowsiness, dyspepsia, fever, headache, hyperglycemia, hypotension, QT prolongation, weight gain INTERACTIONS Antihypertensives, QT-prolonging drugs, St. John's wort NC/PT Obtain baseline, periodic ECG; monitor serum glucose, weight. Not for use in pregnancy (contraceptives advised). Pt should take safety precautions w/ CNS effects, avoid St. John's wort, report palpitations, sx return.

ziv-aflibercept (Zaltrap)
CLASS Antineoplastic, ligand binding factor
PREG/CONT C/NA

BBW Risk of hemorrhage; do not administer w/ active bleeding. Risk of GI perforation, compromised wound healing. Stop at least 4 wk before elective surgery; do not start until all surgical wounds healed.
IND & DOSE Tx of metastatic colorectal cancer resistant to oxaliplatin, w/ 5-FU, leucovorin, irinotecan. *Adult:* 4 mg/kg IV over 1 hr q 2 wk.
ADV EFF Abd pain, anorexia, dehydration, diarrhea, dysphonia, epistaxis, fatigue, headache, hepatic impairment, hypertension, neutropenia, proteinuria, RPLS, thrombotic events
NC/PT Not for use w/ active bleeding; do not use within 4 wk of surgery. Monitor urine protein, BP, hydration status; watch for s&sx of CV events. Not for use in pregnancy (barrier contraceptives advised for men, women during and for 3 mo after tx), breast-feeding. Pt should mark calendar for infusion dates; avoid exposure to infection; report

chest pain, fever, s&sx of infection, difficulty breathing, numbness/tingling, severe diarrhea.

zoledronic acid (Reclast, Zometa)
CLASS Bisphosphonate, calcium regulator
PREG/CONT D/NA

IND & DOSE Tx of hypercalcemia of malignancy; bone metastases w/ multiple myeloma. *Adult:* 4 mg IV as single-dose infusion of not less than 15 min for hypercalcemia of malignancy w/ albumin-corrected serum calcium of 12 mg/dL or more. May retreat w/ 4 mg IV if needed. Minimum of 7 days should elapse between doses w/ careful monitoring of serum creatinine. Pts w/ solid tumors should receive 4 mg IV q 3–4 wk to treat bone metastasis (Zometa). Tx of Paget disease, postmenopausal osteoporosis, osteoporosis in men; px of new clinical fractures in pts w/ low-trauma hip fractures; tx, px of glucocorticoid-induced osteoporosis; px of osteoporosis in postmenopausal women. *Adult:* 5 mg IV infused via vented infusion line over at least 15 min. May consider retreatment as needed once q 2 yr for osteoporosis (Reclast).
ADJUST DOSE Renal impairment
ADV EFF Constipation; coughing; decreased phosphate, magnesium, potassium, calcium levels; dyspnea; fever; hypotension; infections; insomnia, nephrotoxicity, osteonecrosis of the jaw
INTERACTIONS Aminoglycosides, loop diuretics, nephrotoxic drugs
NC/PT Do not confuse Reclast, Zometa; dosage varies. Pt should have dental exam before tx; mark calendar of infusion dates; drink plenty of fluids; take supplemental vitamin D, calcium; avoid exposure to infection; report difficulty breathing, swelling, jaw pain.

352   zolmitriptan

zolmitriptan (Zomig)
CLASS Antimigraine drug, triptan
PREG/CONT C/NA

IND & DOSE Tx of acute migraine attacks. *Adult:* 2.5 mg PO at onset of headache or w/ beginning of aura; may repeat if headache persists after 2 hr. Max, 10 mg/24 hr. Or, 1 spray in nostril at onset of headache or beginning of aura; may repeat in 2 hr if needed. Max, 10 mg/24 hr (2 sprays).
ADJUST DOSE Hepatic impairment
ADV EFF BP changes, burning/pressure sensation, chest pain, dizziness, drowsiness, numbness, QT prolongation, vertigo, weakness
INTERACTIONS Cimetidine, ergots, hormonal contraceptives, MAOIs, QT-prolonging drugs, sibutramine
NC/PT For acute attack, not for px. Not for use in pregnancy (may make hormonal contraceptives ineffective; barrier contraceptives advised). Pt should use right after removing from blister pack; not break, crush, or chew tablet; place orally disintegrating tablet on tongue, let dissolve; use one spray only if using nasal spray (may repeat after 2 hours if needed); take safety precautions w/ CNS effects; report chest pain, swelling, palpitations.

zolpidem tartrate (Ambien, Edluar, Intermezzo, Zolpimist)
CLASS Sedative-hypnotic
PREG/CONT C/C-IV

BBW Risk of suicidality; limit amount dispensed to depressed or suicidal pt.
IND & DOSE Short-term tx of insomnia. *Adult:* 10 mg PO at bedtime; max, 10 mg/day. ER tablets, 12.5 mg/day PO. Oral spray, two to three sprays in mouth, over tongue at bedtime. **Short-term tx of insomnia w/ middle-of-night awakening when pt has at least 4 hr of bedtime left** *(Intermezzo).* *Adult:* 1.75 mg (women) or 3.5 mg (men) sublingually; limit to 1.75 mg if also on CNS depressants.
ADJUST DOSE Elderly pts
ADV EFF Anaphylaxis, angioedema, dizziness, drowsiness, hangover, headache, sleep disorders, suicidality, suppression of REM sleep, vision disorders
NC/PT Limit amount of drug given to depressed pts. Withdraw gradually after long-term use. Review proper administration of various forms. Pt should take safety precautions w/ CNS effects, report difficulty breathing, swelling, thoughts of suicide.

zonisamide (Zonegran)
CLASS Antiepileptic
PREG/CONT C/NA

BBW Increased risk of suicidal ideation, suicidality; monitor accordingly.
IND & DOSE Adjuvant tx for partial seizures. *Adult, child 16 and over:* 100 mg PO daily as single dose, not divided; may divide subsequent doses. May increase by 100 mg/day q 2 wk to achieve control. Max, 600 mg/day.
ADJUST DOSE Renal impairment
ADV EFF Anorexia, ataxia, decrease in mental functioning, dizziness, dry mouth, metabolic acidosis, nausea, renal calculi, suicidality, unusual taste
INTERACTIONS Carbamazepine, phenobarbital, phenytoin, primidone
NC/PT Withdraw gradually after long-term use. Pt should drink plenty of fluids, take safety precautions w/ CNS effects, wear medical ID, report flank pain, urine/stool color changes, thoughts of suicide.

Patient Safety and Medication Administration

The seven rights of medication administration

In the clinical setting, the monumental task of ensuring medication safety can be managed by consistently using the seven rights of drug administration: right drug, right route, right dose, right time, right patient, right response, and right documentation.

Right drug: Always review a drug order before administering the drug.

- Do not assume that a computer system is always right. Always double-check.
- Make sure the drug name is correct. Ask for a brand name and a generic name; the chance of reading the name incorrectly is greatly reduced if both generic and brand names are used.
- Avoid taking verbal or telephone orders whenever possible. If you must, have a second person listen in to verify and clarify the order.
- Consider whether the drug makes sense for the patient's diagnosis.

Right route: Review the available forms of a drug to make sure the drug can be given according to the order.

- Check the routes available and the appropriateness of the route.
- Make sure the patient is able to take the drug by the route indicated.
- Do not use abbreviations for routes.

Right dose: Make sure the dose about to be delivered is the dose the prescriber ordered.

- There should always be a 0 to the left of a decimal point, and there should never be a 0 to the right of a decimal point. If you see an ordered dose that starts with a decimal point, question it. And if a dose seems much too big, question that.
- Double-check drug calculations, even if a computer did the calculations.
- Check the measuring devices used for liquid drugs. Advise patients not to use kitchen teaspoons or tablespoons to measure drug doses.
- Do not cut tablets in half to get the correct dose without checking the warnings that come with the drug.

Right time

- Ensure the timely delivery of the patient's drugs by scheduling dosing with other drugs, meals, or other consistent events to maintain the serum level.
- Teach patients the importance of timing critical drugs. As needed, make detailed medication schedules and prepare pill boxes.

Right patient: Check the patient's identification even if you think you know who the patient is.

- Review the patient's diagnosis, and verify that the drug matches the diagnosis.
- Make sure all allergies have been checked before giving a drug.

- Ask patients specifically about OTC drugs, vitamin and mineral supplements, herbal remedies, and routine drugs that they may not think to mention.
- Review the patient's drug regimen to prevent potential interactions between the drug you are about to give and drugs the patient already takes.

Right response

Monitor the patient's response to the drug administered to make sure that the response is what is anticipated.

Right Documentation: Document according to facility policy.

- Include the drug name, dose, route, and time of administration.
- Note special circumstances, such as the patient having difficulty swallowing or the site of the injection.
- Include the patient's response to the drug and any special nursing interventions that were used.
- Remember, "if it isn't written, it didn't happen." Accurate documentation provides continuity of care and helps prevent medication errors.

The bottom line in avoiding medication errors is simple: "If in doubt, check it out." A strange abbreviation, a drug or dosage that is new to you, and a confusing name are all examples that signal a need for follow-up. Look up the drug in your drug guide or call the prescriber or the pharmacy to double-check. Never give a drug until you have satisfied yourself that it is the right drug, given by the right route, at the right dose, at the right time, and to the right patient.

Keeping patients safe

Patient and family teaching

In today's world, the patient is usually left to manage on his or her own. The most important safety check after all is said and done is the patient. Only the patient actually knows what health care providers he or she is seeing; what prescription drugs, OTC drugs, and herbal remedies are actually being used; and how they are being used. Today's patient needs to be educated about all drugs being taken and empowered to speak up and protect himself or herself against medication errors.

Medication errors present a constant risk, particularly for patients who take multiple drugs prescribed by multiple health care providers. Educating the patient is key to preventing errors.

Patient teaching to prevent medication errors

When being prescribed medications, patients should learn these key points to reduce the risk of medication errors.

- **Keep a list:** Keep a written list of all the drugs you take, including over-the-counter drugs, herbal products, and other supplements; carry this list with you and show it to all your health care providers, including dentists and emergency personnel. If traveling in a different country, the brand name you are using may be used for a very different drug; it is important to known the generic name as well as the brand name. Refer to your list for safety.

- **Know your drugs:** Make sure you know why you take each of your drugs.

- **Follow the directions:** Carefully read the label of each of your drugs, and follow the directions for taking it safely. Do not stop taking a drug without first consulting the prescriber. Make a calendar if you take drugs on alternating days. Using a weekly pillbox may also help to keep things straight.

- **Store carefully:** Always store drugs in a dry place safely out of the reach of children and pets and away from humidity and heat (the bathroom is a bad storage area). Make sure to keep all drugs in their original, labeled containers.

- **Speak up:** You, the patient, are the most important member of your health care team. *Never be afraid to ask questions* about your health or your treatments.

Special populations

Keeping children safe

Children present unique challenges related to medication errors. Advise the child's caregiver to take these steps to prevent medication errors:

- Keep a list of all medications you are giving your child, including prescription, over-the-counter, and herbal medications. Share this list with any health care provider who cares for your child.
- Never use adult medications to treat a child.
- Read all labels before giving your child a drug. Check the ingredients and dosage to avoid overdose.
- Measure liquid medications using appropriate measuring devices.
- Call your health care provider immediately if your child seems to get worse or seems to be having trouble with a drug.
- When in doubt, do not hesitate to ask questions. You are your child's best advocate.

Protecting elderly patients

The elderly population is the most rapidly growing group in our country. Frequently, these patients have chronic diseases, are on multiple drugs, and have increasing health problems that can be a challenge to following a drug regimen. They are also more likely to suffer adverse reactions to drugs and drug combinations.

- Advise them to keep a medication list with them to share with all health care providers and to post a list somewhere in their home for easy access by emergency personnel.
- Prepare drug boxes for the week, draw up injectables (if stable) for the week, and provide daily reminders to take their medications.
- Be an advocate for elderly patients by asking questions, supplying information to providers, and helping elderly patients stay on top of their drug regimen and monitor their response.

Protecting women of childbearing age

As a general rule, it is best to avoid taking any drugs while pregnant.

- Advise women who may be pregnant to avoid Pregnancy Category X drugs (statins, hormones) that could cause serious harm to the fetus.
- Advise pregnant women to avoid all over-the-counter drugs and herbal therapies until they have checked with the obstetrician for safety.
- Advise pregnant women to question all prescribed drugs and to check carefully to make sure that the drugs are safe for the fetus.
- Advise breast-feeding women to question the safety of prescribed drugs, over-the-counter drugs, or herbal therapies to make sure that the drugs or therapies will not adversely affect the baby.
- Encourage pregnant women to ask questions. Supply information and be an advocate for the fetus or newborn child.

Avoiding dangerous abbreviations

Although abbreviations can save time, they also raise the risk of misinterpretation, which can lead to potentially disastrous consequences, especially when dealing with drug administration. To help reduce the risk of being misunderstood, always take the time to write legibly and to spell out anything that could be misread. This caution extends to how you write numbers as well as drug names and other drug-related instructions. The Joint Commission is enforcing a growing list of abbreviations that should not be used in medical records to help alleviate this problem. It is important to be familiar with the abbreviations used in your clinical area and to avoid the use of any other abbreviations.

Common dangerous abbreviations

Try to avoid these common—and dangerous—abbreviations, especially those that appear in **bold**.

Abbreviation	Intended use	Potential misreading	Preferred use
BT	bedtime	May be read as "bid" or twice daily	Spell out "bedtime."
cc	cubic centimeters	May be read as "u" or units	Use "milliliters," abbreviated as "mL" or "ml."
D/C	discharge or discontinue	May lead to premature discontinuation of drug therapy or premature discharge	Spell out "discharge" or "discontinue."
hs	at bedtime	May be read as "half-strength"	Spell out "at bedtime."
HS	half-strength	May be read as "at bedtime"	Spell out "half-strength."
IJ	injection	May be read as "IV"	Spell out "injection."
IN	intranasal	May be read as "IM" or "IV"	Spell out "intranasal" or use "NAS."
IU	international unit	May be read as "IV" or "10"	Spell out "international unit."
µg	microgram	May be read as "mg"	Use "mcg."
o.d. or O.D.	once daily	May be read as "right eye"	Spell out "once daily."
per os	by mouth	May be read as "left eye"	Use "PO" or spell out "orally."

Abbreviation	Intended use	Potential misreading	Preferred use
q.d. or QD	daily	May be read as "qid"	Spell out "daily."
q1d	once daily	May be read as "qid"	Spell out "once daily."
qhs	every bedtime	May be read as "qhr" (every hour)	Spell out "nightly" or "at bedtime."
qn	every night	May be read as "qh" (every hour)	Spell out "nightly" or "at bedtime."
q.o.d. or QOD	every other day	May be read as "q.d." (daily) or "q.i.d." (four times daily)	Spell out "every other day."
SC, SQ	subcutaneous	May be read as "SL" (sublingual) or "5 every"	Spell out "subcutaneous" or use "subcut."
U or u	unit	May be read as "0" (100 instead of 10U)	Spell out "unit."
×7d	for 7 days	May be read as "for seven doses"	Spell out "for 7 days."
°	hour	May be read as a zero	Spell out "hour" or use "hr."

Reporting medication errors

Due to increases in the number of drugs available, the aging population, and more people taking many drugs, the possibilities for medication errors seem to be increasing. Institutions have adopted policies for reporting errors, but it is also important to submit information about errors to national programs. These national programs, coordinated by the US Pharmacopeia (USP), help to gather and disseminate information about errors, to prevent their recurrence at other sites and by other providers.

Witnessing an error

If you witness or participate in an actual or potential medication error, it is important to report that error to the national clearinghouse to ultimately help other professionals avoid similar errors. The USP maintains one central reporting center, from which it disseminates information to the FDA, drug manufacturers, and the Institute for Safe Medication Practices (ISMP). You can report an actual error or potential error by calling 1-800-23-ERROR, the USP Medication Errors Reporting Program. This office will send you a mailer to fill out and return to them. Or, you can log on to www.usp.org to report an error online or to print out the form to mail or fax back to the USP. You may request to remain anonymous. If you are not sure about what you want to report, you may report errors to the USP through the ISMP website at www.ismp.org, which also offers a discussion forum on medication errors.

What kind of errors should be reported?

Errors (or potential errors) to report include administration of the wrong drug or the wrong strength or dose of a drug, incorrect routes of administration, miscalculations, misuse of medical equipment, mistakes in prescribing or transcribing (misunderstanding of verbal orders), and errors resulting from sound-alike or look-alike names. In your report, you will be asked to include the following:

1. A description of the error or preventable adverse drug reaction. What went wrong?
2. Was this an actual medication accident or are you expressing concern about a potential error or writing about an error that was discovered before it reached the patient?
3. Patient outcome. Did the patient suffer any adverse effects?
4. Type of practice site where the event occurred
5. Generic and brand names of all products involved
6. Dosage form, concentration or strength, and so forth
7. If the error was based on a communication problem, is a sample of the order available? Are package label samples or pictures available if requested?
8. Your recommendations for error prevention.

The ISMP publishes case studies and publicizes warnings and alerts based on clinician reports of medication errors. Their efforts have helped to increase recognition of the many types of errors, such as those involving sound-alike names, look-alike names and packaging, instructions on equipment and delivery devices, and others.

Guidelines for safe disposal of medications

The White House Office of National Drug Control Policy, the Department of Health and Human Services, and the Environmental Protection Agency have established guidelines for the proper disposal of unused, unneeded, or expired medications to promote consumer safety, block access to them by potential abusers, and protect the water supply and the environment from possible contamination.

Medical disposal guidelines

Disposing in trash

- Take unused, unneeded, or expired medications out of their original containers.
- Mix the medication with an undesirable substance, such as coffee grounds or used kitty litter, and place it in an impermeable, nondescript container, such as an empty can or a sealable storage bag. These steps help keep the medication from being diverted for illicit use or being accidentally ingested by children or animals.
- Place the closed container in your household trash.

Disposing in toilet

- Flush prescription drugs down the toilet **only** if the accompanying patient information specifically instructs you to do so.

Disposing at a hospital or government-sponsored site

- You may be able to return unused, unneeded, or expired prescription drugs to a pharmaceutical take-back location that offers safe disposal. Check with your local hospital, health department, or local government for a site near you.

Appendices

Alternative and complementary therapies

Many pts are now using herbs and alternative therapies. Some of these products may contain ingredients that interact with prescribed drugs. Pt hx of alternative therapy use may explain unexpected reactions to some drugs. In the chart below, drugs that the substance interacts with are in **bold**.

Substance	Reported uses, possible risks
acidophilus (probiotics)	*Oral:* px, tx of uncomplicated diarrhea; restoration of intestinal flora. RISK: **warfarin.**
alfalfa	*Topical:* healing ointment, relief of arthritis pain. *Oral:* tx of arthritis, hot flashes; strength giving; to reduce cholesterol level. RISK: **warfarin, chlorpromazine, antidiabetics, hormonal contraceptives, hormone replacement.**
allspice	*Topical:* anesthetic for teeth, gums; soothes sore joints, muscles. *Oral:* tx of indigestion, flatulence, diarrhea, fatigue. RISK: **iron.**
aloe leaves	*Topical:* tx of burns, healing of wounds. *Oral:* tx of chronic constipation. RISK: hypokalemia; spontaneous abortion if used in third trimester.
androstenedione	*Oral, spray:* anabolic steroid to increase muscle mass/ strength. RISK: CV disease, certain cancers.
angelica	*Oral:* "cure all" for gynecologic problems, headaches, backaches, appetite loss, GI spasms; increases circulation in periphery. RISK: **anticoagulants.**
anise	*Oral:* relief of dry cough, tx of flatulence, bloating. RISK: **iron.**
apple	*Oral:* blood glucose control, constipation, cancer, heart problems. RISK: **antidiabetics, fexofenadine.**
arnica	*Topical:* relief of pain from muscle, soft-tissue injury. *Oral:* immune system stimulant; very toxic to children. RISK: **antihypertensives, anticoagulants, antiplatelet drugs.**

Substance	Reported uses, possible risks
ashwagandha	*Oral:* to improve mental, physical functioning; general tonic; to protect cells during cancer chemotherapy, radiation therapy. RISK: **anticoagulants; thyroid replacement.**
astragalus	*Oral:* to increase stamina, energy; to improve immune function, resistance to disease; tx of URI, common cold. RISK: **antihypertensives.**
barberry	*Oral:* antidiarrheal, antipyretic, cough suppressant. RISK: **antihypertensives, antiarrhythmics;** spontaneous abortion if taken during pregnancy.
basil	*Oral:* analgesic, anti-inflammatory, hypoglycemic. RISK: **antidiabetics.**
bayberry	*Topical:* to promote wound healing. *Oral:* stimulant, emetic, antidiarrheal. RISK: **antihypertensives.**
bee pollen	*Oral:* to treat allergies, asthma, ED, prostatitis; suggested use to decrease cholesterol levels, premenstrual syndrome. RISK: **antidiabetics;** bee allergy.
betel palm	*Oral:* mild stimulant, digestive aid. RISK: **MAOIs; beta blockers, digoxin, antiglaucoma drugs.**
bilberry	*Oral:* tx of diabetes, diabetic retinopathy, CV problems, cataracts, night blindness; lowers cholesterol, triglycerides. RISK: **anticoagulants, alcohol.**
birch bark	*Topical:* tx of infected wounds, cuts; very toxic to children. *Oral:* as tea for relief of stomachache.
blackberry	*Oral:* generalized healing; tx of diabetes. RISK: **antidiabetics.**
black cohosh root	*Oral:* tx of PMS, menopausal disorders, rheumatoid arthritis. Contains estrogen-like components. RISK: **hormone replacement, hormonal contraceptives, sedatives, antihypertensives, anesthetics, immunosuppressants.**
bromelain	*Oral:* tx of inflammation, sports injuries, URI, PMS; adjunct in cancer treatment. RISK: **n/v/d, menstrual disorders.**
burdock	*Oral:* tx of diabetes; atropine-like adverse effects; uterine stimulant. RISK: **antidiabetics.**

Substance	Reported uses, possible risks
capsicum	*Topical*: external analgesic. *Oral*: tx of bowel disorders, chronic laryngitis, peripheral vascular disease. RISK: **warfarin, aspirin, ACE inhibitors, MAOIs, sedatives.**
catnip leaves	*Oral*: tx of bronchitis, diarrhea.
cat's claw	*Oral*: tx of allergies, arthritis; adjunct in tx of cancers, AIDS. Discourage use by transplant recipients, during pregnancy, breast-feeding. RISK: **oral anticoagulants, antihypertensives.**
cayenne pepper	*Topical*: tx of burns, wounds; relief of toothache.
celery	*Oral*: lowers blood glucose, acts as diuretic; may cause potassium depletion. RISK: **antidiabetics.**
chamomile	*Topical*: tx of wounds, ulcers, conjunctivitis. *Oral*: tx of migraines, gastric cramps; relief of anxiety, inflammatory diseases. Contains coumarin; closely monitor pts taking anticoagulants. RISK: **antidepressants;** ragweed allergies.
chaste-tree berry	*Oral*: tx of PMS, menopausal problems; to stimulate lactation. Progesterone-like effects. RISK: **hormone replacement, hormonal contraceptives.**
chicken soup	*Oral*: breaks up respiratory secretions; bronchodilator; relieves anxiety.
chicory	*Oral*: tx of digestive tract problems, gout; stimulates bile secretions.
Chinese angelica (dong quai)	*Oral*: general tonic; tx of anemias, PMS, menopausal sx, antihypertensive, laxative. Use caution with flu, hemorrhagic diseases. RISK: **antihypertensives, vasodilators, anticoagulants, hormone replacement.**
chondroitin	*Oral*: tx of osteoarthritis, related disorders (usually w/ glucosamine). RISK: **anticoagulants.**
chong cao fungi	*Oral*: antioxidant; promotes stamina, sexual function.
Coleus forskohlii	*Oral*: tx of asthma, hypertension, eczema. RISK: **antihypertensives, antihistamines;** peptic ulcer.
comfrey	*Topical*: tx of wounds, cuts, ulcers. *Oral*: gargle for tonsillitis. RISK: **eucalyptus;** monitor LFTs.

Substance	Reported uses, possible risks
coriander	*Oral:* weight loss, lowers blood glucose. RISK: **antidiabetics.**
creatine monohydrate	*Oral:* to enhance athletic performance. RISK: **insulin, caffeine.**
dandelion root	*Oral:* tx of liver, kidney problems; decreases lactation (after delivery, w/ weaning); lowers blood glucose. RISK: **antidiabetics, antihypertensives, quinolone antibiotics.**
DHEA	*Oral:* slows aging, improves vigor ("Fountain of Youth"); androgenic side effects. RISK: **alprazolam, calcium channel blockers, antidiabetics.**
di huang	*Oral:* tx of diabetes mellitus. RISK: **antidiabetics.**
dried root bark of *Lycium chinense* Miller	*Oral:* lowers cholesterol, blood glucose. RISK: **antidiabetics.**
echinacea (cone flower)	*Oral:* tx of colds, flu; stimulates immune system, attacks viruses; causes immunosuppression if used long-term. May be hepatotoxic; discourage use for longer than 12 wk. Discourage use by patients with SLE, TB, AIDS. RISK: **hepatotoxic drugs, immunosuppressants, antifungals.**
elder bark and flowers	*Topical:* gargle for tonsillitis/pharyngitis. *Oral:* tx of fever, chills.
ephedra	*Oral:* increases energy, relieves fatigue. RISK: **serious complications, including death; increased risk of hypertension, stroke, MI; interacts w/ many drugs; banned by FDA.**
ergot	*Oral:* tx of migraine headaches, menstrual problems, hemorrhage. RISK: **antihypertensives.**
eucalyptus	*Topical:* tx of wounds. *Oral:* decreases respiratory secretions; suppresses cough. Very toxic in children. RISK: **comfrey.**
evening primrose	*Oral:* tx of PMS, menopause, rheumatoid arthritis, diabetic neuropathy. Discourage use by pts with epilepsy, schizophrenia. RISK: **phenothiazines, antidepressants.**
false unicorn root	*Oral:* tx of menstrual, uterine problems. Not for use in pregnancy, breast-feeding.

Substance	Reported uses, possible risks
fennel	*Oral:* tx of colic, gout, flatulence; enhances lactation. RISK: **ciprofloxacin.**
fenugreek	*Oral:* lowers cholesterol level; reduces blood glucose; aids in healing. RISK: **antidiabetics, anticoagulants.**
feverfew	*Oral:* tx of arthritis, fever, migraine. Not for use if surgery planned. RISK: **anticoagulants.**
fish oil	*Oral:* tx of coronary diseases, arthritis, colitis, depression, aggression, attention deficit disorder.
garlic	*Oral:* tx of colds; diuretic; px of CAD; intestinal antiseptic; lowers blood glucose; anticoagulant effects; decreases BP; anemia. RISK: **antidiabetics.**
ginger	*Oral:* tx of nausea, motion sickness, postop nausea (may increase risk of miscarriage). RISK: **anticoagulants.**
ginkgo	*Oral:* vascular dilation; increases blood flow to brain, improving cognitive function; tx of Alzheimer disease; antioxidant. Can inhibit blood clotting. Seizures reported w/ high doses. RISK: **anticoagulants, aspirin, NSAIDs, phenytoin, carbamazepine, phenobarbital, TCAs, MAOIs, antidiabetics.**
ginseng	*Oral:* aphrodisiac, mood elevator, tonic; antihypertensive; decreases cholesterol levels; lowers blood glucose; adjunct in cancer chemotherapy, radiation therapy. May cause irritability if used w/ caffeine. Inhibits clotting. RISK: **anticoagulants, aspirin, NSAIDs, phenelzine, MAOIs, estrogens, corticosteroids, digoxin, antidiabetics.**
glucosamine	*Oral:* tx of osteoarthritis, joint diseases; usually w/ chondroitin. RISK: diabetic pts.
goldenrod leaves	*Oral:* tx of renal disease, rheumatism, sore throat, eczema. RISK: **diuretics.**
goldenseal	*Oral:* lowers blood glucose, aids healing; tx of bronchitis, colds, flulike sx, cystitis. May cause false-negative results in pts using drugs such as marijuana, cocaine. Large amounts may cause paralysis; overdose can cause death. RISK: **anticoagulants, antihypertensives, acid blockers, barbiturates, sedatives.**

Substance	Reported uses, possible risks
gotu kola	*Topical:* chronic venous insufficiency. RISK: **antidiabetics, cholesterol-lowering drugs, sedatives.**
grape seed extract	*Oral:* tx of allergies, asthma; improves circulation; decreases platelet aggregation. RISK: **anticoagulants.**
green tea leaf	*Oral:* antioxidant; to prevent cancer, CV disease; to increase cognitive function (caffeine effects). RISK: **anticoagulants, milk.**
guarana	*Oral:* decreases appetite; promotes weight loss; increases BP, risk of CV events.
guayusa	*Oral:* lowers blood glucose; promotes weight loss. RISK: **antihypertensives, iron, lithium.**
hawthorn	*Oral:* tx of angina, arrhythmias, BP problems; decreases cholesterol. RISK: **digoxin, ACE inhibitors, CNS depressants.**
hop	*Oral:* sedative; aids healing; alters blood glucose. RISK: **CNS depressants, antipsychotics.**
horehound	*Oral:* expectorant; tx of respiratory problems, GI disorders. RISK: **antidiabetics, antihypertensives.**
horse chestnut seed	*Oral:* tx of varicose veins, hemorrhoids, venous insufficiency. RISK: **anticoagulants.**
hyssop	*Topical:* tx of cold sores, genital herpes, burns, wounds. *Oral:* tx of coughs, colds, indigestion, flatulence. Toxic in children, pets. RISK: pregnancy, pts w/ seizures.
jambul	*Oral:* tx of diarrhea, dysentery; lowers blood glucose. RISK: **CNS depressants, Java plum.**
Java plum	*Oral:* tx of diabetes mellitus. RISK: **antidiabetics.**
jojoba	*Topical:* promotion of hair growth; relief of skin problems. Toxic if ingested.
juniper berries	*Oral:* increases appetite, aids digestion; diuretic; urinary tract disinfectant; lowers blood glucose. RISK: **Antidiabetics;** pregnancy.
kava	*Oral:* tx of nervous anxiety, stress, restlessness; tranquilizer. Warn against use with alprazolam; may cause coma. Advise against use with Parkinson disease, hx of stroke. Risk of serious hepatotoxicity. RISK: **St. John's wort, anxiolytics, alcohol.**

Substance	Reported uses, possible risks
kudzu	*Oral:* reduces alcohol craving (undergoing research for use w/ alcoholics). RISK: **anticoagulants, aspirin, antidiabetics, CV drugs.**
lavender	*Topical:* astringent for minor cuts, burns. Oil potentially poisonous. *Oral:* tx of insomnia, restlessness. RISK: **CNS depressants.**
ledum tincture	*Topical:* tx of insect bites, puncture wounds; dissolves some blood clots, bruises.
licorice	*Oral:* px of thirst; soothes coughs; treats "incurable" chronic fatigue syndrome; tx of duodenal ulcer. Acts like aldosterone. Blocks spironolactone effects. Can lead to digoxin toxicity because of aldosterone-lowering effects; advise extreme caution. RISK: **thyroid drugs, antihypertensives, hormonal contraceptives;** renal/liver disease, hypertension, CAD, pregnancy, breast-feeding.
ma huang	*Oral:* tx of colds, nasal congestion, asthma. Contains ephedrine. RISK: **antihypertensives, antidiabetics, MAOIs, digoxin.**
mandrake root	*Oral:* tx of fertility problems.
marigold leaves and flowers	*Oral:* relief of muscle tension; increases wound healing. RISK: pregnancy, breast-feeding.
melatonin	*Oral:* relief of jet lag; tx of insomnia. RISK: **antihypertensives, benzodiazepines, beta blockers, methamphetamine.**
milk thistle	*Oral:* tx of hepatitis, cirrhosis, fatty liver caused by alcohol/drug use. RISK: **drugs using CP450, CYP3A4, CYP2C9 systems.**
milk vetch	*Oral:* improves resistance to disease; adjunct in cancer chemotherapy, radiation therapy.
mistletoe leaves	*Oral:* promotes weight loss; relief of s&sx of diabetes. RISK: **antihypertensives, CNS depressants, immunosuppressants.**
Momordica charantia (Karela)	*Oral:* blocks intestinal absorption of glucose; lowers blood glucose; weight loss. RISK: **antidiabetics.**
nettle	*Topical:* stimulation of hair growth, tx of bleeding. *Oral:* tx of rheumatism, allergic rhinitis; antispasmodic; expectorant. RISK: **diuretics;** pregnancy, breast-feeding.

Substance	Reported uses, possible risks
nightshade leaves and roots	*Oral:* stimulates circulatory system; tx of eye disorders.
octacosanol	*Oral:* tx of parkinsonism, enhancement of athletic performance. RISK: **carbidopa-levodopa; pregnancy, breast-feeding.**
parsley seeds and leaves	*Oral:* tx of jaundice, asthma, menstrual difficulties, urinary infections, conjunctivitis. RISK: **SSRIs, lithium, opioids, antihypertensives.**
passionflower vine	*Oral:* sedative-hypnotic. RISK: **CNS depressants, MAOIs, alcohol, anticoagulants.**
peppermint leaves	*Topical:* rubbed on forehead to relieve tension headaches. *Oral:* tx of nervousness, insomnia, dizziness, cramps, coughs.
psyllium	*Oral:* tx of constipation; lowers cholesterol. Can cause severe gas, stomach pain. May interfere w/ nutrient absorption. RISK: **warfarin, digoxin, lithium, oral drugs, laxatives.**
raspberry	*Oral:* healing of minor wounds; control, tx of diabetes, GI disorders, upper respiratory disorders. RISK: **antidiabetics; alcohol.**
red clover	*Oral:* estrogen replacement in menopause; suppresses whooping cough; asthma. RISK: **anticoagulants, antiplatelets; pregnancy.**
red yeast rice	*Oral:* lowers cholesterol. RISK: **cyclosporine, fibric acid, niacin, lovastatin, grapefruit juice.**
rose hips	*Oral:* laxative; to boost immune system, prevent illness. RISK: **estrogens, iron, warfarin.**
rosemary	*Topical:* relief of rheumatism, sprains, wounds, bruises, eczema. *Oral:* gastric stimulation; relief of flatulence, colic; stimulation of bile release. RISK: **alcohol.**
rue extract	*Topical:* relief of pain associated w/ sprains, groin pulls, whiplash. RISK: **antihypertensives, digoxin, warfarin.**
saffron	*Oral:* tx of menstrual problems; abortifacient.
sage	*Oral:* lowers BP, blood glucose. RISK: **antidiabetics, anticonvulsants, alcohol.**

Substance	Reported uses, possible risks
SAM-e (adomet)	*Oral:* promotion of general well-being, health. May cause frequent GI complaints, headache. RISK: **antidepressants.**
sarsaparilla	*Oral:* tx of skin disorders, rheumatism. RISK: **anticonvulsants.**
sassafras	*Topical:* tx of local pain, skin eruptions. *Oral:* enhancement of athletic performance, "cure" for syphilis. **Oil may be toxic to fetus, children, adults when ingested. Interacts with many drugs.**
saw palmetto	*Oral:* tx of BPH. RISK: **estrogen-replacement, hormonal contraceptives, iron, finasteride.**
schisandra	*Oral:* health tonic, liver protectant; adjunct in cancer chemotherapy, radiation therapy. RISK: **drugs metabolized in liver;** pregnancy (causes uterine stimulation).
squaw vine	*Oral:* diuretic, tonic; aid in labor, delivery; tx of menstrual problems. RISK: **digoxin, alcohol.**
St. John's wort	*Topical:* tx of puncture wounds, insect bites, crushed fingers/toes. *Oral:* tx of depression, PMS symptoms; antiviral. Discourage tyramine-containing foods; hypertensive crisis possible. Thrombocytopenia has occurred. Can increase light sensitivity; advise against taking w/ drugs causing photosensitivity. Severe photosensitivity possible in light-skinned people. RISK: **SSRIs, MAOIs, kava, digoxin, theophylline, AIDS antivirals, sympathomimetics, antineoplastics, hormonal contraceptives.**
sweet violet flowers	*Oral:* tx of respiratory disorders; emetic. RISK: **laxatives.**
tarragon	*Oral:* weight loss; prevents cancer; lowers blood glucose. RISK: **antidiabetics.**
tea tree oil	*Topical:* antifungal, antibacterial; tx of burns, insect bites, irritated skin, acne; mouthwash.
thyme	*Topical:* liniment, gargle; tx of wounds. *Oral:* antidiarrheal; relief of bronchitis, laryngitis. May increase light sensitivity; warn against using w/ photosensitivity-causing drugs. RISK: **MAOIs, SSRIs.**

Substance	Reported uses, possible risks
turmeric	*Oral:* antioxidant, anti-inflammatory; tx of arthritis. May cause GI distress. Warn against use w/ known biliary obstruction. RISK: **oral anticoagulants, NSAIDs, immunosuppressants.**
valerian	*Oral:* sedative-hypnotic; reduces anxiety, relaxes muscles. Can cause severe liver damage. RISK: **barbiturates, alcohol, CNS depressants, benzodiazepines, antihistamines.**
went rice	*Oral:* cholesterol-, triglyceride-lowering effects. Warn against use in pregnancy, liver disease, alcoholism, acute infection.
white willow bark	*Oral:* tx of fevers. RISK: **anticoagulants, NSAIDs, diuretics.**
xuan shen	*Oral:* lowers blood glucose; slows heart rate; tx of HF. RISK: **antidiabetics.**
yohimbe	*Oral:* tx of ED. Can affect BP; CNS stimulant. Has cardiac effects. Manic episodes have occurred in psychiatric pts. RISK: **SSRIs, tyramine-containing foods, TCAs.**

Appendix B

Topical drugs

Topical drugs are intended for surface use, not ingestion or injection. They may be toxic if absorbed into the system, but they serve several purposes when used topically.

PREG/CONT C

ADV EFF Burning, dermatitis, local irritation (common), stinging, toxic effects if absorbed systemically

NC/PT Apply sparingly to affected area as directed. Do not use w/ open wounds, broken skin. Avoid contact w/ eyes. Pt should report local irritation, allergic reaction, worsening of condition.

Acne, rosacea, melasma products

adapalene (Differin): Not for use under 12 yr. Avoid use on sunburned skin, w/ other products, sun exposure. Apply thin film to affected area after washing q night at bedtime. Available as cream, gel; 0.1%, 0.3% conc.

alitretinoin (Panretin): Tx of lesions of Kaposi sarcoma (1% gel). Apply as needed bid to cover lesions. Photosensitivity common. Inflammation, peeling, redness possible. Pregnancy Category D.

azelaic acid (Azelex, Finacea): Wash, dry skin. Massage thin layer into affected area bid. Wash hands thoroughly after applying. Improvement usually within 4 wk. Initial irritation usual; passes with time.

brimonidine (Mirvaso): Tx of persistent facial erythema of rosacea in adult. Apply pea-size amount to forehead, chin, cheeks daily. Risk of vascular insufficiency. Wash hands immediately after application; do not ingest.

clindamycin (Clindesse, Evoclin): Tx of bacterial vaginitis (2% vaginal cream): One applicatorful (100 mg) vaginally at any time of day. Tx of acne vulgaris (1% foam): Apply once daily to affected areas that have been washed, are fully dry.

clindamycin/benzoyl peroxide (Acanya, BenzaClin): Apply gel to affected areas bid. Wash area, pat dry before applying.

clindamycin/tretinoin (Veltin, Ziana): Rub pea-size amount over entire face once daily at bedtime. Not for use in colitis. Avoid sun exposure.

dapsone (Aczone Gel): Apply thin layer to affected areas bid. Closely follow Hgb, reticulocyte count in pts w/ G6PD deficiencies.

fluocinolone acetonide/hydroquinone/tretinoin (Tri-Luma): Do not use in pregnancy. Apply to depigmented area of melasma once each p.m. at least 30 min before bedtime after washing, patting dry; avoid occlusive dressings. Use sunscreen, protective clothing if outside (skin dryness, peeling possible).

ingenol mebutate (Picato): Tx of acne: Apply 0.015% gel once daily to face/scalp for 5 days. Apply 0.05% gel once daily to trunk/extremities for 2 days.

metronidazole (MetroCream, MetroGel, MetroLotion, Noritate): Tx of rosacea. Apply cream to affected area bid.

sodium sulfacetamide (Klaron): Apply thin film to affected area bid. Wash affected area w/ mild soap, water; pat dry. Avoid use in denuded, abraded areas.

tazarotene (Fabior, Tazorac): Tx of psoriasis. Avoid use in pregnancy. Apply thin film once daily in p.m. Do not use with irritants, products w/ high alcohol content. Drying causes photosensitivity.

tretinoin 0.025% cream (Avita): Apply thin layer once daily. Discomfort, peeling, redness possible first 2–4 wk. Worsened acne possible in first few wk.

tretinoin 0.05% cream (Renova): To remove fine wrinkles. Apply thin coat in p.m.

tretinoin gel (Retin-A* Micro): Apply to cover once daily after washing. Inflammation exacerbation possible initially. Therapeutic effects usually seen in first 2 wk.

Analgesics

capsaicin (Axsain, Capsin, Capzasin, Icy Hot PM, No Pain-HP, Pain Doctor, Zostrix, Zostrix-HP): Local pain relief for osteoarthritis, rheumatoid arthritis, neuralgias. Apply no more than tid–qid. Do not bandage tightly. Consult physician if condition worsens or persists after 14–28 days. **Qutenza:** Apply patch to relieve postherpetic neuralgia pain.

Antibiotics

ciprofloxacin/dexamethasone (Ciprodex), ciprofloxacin/hydro-

cortisone (Cipro-HC Otic Drops): Apply to ears of child w/ acute otitis media and tympanostomy tubes; apply to outer ear canal for acute otitis externa. Use bid for 7 days.

mupirocin (Bactroban, Centany): Tx of impetigo caused by susceptible strains. Apply small amt to affected area tid; may cover with gauze dressing. Risk of superinfection.

mupirocin calcium (Bactroban Nasal): To eradicate nasal colonization of MRSA. Apply ½ of oint from single-use tubes between nostrils bid for 5 days.

retapamulin (Altabax): Tx of impetigo in pts 9 mo and older. Apply thin layer to affected area bid for 5 days.

Anti-diaper-rash drug

miconazole/zinc oxide/petrolatum (Vusion): Culture for *Candida* before tx. Apply gently for 7 days; change diapers frequently, wash gently.

Antifungals

butenafine hydrochloride (Mentax): Tx of athlete's foot; tinea corporis, cruris; ringworm. Apply once/day for 4 wk.

ciclopirox (Loprox, Penlac Nail Lacquer): Tx of onychomycosis of fingernails, toenails in immunosuppressed pts. Apply directly to nails.

clotrimazole (Cruex, Desenex, Lotrimin, Mycelex): Clean area; gently massage in up to bid for max 4 wk.

econazole (Spectazole): Apply daily or bid for 2–4 wk. Clean area before applying. Change socks at least once/day for athlete's foot.

gentian violet (generic): Apply locally up to bid. Do not apply to active lesions. Will stain skin, clothing.

ketoconazole (Extina, Nizoral, Xolegel): Available as cream, foam, gel, shampoo. Use as shampoo daily.

luliconazole (Luzu): Tx of tinea cruris, tinea corporis. Apply to affected area once a day for 1 wk, 2 wk for interdigital tinea pedis.

naftifine hydrochloride (Naftin): Gently massage in bid for no more than 4 wk. Avoid occlusive dressings. Wash hands thoroughly after applying.

oxiconazole (Oxistat): Apply q day to bid for max 1 mo.

sertaconazole (Ertaczo): Apply between toes, to surrounding tissue bid for 4 wk.

terbinafine (Lamisil): Apply bid for 1–4 wk. Avoid occlusive dressings. Stop if local irritation.

tolnaftate (Absorbine, Tinactin): Apply small amount bid for 2–3 wk; 4–6 wk if skin very thick. Clean, dry area before use. Change socks qid.

Antihistamine

azelastine hydrochloride (Astelin, Astepro): 2 sprays/nostril bid. Do not use w/ alcohol, OTC antihistamines; dizziness, sedation possible.

Antipsoriatics

anthralin (Balnetar, Dritho-Cream HP, Fototar, Zithranol): Apply daily; use protective dressings. Avoid contact w/ eyes. May stain fabric, skin, hair, fingernails.

calcipotriene (Dovonex): Apply thin layer q day or bid. Monitor calcium with extended use.

calcipotriene/betamethasone (Taclonex, Taclonex Scalp): Apply q day for 4 wk. Max, 100 g/wk. Avoid occlusive dressings. Limit to 30% of body area.

Antiseborrheic

selenium sulfide (Selsun Blue): Massage 5–10 mL into scalp, leave on 2–3 min, rinse; repeat. May damage jewelry.

Antiseptics

benzalkonium chloride (Benza, Mycocide NS, Zephiran): Mix in sol. Spray preop area; store instruments in sol (add antirust tablets). Rinse detergents, soaps from skin before use.

chlorhexidine gluconate (BactoShield, Dyna-Hex, Exidine, Hibistat): For surgical scrub, preop skin prep, wound cleansing. Scrub, leave on for 15 sec (3 min for surgical scrub), rinse.

hexachlorophene (pHisoHex): For surgical wash, scrub. Do not use on mucous membranes, w/ burns. Rinse thoroughly. Not for routine bathing of infants.

iodine (generic): Wash area w/ sol. Highly toxic. Avoid occlusive dressings. Stains skin, clothing.

povidone iodine (ACU-Dyne, Betadine, Betagen, Exodine, Iodex, Minidyne, Operand, Polydine): Less irritating than iodine. May bandage area. May inactivate HIV.

sodium hypochlorite (Dakin's solution): Apply as antiseptic. Chemical burns possible.

Antivirals

acyclovir (Zovirax): Apply 0.5-inch ribbon, rub in gently six times/day for 7 days.

acyclovir/hydrocortisone (Xerese): Tx of cold sores in pts 6 yr and older. Apply five times/day for 5 days.

docosanol (Abreva): Tx of oral, facial herpes simplex cold sores. Apply five times/day for 10 days. Do not overuse.

imiquimod (Aldara): Tx of external genital, perianal warts: Apply thin layer three times/week at bedtime for up to 16 wk; remove with soap, water after 6–10 hr. Tx of nonhyperkeratotic actinic keratosis on face, scalp in immunosuppressed pts: Apply before bed for 16 wk. Tx of superficial basal cell carcinoma in immunosuppressed pts: 10–40 mg applied to lesion five times/wk at bedtime for 6 wk.

imiquimod (Zyclara): Tx of nonhyperkeratotic, nonhypertrophic actinic keratoses on face, balding scalp: Apply daily at bedtime for 2 wk, then 2 wk of no tx. May repeat. Tx of genital, perianal warts in pts 12 yr and older: Apply daily.

kunecatechins (Veregen): External tx of genital, perianal warts in pts 18 yr and older. Apply to each wart tid for 16 wk. Do not cover tx area.

penciclovir (Denavir): Tx of cold sores on lips, face. Apply thin layer q 2 hr while awake for 4 days.

Burn tx

mafenide (Sulfamylon): Apply to clean, dry, debrided wound q day or bid. Cover at all times w/ drug. Monitor for infection, acidosis. Pretreat for pain.

silver sulfadiazine (Silvadene, SSD Cream, Thermazene): Apply q day to bid using 1/16-inch thickness. Dressings not necessary. Monitor for fungal infection.

Corticosteroids for inflammatory disorders

alclometasone dipropionate (Aclovate): 0.05% oint, cream

beclomethasone (Beconase AQ, Qnasl): Nasal spray for rhinitis

betamethasone dipropionate: 0.05% oint, cream, gel, lotion, aerosol

betamethasone dipropionate augmented (Diprolene, Diprolene AF): 0.05% oint, cream, lotion

betamethasone valerate (Beta-Val, Luxiq, Valisone): 0.1% oint, cream, lotion; 0.12% foam

ciclesonide (Alvesco, Omnaris, Zetonna): 80 or 160 mcg/actuation as nasal spray or for inhalation

clobetasol propionate (Clobex, Cormax, Olux, Temovate): 0.05% spray, oint, cream, foam, gel

clocortolone pivalate (Cloderm): 0.1% cream

desonide (DesOwen, Verdeso): 0.05% oint, lotion, cream, foam

desoximetasone (Topicort): 0.25% oint, cream

dexamethasone (Aeroseb-Dex): 0.05% cream, gel

diflorasone diacetate (Florone, Florone E, Maxiflor, Psorcon E): 0.1% cream

fluocinolone acetate (Fluonid, Synalar): 0.05% oint, cream; 0.01% sol

fluocinonide (Fluonex, Lidex, Vanos): 0.025% cream, oint; 0.01% cream; 0.05% cream, oint, gel, sol, 0.1% cream

flurandrenolide (generic): 0.05% cream, lotion, oint; tape, 4 mcg/cm²

fluticasone fumarate (Veramyst): 35 mcg/spray nasal spray

fluticasone propionate (Cutivate): 0.05% cream, 0.005% oint

halcinonide (Halog): 0.1% oint, cream, sol

halobetasol propionate (Ultravate): 0.05% cream, oint

hydrocortisone (Bactine Hydrocortisone, Cort-Dome, Dermolate, Dermtex HC, Cortizone-10, Hycort, Tegrin-HC, Hytone): 0.25%, 0.5%, 1%, 2%, 2.5 % cream, lotion, oint, sol

hydrocortisone acetate (Anusol-HCL, Cortaid, Cortaid with Aloe, Gynecort, Lanacort-5): 0.5%, 1% cream, oint

hydrocortisone buteprate (generic): 0.1% cream

hydrocortisone butyrate (Locoid): 0.1% oint, cream

hydrocortisone valerate (Westcort): 0.2% oint, cream

mometasone furoate (Asmanex Twisthaler, Elocon, Nasonex): 220 mcg/actuation powder for oral inhalation; 0.1% oint, cream, lotion; 0.2% nasal spray

prednicarbate (Dermatop): 0.1% cream

triamcinolone acetonide (Triacet, Triderm): 0.1% cream, lotion; 0.025% lotion

Emollients

dexpanthenol (Panthoderm): To relieve itching, aids in healing skin irritation; q day to bid.

urea (Aquacare; Carmol 10, 20, 40; Gordon's Urea 40%; Nutraplus; Ureacin 10, 20): Rub in bid–qid.

vitamins A, D (generic): To relieve minor burns, chafing, skin irritation. bid–qid for up to 7 days.

zinc oxide (Borofax Skin Protectant): To relieve burns, abrasions, diaper rash. Apply PRN.

Estrogen

estradiol hemihydrate (Vagifem): Tx of atrophic vaginitis. One tablet/day vaginally for 2 wk, then 1 tablet two times/wk. Taper over 3–6 mo.

Growth factor

becaplermin (Regranex): Adjunct tx of diabetic foot ulcers. Must have adequate blood supply. Risk of cancer with long-term use.

Hair removal product

eflornithine (Vaniqa): For women only. Apply to unwanted facial hair bid for 24 wk; do not wash treated area for 4 hr.

Hemostatics

absorbable gelatin (Gelfoam): Add 3–4 mL sterile saline to contents of jar; smear or press to cut surface. Assess for infection; do not use if area infected.

absorbable fibrin sealant (TachoSil): For CV surgery when usual techniques to control bleeding ineffective. Apply yellow side of patches directly to bleeding area. Do not use intravascularly or with known hypersensitivity to human blood products, horse protein.

human fibrin sealant (Artiss, Evicel, Tisseel): Adjunct to decrease bleeding in vascular, liver surgery; to adhere autologous skin grafts for burns. Spray or drip onto tissue in short bursts to produce thin layer; may use second layer.

microfibrillar collagen (Hemopad): Apply dry directly to bleeding source. Monitor for infection. Remove any excess material once bleeding stopped.

thrombin (Thrombinar, Thrombostat): 100–1,000 units/mL. Prepare in sterile distilled water or isotonic saline. Mix freely with blood on surface of injury; watch for allergic reactions.

thrombin, recombinant (Recothrom): Apply directly to bleeding site w/ absorbable gelatin sponge; reserve for minor bleeds. Not for use w/ hamster, snake protein allergies.

Immunomodulator

pimecrolimus (Elidel): Tx of mild to moderate atopic dermatitis in nonimmunosuppressed pts over 2 yr. Apply bid.

Keratolytics

podofilox (Condylox): Apply to dry skin q 12 hr for 3 days.

podophyllum resin (Podocon-25, Podofin): Use minimum possible for wart removal; very toxic.

Local anesthetic

lidocaine/tetracaine (Synera): Dermal analgesia for superficial venous access, dermatologic procedures. Apply one patch to intact skin 20–30 min before procedure.

Lotions, solutions

Burow's solution aluminum acetate (Domeboro Powder): Astrin-

gent wet dressing for inflammatory conditions, insect bites, athlete's foot, bruises. Dissolve packet, tablet in pint of water; apply q 15–30 min for 4–8 hr.

calamine lotion (generic): To relieve topical itching. Apply tid–qid.

hamamelis water (A-E-R, Witch Hazel): To relieve itching of vaginal infection, hemorrhoids; post-episiotomy, post hemorrhoidectomy care. Apply locally six times/day.

Nasal corticosteroid

fluticasone propionate (Flonase, Flovent Diskus, Flovent HFA): Px of asthma in pts over 4 yr. Two sprays/nostril/day or 88–220 mcg bid using inhalation device, nasal inhalation.

Oral preparation

amlexanox (Aphthasol): Apply sol or mucoadhesive disc to each aphthous ulcer qid for 10 days. Consult dentist if not healed in 10 days.

Pediculicides, scabicides

benzyl alcohol (generic): Tx of head lice in pts 6 mo and older. Apply 5% lotion to scalp, hair near scalp.

crotamiton (Eurax): Massage into skin of entire body; repeat in 24 hr. Bathe 48 hr after use. Change bed linens, clothing; wash in hot water, dry clean.

ivermectin (Sklice): Tx of head lice in pts 6 mo and older. Apply 0.5% lotion once to head for 10 min; no need for nit picking.

lindane (generic): Apply thin layer to entire body, leave on 8–12 hr, then wash thoroughly. For shampoo, 2 oz into dry hair, leave on 4 min, then rinse. Reapply in 7 days if needed.

malathion (Ovide Lotion): Apply to dry hair, leave on 8–12 hr, rinse. Repeat in 7–9 days. Contains flammable alcohol.

permethrin (Acticin, Elimite, Nix): Thoroughly massage into skin, wash off after 8–14 hr. For shampoo, work into freshly washed, towel-dried hair, leave on 10 min, then rinse.

spinosad (Natroba): Tx of head lice in pts 4 yr and older. Apply to dry scalp, leave on 10 min, rinse. May repeat q 7 days.

Ophthalmic drugs

Ophthalmic drugs are intended for direct administration into the conjunctiva of the eye.

IND & DOSE Tx of glaucoma; to aid in dx of eye problems; tx of local ophthalmic infection, inflammation; to relieve s&sx of allergic reactions.
Adult, child: 1–2 drops to each eye bid–qid, or 0.25–0.5 inch oint to each eye.

PREG/CONT C/NA

ADV EFF Blurred vision (prolonged w/ oint), burning, local irritation, stinging, tearing; headache

NC/PT Sol, drops: Wash hands thoroughly before giving; do not touch dropper to eye or other surface; have pt tilt head back or lie down and stare upward. Gently grasp lower eyelid; pull eyelid away from eyeball. Instill drop(s) into pouch formed by eyelid; release lid slowly. Have pt close eye, look downward. Apply gentle pressure to inside corner of eye for 3–5 min to retard drainage. Pt should not rub eyes, rinse eyedropper; avoid eyedrops that have changed color; separate administration by 5 min if more than one type of eyedrop used.
Oint: Wash hands thoroughly before giving; hold tube between hands for several min to warm; discard first cm of oint when opening tube for first time. Have pt tilt head back or lie down and stare upward. Gently pull out lower lid to form pouch; place 0.25–0.5 inch oint inside lower lid. Have pt close eyes for 1–2 min, roll eyeball in all directions. Remove excess oint from around eye. Separate administration by 10 min if using more than one kind of oint. Transient stinging, burning, blurred vision possible; pt should take appropriate safety measures. Sun sensitivity w/ mydriatic agents (pupils will dilate); pt may need sunglasses. Pt should report severe eye discomfort, palpitations, nausea, headache.

alcaftadine (Lastacaft): Px of itching associated w/ allergic conjunctivitis. 1 drop in each eye daily. Remove contacts. Not for tx of contact lens irritation.

apraclonidine (Iopidine): To control, prevent postop IOP elevation after argon-laser surgery; short-term adjunct tx in pts on max tolerated tx who need additional IOP reduction. Monitor for possible vasovagal attack. Do not give to pts w/ clonidine allergy.

azelastine hydrochloride (Optivar): Tx of ocular itching associated w/ allergic conjunctivitis in pts 3 yr and older. Antihistamine, mast cell stabilizer. 1 drop bid. Rapid onset, 8-hr duration.

azithromycin (Azasite): Tx of bacterial conjunctivitis in pts 1 yr and older. 1 drop bid 8–12 hr apart for 2 days, then once/day for 5 days.

bepotastine besilate (Bepreve): Tx of ocular itching from allergic rhinitis in pts 2 yr and older. Apply bid.

besifloxacin (Besivance): Tx of pink eye: 1 drop tid for 7 days *(Besivance)*.

bimatoprost (Latisse, Lumigan): Tx of open-angle glaucoma, ocular hypertension: 1 drop daily in p.m. Tx of hypertrichosis of eyelashes: 1 drop each p.m.; iris darkening possible *(Latisse).*

brimonidine tartrate (Alphagan P): Tx of open-angle glaucoma, ocular hypertension. 1 drop tid. May stain contacts. Do not use w/ MAOIs.

brimonidine/timolol (Combigan): Tx of increased IOP. 1 drop q 12 hr. Do not wear contacts.

brinzolamide (Azopt): To decrease IOP in open-angle glaucoma. 1 drop tid; give 10 min apart from other drops.

bromfenac (Bromday, Xibrom): Tx of postop inflammation, pain after cataract extraction. 1 drop bid starting 24 hr after surgery and for 2 wk; once/day w/ *Bromday.*

carbachol (Miostat): Tx of glaucoma, miosis during surgery. 1–2 drops tid for glaucoma, one dose before surgery.

carteolol (generic): Tx of elevated IOP in open-angle glaucoma. 1 drop bid; monitor IOP closely.

ciprofloxacin (Ciloxan): Tx of ocular infections, conjunctivitis: Apply ¼-inch ribbon to eye sac tid for 2 days, then bid for 5 days, or 1–2 drops q 2 hr while awake for 2 days, then q 4 r for 5 days.

cyclopentolate (AK-Pentolate, Cyclogyl, Paremyd): Diagnostic procedures. Pts w/ dark irises may need higher doses. Compress lacrimal sac for 2–3 min after giving.

cyclosporine emulsion (Restasis): To increase tear production. 1 drop in each eye bid approximately 12 hr apart. Remove contacts before use.

dexamethasone intravitreal (Ozurdex): Tx of macular edema after branch retinal artery, central retinal vein occlusion; tx of noninfectious uveitis of posterior segment of eye. Intravitreal injection. Monitor for infection, retinal detachment.

diclofenac sodium (Voltaren): Tx of photophobia in pts undergoing incisional refractive surgery; tx of postop ocular inflammation. 1 drop qid starting 24 hr after surgery and for 2 wk, or 1–2 drops within 1 hour of corneal surgery, then 1–2 drops 15 min after surgery, then qid for max 3 days.

difluprednate (Durezol): Tx of postop ocular pain, inflammation: 1 drop qid starting 24 after surgery and for 2 wk.

dorzolamide (Trusopt): Tx of increased IOP, open-angle glaucoma. 1 drop tid.

dorzolamide/timolol (Cosopt): To reduce IOP. 1 drop bid. Monitor for HF if absorbed systemically.

echothiophate (generic): Tx of open-angle glaucoma, accommodative estropia. Give q day or bid. Long-acting irreversible cholinesterase inhibitor; tolerance possible.

emedastine (Emadine): To relieve s&sx of allergic conjunctivitis in pts 3 yr and older. 1 drop q day to qid. Do not wear contacts. May cause headache, blurred vision.

epinastine hydrochloride (Elestat): Px of allergic conjunctivitis itching. 1 drop bid for entire time of exposure. Remove contacts.

fluocinolone acetonide (Retisert): Tx of chronic noninfectious uveitis of posterior segment of eye. 1 surgically implanted insert replaced after 30 mo if needed.

fluorometholone (Flarex, Fluor-Op, FML): Tx of inflammatory eye conditions. Stop if swelling; monitor IOP after 10 days.

ganciclovir (Zirgan): Tx of acute herpetic keratitis. 1 drop five times/day until ulcer heals, then 1 drop tid for 7 days.

gatifloxacin (Zymar, Zymaxid): Tx of conjunctivitis caused by susceptible strains. 1 drop q 2 hr while awake up to eight times/day on days 1 and 2; then 1 drop q 4 hr while awake up to four times/day for 5 days. Pt should not wear contact lenses; may cause blurred vision.

homatropine (Homatropine HBr, Isopto-Homatropine): Refraction; tx of inflammatory conditions, preop and postop when mydriasis needed. 5–10 min needed for refraction; dark irises may require bigger doses.

ketorolac (Acuvail): Tx of pain, inflammation after cataract surgery. 1 drop bid.

ketotifen (Alaway, Zaditor): Temporary relief of itching due to allergic conjunctivitis in pts 3 yr and older. 1 drop q 8–12 hr; remove contacts for 10 min.

latanoprost (Xalatan): Tx of open-angle glaucoma, ocular hypertension. Remove contacts before and for 15 min after drops. Allow 5 min between this and other drops.

levobunolol (AKBeta, Betagon Liquifilm): Tx of bacterial conjunctivitis caused by susceptible strains. 1–2 drops q 2 hr while awake on days 1, 2; then q 4 hr while awake on days 3–7.

levofloxacin (Quixin): Tx of conjunctivitis caused by susceptible strains. 1 or 2 drops q 2 hr while awake up to eight times/day on days 1 and 2; then 1 drop q 4 hr while awake up to four times/day for 3–7 days.

lodoxamide tromethamine (Alomide): Tx of vernal conjunctivitis, keratitis in pts over 2 yr. Do not wear contacts. Stop if stinging, burning persists.

loteprednol etabonate (Alrex, Lotemax): Tx of postop inflammation, ocular disease. 1–2 drops qid. Discard after 14 days. Prolonged use can cause eye nerve damage.

loteprednol etabonate/tobramycin (Zylet): Tx of ocular conditions w/ risk of bacterial ocular infection. 1–2 drops q 4–6 hr for 24–48 hr.

metipranolol (OptiPranolol): Tx of chronic open-angle glaucoma, ocular hypertension. Vision changes possible; may need to use w/ other drugs.

mitomycin-C (Mitosol): Adjunct to ab externo glaucoma surgery. Apply fully saturated sponges to tx area for 2 min. Topical only; biohazard disposal.

moxifloxacin (Moxeza, Vigamox): Tx of bacterial conjunctivitis caused by susceptible strains. *Moxeza* (pts 4 mo and older), 1 drop bid for 7 days. *Vigamox* (pts 1 yr and older), 1 drop tid for 7 days. Do not wear contacts. Can cause blurred vision.

natamycin (Natacyn): Tx of fungal blepharitis, conjunctivitis, keratitis. 1–2 drops/day for 7 days.

nedocromil sodium (Alocril): Tx of allergic conjunctivitis itching. 1–2 drops bid through entire allergy season.

olopatadine hydrochloride (Pataday, Patanol): Tx of allergic conjunctivitis itching in pts 3 yr and older.

1–2 drops q 6–8 hr. Not for use
w/ contacts. Headache common.

pemirolast potassium (Alamast):
Tx of allergic conjunctivitis itching.
1–2 drops qid.

**pilocarpine (Adsorbocarpine,
Piloptic, Pilostat):** Tx of chronic,
acute glaucoma; mydriasis caused by
drugs. 1–2 drops up to six times/day.

**polydimethylsiloxane (AdatoSil
5000):** Tx of retinal detachment.
Inject into aqueous humor. Monitor
for cataract.

rimexolone (Vexol): Tx of anterior
uveitis; postop. Corticosteroid.
Monitor for systemic absorption.

sulfacetamide (Bleph-10): Tx of
ocular infections. 1–2 drops q
2–3 hr; gradually taper over
7–10 days.

tafluprost (Zioptan): Tx of elevated IOP in open-angle glaucoma/oc-
ular hypertension. 1 drop in p.m.;
permanent changes in eyelashes,
iris color.

timolol maleate (Timoptic XE): Tx
of increased IOP. 1 drop/day in a.m.

travoprost (Travatan Z): Tx of
open-angle glaucoma, ocular hypertension. 1 drop each p.m.; iris darkening, eyelash growth common.

trifluridine (Viroptic): Tx of kerato-
conjunctivitis, recurrent epithelial
keratitis due to herpes simplex 1, 2.
Max, 9 drops/day in affected eye(s)
no longer than 21 days.

**tropicamide (Mydral, Mydriacyl,
Tropicacyl):** Refraction. 1–2 drops,
repeat in 5 min. May repeat again in
30 min if needed.

Laxatives

Laxative use has been replaced by proper diet and exercise in many clinical situations. Most laxatives are available as OTC preparations and are often abused by people who become dependent on them for GI movement.

IND & DOSE Short-term relief of constipation; to prevent straining; to evacuate bowel for diagnostic procedures; to remove ingested poisons from lower GI tract; as adjunct in anthelmintic tx.

PREG/CONT C/NA

ADV EFF Abd cramps, cathartic dependence, dizziness, excessive bowel activity, perianal irritation, weakness

NC/PT Use as temporary measure. Swallow tablets whole. Do not take within 1 hr of other drugs. Report sweating, flushing, muscle cramps, excessive thirst.

bisacodyl (Bisa-Lax, Correctol, Dulcolax): Stimulant. 5–15 mg PO; 2.5 g in water via enema. Onset, 6–12 hr; rapid. Tartrazine in *Dulcolax* tablets. May discolor urine. Not for child under 6 yr.

cascara: Stimulant. 325 mg–6 g PO. Onset, 6–10 hr. Use caution if pt taking prescription drugs. May discolor urine. Not for children younger than 18 yr.

castor oil: Stimulant. 15–60 mL PO. Onset, 2–6 hr. May be very vigorous; may cause abd cramping.

docusate (Colace, Ex-Lax Stool Softener, Genasoft, Phillips' Liqui-Gels, Silace): Detergent, softener. 50–300 mg PO. Onset, 12–72 hr. Gentle; beneficial w/ painful anorectal conditions, dry or hard feces.

glycerin (Fleet Babylax, Fleet Liquid Glycerin Suppository, Sani-Supp): Hyperosmolar agent. Rectal suppository; 4 mL liquid by rectum (child rectal liquid). Onset, 15–60 min. Insert suppository high into rectum, retain 15 min. Insert liquid dispenser. Apply gentle, steady pressure until all liquid gone; then remove.

lactulose (Constilac, Constulose): Hyperosmolar agent. 15–30 mL PO. Onset, 24–48 hr. Also used for tx of portal system encephalopathy. More palatable if mixed w/ fruit juice, milk, water.

lubiprostone (Amitiza): Chloride channel activator. 24 mcg PO bid w/ food, water. Onset, 1–2 hr. Also used for tx of women w/ IBS w/ constipation. Contains sorbitol; may cause nausea, diarrhea.

magnesium citrate (Citrate of Magnesia): Saline. 1 glassful PO. Onset, 0.5–3 hr. For child dose, reduce by half.

magnesium (Milk of Magnesia, MOM, Phillip's MOM): Saline. 30–60 mL PO at bedtime; 15–30 mL of conc PO. Onset, 0.5–3 hr. Take w/ liquids. Flavored forms available.

magnesium sulfate (Epsom Salts): Saline. 5–10 mL PO. Onset, 0.5–3 hr. Take mixed w/ full glass of water. Child dose, reduce to 2.5–5 mL PO in ½ glass water.

mineral oil (Kondremul Plain): Emollient. 5–45 mL PO. Onset, 6–8 hr. May decrease absorption of fat-soluble vitamins. Child 6 yr and older, reduce dose to 5–15 mL.

polycarbophil (Equalactin, Fiber-Con, Konsyl Fiber): Bulk. 1–2 tablets PO up to qid. Onset, 12–72 hr. Good w/ IBS, diverticulitis. Swallow w/ full glass of water to prevent sticking in esophagus, choking.

polyethylene glycol (MiraLax): Bulk. 17 g PO in 8 oz water daily for up to 2 wk. Onset, 48–72 hr. Do not use w/ bowel obstruction. Diarrhea common.

polyethylene glycolelectrolyte solution (CoLyte, GoLytely, Nu-Lytely): Bulk. 4 L oral sol PO before exam. Onset, 1 hr. Used as bowel evacuant before exam. Do not use w/ GI obstruction, megacolon.

polyethylene glycol, sodium sulfate, sodium chloride, potassium chloride, sodium ascorbate, ascorbic acid (MoviPrep): Osmotic. 1 L PO, then 16 oz fluid pm before colonoscopy. Or, 2 L PO, then 32 oz fluid p.m. before colonoscopy. Onset, 1 hr. Maintain hydration. Monitor pt w/ hx of seizures.

psyllium (Fiberall, Hydrocil Instant, Konsyl, Metamucil): Bulk. 1 tsp or packet in water, juice 1–3 times/day PO. Onset, 12–72 hr. Swallow w/ full glass of water to prevent esophageal sticking, choking.

senna (Agoral, Black Draught, Fletcher's Castoria, Senna-Gen, Senokot): Stimulant. 1–8 tablets/day PO at bedtime; suppository/syrup, 10–30 mL PO. Onset, 6–10 hr. May cause abd cramps, discomfort.

sodium picosulfate, magnesium oxide, anhydrous citric acid (Prepopik): Bowel cleansing before colonoscopy. Reconstitute w/ cold water, swallow immediately, follow w/ clear liquids; repeat. Risk of fluid/ electrolyte abnormalities.

Appendix E

Combination products by therapeutic class

AMPHETAMINES

▶ dextroamphetamine and amphetamine
CONTROLLED SUBSTANCE C-II
Adderall, Adderall XR

Tablets: 1.25 mg (5-mg tablet), 2.5 mg (10-mg tablet), 5 mg (20-mg tablet), 7.5 mg (30-mg tablet) each of dextroamphetamine sulfate and saccharate, amphetamine aspartate, and sulfate.
ER capsules: 1.25 mg (5-mg capsule), 1.875 (7.5-mg tablet), 2.5 mg (10-mg capsule), 3.125 (12.5-mg tablet), 3.75 mg (15-mg capsule), 5 mg (20-mg capsule), 6.25 mg (25-mg capsule), 7.5 mg (30-mg capsule) of each component.
Usual adult, child dose: 5–60 mg/day PO in divided doses to control sx of narcolepsy, ADHD. ER capsules: 10–30 mg/day.

ANALGESICS

▶ acetaminophen and codeine
CONTROLLED SUBSTANCE C-III
Tylenol with Codeine

Elixir: 12 mg codeine, 120 mg acetaminophen/5 mL.
Tablets: No. 2: 15 mg codeine, 300 mg acetaminophen. No. 3: 30 mg codeine, 300 mg acetaminophen. No. 4: 60 mg codeine, 300 mg acetaminophen.

Usual adult dose: 1 or 2 tablets PO q 4–6 hr as needed, or 15 mL q 4–6 hr.

▶ aspirin and codeine
CONTROLLED SUBSTANCE C-III
Empirin with Codeine

Tablets: No. 3: 30 mg codeine, 325 mg aspirin. No. 4: 60 mg codeine, 325 mg aspirin.
Usual adult dose: 1 or 2 tablets PO q 4–6 hr as needed.

▶ codeine, aspirin, caffeine, and butalbital
CONTROLLED SUBSTANCE C-III
Fiorinal with Codeine

Capsules: 30 mg codeine, 325 mg aspirin, 40 mg caffeine, 50 mg butabarbital.
Usual adult dose: 1 or 2 capsules PO q 4 hr as needed for pain, up to 6/day.

▶ diclofenac sodium and misoprostol
PREGNANCY CATEGORY X
Arthrotec

Tablets: '50': 50 mg diclofenac, 200 mcg misoprostol. '75': 75 mg diclofenac, 200 mcg misoprostol.
Usual adult dose: *Osteoarthritis:* Arthrotec 50, PO tid. Arthrotec 50 or 75, PO bid. *Rheumatoid arthritis:* Arthrotec 50, PO tid or qid; Arthrotec 50 or 75, PO bid.

▶ famotidine and ibuprofen
Duexis

Tablets: 26.6 mg famotidine, 800 mg ibuprofen.
Usual adult dose: 1 tablet PO daily for arthritis pain.

▶ hydrocodone and aspirin
CONTROLLED SUBSTANCE C-III
Damason-P

Tablets: 5 mg hydrocodone, 500 mg aspirin.
Usual adult dose: 1 tablet PO q 4–6 hr as needed.

▶ hydrocodone bitartrate and acetaminophen
CONTROLLED SUBSTANCE C-III
Lortab Tablets, Norco, Stagesic, Zydone

Elixir: 2.5 mg hydrocodone, 167 mg acetaminophen/5 mL.
Capsules, tablets: 2.5 mg hydrocodone, 500 mg acetaminophen; 5 mg hydrocodone, 500 mg acetaminophen; 5, 7.5, 10 mg hydrocodone, 400 mg acetaminophen; 7.5 mg hydrocodone, 500 mg acetaminophen; 7.5 mg hydrocodone, 650 mg acetaminophen; 10 mg hydrocodone, 650 mg acetaminophen.
Norco tablets: 5 mg hydrocodone, 325 mg acetaminophen; 7.5 mg hydrocodone, 325 mg acetaminophen; 10 mg hydrocodone, 325 mg acetaminophen.
Usual adult dose: Check brand-name products to determine specific dose combinations available. One or two tablets, capsules PO q 4–6 hr, up to 8/day.

▶ hydrocodone and ibuprofen
CONTROLLED SUBSTANCE C-III
Reprexain, Vicoprofen

Tablets: 2.5 mg hydrocodone, 200 mg ibuprofen; 7.5 mg hydrocodone, 200 mg ibuprofen; 10 mg hydrocodone, 200 mg ibuprofen.
Usual adult dose: 1 tablet PO q 4–6 hr as needed.

▶ methylsalicylate and menthol
Salonpas

Dermal patch: 10% methylsalicylate, 3% menthol.
Usual adult dose: Apply 1 patch to clean, dry affected area; leave on for 8–12 hr. Remove patch, apply another as needed. To relieve pain from sprains, bruises, strains, backache.

▶ morphine and naltrexone
CONTROLLED SUBSTANCE C-II
Embeda

ER capsules: 20 mg morphine, 0.8 mg naltrexone; 30 mg morphine, 1.2 mg naltrexone; 50 mg morphine, 2 mg naltrexone; 60 mg morphine, 2.4 mg naltrexone; 80 mg morphine, 3.2 mg naltrexone; 100 mg morphine, 4 mg naltrexone.
Usual adult dose: 1 or 2 tablets PO daily when continuous, around-the-clock analgesic needed long-term. May open capsules, sprinkle over applesauce. Pt should not cut, crush, or chew capsule.

▶ naproxen and esomeprazole
Vimovo

DR tablets: 375 mg naproxen, 20 mg esomeprazole; 500 mg naproxen, 20 mg esomeprazole.

Usual adult dose: 1 tablet PO bid. Not recommended in moderate to severe renal insufficiency, severe hepatic insufficiency; reduce w/ mild to moderate hepatic insufficiency.

▶ oxycodone and acetaminophen
CONTROLLED SUBSTANCE C-II
Percocet, Roxicet, Roxilox, Tylox

Tylox capsules: 5 mg oxycodone, 500 mg acetaminophen.
Tablets: 2.25, 4.5, 5 mg oxycodone, 325 mg acetaminophen.
Usual adult dose: 1 or 2 tablets PO q 4–6 hr as needed.

▶ oxycodone and aspirin
CONTROLLED SUBSTANCE C-II
Percodan, Roxiprin

Tablets: 4.5 mg oxycodone, 325 mg aspirin.
Usual adult dose: 1 or 2 tablets PO q 6 hr as needed.

▶ oxycodone and ibuprofen
CONTROLLED SUBSTANCE C-II
generic

Tablets: 5 mg oxycodone, 400 mg ibuprofen.
Usual adult dose: 1 tablet PO q 6 hr as needed for moderate to severe pain. Max, 4 tablets/24 hr for no more than 7 days.

▶ pentazocine and acetaminophen
CONTROLLED SUBSTANCE C-IV
generic

Tablets: 25 mg pentazocine, 650 mg acetaminophen.
Usual adult dose: 1 tablet PO q 4 hr; max, 6 tablets/day.

▶ tramadol hydrochloride and acetaminophen
Ultracet

Tablets: 37.5 mg tramadol, 325 mg acetaminophen.
Usual adult dose: 2 tablets PO q 4–6 hr as needed; max, 8 tablets/day. Reduce in elderly/renally impaired pts.

ANTIACNE DRUGS

▶ ethinyl estradiol and norethindrone
Estrostep Fe

Tablets: 1 mg norethindrone, 20 mcg ethinyl estradiol; 1 mg norethindrone, 30 mcg ethinyl estradiol; 1 mg norethindrone, 35 mcg ethinyl estradiol.
Usual adult dose: 1 tablet PO each day (21 tablets have active ingredients; 7 are inert).

▶ norgestimate and ethinyl estradiol
Ortho Tri-Cyclen

Tablets: 0.18 mg norgestimate, 35 mcg ethinyl estradiol (7 tablets); 0.215 mg norgestimate, 35 mcg ethinyl estradiol (7 tablets); 0.25 mg norgestimate, 35 mcg ethinyl estradiol (7 tablets).
Usual adult dose: For women over 15 yr, 1 tablet/day PO. Birth control agent used cyclically (21 tablets have active ingredients, 7 are inert).

ANTIBACTERIALS

▶ amoxicillin and clavulanic acid
Augmentin, Augmentin ES-600, Augmentin XR

Tablets: '250': 250 mg amoxicillin, 125 mg clavulanic acid; '500': 500 mg amoxicillin, 125 mg clavulanic acid; '875': 875 mg amoxicillin, 125 mg clavulanic acid.

Powder for oral suspension:
'125': 125 mg amoxicillin, 31.25 mg clavulanic acid; '250': 250 mg amoxicillin, 62.5 mg clavulanic acid; '400': 400 mg amoxicillin, 57 mg clavulanic acid. Sol (Augmentin ES-600): 600 mg amoxicillin, 42.9 mg clavulanic acid/5 mL.

Chewable tablets: '125': 125 mg amoxicillin, 31.25 mg clavulanic acid; '200': 200 mg amoxicillin, 28.5 mg clavulanic acid; '400': 400 mg amoxicillin, 57 mg clavulanic acid.

XR tablets: 1,000 mg amoxicillin, 62.5 mg clavulanic acid.

Usual adult dose: 1 250-mg tablet or one 500-mg tablet PO q 8 hr. For severe infections, 875-mg tablet PO q 12 hr. W/ difficulty swallowing, substitute 125-mg/5 mL or 250-mg/5 mL for 500-mg tablet, or 200-mg/5 mL or 400-mg/5 mL for 875-mg tablet.

Usual child dose: Under 40 kg, 20–40 mg amoxicillin/kg/day PO in divided doses q 8 hr (dose based on amoxicillin content) or q 12 hr; 90 mg/kg/day PO oral sol divided q 12 hr (Augmentin ES-600).

► **co-trimoxazole (TMP-SMZ)**
Bactrim, Bactrim DS, Septra, Septra DS, Sulfatrim Pediatric

Tablets: 80 mg trimethoprim (TMP), 400 mg sulfamethoxazole (SMZ); 160 mg TMP, 800 mg SMZ.

Oral suspension: 40 mg TMP, 200 mg SMZ/5 mL.

Usual adult dose: UTIs, shigellosis, acute otitis media: 160 mg TMP/800 mg SMZ PO q 12 hr. Up to 14 days (UTI) or 5 days (shigellosis). Acute exacerbations of chronic bronchitis: 160 mg TMP/800 mg SMZ PO q 12 hr for 14 days. Pneumocystis jiroveci pneumonitis: 20 mg/kg TMP/100 mg/kg SMZ q 24 hr PO in divided doses q 6 hr for 14 days. Traveler's diarrhea:

160 mg TMP/800 mg SMZ PO q 12 hr for 5 days.

Usual child dose: UTIs, shigellosis, acute otitis media: 8 mg/kg/day TMP/40 mg/kg/day SMZ PO in two divided doses q 12 hr. For 10–14 days (UTIs, acute otitis media), 5 days (shigellosis). Pneumocystis jiroveci pneumonitis: 20 mg/kg TMP/100 mg/kg SMZ q 24 hr PO in divided doses q 6 hr for 14 days.

► **erythromycin and sulfisoxazole**
generic

Granules for oral suspension:
Erythromycin ethylsuccinate (equivalent of 200 mg erythromycin activity) and 600 mg sulfisoxazole/5 mL when reconstituted according to manufacturer's directions.

Usual child dose: Otitis media: 50 mg/kg/day erythromycin and 150 mg/kg/day sulfisoxazole PO in divided doses qid for 10 days. Give without regard to meals. Refrigerate after reconstitution; use within 14 days.

► **imipenem and cilastatin**
Primaxin

Powder for injection (IV): 250 mg imipenem, 250 mg cilastatin; 500 mg imipenem, 500 mg cilastatin.

Powder for injection (IM): 500 mg imipenem, 500 mg cilastatin. Follow manufacturer's instructions for reconstituting, diluting drug. Give each 250- to 500-mg dose by IV infusion over 20–30 min; infuse each 1-g dose over 40–60 min. Give 500–750 mg IM q 12 hr. Max, 1,500 mg/day.

Usual adult dose: Dose recommendations based on imipenem. Initially based on type, severity of infection; later on illness severity, degree of susceptibility of pathogens, and age, weight, CrCl. For adults w/ normal renal function, 250 mg–1 g IV q 6–8 hr. Max,

50 mg/kg/day or 4 g/day, whichever less. Adjust in renal impairment.

▶ piperacillin sodium and tazobactam sodium
Zosyn

Powder for injection: 2 g piperacillin, 0.25 g tazobactam; 3 g piperacillin, 0.375 g tazobactam; 4 g piperacillin, 0.5 g tazobactam.
Usual adult dose: 12 g/1.5 g IV as 3.375 g q 6 hr over 30 min. Recommended for appendicitis; peritonitis; postpartum endometritis, PID; community-acquired pneumonia; nosocomial pneumonia if agent responsive in sensitivity testing. Adjust in renal impairment.

▶ quinupristin and dalfopristin
Synercid

Streptogramin antibiotics available only in combination.
Sol for IV use: 500-mg/10-mL vial (150 mg quinupristin, 350 mg dalfopristin).
Dose in pts over 16 yr: *Complicated skin infections due to* Staphylococcus. aureus, Streptococcus pyogenes: 7.5 mg/kg IV q 12 hr for 7 days. *Tx of life-threatening, susceptible infections associated w/ VREF:* 7.5 mg/kg IV q 8 hr. Dangerous when used w/ QT-prolonging drugs.

▶ sulbactam and ampicillin
Unasyn

Powder for injection: 1.5-g vial (1 g ampicillin, 0.5 g sulbactam); 3-g vial (2 g ampicillin, 1 g sulbactam).
Usual adult dose: 0.5–1 g sulbactam w/ 1–2 g ampicillin IM or IV q 6–8 hr.
Usual child dose: 40 kg or more, adult dosage; max, 4 g/day. Under

40 kg, 300 mg/kg/day IV in divided doses q 6 hr.

▶ ticarcillin and clavulanic acid
Timentin

Powder, sol for injection: 3.1-g vial (3 g ticarcillin, 0.1 g clavulanic acid).
Usual adult dose: 60 kg, 3.1 g (3 g ticarcillin, 0.1 g clavulanic acid) IV over 30 min q 4–6 hr. Under 60 kg, 200–300 mg ticarcillin/kg/day IV over 30 min in divided doses q 4–6 hr. *UTIs:* 3.1 g (3 g ticarcillin, 0.1 g clavulanic acid) IV q 8 hr.
Child 3 mo and over: 3.1 g (3 g ticarcillin, 0.1 g clavulanic acid) IV over 30 min q 4–6 hr, or 200–300 mg/kg/day IV in divided doses q 4–6 hr. Adjust in elderly pts, pts w/ renal impairment.

ANTI–CORONARY ARTERY DISEASE DRUG

▶ amlodipine besylate and atorvastatin calcium
Caduet

Tablets: 2.5 mg amlodipine w/ 10, 20, 40 mg atorvastatin; 5 mg amlodipine w/ 10, 20, 40, 80 mg atorvastatin; 10 mg amlodipine w/ 10, 20, 40, 80 mg atorvastatin.
Usual adult dose: 1 tablet PO daily in p.m. Adjust using individual products, then switch to appropriate combination product.

ANTIDEPRESSANTS

▶ chlordiazepoxide and amitriptyline
CONTROLLED SUBSTANCE C-IV
Limbitrol, Limbitrol DS 10–25

Tablets: 5 mg chlordiazepoxide, 12.5 mg amitriptyline; 10 mg chlordiazepoxide, 25 mg amitriptyline.

Usual adult dose: 10 mg chlordiazepoxide w/ 25 mg amitriptyline PO tid–qid up to six times/day. For pts intolerant of higher doses, 5 mg chlordiazepoxide w/ 12.5 mg amitriptyline PO tid–qid.

▶ olanzapine and fluoxetine
Symbyax

Capsules: 6 mg olanzapine, 25 mg fluoxetine; 6 mg olanzapine, 50 mg fluoxetine; 12 mg olanzapine, 25 mg fluoxetine; 12 mg olanzapine, 50 mg fluoxetine.
Usual adult dose: 1 capsule PO daily in p.m.

▶ perphenazine and amitriptyline
Etrafon, Etrafon-A, Etrafon-Forte

Tablets: 2 mg perphenazine, 10 mg amitriptyline; 2 mg perphenazine, 25 mg amitriptyline; 4 mg perphenazine, 10 mg amitriptyline; 4 mg perphenazine, 25 mg amitriptyline; 4 mg perphenazine, 50 mg amitriptyline.
Usual adult dose: 2–4 mg perphenazine w/ 10–50 mg amitriptyline PO tid–qid.

ANTIDIABETICS

▶ alogliptin and metformin
Kazano

Tablets: 12.5 mg alogliptin, 500 mg metformin; 12.5 mg alogliptin, 1,000 mg metformin.
Usual adult dose: Base on pt response, PO bid w/ food; max, 25 mg alogliptin, 2,000 mg metformin/day.

▶ alogliptin and pioglitazone
Oseni

Tablets: 12.5 mg alogliptin, 15 mg pioglitazone; 12.5 mg alogliptin, 30 mg pioglitazone; 12.5 mg alogliptin, 45 mg pioglitazone; 25 mg alogliptin, 15 mg pioglitazone; 25 mg alogliptin, 30 mg pioglitazone; 25 mg alogliptin, 45 mg pioglitazone. Usual adult dose: Base on pt response, PO once daily. Max, 25 mg alogliptin, 45 mg pioglitazone. Limit w/ HF, renal impairment.

▶ glyburide and metformin
Glucovance

Tablets: 1.25 mg glyburide, 250 mg metformin; 2.5 mg glyburide, 500 mg metformin; 5 mg glyburide, 500 mg metformin.
Usual adult dose: 1 tablet/day PO w/ meal, usually in a.m.

▶ linagliptin and metformin
Jentadueto

Tablets: 2.5 mg linagliptin, 500 mg metformin; 2.5 mg linagliptin, 850 mg metformin; 2.5 mg linagliptin, 1,000 mg metformin.
Usual adult dose: Base on current use of each drug, PO bid w/ meals.

▶ pioglitazone and glimepiride
Duetact

Tablets: 30 mg pioglitazone w/ 2 or 4 mg glimepiride.
Usual adult dose: 1 tablet/day PO w/ first meal of day.

▶ pioglitazone and metformin
ActoPlus Met, ActoPlus Met XR

Tablets: 15 mg pioglitazone, 500 mg metformin; 15 mg pioglitazone, 850 mg metformin.
ER tablets: 5 mg pioglitazone, 1,000 mg metformin; 30 mg pioglitazone, 1,000 mg metformin.
Usual adult dose: 1 tablet PO once/day or bid w/ meals; ER tablets, once/day.

▶ repaglinide and metformin
PrandiMet

Tablets: 1 mg repaglinide, 500 mg metformin; 2 mg repaglinide, 500 mg metformin.
Usual adult dose: 1 tablet PO once/day or in divided doses.

▶ rosiglitazone and glimepiride
Avandaryl

Tablets: 4 mg rosiglitazone, 1 mg glimepiride; 4 mg rosiglitazone, 2 mg glimepiride; 4 mg rosiglitazone, 4 mg glimepiride; 8 mg rosiglitazone, 2 mg glimepiride; 8 mg rosiglitazone, 4 mg glimepiride.
Usual adult dose: 4 mg rosiglitazone w/ 1 or 2 mg glimepiride PO once/day w/ first meal of day. Available through limited-access program only.

▶ rosiglitazone and metformin
Avandamet

Tablets: 1 mg rosiglitazone, 500 mg metformin; 2 mg rosiglitazone, 500 mg metformin; 2 mg rosiglitazone, 1 g metformin; 4 mg rosiglitazone, 500 mg metformin; 4 mg rosiglitazone, 1 g metformin.
Usual adult dose: 4 mg rosiglitazone w/ 500 mg metformin PO once/day or in divided doses. Available through limited-access program only.

▶ saxagliptin and metformin
Kombiglyze XR

Tablets: 5 mg saxagliptin, 500 mg metformin; 5 mg saxagliptin, 1,000 mg metformin; 2.5 mg saxagliptin, 1,000 mg metformin.
Usual adult dose: 1 tablet PO daily. Do not cut, crush, or allow pt to chew tablets.

▶ sitagliptin and metformin
Janumet, Janumet XR

Tablets: 50 mg sitagliptin, 500 or 1,000 mg metformin.
ER tablets: 50 mg sitagliptin, 500 mg or 1 g metformin; 100 mg sitagliptin, 1 g metformin.
Usual adult dose: 1 tablet PO bid w/ meals; max, 100 mg sitagliptin, 2,000 mg metformin/day.

ANTIDIABETIC/LIPID-LOWERING DRUG

▶ sitagliptin and simvastatin
Juvisync

Tablets: 100 mg sitagliptin, 10 mg simvastatin; 100 mg sitagliptin, 20 mg simvastatin; 100 mg sitagliptin, 40 mg simvastatin.
Usual adult dose: Initially, 100 mg sitagliptin/40 mg simvastatin PO in p.m. Use w/ diet, exercise program.

ANTIDIARRHEAL

▶ diphenoxylate hydrochloride and atropine sulfate

CONTROLLED SUBSTANCE C-V
Logen, Lomanate, Lomotil, Lonox

Tablets: 2.5 mg diphenoxylate hydrochloride, 0.025 mg atropine sulfate.
Liquid: 2.5 mg diphenoxylate hydrochloride, 0.025 mg atropine sulfate/5 mL.
Usual adult dose: 5 mg PO qid.
Usual child dose (use only liquid in child 2–12 yr): 0.3–0.4 mg/kg PO daily in four divided doses.

ANTIHYPERTENSIVES

▶ aliskiren and amlodipine

Tekamlo

Tablets: 150 mg aliskiren, 5 mg amlodipine; 150 mg aliskiren, 10 mg amlodipine; 300 mg aliskiren, 5 mg amlodipine; 300 mg aliskiren, 10 mg amlodipine.
Usual adult dose: 1 tablet/day PO; may give w/ other antihypertensives.

▶ aliskiren and amlodipine and hydrochlorothiazide

Amturnide

Tablets: 150 mg aliskiren, 5 mg amlodipine, 12.5 mg hydrochlorothiazide; 300 mg aliskiren, 5 mg amlodipine, 12.5 mg hydrochlorothiazide; 300 mg aliskiren, 5 mg amlodipine, 25 mg hydrochlorothiazide; 150 mg aliskiren, 10 mg amlodipine, 12.5 mg hydrochlorothiazide; 150 mg aliskiren, 10 mg amlodipine, 25 mg hydrochlorothiazide.
Usual adult dose: 1 tablet/day PO.

▶ aliskiren and hydrochlorothiazide

Tekturna HCT

Tablets: 150 mg aliskiren, 12.5 mg hydrochlorothiazide; 150 mg aliskiren, 25 mg hydrochlorothiazide; 300 mg aliskiren, 12.5 mg hydrochlorothiazide; 300 mg aliskiren, 25 mg hydrochlorothiazide.
Usual adult dose: 1 tablet/day PO.

▶ aliskiren and valsartan

Valturna

Tablets: 150 mg aliskiren, 160 mg valsartan; 300 mg aliskiren, 320 mg valsartan.
Usual adult dose: 1 tablet/day PO.

▶ amlodipine and benazepril

Lotrel

Capsules: 2.5 mg amlodipine, 10 mg benazepril; 5 mg amlodipine, 10 mg benazepril; 5 mg amlodipine, 20 mg benazepril; 5 mg amlodipine, 40 mg benazepril; 10 mg amlodipine, 20 mg benazepril; 10 mg amlodipine, 40 mg benazepril.
Usual adult dose: 1 tablet/day PO in a.m.

▶ amlodipine and olmesartan

Azor

Tablets: 5 mg amlodipine, 20 mg olmesartan; 10 mg amlodipine, 20 mg olmesartan; 5 mg amlodipine, 40 mg olmesartan; 10 mg amlodipine, 40 mg olmesartan.
Usual adult dose: 1 tablet/day PO.

► amlodipine and valsartan
Exforge

Tablets: 5 mg amlodipine, 160 mg valsartan; 5 mg amlodipine, 320 mg valsartan; 10 mg amlodipine, 160 mg valsartan; 10 mg amlodipine, 320 mg valsartan.
Usual adult dose: 1 tablet/day PO.

► amlodipine, valsartan, and hydrochlorothiazide
Exforge HCT

Tablets: 5 mg amlodipine, 160 mg valsartan, 12.5 mg hydrochlorothiazide; 10 mg amlodipine, 160 mg valsartan, 12.5 mg hydrochlorothiazide; 5 mg amlodipine, 160 mg valsartan, 25 mg hydrochlorothiazide; 10 mg amlodipine, 320 mg valsartan, 25 mg hydrochlorothiazide.
Usual adult dose: 1 tablet /day PO.

► atenolol and chlorthalidone
Tenoretic

Tablets: 50 mg atenolol, 25 mg chlorthalidone; 100 mg atenolol, 25 mg chlorthalidone.
Usual adult dose: 1 tablet/day PO in a.m.

► azilsartan and chlorthalidone
Edarbyclor

Tablets: 40 mg azilsartan, 12.5 mg chlorthalidone; 40 mg azilsartan, 25 mg chlorthalidone.
Usual adult dose: 1 tablet/day PO. Not for use in pregnancy, renal failure. Monitor potassium level.

► bisoprolol and hydrochlorothiazide
Ziac

Tablets: 2.5 mg bisoprolol, 6.25 mg hydrochlorothiazide; 5 mg bisoprolol, 6.25 mg hydrochlorothiazide; 10 mg bisoprolol, 6.25 mg hydrochlorothiazide.
Usual adult dose: 1 tablet/day PO in a.m. Initially, 2.5/6.25-mg tablet/day PO. May need 2–3 wk for optimal antihypertensive effect.

► candesartan and hydrochlorothiazide
Atacand HCT

Tablets: 16 mg candesartan, 12.5 mg hydrochlorothiazide; 32 mg candesartan, 12.5 mg hydrochlorothiazide.
Usual adult dose: 1 tablet/day PO in a.m.

► chlorthalidone and clonidine
Clorpres

Tablets: 15 mg chlorthalidone, 0.1 mg clonidine hydrochloride; 15 mg chlorthalidone, 0.2 mg clonidine hydrochloride; 15 mg chlorthalidone, 0.3 mg clonidine hydrochloride.
Usual adult dose: 1 or 2 tablets/day PO in a.m.; may give once/day or bid.

► enalapril and hydrochlorothiazide
Vaseretic

Tablets: 5 mg enalapril maleate, 12.5 mg hydrochlorothiazide; 10 mg enalapril maleate, 25 mg hydrochlorothiazide.
Usual adult dose: 1 or 2 tablets/day PO in a.m.

▶ eprosartan and hydrochlorothiazide
Teveten HCT

Tablets: 600 mg eprosartan, 12.5 mg hydrochlorothiazide; 600 mg eprosartan, 25 mg hydrochlorothiazide.
Usual adult dose: 1 tablet/day PO.

▶ fosinopril and hydrochlorothiazide
Monopril-HCT

Tablets: 10 mg fosinopril, 12.5 mg hydrochlorothiazide; 20 mg fosinopril, 12.5 mg hydrochlorothiazide.
Usual adult dose: 1 tablet/day PO in a.m.

▶ hydrochlorothiazide and benazepril
Lotensin HCT

Tablets: 6.25 mg hydrochlorothiazide, 5 mg benazepril; 12.5 mg hydrochlorothiazide, 10 mg benazepril; 12.5 mg hydrochlorothiazide, 20 mg benazepril; 25 mg hydrochlorothiazide, 20 mg benazepril.
Usual adult dose: 1 tablet/day PO in a.m.

▶ hydrochlorothiazide and captopril
generic

Tablets: 15 mg hydrochlorothiazide, 25 mg captopril; 15 mg hydrochlorothiazide, 50 mg captopril; 25 mg hydrochlorothiazide, 25 mg captopril; 25 mg hydrochlorothiazide, 50 mg captopril.
Usual adult dose: 1 or 2 tablets/day PO 1 hr before or 2 hr after meals.

▶ hydrochlorothiazide and propranolol
generic

Tablets: 25 mg hydrochlorothiazide, 40 mg propranolol; 25 mg hydrochlorothiazide, 80 mg propranolol.
Usual adult dose: 1 or 2 tablets PO bid.

▶ irbesartan and hydrochlorothiazide
Avalide

Tablets: 150 mg irbesartan, 12.5 mg hydrochlorothiazide; 300 mg irbesartan, 12.5 mg hydrochlorothiazide; 300 mg irbesartan, 25 mg hydrochlorothiazide.
Usual adult dose: 1 or 2 tablets/day PO.

▶ lisinopril and hydrochlorothiazide
(Prinzide, Zestoretic)

Tablets: 10 mg lisinopril, 12.5 mg hydrochlorothiazide; 20 mg lisinopril, 12.5 mg hydrochlorothiazide; 20 mg lisinopril, 25 mg hydrochlorothiazide.
Usual adult dose: 1 tablet/day PO in a.m.

▶ losartan and hydrochlorothiazide
Hyzaar

Tablets: 50 mg losartan, 12.5 mg hydrochlorothiazide; 100 mg losartan, 12.5 mg hydrochlorothiazide; 100 mg losartan, 25 mg hydrochlorothiazide.
Usual adult dose: 1 tablet/day PO in a.m. Also used to reduce stroke incidence in hypertensive pts w/ left ventricular hypertrophy (not effective for this use in black pts).

► **metoprolol and hydrochlorothiazide**
Dutoprol, Lopressor HCT

Tablets: 50 mg metoprolol, 25 mg hydrochlorothiazide; 100 mg metoprolol, 25 mg hydrochlorothiazide; 100 mg metoprolol, 50 mg hydrochlorothiazide.
ER tablets: 25 mg metoprolol, 12.5 mg hydrochlorothiazide; 50 mg metoprolol, 12.5 mg hydrochlorothiazide; 100 mg metoprolol, 12.5 mg hydrochlorothiazide.
Usual adult dose: 1 tablet/day PO. Pt should not cut, crush, or chew ER form (*Dutoprol*).

► **moexipril and hydrochlorothiazide**
Uniretic

Tablets: 7.5 mg moexipril, 12.5 mg hydrochlorothiazide; 15 mg moexipril, 25 mg hydrochlorothiazide.
Usual adult dose: 1 or 2 tablets/day PO 1 hr before or 2 hr after meal.

► **nadolol and bendroflumethiazide**
Corzide

Tablets: 40 mg nadolol, 5 mg bendroflumethiazide; 80 mg nadolol, 5 mg bendroflumethiazide.
Usual adult dose: 1 tablet/day PO in a.m.

► **olmesartan, amlodipine, and hydrochlorothiazide**
Tribenzor

Tablets: 40 mg olmesartan, 10 mg amlodipine, 25 mg hydrochlorothiazide.
Usual adult dose: 1 tablet/day PO.

► **olmesartan medoxomil and hydrochlorothiazide**
Benicar HCT

Tablets: 20 mg olmesartan, 12.5 mg hydrochlorothiazide; 40 mg olmesartan, 12.5 mg hydrochlorothiazide; 40 mg olmesartan, 25 mg hydrochlorothiazide.
Usual adult dose: 1 tablet/day PO in a.m.

► **quinapril and hydrochlorothiazide**
Accuretic

Tablets: 10 mg quinapril, 12.5 mg hydrochlorothiazide; 20 mg quinapril, 12.5 mg hydrochlorothiazide.
Usual adult dose: 1 tablet/day PO in a.m.

► **telmisartan and amlodipine**
Twynsta

Tablets: 40 mg telmisartan, 5 mg amlodipine; 40 mg telmisartan, 10 mg amlodipine; 80 mg telmisartan, 5 mg amlodipine; 80 mg telmisartan, 10 mg amlodipine.
Usual adult dose: 1 tablet/day PO.

► **telmisartan and hydrochlorothiazide**
Micardis HCT

Tablets: 40 mg telmisartan, 12.5 mg hydrochlorothiazide; 80 mg telmisartan, 12.5 mg hydrochlorothiazide; 80 mg telmisartan, 25 mg hydrochlorothiazide.
Usual adult dose: 1 tablet/ day PO; max, 160 mg telmisartan and 25 mg hydrochlorothiazide/day.

▶ trandolapril and verapamil
Tarka

Tablets: 1 mg trandolapril, 240 mg verapamil; 2 mg trandolapril, 180 mg verapamil; 2 mg trandolapril, 240 mg verapamil; 4 mg trandolapril, 240 mg verapamil.
Usual adult dose: 1 tablet/day PO w/ food. Pt should not cut, crush, or chew tablet.

▶ valsartan and hydrochlorothiazide
Diovan HCT

Tablets: 80 mg valsartan, 12.5 mg hydrochlorothiazide; 160 mg valsartan, 12.5 mg hydrochlorothiazide; 160 mg valsartan, 25 mg hydrochlorothiazide; 320 mg valsartan, 12.5 mg hydrochlorothiazide; 320 mg valsartan, 25 mg hydrochlorothiazide.
Usual adult dose: 1 tablet/day PO.

ANTIMIGRAINE DRUGS

▶ acetaminophen, caffeine, and isometheptene
MigraTen

Capsules: 325 mg acetaminophen, 100 mg caffeine.
Usual adult dose: 2 capsules PO at onset of migraine, then 1 capsule PO q hr until resolved; max, 5 capsules in 12 hr. For tension headache, 1–2 capsules PO q 4 hr; max, 8 capsules/day.

▶ ergotamine and caffeine
Cafergot, Migergot

Tablets: 1 mg ergotamine tartrate, 100 mg caffeine.
Suppositories: 2 mg ergotamine tartrate, 100 mg caffeine.

Usual adult dose: 2 tablets PO at first sign of attack, then 1 tablet q 30 min, if needed. Max, 6/attack, 10/wk. Or, 1 suppository at first sign of attack, then second dose after 1 hr, if needed. Max, 2/attack, 5/wk. Do not use w/ ritonavir, nelfinavir, indinavir, erythromycin, clarithromycin, troleandomycin; serious vasospasm possible.

▶ sumatriptan and naproxen sodium
Treximet

Tablets: 85 mg sumatriptan, 500 mg naproxen.
Usual adult dose: 1 tablet PO at onset of acute migraine.

ANTINAUSEA DRUG

▶ doxylamine and pyridoxine
Diclegis

DR tablets: 10 mg doxylamine, 10 mg pyridoxine.
Usual adult dose: 1 tablet PO at bedtime; max 4 tablets/day. Tx of n/v in pregnancy in pts not responding to other tx.

ANTIPARKINSONIANS

▶ levodopa and carbidopa
Parcopa, Sinemet, Sinemet CR

Tablets: 100 mg levodopa, 10 mg carbidopa; 100 mg levodopa, 25 mg carbidopa; 250 mg levodopa, 25 mg carbidopa.
Orally disintegrating tablets: 100 mg levodopa, 10 mg carbidopa; 100 mg levodopa, 25 mg carbidopa; 250 mg levodopa, 25 mg carbidopa.
CR tablets: 100 mg levodopa, 25 mg carbidopa; 200 mg levodopa, 50 mg carbidopa.

Usual adult dose: Start w/ lowest dose; titrate based on response, tolerance.

▶ levodopa, carbidopa, and entacapone
Stalevo 50, Stalevo 75, Stalevo 100, Stalevo 125, Stalevo 150, Stalevo 200

Tablets: 50 mg levodopa, 12.5 mg carbidopa, 200 mg entacapone; 75 mg levodopa, 18.75 mg carbidopa, 200 mg entacapone; 100 mg levodopa, 25 mg carbidopa, 200 mg entacapone; 125 mg levodopa, 31.25 mg carbidopa, 200 mg entacapone; 150 mg levodopa, 37.5 mg carbidopa, 200 mg entacapone; 200 mg levodopa, 50 mg carbidopa, 200 mg entacapone.
Usual adult dose: 1 tablet PO q 3–8 hr.

ANTIPLATELET

▶ aspirin and dipyridamole
Aggrenox

Capsules: 25 mg aspirin, 200 mg dipyridamole.
Usual adult dose: 1 capsule PO bid to decrease risk of stroke in pts w/ known cerebrovascular disease.

ANTIULCER DRUGS

▶ bismuth subsalicylate, metronidazole, and tetracycline
Helidac

Tablets: 262.4 mg bismuth subsalicylate, 250 mg metronidazole, 500 mg tetracycline hydrochloride.
Usual adult dose: 1 tablet PO qid for 14 days w/ prescribed histamine-2 antagonist. For tx of active duodenal ulcers associated w/ *Helicobacter pylori* infection. Do not use

in pregnancy, breast-feeding, children.

▶ lansoprazole, amoxicillin, and clarithromycin
Prevpac

Daily administration pack: Two 30-mg lansoprazole capsules, four 500-mg amoxicillin capsules, two 500-mg clarithromycin tablets.
Usual adult dose: Divide pack equally to take PO bid, a.m. and p.m., for 10–14 days.

ANTIVIRALS

▶ abacavir and lamivudine
Epzicom

Tablets: 600 mg abacavir w/ 300 mg lamivudine.
Usual adult dose: 1 tablet PO daily w/ other antiretrovirals for tx of HIV infection.

▶ abacavir, zidovudine, and lamivudine
Trizivir

Tablets: 300 mg abacavir, 300 mg zidovudine, 150 mg lamivudine.
Usual adult dose: 1 tablet PO bid for tx of HIV infection. Carefully monitor for hypersensitivity reactions; potential increased risk of MI.

▶ efavirenz, emtricitabine, and tenofovir
Atripla

Tablets: 600 mg efavirenz, 200 mg emtricitabine, 300 mg tenofovir.
Usual adult dose: 1 tablet PO at bedtime on empty stomach for tx of HIV infection. Not recommended

w/ moderate or severe renal impairment.

▶ elvitegravir, cobicistat, emtricitabine, and tenofovir
Stribild

Tablets: 150 mg elvitegravir, 150 mg cobicistat, 200 mg emtricitabine, 300 mg tenofovir.
Usual adult dose: 1 tablet PO/day for pts never treated for HIV.

▶ emtricitabine, rilpivirine, and tenofovir
Complera

Tablets: 200 mg emtricitabine, 25 mg rilpivirine, 300 mg tenofovir.
Usual adult dose: 1 tablet/day PO for tx of HIV infection in tx-naive pts.

▶ emtricitabine and tenofovir disoproxil fumarate
Truvada

Tablets: 200 mg emtricitabine w/ 300 mg tenofovir.
Usual adult dose: 1 tablet PO daily w/ other antiretrovirals for tx of HIV infection.

▶ lamivudine and zidovudine
Combivir

Tablets: 150 mg lamivudine, 300 mg zidovudine.
Usual adult dose: 1 tablet PO bid for tx of HIV infection. Not recommended for adult, child under 50 kg.

BPH DRUG

▶ dutasteride and tamsulosin
Jalyn

Capsules: 0.5 mg dutasteride, 0.4 mg tamsulosin.
Usual adult dose: 1 capsule/day PO.

DIURETICS

▶ amiloride and hydrochlorothiazide
Moduretic

Tablets: 5 mg amiloride, 50 mg hydrochlorothiazide.
Usual adult dose: 1 or 2 tablets/day PO w/ meals.

▶ hydrochlorothiazide and triamterene
Dyazide

Capsules: 25 mg hydrochlorothiazide, 37.5 mg triamterene.
Usual adult dose: 1 or 2 capsules PO once/day or bid after meals.

▶ hydrochlorothiazide and triamterene
Maxzide, Maxzide-25

Tablets: 25 mg hydrochlorothiazide, 37.5 mg triamterene; 50 mg hydrochlorothiazide, 75 mg triamterene.
Usual adult dose: 1 or 2 tablets/day PO.

▶ spironolactone and hydrochlorothiazide
Aldactazide

Tablets: 25 mg spironolactone, 25 mg hydrochlorothiazide; 50 mg spironolactone, 50 mg hydrochlorothiazide.

Usual adult dose: 1–8 tablets/day PO (25/25). 1–4 tablets/day PO (50/50).

HF DRUG

▶ isosorbide dinitrate and hydralazine hydrochloride
BiDil

Tablets: 20 mg isosorbide dinitrate, 37.5 mg hydralazine.
Usual adult dose: 1 tablet PO tid; may increase to 2 tablets tid. For adjunct tx in self-identified black pts to improve functional survival.

LIPID-LOWERING DRUGS

▶ ezetimibe and atorvastatin
Liptruzet

Tablets: 10 mg ezetimibe w/ 10, 30, 40, or 80 mg atorvastatin
Usual adult dose: 1 tablet PO in p.m. w/ diet, exercise. If using bile acid sequestrant, give this drug 2 hr before or 4 hr after bile acid sequestrant.

▶ ezetimibe and simvastatin
Vytorin

Tablets: 10 mg ezetimibe, 10 mg simvastatin; 10 mg ezetimibe, 20 mg simvastatin; 10 mg ezetimibe, 40 mg simvastatin; 10 mg ezetimibe, 80 mg simvastatin.
Usual adult dose: 1 tablet/day PO in p.m. w/ cholesterol-lowering diet, exercise. Must give at least 2 hr before or 4 hr after bile sequestrant (if used).

▶ niacin and lovastatin
Advicor

Tablets: 500 mg niacin, 20 mg lovastatin; 750 mg niacin, 20 mg lovastatin; 1,000 mg niacin, 20 mg lovastatin.
Usual adult dose: 1 tablet/day PO in p.m.

▶ simvastatin and niacin
Simcor

Tablets: 20 mg simvastatin, 500 mg niacin; 20 mg simvastatin, 750 mg niacin; 20 mg simvastatin, 1,000 mg niacin.
Usual adult dose: 1 tablet/day PO. Max, 2,000 mg niacin w/ 40 mg simvastatin/day.

MENOPAUSE DRUGS

▶ conjugated estrogen and bazedoxifene
Duavee

Tablets: 0.45 mg conjugated estrogen, 20 mg bazedoxifene
Usual adult dose: 1 tablet/day PO.
BBW Risk of endometrial cancer, stroke, DVT, dementia. Not for use to decrease CAD.

▶ drospirenone and estradiol
Angeliq

Tablets: 0.5 mg drospirenone, 1 mg estradiol.
Usual adult dose: 1 tablet/day PO. Monitor potassium level closely.

▶ drospirenone and ethinyl estradiol
YAZ

Tablets: 3 mg drospirenone, 0.02 mg ethinyl estradiol.

Usual adult dose: 1 tablet/day PO. Monitor potassium level closely.

▶ estradiol and norethindrone (transdermal)
CombiPatch

Patch: 0.05 mg/day estradiol, 0.14 mg/day norethindrone; 0.05 mg/day estradiol, 0.25 mg/day norethindrone.
Usual adult dose: Change patch twice/wk.

▶ estradiol and norethindrone (oral)
Activella

Tablets: 0.5 mg estradiol, 0.1 mg norethindrone; 1 mg estradiol, 0.5 mg norethindrone.
Usual adult dose: 1 tablet/day PO.

▶ estradiol and norgestimate
Ortho-Prefest

Tablets: 1 mg estradiol, 0.09 mg norgestimate.
Usual adult dose: 1 tablet/day PO (3 days of pink tablets [estradiol alone], then 3 days of white tablets [estradiol and norgestimate combination]); continue cycle uninterrupted.

▶ estrogens, conjugated, and medroxyprogesterone
Premphase

Tablets: 0.625 mg conjugated estrogens, 5 mg medroxyprogesterone.
Usual adult dose: 1 tablet/day PO. Use in women w/ intact uterus.

▶ estrogens, conjugated, and medroxyprogesterone
Prempro

Tablets: 0.3 mg conjugated estrogen, 1.5 mg medroxyprogesterone; 0.45 mg conjugated estrogen, 1.5 mg medroxyprogesterone; 0.625 mg conjugated estrogen, 2.5 mg medroxyprogesterone; 0.625 mg conjugated estrogen, 5 mg medroxyprogesterone.
Usual adult dose: 1 tablet/day PO. Use in women w/ intact uterus.

▶ ethinyl estradiol and norethindrone acetate
Femhrt

Tablets: 2.5 mcg ethinyl estradiol, 0.5 mg norethindrone acetate; 5 mcg ethinyl estradiol, 1 mg norethindrone acetate.
Usual adult dose: 1 tablet/day PO. Use in women w/ intact uterus.

OPIOID AGONISTS

▶ buprenorphine and naloxone
CONTROLLED SUBSTANCE C-III
Suboxone

Sublingual tablets: 2 mg buprenorphine, 0.5 mg naloxone; 8 mg buprenorphine, 2 mg naloxone.
Usual adult dose: 12–16 mg/day sublingually after induction w/ sublingual buprenorphine for tx of opioid dependence.

▶ buprenorphine and naloxone
Zubsolv

Sublingual tablets: 1.4 mg buprenorphine, 0.36 mg naloxone; 5.7 mg buprenorphine, 1.4 mg naloxone.
Usual adult dose: 1 tablet/day sublingually.

PSYCHIATRIC DRUG

▶ **dextromethorphan and quinidine**
Nuedexta

Capsules: 20 mg dextromethorphan, 10 mg quinidine.
Usual adult dose: 1 capsule/day PO for 7 days; maint, 1 capsule PO q 12 hr. For tx of pseudobulbar affect associated w/ neurologic conditions.

RESPIRATORY DRUGS

▶ **azelastine and fluticasone**
Dymista

Nasal spray: 137 mcg azelastine, 50 mcg fluticasone.
Usual dose in pts 12 yr and older: 1 spray in each nostril bid for relief of sx of seasonal allergic rhinitis.

▶ **budesonide and formoterol fumarate**
Symbicort 80/4.5, Symbicort 160/4.5

Inhalation: 80 mcg budesonide, 4.5 mcg formoterol fumarate; 160 mcg budesonide, 4.5 mcg formoterol fumarate.
Usual dose in pts 12 yr and older: Two inhalations bid, a.m. and p.m. For long-term maint of asthma, not for acute attacks.

▶ **fluticasone and salmeterol**
Advair Diskus, Advair HFA

Inhalation: 100 mcg fluticasone, 50 mcg salmeterol; 250 mcg fluticasone, 50 mcg salmeterol; 500 mcg fluticasone, 50 mcg salmeterol.
Usual dose in pts 12 yr and older: 1 inhalation bid to manage asthma.

Usual dose in child 4–11 yr: 1 inhalation (100 mcg fluticasone, 50 mcg salmeterol) bid, a.m. and p.m. about 12 hr apart.

▶ **fluticasone and vilanterol**
Breo Ellipta

Powder for inhalation: 100 mcg fluticasone, 25 mcg vilanterol.
Usual adult dose: One oral inhalation daily. **BBW** Long-acting beta agonists are associated with asthma-related deaths; not for use in asthma or tx of acute bronchospasm.

▶ **hydrocodone and chlorpheniramine**
Vituz

Oral sol: 5 mg hydrocodone, 4 mg chlorpheniramine/5-mL sol.
Usual adult dose: 5 mL PO q 4–6 hr; max, four doses/day.

▶ **hydrocodone and pseudoephedrine**
Rezira

Oral sol: 5 mg hydrocodone, 60 mg pseudoephedrine/5-mL sol.
Usual adult dose: 5 mL PO q 4–6 hr as needed; max, four doses in 24 hr.

▶ **hydrocodone and pseudoephedrine and chlorpheniramine**
Zutripro

Oral sol: 5 mg hydrocodone, 60 mg pseudoephedrine, 4 mg chlorpheniramine in 5-mL sol.
Usual adult dose: 5 mL PO q 4–6 hr as needed; max, four doses in 24 hr.

▶ ipratropium and albuterol
Combivent

Metered-dose inhaler: 18 mcg ipratropium bromide, 90 mcg albuterol.
Usual adult dose: 2 inhalations four times/day. Not for use during acute attack. Use caution w/ known sensitivity to atropine, soy beans, soya lecithin, peanuts.

▶ loratadine and pseudoephedrine
Claritin-D

ER tablets: 5 mg loratadine, 120 mg pseudoephedrine.
Usual adult dose: 1 tablet PO q 12 hr.

▶ loratadine and pseudoephedrine
Claritin-D 24 Hour

ER tablets: 10 mg loratadine, 240 mg pseudoephedrine.
Usual adult dose: 1 tablet/day PO.

▶ mometasone and formoterol
Dulera 100/5, Dulera 200/5

Metered aerosol inhaler: 100 mcg mometasone, 5 mcg formoterol; 200 mcg mometasone, 5 mcg formoterol.
Usual adult dose: For maint tx of asthma, 2 inhalations bid, a.m. and p.m. Rinse mouth after use. Not for children.

▶ umeclidinium and vilanterol
Anoro Ellipta

Inhalation powder: 62.5 mcg umeclidinium, 25 mcg vilanterol.
Usual adult dose: One oral inhalation/day for maint of COPD.
BBW Long-acting beta agonists associated with asthma-related deaths, not for use in asthma or acute bronchospasm.

TENSION HEADACHE DRUG

▶ butalbital, acetaminophen, and caffeine
Esgic-Plus

Capsules: 50 mg butalbital, 500 mg acetaminophen, 40 mg caffeine.
Usual adult dose: 1 capsule PO q 4 hr as needed; max, 6/day. May be habit-forming; pt should avoid driving, dangerous tasks.

WEIGHT LOSS DRUGS

▶ phentermine and topiramate
Qsymia

Capsules: 3.75 mg phentermine, 23 mg topiramate; 7.5 mg phentermine, 46 mg topiramate; 11.25 mg phentermine, 69 mg topiramate; 15 mg phentermine, 92 mg topiramate.
Usual adult dose: 1 capsule/day PO in a.m. w/ diet/exercise. Hormonal contraceptives may be ineffective; cardiac issues, suicidality.

Appendix F

Hormonal contraceptives

IND & DOSE Take 1 tablet PO daily for 21 days, starting within 5 days of first day of menstrual bleeding (day 1 of cycle is first day of menstrual bleeding). Take inert tablets or no tablets for next 7 days. Then start new course of 21 days. Sunday start: Take first tablet on first Sunday after menstruation begins.

NC/PT Suggested measures for missed doses: One tablet missed: Take tablet as soon as possible, or take 2 tablets next day. Two consecutive tablets missed: Take 2 tablets daily for next 2 days, then resume regular schedule. Three consecutive tablets missed: If Sunday starter, take 1 pill q day until Sunday; then discard pack and start new pack on that day. If day 1 starter, discard rest of pack and start new pack that same day. Use additional birth control method until start of next menstrual period. Increased risk of thromboembolic events if combined w/ smoking.

Postcoital contraception ("morning after" pills): Safe, effective for emergency contraception. Regimen starts within 72 hr of unprotected intercourse w/ follow-up dose of same number of pills 12 hr after first dose. *Ovral:* 2 white tablets. *Nordette:* 4 light orange tablets. *Lo/Ovral:* 4 white tablets. *Plan B:* 0.75 mg levonorgestrel; take 1 tablet within 72 hr of sexual intercourse, take second tablet 12 hr later. *Plan B One-Step:* 1.5 mg levonorgestrel; take 1 tablet within 72 hr of unprotected sexual intercourse. Available OTC. *Ella* (ulipristal; progesterone agonist/antagonist): 30 mg tablet; take within 5 days of unprotected sexual intercourse.

ORAL CONTRACEPTIVES

Trade name	Combination
MONOPHASIC	
Aviane, Lessina, Lutera, Orsythia, Sronyx	20 mcg ethinyl estradiol/0.10 mg levonorgestrel
Altavera, Jolessa, Levora 0.15/30, Nordette, Portia	30 mcg ethinyl estradiol/0.15 mg levonorgestrel
Apri, Desogen, Emoquette, Ortho-Cept, Reclipsen, Solia	30 mcg ethinyl estradiol/0.15 mg desogestrel
Balziva, Femcon Fe chewable tablets, Ovcon-35, Zenchent	35 mcg ethinyl estradiol/0.4 mg norethindrone
Beyaz	3 mg drospirenone/20 mcg ethinyl estradiol/0.45 mg levomefolate; must monitor potassium levels.

Trade name	Combination
Brevicon, Modicon, Necon 0.5/35, Zenchent	35 mcg ethinyl estradiol/0.5 mg norethindrone
Cryselle, Lo/Ovral, Low-Ogestrel	30 mcg ethinyl estradiol/0.3 mg norgestrel
Estarylla, Mononessa, Ortho-Cyclen, Previfem, Sprintec	35 mcg ethinyl estradiol/0.25 mg norgestimate
Gianvi, Loryna, Yaz	30 mcg drospirenone/20 mcg ethinyl estradiol
Kelnor 1/35, Zovia 1/35E	35 mcg ethinyl estradiol/1 mg ethynodiol diacetate
Junel Fe 1/20, Junel 21 Day 1/20, Loestrin 21 1/20, Loestrin Fe 21 1/20, Loestrin 24 Fe, Microgestin Fe 1/20, Minastrin 24 FE	20 mcg ethinyl estradiol/1 mg norethindrone
Junel Fe 1.5/30, Junel 21 Day 1.5/30, Loestrin 21 1.5/30, Loestrin Fe 1.5/30, Microgestin Fe 1.5/30	30 mcg ethinyl estradiol/1.5 mg norethindrone acetate
Lybrel	0.09 mg levonorgestrel/20 mcg ethinyl estradiol in continual use to eliminate menstrual periods
Necon 1/35, Norinyl 1+35, Ortho-Novum 1/35	35 mcg ethinyl estradiol/1 mg norethindrone
Necon 1/50, Norinyl 1+50	50 mcg mestranol/1 mg norethindrone
Ocella, Syeda, Yasmin, Zaran	3 mg drospirenone/30 mcg ethinyl estradiol; must monitor potassium level
Ogestrel, Ovral-28	50 mcg ethinyl estradiol/0.5 mg norgestrel
Ovcon-50	50 mcg ethinyl estradiol/1 mg norethindrone acetate
Quasense, Seasonale, Seasonique	0.15 levonorgestrel/30 mcg ethinyl estradiol taken as 84 days active tablets, 7 days inactive
Safyral	3 mg drospirenone/30 mcg ethinyl estradiol/45 mcg levomefolate

Trade name	Combination
Zovia 1/50E	50 mcg ethinyl estradiol/1 mg ethynodiol diacetate

BIPHASIC

Azurette, Kariva, Mircette	**phase 1:** 21 tablets, 0.15 mg desogestrel/ 20 mcg ethinyl estradiol. **phase 2:** 5 tablets, 10 mcg ethinyl estradiol
Lo Loestrin Fe	**phase 1:** 24 tablets, 1 mg norethindrone/ 10 mcg ethinyl estradiol. **phase 2:** 2 tablets, 10 mcg ethinyl estradiol
LoSeasonique	**phase 1:** 84 tablets, 0.15 mg levonorgestrel/20 mcg ethinyl estradiol. **phase 2:** 7 tablets, 10 mcg ethinyl estradiol
Seasonique	**phase 1:** 84 tablets, 0.15 mg levonorgestrel/30 mcg ethinyl estradiol. **phase 2:** 7 tablets, 10 mcg ethinyl estradiol
Necon 10/11	**phase 1:** 10 tablets, 0.5 mg norethindrone/ 35 mcg ethinyl estradiol. **phase 2:** 11 tablets, 1 mg norethindrone/ 35 mcg ethinyl estradiol

TRIPHASIC

Aranelle, Leena, Tri-Norinyl	**phase 1:** 7 tablets, 0.5 mg norethindrone (progestin)/35 mcg ethinyl estradiol (estrogen). **phase 2:** 9 tablets, 1 mg norethindrone (progestin)/35 mcg ethinyl estradiol (estrogen). **phase 3:** 5 tablets, 0.5 mg norethindrone (progestin)/35 mcg ethinyl estradiol (estrogen)
Caziant, Cesia, Cyclessa, Velivet	**phase 1:** 7 tablets, 0.1 mg desogestrel/ 25 mcg ethinyl estradiol. **phase 2:** 7 tablets, 0.125 mg desogestrel/ 25 mcg ethinyl estradiol. **phase 3:** 7 tablets, 0.15 mg desogestrel/ 25 mcg ethinyl estradiol

Trade name	Combination
Enpresse	**phase 1:** 6 tablets, 0.05 mg levonorgestrel (progestin)/30 mcg ethinyl estradiol (estrogen). **phase 2:** 5 tablets, 0.075 mg levonorgestrel (progestin)/40 mcg ethinyl estradiol (estrogen). **phase 3:** 10 tablets, 0.125 mg levonorgestrel (progestin)/30 mcg ethinyl estradiol (estrogen)
Estrostep Fe, Tilia Fe, Tri-Legest Fe	**phase 1:** 5 tablets, 1 mg norethindrone/ 20 mcg ethinyl estradiol; w/ 75 mg ferrous fumarate. **phase 2:** 7 tablets, 1 mg norethindrone/ 30 mcg ethinyl estradiol; w/ 75 mg ferrous fumarate. **phase 3:** 9 tablets, 1 mg norethindrone/ 35 mcg ethinyl estradiol; w/ 75 mg ferrous fumarate
Ortho-Novum 7/7/7, Necon 7/7/7	**phase 1:** 7 tablets, 0.5 mg norethindrone (progestin)/35 mcg ethinyl estradiol (estrogen). **phase 2:** 7 tablets, 0.75 mg norethindrone (progestin)/35 mcg ethinyl estradiol (estrogen). **phase 3:** 7 tablets, 1 mg norethindrone (progestin)/35 mcg ethinyl estradiol (estrogen)
Ortho Tri-Cyclen, Tri-Estarylla, TriNessa, Tri-Previfem, Tri-Sprintec	**phase 1:** 7 tablets, 0.18 mg norgestimate/ 35 mcg ethinyl estradiol. **phase 2:** 7 tablets, 0.215 mg norgestimate/ 35 mcg ethinyl estradiol. **phase 3:** 7 tablets, 0.25 mg norgestimate/ 35 mcg ethinyl estradiol
Ortho Tri-Cyclen Lo	**phase 1:** 7 tablets, 0.18 mg norgestimate/ 25 mcg ethinyl estradiol. **phase 2:** 7 tablets, 0.215 mg norgestimate/ 25 mcg ethinyl estradiol. **phase 3:** 7 tablets, 0.25 mg norgestimate/ 25 mcg ethinyl estradiol
Tri-Legest	**phase 1:** 5 tablets, 1 mg norethindrone/ 20 mcg ethinyl estradiol. **phase 2:** 7 tablets, 1 mg norethindrone/ 30 mcg ethinyl estradiol. **phase 3:** 9 tablets, 1 mg norethindrone/ 35 mcg ethinyl estradiol

Trade name	Combination
Trivora-28	**phase 1:** 6 tablets, 0.5 mg levonorgestrel (progestin)/30 mcg ethinyl estradiol (estrogen). **phase 2:** 5 tablets, 0.075 mg levonorgestrel (progestin)/40 mcg ethinyl estradiol (estrogen). **phase 3:** 10 tablets, 0.125 mg levonorgestrel (progestin)/30 mcg ethinyl estradiol (estrogen)

4-Phasic

Natazia	**phase 1:** 2 tablets, 3 mg estradiol valerate. **phase 2:** 5 tablets, 2 mg estradiol valerate/ 2 mg dienogest. **phase 3:** 17 tablets, 2 mg estradiol valerate/3 mg dienogest. **phase 4:** 2 tablets, 1 mg estradiol valerate
Quartette	**phase 1:** 42 tablets, 0.15 mg levonorgestrel, 0.02 mg ethinyl estradiol **phase 2:** 21 tablets, 0.15 mg levonorgestrel, 0.025 mg ethinyl estradiol **phase 3:** 21 tablets, 0.15 mg levonorgestrel, 0.03 mg ethinyl estradiol **phase 4:** 7 tablets, 0.01 mg ethinyl estradiol

Progestin only

Camila, Errin, Heather	0.35 mg norethindrone

Implantable System

Trade name	Combination
Implanon, Nexplanon	68 mg etonogestrel implanted subdermally in inner aspect of nondominant upper arm. Left in place for no longer than 3 yr, then must be removed. May then insert new implants.

Injectable Contraceptives

Trade name	Combination
Depo-Provera	150, 400 mcg/mL medroxyprogesterone. Give 1-mL injection deep IM; repeat every 3 mo. **BBW** Risk of significant bone loss.

Trade name	Combination
depo-sub Q provera 104	104 mg medroxyprogesterone. Give 0.65 mL subcut into anterior thigh, abdomen. **BBW** Risk of significant bone loss.

INTRAUTERINE SYSTEM

Trade name	Combination
Mirena	52 mg levonorgestrel inserted into uterus for up to 5 yr. (Also approved to treat heavy menstrual bleeding in women using intrauterine system for contraception.) Releases 20 mcg/day.
Skyla	13.5 mg levonorgestrel inserted into uterus for up to 3 yr.

TRANSDERMAL SYSTEM

Trade name	Combination
Ortho Evra	**BBW** Higher risk of thromboembolic events, death if combined w/ smoking. 6 mg norelgestromin/0.75 ethinyl estradiol in patch form; releases 150 mcg norelgestromin/20 mcg ethinyl estradiol each 24 hr for 1 wk. Patch applied on same day of wk for 3 consecutive wk, followed by patch-free wk.

VAGINAL RING

Trade name	Combination
NuvaRing	0.12 mg etonogestrel (progestin)/0.015 mg ethinyl estradiol (estrogen)/day. Insert into vagina on or before 5th day of menstrual period; remove after 3 wk. Insert new ring after 1-wk rest.

Commonly used biologicals

IND & DOSE Vaccines provide inactivated or attenuated antigens to stimulate production of antibodies; provides active immunity. Immune globulin provides acute, passive immunity by providing preformed antibodies to specific antigen; not long-term protection.

ADV EFF Anorexia, drowsiness, injection-area edema (w/ redness, swelling, induration, pain that may persist for few days), fretfulness, generalized aches/pains, hypersensitivity reactions, malaise, transient fever, vomiting

NC/PT Pregnancy Category C. Use caution in pregnancy; safety not established. Defer administration of routine immunizing or booster doses if acute infection present. Usually not indicated for pts on immunosuppressants or w/ cancer, active infections. Have epinephrine 1:1,000 on hand during injection for hypersensitivity reactions. Provide comfort measures for discomforts of injection. Give pt written record of immunization, booster reminder if needed.

▶ **diphtheria and tetanus toxoids and acellular pertussis vaccine, adsorbed (DTaP, Tdap)**
Adacel, Boostrix, Daptacel, Infanrix, Tripedia

Primary immunization: 3 IM doses of 0.5 mL at 4- to 8-wk intervals. Start doses by 6–8 wk of age; finish by 7th birthday. Use same vaccine for all three doses. *Fourth dose:* 0.5 mL IM at 15–20 mo at least 6 mo after previous dose. *Fifth dose:* 0.5 mL IM at 4–6 yr or preferably before entry into school *(Infanrix, Daptacel, Tripedia).* If fourth dose given after 4-yr birthday, may omit preschool dose. *Booster injections:* 11–64 yr *(Adacel),* 0.5 mL IM. 10 yr and older *(Boostrix),* 0.5 mL IM. Allow at least 5 yr between last of series and booster dose.

▶ **diphtheria and tetanus toxoids and acellular pertussis adsorbed, hepatitis B (recombinant), and inactivated poliovirus vaccine combined (DTaP-HePB-IPV)**
Pediarix

Infants w/ hepatitis B surface antigen (HBsAG)–negative mothers: Three 0.5-mL doses IM at 6- to 8-wk intervals (preferably 8) stating at 2 mo. *Children previously vaccinated w/ one dose of hepatitis B vaccine:* Should receive three-dose series. *Children previously vaccinated w/ one or more doses of Infanrix or IPV:* May use *Pediarix* to complete series.

▶ **diphtheria and tetanus toxoids and acellular pertussis adsorbed and inactivated poliovirus vaccine (DTaP-IIPV)**
Kinrix

Fifth dose in diphtheria, tetanus, acellular pertussis series and fourth dose in inactivated poliovirus series in children 4–6 yr whose previous immunizations have been w/ *Infanrix* or *Pediarix* for first three doses and *Infanrix* for fourth dose. One IM injection of 0.5 mL.

▶ **diphtheria and tetanus toxoids and acellular pertussis adsorbed, inactivated poliovirus vaccine, and *Haemophilus* b conjugate (tetanus toxoid conjugate) vaccine (DTaP-IPV/Hib)**
Pentacel

Four-dose series of IM injections of 0.5 mL at 2, 4, and 6 mo, followed by booster at 18 mo. Give between 6 wk and 4 yr.

▶ **Haemophilus b conjugate vaccine**
ActHIB, Hiberix, Liquid PedvaxHIB

Active immunization of infants, children against *H. influenzae* b for primary immunization, routine recall; 2–71 mo (*PedvaxHIB*), 2–18 mo (*ActHIB w/ DPT*), or 15–18 mo (*ActHIB, Hiberix w/ Tripedia*).
ActHIB: Reconstitute w/ DTP, *Tripedia*, or saline. 2–6 mo, 3 IM injections of 0.5 mL at 2, 4, and 6 mo;

0.5 mL at 15–18 mo and DPT alone at 4–6 yr. 7–11 mo, 2 IM injections of 0.5 mL at 8-wk intervals; booster dose at 15–18 mo. 12–14 mo, 0.5 mL IM w/ a booster 2 mo later. 15–18 mo, 0.5 mL IM, booster of *Tripedia* at 4–6 yr.
Hiberix: 15 mo–4 yr, booster dose of 0.5 mL IM as single dose. Booster dose at 15 mo or older but not less than 2 mo from last dose. Unvaccinated children 15–71 mo, 0.5 mL IM.
PedvaxHIB: 2–14 mo, 2 IM injections of 0.5 mL at 2 mo and 2 mo later; 0.5-mL booster at 12 mo (if two doses complete before 12 mo, not less than 2 mo after last dose). 15 mo or older, 0.5 mL IM single injection.

▶ *Haemophilus* b **conjugate vaccine w/ hepatitis B surface antigen (recombinant)**
Comvax

Infants w/ hepatitis B surface antigen (HBsAg)–negative mothers: Three 0.5-mL IM doses at 2, 4, and 12–15 mo. *Children previously vaccinated w/ one or more doses of hepatitis B vaccine or Haemophilus b vaccine:* 0.5-mL IM doses at 2, 4, and 12–15 mo. Give only to children of HBsAg-negative mothers.

▶ **hepatitis A vaccine, inactivated**
Havrix, Vaqta

Adult: *Havrix,* 1,440 ELISA units (1 mL) IM; same dose booster in 6–12 mo. *Vaqta,* 50 units (1 mL) IM; same dose booster in 6–18 mo.
Child 12 mo–18 yr: *Vaqta,* 25 units /0.5 mL IM, w/ repeat dose in 6–18 mo. *Havrix,* 720 ELISA units

(0.5 mL) IM; repeat dose in 6–12 mo.

▶ hepatitis A inactivated and hepatitis B recombinant vaccine
Twinrix

Three doses (1 mL by IM injection) on 0-, 1-, and 6-month schedule. *Accelerated dosage:* Four doses (1 mL by IM injection) on days 0, 7, 21, 30, followed by booster dose at 12 mo. Safety in pts under 18 yr not established.

▶ hepatitis B immune globulin (HBIG)
HepaGam B, HyperHEP B S/D, Nabi-HB

Perinatal exposure: 0.5 mL IM within 12 hr of birth; repeat dose at 1 mo and 6 mo after initial dose. *Percutaneous exposure:* 0.06 mL/kg IM immediately (within 7 days); repeat 28–30 days after exposure. Usual adult dose, 3–5 mL. *Pts at high risk for infection:* 0.06 mL/kg IM at same time (but at different site) as hepatitis B vaccine is given. *HepaGam B after liver transplant:* 20,000 international units IV at 2 mL/min. Give first dose w/ liver transplant, then daily on days 1–7, q 2 wk from day 14 through 12 wk, and monthly from mo 4 onward. *Sexual exposure:* Single dose of 0.06 mL/kg IM within 14 days of last sexual contact.

▶ hepatitis B vaccine
Engerix-B, Recombivax HB

Adults: Initial dose, 1 mL IM, then 1 mL IM at 1 mo and 6 mo after initial dose, all types. *Child 11–19 yr:* 1 mL IM, then 1 mL IM at 1 mo and 6 mo after initial dose. *Birth–10 yr:* Initial dose, 0.5 mL IM, then 0.5 mL IM at 1 mo and 6 mo after initial dose. *Dialysis, predialysis pts:* Initial dose, 40 mcg (2 mL) IM; repeat at 1, 2, and 6 mo after initial dose *(Engerix-B).* Or, 40 mcg (1 mL) IM; repeat at 1 and 6 mo *(Recombivax HB).* **Revaccination** (consider booster dose w/ anti-HBs level under 10 milli-international units/mL 1–2 mo after third dose). *Adult, child older than 10 yr:* 20 mcg. *Child under 10 yr:* 10 mcg. *Hemodialysis pts (when antibody testing indicates need):* Two 20-mcg doses.

▶ human papillomavirus recombinant vaccine, bivalent types 16 and 18
(Cervarix)

Young girls, women 10–25 yr: Three doses of 0.5 mL IM at 0, 1, and 6 mo.

▶ human papillomavirus recombinant vaccine, quadrivalent
Gardasil

Pts 9–26 yr: Three separate IM injections of 0.5 mL each, second dose 2 mo after initial dose, last dose 6 mo after first dose. For px of cervical cancer, precancerous genital lesions, genital warts, vaginal/vulvar/anal cancer in women; px of genital warts, anal cancer, precancerous lesions in males.

▶ immune globulin intramuscular (IG; gamma globulin; IGIM)
GamaSTAN S/D

▶ immune globulin intravenous (IGIV)
Carimune NF, Flebogamma 5%, Flebogamma 10%, Gammagard Liquid, Privigen

▶ immune globulin subcutaneous (IGSC, SCIG)

Gamunex-C, Hizentra, Vivaglobin

BBW Risk of renal dysfunction, renal failure, death; monitor accordingly. *Hepatitis A:* 0.02 mL/kg IM for household, institutional contacts. Persons traveling to areas where hepatitis A common, 0.02 mL/kg IM if staying less than 2 mo; 0.06 mL/kg IM repeated q 5 mo for prolonged stay. *Measles (rubeola):* 0.25 mL/kg IM if exposed less than 6 days previously; immunocompromised child exposed to measles, 0.5 mL/kg to max 15 mL IM immediately. *Varicella:* 0.6–1.2 mL/kg IM promptly if zoster immune globulin unavailable. *Rubella:* 0.55 mL/kg IM to pregnant women exposed to rubella but not considering therapeutic abortion; may decrease likelihood of infection, fetal damage. *Immunoglobulin deficiency:* Initially, 1.3 mL/kg IM, followed in 3–4 wk by 0.66 mL/kg IM q 3–4 wk; some pts may need more frequent injections. *Carimune NF:* 0.4–0.8 g/kg by IV infusion q 3–4 wk. *Flebogamma:* 300–600 mg/kg IV q 3–4 wk. *Primary immune deficiency, idiopathic thrombocytopenic purpura, chronic inflammatory demyelinating polyneuropathy:* 100–200 mg/kg subcut q wk. Or initially, 1.37 × previous IGIV dose (grams)/number of wk between IGIV doses (Gamunex-C). Adjust based on response.

▶ influenza type A (H5N1) virus monovalent vaccine, adjuvanted

generic

Adult: 0.5 mL IM into deltoid muscle; then 0.5 mL IM 21 days later. Prepare by mixing one vial AS03 adjuvant with one vial H5N1 adjuvant just before administration; do not mix in syringe w/ other vaccines. Virus grown in chicken eggs; use caution w/ chicken allergies. Use caution in pregnancy. Give pt written record.

▶ influenza type A and B virus vaccine

Afluria, Agriflu, Fluarix, FluLaval, Fluvirin, Fluzone, Fluzone High Dose, Fluzone Quadrivalent

Do not give w/ sensitivity to eggs, chicken, chicken feathers, chicken dander; hypersensitivity to vaccine components; hx of Guillain-Barré syndrome. Do not give to infants, children at same time as diphtheria, tetanus toxoid, pertussis vaccine (DTP) or within 14 days after measles virus vaccine. *6–35 mo:* 0.25 mL IM; repeat in 4 wk (Afluria, Fluzone). *3 yr and older:* 0.5 mL IM (Afluria, Fluzone, Fluarix). If under 9 yr and receiving vaccine for first time or received only one dose last year, give repeat dose in 4 wk. *4 yr and older:* 0.5 mL IM (Fluvirin). If under 8 yr and receiving vaccine for first time or received only one dose last year, give repeat dose in 4 wk. *18 yr and older:* 0.5 mL IM. Shake prefilled syringe before use (Agriflu, Afluria, Fluarix, FluLaval, Fluzone, Fluvirin). *18–64 yr:* 0.1 mL intradermally (Fluzone Intradermal). *65 yr and older:* 0.5 mL IM (Fluzone High Dose).

▶ influenza type A and B virus vaccine, live, intranasal

FluMist

2–8 yr, not previously vaccinated: Two doses (0.2 mL each) intranasally as one spray (0.1 mL)/nostril at least 1 mo apart. *2–8 yr, previously vaccinated:* One dose (0.2 mL) intranasally as one spray (0.1 mL)/nostril. *9–49 yr:* One dose of one spray

(0.1 mL) in each nostril/flu season.
*5–8 yr not previously vaccinated
w/ FluMist:* Two doses (0.5 mL each)
60 days apart ± 14 days. *5–8 yr previously vaccinated w/ FluMist:* One
dose (0.5 mL)/flu season.

► influenza virus vaccine, H5N1
H5N1

Adult 18–64 yr: 1 mL IM into deltoid
muscle of upper arm, then 1 mL IM
21–35 days later. Virus grown in
chicken eggs; use caution in pts w/
chicken allergy.

► measles (rubeola) virus vaccine, live, attenuated
Attenuvax

Inject total volume of reconstituted
vaccine or 0.5 mL of multidose vial
subcut into outer aspect of upper
arm; dose same for all pts. Recommended age for primary vaccination,
12–15 mo. Use caution if giving to pt
w/ hx of sensitivity to eggs, chicken,
chicken feathers. Do not give within
1 mo of immunization w/ other live
virus vaccines, mumps vaccine. Do
not give for at least 3 mo after blood,
plasma transfusions or serum immune globulin administration.

► measles, mumps, rubella vaccine, live (MMR)
M-M-R II

Inject 0.5 mL reconstituted vaccine
subcut into outer aspect of upper
arm. Dose same for all pts. Booster
dose recommended on entry into elementary school. Use caution if giving to pt w/ hx of sensitivity to eggs,
chicken, chicken feathers. Do not

give within 1 mo of immunization w/
other live virus vaccines. Do not give
for at least 3 mo after blood, or plasma transfusions or serum immune
globulin administration.

► measles, mumps, rubella, and varicella virus vaccine, live
ProQuad

12 mo–12 yr: 0.5 mL subcut. Allow
1 mo between administration of vaccines containing measles antigens
and administration of *ProQuad*. If
second varicella vaccine needed, allow 3 mo between administration of
the two doses.

► meningococcal groups C and Y, *Haemophilus* b tetanus toxoid conjugate vaccine
MenHibrix

Four doses, 0.5 mL IM each; first as
early as 6 wk, 4th as late as 18 mo.
Usual timing, 2, 4, 6, and 12–15 mo.

► meningococcal vaccine
Menactra, Menomune A/C/
Y/W-135, Menveo

Menactra: 9 mo–55 yr, 0.5 mL IM in
deltoid region as one dose. *Menomune:* 2–55 yr, 0.5 mL IM; may give
booster in 3–5 yr. *Menveo:* 2 mo–
55 yr, 0.5 mL IM as one dose. Children 2–5 yr may receive second
dose 2 mo after first dose.

► pneumococcal vaccine, polyvalent
Pneumovax 23

One 0.5-mL dose subcut, IM. Not recommended for children under 2 yr. Give at least 2 wk before initiation of cancer chemotherapy, other immunosuppressive therapy.

► **pneumococcal 13-valent conjugate vaccine (diphtheria CRM$_{197}$ protein)**
Prevnar-13

0.5 mg IM, preferably in anterolateral aspect of thigh in infants, deltoid muscle of upper arm in older children. *6 wk–5 yr:* Four-dose series given 4–8 wk apart at 2, 4, 6 mo; then at 12–15 mo. *Catch-up schedule for children 7 mo and older:* 7–11 mo, three doses, first two doses at least 4 wk apart; third dose after first birthday. 12–23 mo, two doses at least 2 mo apart. 24 mo–5 yr, one dose (before 6th birthday).

► **poliovirus vaccine, inactivated (IPV, Salk)**
IPOL

Do not give w/ known hypersensitivity to streptomycin, neomycin (each dose contains under 25 mcg of each). *Adults:* Not usually needed in adults in United States. Recommended if unimmunized adult is exposed, traveling to high-risk area, or household contact of children receiving IPV. Give 0.5 mL subcut: two doses at 1- to 2-mo intervals, third dose 6–12 mo later. Previously vaccinated adults at risk for exposure should receive 0.5-mL dose. *Children:* 0.5 mL subcut at 2, 4, and 6–18 mo. Booster dose needed at time of entry into elementary school.

► **RHo (D) immune globulin**
HyperRHO S/D Full Dose, RhoGAM, Ultra-Filtered Plus

► **RHo (D) immune globulin micro-dose**
HyperRHO S/D minidose, MICRhoGAM, Ultra-Filtered Plus

► **RHo (D) immune globulin IV (human) (RHo D IGIV)**
Rhophylac, WinRho SDF

BBW Risk of intravascular hemolysis, death when used for idiopathic thrombocytopenia purpura (ITP; *WinRho*). monitor dipstick urinalysis at baseline, then at 2, 4, 8 hr. Ask pt to report back pain, chills, discolored urine.

Postpartum prophylaxis: 1 vial IM, IV (*WinRho SDF*) within 72 hr of delivery. *Antepartum prophylaxis:* 1 vial IM, IV (*WinRho SDF*) at 26–28 wk' gestation; 1 vial within 72 hr after Rh-incompatible delivery to prevent Rh isoimmunization during pregnancy. *After amniocentesis, miscarriage, abortion, ectopic pregnancy at or beyond 13 wk' gestation:* 1 vial IM, IV. *Transfusion accidents:* Multiply volume in mL of Rh-positive whole blood given by Hct of donor unit; divide this volume (in mL) by 15 to obtain number of vials to be given. If results of calculation are fraction, give next whole number of vials. *ITP:* 250 international units/kg IV at 2 mL/ 15–60 sec. *Spontaneous/induced abortion, termination of ectopic pregnancy up to and including 12 wk' gestation (unless father Rh negative):* 1 vial microdose IM as soon as possible after pregnancy termination.

► rotavirus vaccine, live, oral pentavalent
Rotarix, RotaTeq

Three ready-to-use liquid pouch doses (2 mL each) PO starting at age 6–12 wk, w/ subsequent doses at 4- to 10-wk intervals (do not give third dose after age 32 wk) (RotaTeq). Two doses of 1 mL each PO starting at age 6 wk. Allow 4 wk before second dose. Must complete Series by age 24 wk (Rotarix).

► typhoid vaccine
Typhim Vi, Vivotif Berna

Complete vaccine regimen 1–2 wk before potential exposure.
Parenteral *Older than 10 yr:* 2 doses of 0.5 mL subcut at intervals of 4 wk or longer. *10 yr or younger:* Two doses of 0.25 mL subcut at intervals of 4 wk or longer.
Booster dose. Given q 3 yr in cases of continued exposure. *Older than 10 yr:* 0.5 mL subcut or 0.1 mL intradermally. *6 mo–10 yr:* 0.25 mL subcut or 0.1 mL intradermally.

Parenteral *(Typhim Vi). Children 2 yr and older:* 0.5 mL IM. Booster dose q 2 yr; 0.5 mL IM.
Oral *(Vivotif Berna). Pts over 6 yr:* 1 capsule on days 1, 3, 5, 7 1 hr before meal w/ cold, lukewarm drink. No data on need for booster dose; 4 capsules on alternating days once q 5 yr suggested.

► varicella virus vaccine, live
Varivax

Adult, child 13 yr and older: 0.5 mL subcut in deltoid area, then 0.5 mL 4–8 wk later. *Child 1–12 yr:* Single 0.5-mL dose subcut.

► zoster vaccine, live
Zostavax

Adult 50 yr and older: 1 injection of single-dose vaccine subcut in upper arm. Vaccine should be frozen and reconstituted, using supplied diluent, immediately after removal from freezer. Give immediately after reconstituting.

OTHER BIOLOGICALS

Name	Indications	Instructions
IMMUNE GLOBULINS		
anti-thymocyte globulin (Thymoglobulin)	Tx of renal transplant acute rejection w/immunosuppression	1.5 mg/kg/day for 7–14 days as 6-hr IV infusion for first dose and at least 4 hr each subsequent dose. Give through 0.22-micron filter. Store in refrigerator; use within 4 hr of reconstitution.
botulism immune globulin (BabyBIG)	Tx of pts under 1 yr w/ infant botulism caused by toxin A or B	1 mL/kg as single IV infusion as soon as dx made.

Name	Indications	Instructions
cytomegalovirus immune globulin IV (CMV-IGIV) (CytoGam)	Px of CMV disease after renal, lung, liver, pancreas, heart transplant	15 mg/kg IV over 30 min; increase to 30 mg/kg IV for 30 min, then 60 mg/kg IV to max 150 mg/kg. Infuse at 72 hr, 2 wk, then 4, 6, 8, 12, 16 wk. monitor for allergic reactions. Use within 6 hr of entering vial. Give through IV line w/ in-line filter (15 micron).
lymphocyte, immune globulin (Atgam)	Mgt of allograft rejection in renal transplant; tx of aplastic anemia	10–30 mg/kg/day IV adult transplant; 5–25 mg/kg/day IV child transplant; 10–20 mg/kg/day IV for 8–14 days for aplastic anemia. Stable for up to 12 hr after reconstitution. Give skin test before first dose.
rabies immune globulin (HyperRab S/D, Imogam Rabies-HT)	Passive protection against rabies in nonimmunized pts w/ exposure to rabies	20 international units/kg IM as single dose at same time as rabies vaccine. Infuse wound area if possible. Never give in same site as vaccine. Refrigerate vial.
vaccinia immune globulin IV (VIGIV)	Tx, modification of vaccinia infections	2 mL/kg (100 mg/kg) IV.
varicella zoster immune globulin (VZIG)	Decrease severity of chickenpox sx in high-risk pts	125 units/10 kg IV or IM given within 96 hr of exposure.

ANTITOXINS, ANTIVENINS

Name	Indications	Instructions
antivenin (Micrurus fulvius)	Neutralization of venom of U.S. coral snakes	3–5 vials by slow IV injection. Give first 1 to 2 mL over 3–5 min; observe for allergic reaction. Flush w/ IV fluids after antivenin infused. May need up to 100 mL.
black widow spider species antivenin (Antivenin Latrodectus mactans)	Tx of sx of black widow spider bites	2.5 mL IM. May give IV in 10–50 mL saline over 15 min. Ensure supportive tx, muscle relaxant use.
botulism antitoxin (Botulism antitoxin heptavalent [HBAT])	Tx of suspected/known exposure to botulinum neurotoxin	For pts 1 yr and older, base dose on CDC protocol and exposure.

Name	Indications	Instructions
centruroides (scorpion) immune fab *(Anascorp)*	Tx of scorpion stings	Initially, 3 vials infused IV over 10 min; then 1 vial at a time at intervals of 30–60 min until clinically stable. Begin as soon as possible after sting. Severe hypersensitivity reactions, delayed serum sickness reaction possible (contains equine proteins).
crotalidae polyvalent immune fab (ovine) *(CroFab)*	Tx of rattlesnake bites	4–6 vials IV; may repeat based on response. Dilute each vial w/ 10 mL sterile water, then w/ 250 mL 0.9% normal saline. Give each 250 mL over 60 min. Contains specific antibody fragments that bind to four different rattlesnake toxins. Venom removal should be done at once. monitor carefully for hypersensitivity reaction. most effective if given within first 6 hr after snake bite.
varicella zoster immune globulin *(VariZIG)*	Decrease severity of chickenpox; used within 4 days of exposure	1.25 mL diluted IM or 2.5 mL diluted IV over 3–5 min. Do not give w/ varicella vaccine.

BACTERIAL VACCINES

BCG *(TICE BCG)*	Exposure to TB of skin test negative infants and children; tx of groups w/ high rates of TB; travel to areas w/ high endemic TB rates	0.2–0.3 mL percutaneously using sterile multipuncture disc. Refrigerate, protect from light. Keep vaccination site clean until reaction disappears.

VIRAL VACCINES

Japanese encephalitis vaccine *(JE-VAX)*	Active immunization in pts older than 1 yr who will reside, travel in endemic or epidemic areas	3 subcut doses of 1 mL on days 0, 7, 30. Child 1–3 yr, 3 subcut doses of 0.5 mL. Refrigerate vial. Do not remove rubber stopper. Pt should not travel within 10 days of vaccination.

Name	Indications	Instructions
Japanese encephalitis virus (JEV) vaccine, inactivated, adsorbed *(Ixiaro)*	Active immunization in pts 17 yr and older	2 doses of 0.5 mL each IM 28 days apart. Should complete series at least 1 wk before exposure to JEV. Contains protamine sulfate. Use only if clearly needed in pregnancy, breast-feeding.
rabies vaccine *(Imovax Rabies, RabAvert)*	Preexposure rabies immunization for pts in high-risk area; postexposure antirabies regimen w/ rabies immunoglobulin	*Preexposure:* 1 mL IM on days 0, 7, and 21 or 28. *Postexposure:* 1 mL IM on days 0, 3, 7, 14, 28. Refrigerate. If titers low, may need booster.
yellow fever vaccine *(YF-Vax)*	Immunization of pts 9 mo and older living in or traveling to endemic areas	0.5 mL subcut. Booster dose suggested q 10 yr. Use cautiously w/ allergy to chicken, egg products.

Drugs commonly used to treat specific disorders

The list below includes 50 common disorders and the medications most commonly prescribed to treat them.

ADHD

Stimulants
dexmethylphenidate *(Focalin)*
dextroamphetamine *(Dexedrine)*
lisdexamphetamine *(Vyvanse)*
methylphenidate *(Concerta, Ritalin)*
mixed amphetamines *(Adderall)*

Nonstimulants
atomoxetine *(Strattera)*
guanfacine *(Intuniv)*

Alzheimer disease

Cholinergics
donepezil *(Aricept)*
galantamine *(Razadyne)*
rivastigmine *(Exelon)*

NMDA receptor antagonist
memantine *(Namenda)*

Angina

Nitrates
isosorbide dinitrate *(Isordil)*
isosorbide mononitrate *(Imdur)*
nitroglycerin *(Nitro-Bid, Nitrostat, others)*

Beta blockers
metoprolol *(Toprol)*
nadolol *(Corgard)*
propranolol *(Inderal)*

Calcium channel blockers
amlodipine *(Norvasc)*
diltiazem *(Cardizem)*
nicardipine *(Cardene)*
nifedipine *(Adalat)*
verapamil *(Calan)*

Piperazine-acetamide
ranolazine *(Ranexa)*

Anxiety disorder

Benzodiazepines
alprazolam *(Xanax)*
chlordiazepoxide
clonazepam *(Klonopin)*
clorazepate *(Tranxene)*
diazepam *(Valium)*
lorazepam *(Ativan)*
oxazepam

Barbiturates
mephobarbital *(Mebaral)*

Others
buspirone
meprobamate

Arthritis, rheumatoid

Pain relief
aspirin (generic)
capsaicin *(Qutenza)*
celecoxib *(Celebrex)*
diclofenac *(Cataflam)*

Immunomodulators
abatacept *(Orencia)*
adalimumab *(Humira)*
anakinra *(Kineret)*
auranofin *(Ridaura)*
aurothioglucose *(Solganal)*
azathioprine *(Imuran)*
certolizumab *(Cimzia)*
cyclosporine *(Sandimmune)*
etanercept *(Enbrel)*
hydroxychloroquine *(Plaquenil)*
infliximab *(Remicade)*
leflunomide *(Arava)*

methotrexate
penicillamine (*Cuprimine*)
prednisone (*Rayos*)
rituximab (*Rituxan*)

Asthma

Xanthines
aminophylline (*Truphylline*)
diphylline (*Lufyllin*)
theophylline (*Elixophyllin, others*)

Sympathomimetics
albuterol (*Proventil*)
epinephrine (*Adrenaclick*)
formoterol (*Foradil*)
isoetharine
isoproterenol (*Isuprel*)
levalbuterol (*Xopenex*)
metaproterenol (*Alupent*)
pirbuterol (*Maxair*)
salmeterol (*Serevent*)
terbutaline

Inhaled steroids
beclomethasone (*Beclovent*)
budesonide (*Pulmicort*)
ciclesonide (*Alvesco*)
fluticasone (*Flovent*)
triamcinolone (*Azmacort*)

Leukotriene
montelukast (*Singulair*)

Receptor antagonists
zafirlukast (*Accolate*)
zileuton (*Zyflo*)

BPH

Alpha₁ blockers
alfuzosin (*UroXatral*)
doxazosin (*Cardura*)
tamsulosin (*Flomax*)
terazosin (*Hytrin*)

Androgen inhibitors
dutasteride (*Avodart*)
finasteride (*Proscar*)

Cancer, breast

Antineoplastics
anastrozole (*Arimidex*)
capecitabine (*Xeloda*)
cyclophosphamide
docetaxel (*Taxotere*)
doxorubicin
epirubicin (*Ellence*)
eribulin (*Halaven*)
exemestane (*Aromasin*)
fluorouracil (*Efudex, Fluoroplex*)
fulvestrant (*Faslodex*)
gemcitabine (*Gemzar*)
ixabepilone (*Ixempra*)
lapatinib (*Tykerb*)
letrozole (*Femara*)
methotrexate (*Trexall*)
paclitaxel (*Abraxane, Taxol*)
tamoxifen (*Soltamox*)
toremifene (*Fareston*)

Cancer, colon

Antineoplastics
bevacizumab (*Avastin*)
capecitabine (*Xeloda*)
cetuximab (*Erbitux*)
irinotecan (*Camptosar*)
leucovorin (*Fusilev*)
oxaliplatin (*Eloxatin*)
panitumumab (*Vectibix*)

Cancer, lung

Antineoplastics
bevacizumab (*Avastin*)
carboplatin
cisplatin
docetaxel (*Taxotere*)
erlotinib (*Tarceva*)
etoposide
gemcitabine (*Gemzar*)
irinotecan (*Camptosar*)
paclitaxel (*Taxol*)
pemetrexed (*Alimta*)
vinorelbine (*Navelbine*)

Cancer, prostate

LH-RH agonists
degarelix (*Firmagon*)
goserelin (*Zoladex*)

histrelin (*Vantas*)
leuprolide (*Lupron*)
triptorelin (*Trelstar*)

Anti-androgens
bicalutamide (*Casodex*)
flutamide
nilutamide (*Nilandron*)

Antineoplastics
abiraterone (*Zytiga*)
cabazitaxel (*Jevtana*)

Immunotherapy
sipuleucel-T (*Provenge*)

Constipation

Chemical stimulants
bisacodyl (*Dulcolax*)
cascara
castor oil (*Neolid*)
senna (*Senokot*)

Bulk stimulants
lactulose
magnesium citrate (*Citrate of Magnesia*)
magnesium hydroxide (*Milk of Magnesia*)
magnesium sulfate (*Epsom Salts*)
polycarbophil (*FiberCon*)
polyethylene glycol (*Miralax*)
polyethylene glycol electrolyte solution (*GoLYTELY, others*)
psyllium (*Metamucil*)

Lubricants
docusate (*Colace*)
glycerin (*Sani-Supp*)
mineral oil

COPD

Xanthines
aminophylline
diphylline (*Lufyllin*)
theophylline (*Elixophyllin, others*)

Sympathomimetics
arformoterol (*Brovana*)
indacaterol (*Arcapta*)

Anticholinergics
aclidinium (*Tudorza Pressair*)
ipratropium (*Atrovent*)
tiotropium (*Spiriva*)

Phosphodiesterase inhibitor
roflumilast (*Daliresp*)

Crohn disease

Salicylates
mesalamine (*Apriso, Asacol*)
sulfasalazine (*Azulfidine*)

Antibiotics
ciprofloxacin (*Cipro*)
metronidazole (*Flagyl*)

Corticosteroids
budesonide (*Entocort EC*)
prednisone (*Rayos*)

Immunomodulators
azathioprine (*Imuran*)
mercaptopurine (*Purinethol*)

Monoclonal antibodies
adalimumab (*Humira*)
infliximab (*Remicade*)

Cystic fibrosis

Bronchodilators
albuterol
salmeterol (*Serevent*)

Mucolytic
acetylcysteine

Digestive enzyme
pancrelipase (*Creon, Pancrease*)

Others
dornase alfa: dornase (*Pulmozyme*)

Depression

TCAs
amitriptyline
amoxapine (*Ascendin*)
clomipramine (*Anafranil*)
desipramine (*Norpramin*)
doxepin (*Silenor*)

imipramine *(Tofranil)*
maprotiline
nortriptyline *(Aventyl)*
protriptyline *(Vivactil)*
trimipramine *(Surmontil)*

MAOIs
isocarboxazid *(Marplan)*
phenelzine *(Nardil)*
tranylcypromine *(Parnate)*

SSRIs
citalopram *(Celexa)*
escitalopram *(Lexapro)*
fluoxetine *(Prozac)*
fluvoxamine *(Luvox)*
paroxetine *(Paxil)*
sertraline *(Zoloft)*
vilazodone *(Viibryd)*

Others
bupropion *(Wellbutrin)*
desvenlafaxine *(Pristiq)*
duloxetine *(Cymbalta)*
milnacipran *(Remeron)*
nefazodone
selegiline *(Emsam)*
trazodone *(Desyrel)*
venlafaxine *(Effexor)*

Diabetes mellitus

Insulin
insulin *(Humulin, others)*

Sulfonylureas
chlorpropamide *(Diabinese)*
glimepiride *(Amaryl)*
glipizide *(Glucotrol)*
glyburide *(DiaBeta)*
tolazamide *(Tolinase)*
tolbutamide *(Orinase)*

Alpha-glucosidase inhibitors
acarbose *(Precose)*
miglitol *(Glyset)*

Biguanide
metformin *(Glucophage)*

DPP-4 inhibitors
alogliptin *(Nesina)*
linagliptin *(Tradjenta)*
saxagliptin *(Onglyza)*
sitagliptin *(Januvia)*

Human amylin
pramlintide *(Symlin)*

Incretin mimetics
exenatide *(Bydureon, Byetta)*
liraglutide *(Victoza)*

Meglitinides
nateglinide *(Starlix)*
repaglinide *(Prandin)*

Sodium-glucose transport inhibitors
canagliflozin *(Invokana)*
dapagliflozin *(Forxiga)*

Thiazolidinediones
pioglitazone *(Actos)*
rosiglitazone *(Avandia)*

Diarrhea

Antidiarrheals
bismuth subsalicylate *(Pepto-Bismol)*
loperamide *(Imodium)*
opium derivatives *(Paregoric)*

ED

Prostaglandin
alprostadil *(Caverject)*

Phosphodiesterase inhibitors
avanafil *(Stendra)*
sildenafil *(Viagra)*
tadalafil *(Cialis)*
vardenafil *(Levitra)*

GERD

Antacids
aluminum salts *(ALternaGEL)*
calcium salts *(Tums)*

magnesium salts *(Milk of Magnesia)*
sodium bicarbonate *(Bells/ans)*

Histamine-2 antagonists
cimetidine *(Tagamet)*
famotidine *(Pepcid)*
nizatidine *(Axid)*
ranitidine *(Zantac)*

Proton pump inhibitors
dexlansoprazole *(Dexilant)*
esomeprazole *(Nexium)*
lansoprazole *(Prevacid)*
omeprazole *(Prilosec)*
pantoprazole *(Protonix)*
rabeprazole *(AcipHex)*

Glaucoma

Ophthalmic agents
acetazolamide *(Diamox)*
apraclonidine *(Iopidine)*
betaxolol *(Betoptic)*
bimatoprost *(Lumigan)*
brimonidine *(Alphagan P)*
carteolol *(Ocupress)*
dipivefrin *(Propine)*
dorzolamide *(Trusopt)*
echothiophate *(Phospholine)*
latanoprost *(Xalatan)*
levobunolol *(Betagan)*
metipranolol *(OptiPranolol)*
pilocarpine *(Isopto Carpine)*
timolol *(Timoptic)*
travoprost *(Travatan)*

Hepatitis B

Antivirals
adefovir *(Hepsera)*
entecavir *(Baraclude)*
telbivudine *(Tyzeka)*

Hepatitis C

boceprevir *(Victrelis)*
simeprevir *(Olysio)*
sofosbuvir *(Sovaldi)*
telaprevir *(Incivek)*

HF

Cardiac glycoside
digoxin *(Lanoxin)*

Phosphodiesterase inhibitors
milrinone

Nitrates
isosorbide dinitrate *(Isordil)*
isosorbide mononitrate *(Imdur)*
nitroglycerin *(Nitro-Bid, Nitrostat, others)*

Beta-adrenergic blockers
metoprolol *(Toprol)*
nadolol *(Corgard)*
propranolol *(Inderal)*

ACE inhibitors
benazepril *(Lotensin)*
captopril *(Capoten)*
enalapril *(Vasotec)*
fosinopril *(Monopril)*
lisinopril *(Zestril)*
moexipril *(Univasc)*
perindopril *(Aceon)*
quinapril *(Accupril)*
ramipril *(Altace)*
trandolapril *(Mavik)*

Diuretics
bumetanide *(Bumex)*
furosemide *(Lasix)*
torsemide *(Demadex)*

Natriuretic peptide
nesiritide *(Natrecor)*

HIV/AIDS

Nonnucleoside reverse transcriptase inhibitors
delavirdine *(Rescriptor)*
efavirenz *(Sustiva)*
etravirine *(Intelence)*
nevirapine *(Viramune)*
rilpivirine *(Edurant)*

Nucleoside reverse transcriptase inhibitors
abacavir *(Ziagen)*
didanosine *(Videx)*
emtricitabine *(Emtriva)*
lamivudine *(Epivir)*
stavudine *(Zerit XR)*
tenofovir *(Viread)*
zidovudine *(Retrovir)*

Protease inhibitors
atazanavir *(Reyataz)*
darunavir *(Prezista)*
fosamprenavir *(Lexiva)*
indinavir *(Crixivan)*
lopinavir *(Kaletra)*
nelfinavir *(Viracept)*
ritonavir *(Norvir)*
saquinavir *(Invirase)*
tipranavir *(Aptivus)*

Fusion inhibitor
enfuvirtide *(Fuzeon)*

CCR5 coreceptor antagonist
maraviroc *(Selzentry)*

Integrase inhibitor
raltegravir *(Isentress)*

Hyperlipidemia

Bile acid sequestrants
cholestyramine *(Prevalite)*
colesevelam *(Welchol)*
colestipol *(Colestid)*

Statins
atorvastatin *(Lipitor)*
fluvastatin *(Lescol)*
lovastatin *(Altoprev)*
pitavastatin *(Livalo)*
pravastatin *(Pravachol)*
rosuvastatin *(Crestor)*
simvastatin *(Zocor)*

Cholesterol absorption inhibitor
ezetimibe *(Zetia)*

Fibrates
fenofibrate *(TriCor)*
fenofibric acid *(Trilipix)*
gemfibrozil *(Lopid)*

Vitamin B
niacin *(Niaspan)*

Other
omega-3-acid ethyl esters *(Lovaza)*

Hypertension

ACE inhibitors
benazepril *(Lotensin)*
captopril *(Capoten)*
enalapril *(Vasotec)*
fosinopril
lisinopril *(Zestril)*
moexipril *(Univasc)*
perindopril *(Aceon)*
quinapril *(Accupril)*
ramipril *(Altace)*
trandolapril *(Mavik)*

ARBs
azilsartan *(Edarbi)*
candesartan *(Atacand)*
eprosartan *(Teveten)*
irbesartan *(Avapro)*
losartan *(Cozaar)*
olmesartan *(Benicar)*
telmisartan *(Micardis)*
valsartan *(Diovan)*

Calcium channel blockers
amlodipine *(Norvasc)*
clevidipine *(Cleviprex)*
diltiazem *(Cardizem)*
felodipine *(Plendil)*
isradipine *(DynaCirc)*
nicardipine *(Cardene)*
nifedipine *(Procardia XL)*
nisoldipine *(Sular)*
verapamil *(Calan SR)*

Renin inhibitor
aliskiren *(Tekturna)*

Thiazide diuretics
chlorothiazide *(Diuril)*
hydrochlorothiazide *(HydroDIURIL)*

Adrenergic blockers
acebutolol *(Sectral)*
atenolol *(Tenormin)*
betaxolol
bisoprolol *(Zebeta)*

metoprolol *(Lopressor)*
nadolol *(Corgard)*
nebivolol *(Bystolic)*
propranolol *(Inderal)*
timolol

Infertility

Hormones
cetrorelix *(Cetrotide)*
chorionic gonadotropin
clomiphene *(Clomid)*
follitropin alfa *(Gonal-F)*
follitropin beta *(Follistim)*
ganirelix *(Antagon)*
menotropins *(Repronex)*
urofollitropin *(Bravelle)*

Influenza

Antivirals
amantadine *(Symmetrel)*
oseltamivir *(Tamiflu)*
ribavirin *(Rebetron)*
rimantadine *(Flumadine)*
zanamivir *(Relenza)*

Insomnia

Benzodiazepines
estazolam
flurazepam
quazepam *(Doral)*
temazepam *(Restoril)*
triazolam *(Halcion)*

Other
diphenhydramine *(Benadryl)*
eszopiclone *(Lunesta)*
ramelteon *(Rozerem)*
zaleplon *(Sonata)*
zolpidem *(Ambien)*

Irritable bladder syndrome

Anticholinergics
darifenacin *(Enablex)*
fesoterodine *(Toviaz)*
flavoxate *(Urispas)*
oxybutynin *(Ditropan, Gelnique, Oxytrol)*
solifenacin *(VESIcare)*

tolterodine *(Detrol)*
trospium *(Sanctura)*

Beta agonist
mirabegron *(Myrbetriq)*

Menopause

Estrogens
estradiol *(Estrace)*
estrogens, conjugated *(Premarin)*
estrogens, esterified *(Menest)*
estropipate *(Ortho-Est)*

Progestins
drospirenone *(Yasmin* with ethinyl estradiol)

Estrogen receptor modulator
raloxifene *(Evista)*

MI

Platelet inhibitors
abciximab *(ReoPro)*
aspirin
clopidogrel *(Plavix)*
eptifibatide *(Integrilin)*
prasugrel *(Effient)*
ticagrelor *(Brilinta)*
ticlopidine *(Ticlid)*
tirofiban *(Aggrastat)*

Anticoagulants
dalteparin *(Fragmin)*
enoxaparin *(Lovenox)*
heparin

Pain relief
morphine

Nitrates
isosorbide dinitrate *(Isordil)*
isosorbide mononitrate *(Imdur)*
nitroglycerin *(Nitro-Bid, Nitrostat, others)*

Beta-adrenergic blockers
metoprolol *(Toprol)*
nadolol *(Corgard)*
propranolol *(Inderal)*

Calcium channel blockers
amlodipine *(Norvasc)*
diltiazem *(Cardizem)*
nicardipine *(Cardene)*
nifedipine *(Adalat)*
verapamil *(Calan)*

Migraine headache

Ergots
dihydroergotamine *(Migranal)*
ergotamine *(Ergomar)*

Triptans
almotriptan *(Axert)*
eletriptan *(Relpax)*
frovatriptan *(Frova)*
naratriptan *(Amerge)*
rizatriptan *(Maxalt)*
sumatriptan *(Imitrex)*

Nausea, vomiting

Phenothiazines
chlorpromazine
prochlorperazine
promethazine
perphenazine

Nonphenothiazines
metoclopramide *(Reglan)*

Anticholinergics/antihistamines
meclizine *(Antivert)*

5HT$_3$ receptor blockers
dolasetron *(Anzemet)*
granisetron
ondansetron *(Zofran)*
palonosetron *(Aloxi)*

Substance P/neurokinin 1 receptor antagonist
aprepitant *(Emend)*

Other
dronabinol *(Marinol)*
hydroxyzine *(Vistaril)*
nabilone *(Cesamet)*
trimethobenzamide *(Tigan)*

OCD

TCA
clomipramine *(Anafranil)*

SSRIs
citalopram *(Celexa)*
fluoxetine *(Prozac)*
fluvoxamine *(Luvox)*
paroxetine *(Paxil)*
sertraline *(Zoloft)*

Osteoporosis

Bisphosphonates
alendronate *(Fosamax)*
etidronate *(Didronel)*
ibandronate *(Boniva)*
pamidronate *(Aredia)*
risedronate *(Actonel)*
tiludronate *(Skelid)*
zoledronic acid *(Reclast, Zometa)*

Calcitonin
calcitonin, salmon *(Fortical, Miacalcin)*

Parathyroid hormone
teriparatide *(Forteo)*

Estrogen modulator
raloxifene *(Evista)*

Otitis media

Analgesics
acetaminophen *(Tylenol)*
ibuprofen *(Advil, Motrin)*
benzocaine, topical *(Cylex)*

Antibiotics
amoxicillin *(Amoxil)*
amoxicillin/clavulanate *(Augmentin)*
cefdinir *(Omnicef)*
ofloxacin *(Floxin)*

Parkinson disease

Dopaminergics
amantadine *(Symmetrel)*
apomorphine *(Apokyn)*

bromocriptine *(Parlodel)*
carbidopa/levodopa *(Sinemet)*
levodopa *(Dopar)*
pramipexole *(Mirapex)*
rasagiline *(Azilect)*
ropinirole *(Requip)*
rotigotine *(Neupro)*

Anticholinergics
benztropine *(Cogentin)*
diphenhydramine *(Benadryl)*
trihexyphenidyl

Adjuncts
entacapone *(Comtan)*
selegiline *(Carbex, Eldepryl)*
tolcapone *(Tasmar)*

Peptic ulcers

Histamine-2 antagonists
cimetidine *(Tagamet)*
famotidine *(Pepcid)*
ranitidine *(Zantac)*

Proton pump inhibitors
dexlansoprazole *(Dexilant)*
esomeprazole *(Nexium)*
lansoprazole *(Prevacid)*
omeprazole *(Prilosec)*
pantoprazole *(Protonix)*
rabeprazole *(AcipHex)*

GI protectant
sucralfate *(Carafate)*

Prostaglandin
misoprostol *(Cytotec)*

PTSD

SSRIs
citalopram *(Celexa)*
escitalopram *(Lexapro)*
fluoxetine *(Prozac)*
paroxetine *(Paxil)*
sertraline *(Zoloft)*
venlafaxine *(Effexor)*

TCA
amitriptyline

Antipsychotics
aripiprazole *(Abilify)*
olanzapine *(Zyprexa)*
quetiapine *(Seroquel)*
risperidone *(Risperdal)*
ziprasidone *(Geodon)*

Pulmonary artery hypertension

Endothelin receptor antagonist
ambrisentan *(Letairis)*
bosentan *(Tracleer)*
macitentan *(Opsumit)*
treprostinil *(Remodulin)*

Phosphodiesterase inhibitors
sildenafil *(Revatio)*
tadalafil *(Adcirca)*

Prostaglandin
epoprostenol *(Flolan)*

Prostacyclin
iloprost *(Ventavis)*
riociguat *(Adempas)*

Renal failure

ACE inhibitors
benazepril *(Lotensin)*
captopril *(Capoten)*
enalapril *(Vasotec)*
fosinopril *(Monopril)*
lisinopril *(Zestril)*
moexipril *(Univasc)*
perindopril *(Aceon)*
quinapril *(Accupril)*
ramipril *(Altace)*
trandolapril *(Mavik)*

ARBs
azilsartan *(Edarbi)*
candesartan *(Atacand)*
eprosartan *(Teveten)*
irbesartan *(Avapro)*
losartan *(Cozaar)*
olmesartan *(Benicar)*
telmisartan *(Micardis)*
valsartan *(Diovan)*

Diuretics
bumetanide
furosemide *(Lasix)*

Erythropoietins
darbepoetin *(Aranesp)*
epoetin alfa *(Procrit)*
peginesatide *(Omontys)*

Vitamins
doxercalciferol *(Hectorol)*
paricalcitol *(Zemplar)*

Iron
ferumoxytol *(Feraheme)*
iron sucrose *(Venofer)*
sodium ferric gluconate complex
    (Ferrlecit)

Phosphate binder
lanthanum *(Fosrenol)*

Rhinitis (allergic/seasonal)

Topical nasal decongestants
ephedrine *(Pretz-D)*
tetrahydrozoline *(Tyzine)*

Nasal steroids
beclomethasone *(Becloven, QNASL)*
budesonide *(Pulmicort Flexhaler)*
flunisolide *(AeroBid)*
fluticasone *(Flonase, Flovent)*
triamcinolone *(Azmacort)*

Antihistamines
brompheniramine *(Veltane)*
carbinoxamine *(Karbinal ER)*
chlorpheniramine *(Chlor-Trimeton,*
    others)
clemastine *(Tavist-1)*
cyclizine *(Marezine)*
cyproheptadine
dexchlorpheniramine
dimenhydrinate *(Dimentabs)*
diphenhydramine *(Benadryl)*
hydroxyzine *(Vistaril)*
phenindamine *(Nolahist)*
promethazine *(Phenergan)*
triprolidine *(Zymine)*

Nonsedating antihistamines
azelastine *(Astelin)*
cetirizine *(Zyrtec)*
desloratadine *(Clarinex)*
fexofenadine *(Allegra)*

levocetirizine *(Xyzal)*
loratadine *(Claritin)*

Oral decongestant
pseudoephedrine *(Sudafed 12 Hour)*

Schizophrenia

Typical antipsychotics
chlorpromazine
fluphenazine
haloperidol *(Haldol)*
loxapine
perphenazine
pimozide *(Orap)*
prochlorperazine
thioridazine
thiothixene *(Navane)*
trifluoperazine

Atypical antipsychotics
aripiprazole *(Abilify)*
clozapine *(Clozaril)*
iloperidone *(Fanapt)*
lurasidone *(Latuda)*
olanzapine *(Zyprexa)*
paliperidone *(Invega)*
quetiapine *(Seroquel)*
risperidone *(Risperdal)*
ziprasidone *(Geodon)*

Seizure disorder

Hydantoins
ethotoin *(Peganone)*
fosphenytoin
phenytoin *(Dilantin)*

Barbiturates
phenobarbital *(Solfoton)*
primidone *(Mysoline)*

Benzodiazepines
clobazam *(Onfi)*
clonazepam *(Klonopin)*
diazepam *(Valium)*

Glutamate antagonist
perampanel *(Fycompa)*

Potassium channel blocker
ezogabine *(Potiga)*

Succinimides
ethosuximide *(Zarontin)*
methsuximide *(Celontin)*

GABA modulators
acetazolamide *(Diamox)*
valproic acid *(Depakene)*
zonisamide *(Zonegran)*

Drugs for partial seizures
carbamazepine *(Tegretol)*
clorazepate *(Tranxene)*
felbamate *(Felbatol)*
gabapentin *(Neurontin)*
lacosamide *(Vimpat)*
lamotrigine *(Lamictal)*
levetiracetam *(Keppra)*
oxcarbazepine *(Trileptal)*
pregabalin *(Lyrica)*
rufinamide *(Banzel)*
tiagabine *(Gabitril)*
topiramate *(Topamax)*

Shock

Vasopressors
dobutamine
dopamine
ephedrine
epinephrine *(Adrenalin)*
isoproterenol *(Isuprel)*
norepinephrine *(Levophed)*

TB, first line

Antimycobacterial antibiotics
ethambutol *(Myambutol)*
isoniazid *(Nydrazid)*
pyrazinamide
rifampin *(Rifadin)*
rifapentine *(Priftin)*
streptomycin

TB, second line

Antimycobacterial antibiotics
bedaquiline *(Sirturo)*
capreomycin *(Capastat)*
cycloserine *(Seromycin)*

ethionamide *(Trecator)*
rifabutin *(Mycobutin)*

Thromboembolic disorders

Heparins
dalteparin *(Fragmin)*
enoxaparin *(Lovenox)*
heparin

Oral anticoagulants
apixaban *(Elliquis)*
dabigatran *(Pradaxa)*
rivaroxaban *(Xarelto)*
warfarin *(Coumadin)*

Thyroid dysfx

Replacement
levothyroxine *(Synthroid, Levoxyl, others)*
liothyronine *(Cytomel)*
liotrix *(Thyrolar)*
thyroid, desiccated *(Armour Thyroid)*

Antithyroid
methimazole *(Tapazole)*
propylthiouracil
sodium iodide/potassium iodide *(Thyro-Block)*

UTIs

Anti-infectives
cinoxacin *(Cinobac)*
co-trimoxazole *(Bactrim, Septra)*
fosfomycin *(Monurol)*
methenamine *(Hiprex)*
nitrofurantoin *(Furadantin)*
norfloxacin *(Noraxin)*

Bibliography

Aschenbrenner, D., & Venable, S. (2011). *Drug therapy in nursing* (4th ed.). Philadelphia, PA: Lippincott Williams & Wilkins.

Brunton, L., Chabner, B., & Khollman, B. (2010). *Goodman and Gilman's the pharmacological basis of therapeutics* (12th ed.). New York, NY: McGraw-Hill.

Carpenito-Moyet, L. J. (2012). *Nursing diagnosis: Application to clinical practice* (14th ed.). Philadelphia, PA: Lippincott Williams & Wilkins.

Drug evaluations subscription. (2014). Chicago, IL: American Medical Association.

Drug facts and comparisons. (2014). St. Louis, MO: Facts and Comparisons.

Drug facts update: Physicians on-line. (2014). Multimedia.

Fetrow, C. W., & Avila, J. (2003). *Professional handbook of complementary and alternative medicines* (3rd ed.). Springhouse, PA: Lippincott Williams & Wilkins.

Griffiths, M. C. (Ed.). (2012). *USAN and the USP 2012 dictionary of drug names.* Rockville, MD: United States Pharmacopeial Convention.

Handbook of adverse drug interactions. (2012). New Rochelle, NY: The Medical Letter.

ISMP medication safety alert! (2014). Huntingdon Valley, PA: Institute for Safe Medication Practices.

Karch, A. M. (2013). *Focus on nursing pharmacology* (6th ed.). Philadelphia, PA: Lippincott Williams & Wilkins.

The medical letter on drugs and therapeutics. (2014). New Rochelle, NY: Medical Letter.

PDR for nonprescriptive drugs. (2014). Oradell, NJ: Medical Economics.

PDR for ophthalmic medications. (2014). Oradell, NJ: Medical Economics.

Physicians' desk reference (68th ed.). (2014). Oradell, NJ: Medical Economics.

Smeltzer, S. C., & Bare, B. G. (2009). *Brunner and Suddarth's textbook of medical-surgical nursing* (12th ed.). Philadelphia, PA: Lippincott Williams & Wilkins.

Tatro, D. S. (Ed.). (2014). *Drug interaction facts.* St. Louis, MO: Facts and Comparisons.

Index

*Entries in **boldface** are drug classes.*

Aldosterone antagonist
   spironolactone, 307
Aldosterone receptor blocker
   eplerenone, 113–114
Aldurazyme, 181

Entries in **boldface** *are drug classes.*

*Entries in **boldface** are drug classes.*

*Entries in **boldface** are drug classes.*

Entries in **boldface** *are drug classes.*

*Entries in **boldface** are drug classes.*

Entries in **boldface** are drug classes.

*Entries in **boldface** are drug classes.*

*Entries in **boldface** are drug classes.*

Entries in **boldface** are drug classes.

*Entries in **boldface** are drug classes.*

*Entries in **boldface** are drug classes.*

*Entries in **boldface** are drug classes.*

*Entries in **boldface** are drug classes.*

Entries in boldface are drug classes.

Entries in **boldface** *are drug classes.*

*Entries in **boldface** are drug classes.*

---

*Entries in **boldface** are drug classes.*

*Entries in **boldface** are drug classes.*

*Entries in **boldface** are drug classes.*

---

*Entries in **boldface** are drug classes.*

*Entries in **boldface** are drug classes.*

---

*Entries in **boldface** are drug classes.*

*Entries in **boldface** are drug classes.*

*Entries in **boldface** are drug classes.*

Entries in **boldface** *are drug classes.*

*Entries in **boldface** are drug classes.*

Entries in **boldface** are drug classes.

*Entries in **boldface** are drug classes.*

*Entries in **boldface** are drug classes.*

Entries in **boldface** *are drug classes.*

---

*Entries in **boldface** are drug classes.*

*Entries in **boldface** are drug classes.*

*Entries in **boldface** are drug classes.*

*Entries in **boldface** are drug classes.*

*Entries in **boldface** are drug classes.*

*Entries in **boldface** are drug classes.*

*Entries in **boldface** are drug classes.*

*Entries in **boldface** are drug classes.*

*Entries in **boldface** are drug classes.*

Entries in **boldface** are drug classes.

---

*Entries in **boldface** are drug classes.*

*Entries in **boldface** are drug classes.*

*Entries in **boldface** are drug classes.*